MEDICAL CARE OF THE PREGNANT PATIENT

MEDICAL CARE OF THE PREGNANT PATIENT

EDITED BY

Richard S. Abrams, M.D.

Assistant Clinical Professor of Medicine,
University of Colorado School of Medicine;
Attending Physician, Rose Medical Center;
Consultant, High-Risk Obstetrics Clinic,
University of Colorado Health Sciences Center,
Denver

Paul Wexler, M.D.

Clinical Professor of Obstetrics and Gynecology,
University of Colorado School of Medicine;
Chairman, Department of Obstetrics and Gynecology,
Rose Medical Center, Denver

Forewords by
Robert W. Schrier, M.D.

Professor and Chairman, Department of Medicine,
University of Colorado School of Medicine,
Denver

E. Stewart Taylor, M.D.

Professor Emeritus and Former Chairman,
Department of Obstetrics and Gynecology,
University of Colorado School of Medicine,
Denver

LITTLE, BROWN AND COMPANY
BOSTON/TORONTO

Wife and child
Those precious motives, those
  strong knots of love
—Shakespeare

TO CAROL, BRIAN, KATIE

HILDE, KEITH, JENNIFER, LAURA

CONTENTS

FOREWORD

Medical Care of the Pregnant Patient represents an important interdisciplinary approach to the management of medical problems during pregnancy. This book is directed toward internists, medical subspecialists, and primary care physicians whose clinical training in obstetrics, in most cases, is limited. These physicians are frequently involved directly in the care of pregnant patients and are often asked for advice about specific medical problems.

By gathering the expertise of a very able group of contributors, the editors have produced a unique book, which is a comprehensive and coordinated review of the physiologic changes that occur during gestation and which shows how these changes influence the care of specific medical problems. Some of the important subjects that are discussed include nutrition, principles of teratology, prenatal genetics, and psychiatric problems during pregnancy. Medical problems are organized according to subspecialty areas, and diagnosis and management are covered in each chapter.

It has long been known that pregnancy causes dramatic physiologic changes in a woman. Only in recent years, however, have we learned how dramatically and permanently the fetus can be affected not only by the general health of the mother but also by factors in the mother's environment; by her use or abuse of drugs, alcohol, and cigarettes; and by the various methods used to diagnose and treat illness

Medical Care of the Pregnant Patient fills a void for physicians involved in the care of the obstetric patient by offering some practical guidelines for the management of coexisting or interrelated conditions. It also helps the physician become aware of the often difficult bioethical considerations and decisions associated with a high-risk pregnancy.

In combining the expertise of numerous subspecialists with a complete review of the heretofore scattered literature, this important new text provides a clear and concise guide to help physicians achieve the delicate balance in treatment and approach that will enhance the well-being of both the mother and the child.

Robert W. Schrier

FOREWORD

During the past 25 years most of the advances made in obstetrics have been directed toward improved prenatal results. Many obstetric problems affecting the life and health of the mother, the fetus, and the newborn occur among women with medical and surgical complications of pregnancy or with preexisting disease. With early recognition of medical disease and with modern management of such problems as lupus erythematosus, hypertension, toxemia of pregnancy, cardiovascular disease, and neoplastic disease, it has been possible to improve maternal and perinatal results.

The authors have discussed fetal diagnostic procedures, which have become an important part of modern obstetrics. Prenatal genetic diagnostic procedures, genetic counseling, and ethical considerations within obstetrics are all presented in detail. Each chapter, whether devoted to maternal diabetes, heart disease, thromboembolism, blood diseases, neurologic disease, dermatologic disease, or maternal neoplastic disease, is well documented by references from current authorities in obstetrics, medicine, radiology, and surgery.

There are many medical and surgical complications of pregnancy for which the obstetrician requires the close cooperation of other specialists for proper management. *Medical Care of the Pregnant Patient* provides obstetricians, internists, surgeons, and general physicians with the opportunity to approach the diagnostic and therapeutic problems that occur during pregnancy with a common knowledge. In the past, internists have often felt uncomfortable in the diagnosis and treatment of disease during pregnancy. The obstetrician also may have felt ill equipped to supervise a patient with serious medical disease, but found little help from colleagues. It is well known that the general surgeon in the past has tended to be too conservative in the management of acute appendicitis or partial bowel obstruction when the patient was pregnant. The authors have made it clear that necessary emergency surgery should not be delayed because of pregnancy.

All of the contributors to this book are well-qualified physicians who are active in clinical practice and teaching. I know each of them either as former students or residents or as professional colleagues. This book is the useful result of their cooperative experience.

E. Stewart Taylor

The woman about to become a mother should be the object of trembling care . . . God forbid that any member of the profession to which she trusts her life, doubly precious at that eventful period, should hazard it negligently, unadvisedly, or selfishly.
—Oliver Wendell Holmes

PREFACE

While relatively few chronic medical problems can prevent pregnancy, almost the entire spectrum of medical disease can complicate it. The lives and the health of two patients depend upon an understanding of the physiologic alterations of pregnancy and a knowledge of proper medical management. Increasingly, physicians from various disciplines are collaborating in the care of pregnant patients. The purpose of this book is to provide practical guidelines drawn from recent review articles, important original data, and classic references for the medical care of the pregnant patient. Because the book is intended for internists and family practitioners, we assume a good deal of familiarity with pathophysiology in the nongravid state. We have therefore emphasized the unique interaction between pregnancy and medical disease.

The first section of the book presents a selection of general background topics not usually included in medical training. Some of the legal ramifications of caring for pregnant women are considered, and a template is provided for the increasingly complex ethical dilemmas that confront the clinician daily in this area. Chapters on teratology, pharmacology, and radiation inform the generalist about the potential impact of environmental substances on the fetus and provide a rational basis for the use of drugs and diagnostic radiation during pregnancy. The prenatal genetics chapter presents the basic principles of inheritance. Because of the possibility for in utero treatment of the fetus, it is incumbent upon the primary care physician to obtain the appropriate genetic history before initiating prenatal evaluation. An overview of gestational nutrition is concerned with the impact of poor nutrition on the developing fetus. Historically, this

impact has been minimized because of the misconception that the fetoplacental unit was a true parasite that was capable of extracting all its needs from the mother, regardless of various deficiencies or excesses. Although detailed discussion of purely obstetric considerations is beyond the scope of this book, a separate chapter covers the mechanics, interpretation, and confidence limits of some of the obstetric tests used to assess fetal well-being.

The second section of the book concerns specific medical problems. Chapters are organized by medical subspecialty. The illnesses that are commonly encountered during pregnancy have been given the greatest attention. Each chapter discusses the effect of normal physiologic adaptations of pregnancy on medical disorders and the effect of medical disorders on pregnancy. The diagnostic measures suggested have been carefully evaluated for their appropriateness and safety during pregnancy. Although the book is not intended to be a treatment manual, specific recommendations for drug usage are provided. Tables and charts are used to summarize individual diagnostic or therapeutic principles or to serve as convenient reference sources.

Our experience with the management of medical problems during pregnancy at Rose Medical Center and the University of Colorado Health Sciences Center has clearly demonstrated the advantage of a multidisciplinary team approach. We hope that this volume will assist both the internist and the family physician to apply their clinical skills alongside those of the obstetrician so as to achieve the optimum medical care of the pregnant patient.

R. S. A.
P. W.

ACKNOWLEDGMENTS

The editors gratefully acknowledge the skillful and creative library research of Nancy Simon, Priscilla Rice, and Sara Katsh. We also wish to extend our appreciation and thanks to Loretta Hempstead, Jack Hempstead, Ella Travis, Linza Giamo, Sandee Cooper, Elizabeth Willis, Michelle Espinoza, and Dee Blisset; each played a major part in the compilation of material and word processing. Illustrations were prepared by Sarah Gustafson, Peggy Randall, and Larry Bartz in the Media Center at Rose Medical Center.

We thank our colleagues who took the time to review various chapters and offer their many insightful suggestions: Daniel Citron, M.D.; Harvey Karsh, M.D.; Fred Katz, M.D.; Sue Murahatta, M.D.; Katie O'Keefe, M.D.; Stuart Schneck, M.D.; Karl Sussman, M.D.; Nina Walknowska, Ph.D.; and Elizabeth Willis, M.S.

We are grateful to the entire staff at Little, Brown and Company for diligent and meticulous assistance: Julia Stair, Copyeditor; Brooke O'Neill, Editorial Assistant; Tony Greenberg, Indexer; and Jean Taylor, Proofreader. We owe an immeasurable debt to Curtis Vouwie, Medical Editor, and Priscilla Hurdle, Associate Book Editor, for their guidance, encouragement, and friendship throughout the preparation of this book.

Finally, words are but empty thanks for the love and patience of our wives and children.

ACKNOWLEDGMENTS

CONTRIBUTING AUTHORS

Fredrick R. Abrams, M.D.

Associate Clinical Professor, Department of Obstetrics and Gynecology, University of Colorado School of Medicine; Director, Center for Biomedical Ethics, Rose Medical Center; Attending Physician, Rose Medical Center, Denver

Richard S. Abrams, M.D.

Assistant Clinical Professor of Medicine, University of Colorado School of Medicine; Attending Physician, Rose Medical Center; Consultant, High-Risk Obstetrics Clinic, University of Colorado Health Sciences Center, Denver

Steven J. Ayres, M.D.

Staff Gastroenterologist, St. Anthony and Beth Israel Hospitals, Denver

Robert G. Benedetti, M.D.

Fellow, Division of Nephrology; Assistant Clinical Professor of Medicine, University of Colorado School of Medicine, Denver

William H. Bentley, M.D.

Clinical Instructor, Department of Neurology, University of Colorado School of Medicine; Attending Neurologist, St. Joseph Hospital, Denver

Tomas Berl, M.D.

Associate Professor of Medicine, University of Colorado School of Medicine; Attending Physician, University Hospital, Denver

George D. Dikeou, J.D.

Clinical Instructor, Department of Preventive Medicine, University of Colorado School of Medicine; Special Counsel, Gorsuch, Kirgis, Campbell, Walker and Grover, Denver

Steven L. Dubovsky, M.D.

Associate Professor of Psychiatry, University of Colorado School of Medicine, Denver

William C. Earley, M.D.

Associate Clinical Professor of Radiology, University of Colorado School of Medicine; Radiologist and Head, Division of Nuclear Medicine, Rose Medical Center, Denver

Lawrence E. Feinberg, M.D.

Assistant Professor of Medicine, University of Colorado School of Medicine; Attending Physician, University of Colorado Health Sciences Center, Denver

Alan S. Feiner, M.D.

Assistant Clinical Professor of Medicine, University of Colorado School of Medicine; Chief, Hematology and Medical Oncology, Department of Medicine, Rose Medical Center, Denver

Barry W. Frank

Clinical Professor of Medicine, University of Colorado School of Medicine; Attending Physician, Rose Medical Center, Denver

Gilbert Hermann, M.D.

Clinical Professor of Surgery, University of Colorado School of Medicine; Attending Surgeon, Rose Medical Center, Denver

Walter A. Huttner, M.D.

Associate Clinical Professor of Medicine, University of Colorado School of Medicine; Attending Physician, Rose Medical Center, Denver

Herbert Kaplan, M.D.

Clinical Professor of Medicine, University of Colorado School of Medicine; Attending Physician, Alpert Arthritis Center, Rose Medical Center, Denver

Linda U. Krebs, R.N., M.S.

Clinical Senior Instructor, University of Colorado School of Nursing; Nurse Oncologist, Division of Medical Oncology, University of Colorado Health Sciences Center, Denver

F. Marc LaForce, M.D.

Professor of Medicine, University of Colorado School of Medicine; Chief, Medical Services, Veterans Administration Medical Center, Denver

Mervyn F. Lifschitz, M.D.

Assistant Clinical Professor of Medicine, University of Colorado School of Medicine; Attending Physician, Rose Medical Center, Denver

James A. McGregor, M.D.C.M.

Assistant Professor of Obstetrics and Gynecology, University of Colorado School of Medicine, Denver

Andrew Mallory, M.D.

Associate Clinical Professor of Medicine, University of Colorado School of Medicine; Attending Physician, Rose Medical Center, Denver

David K. Manchester, M.D.

Assistant Professor of Pediatrics and Pharmacology, University of Colorado School of Medicine; Attending Physician, University Hospital, Denver

John E. Meyer, M.D.

Assistant Clinical Professor of Pathology, University of Colorado School of Medicine, Denver; Staff Pathologist, Boulder Community Hospital, Boulder

Gerald A. Niederman, J.D.

Associate, Gorsuch, Kirgis, Campbell, Walker and Grover, Denver

Audrey Hart Nora, M.D., M.P.H.

Associate Clinical Professor of Pediatrics, University of Colorado School of Medicine; Attending Physician, Human Genetics Institute, Rose Medical Center, Denver

James J. Nora, M.D., M.P.H.

Professor of Genetics, Preventive Medicine, and Pediatrics, University of Colorado School of Medicine; Director, Human Genetics Institute, Rose Medical Center, Denver

David S. Pearlman, M.D.

Clinical Professor of Pediatrics, University of Colorado School of Medicine; Senior Staff Physician, Department of Pediatrics, National Jewish Hospital and Research Center/National Asthma Center, Denver

William A. Robinson, M.D., Ph.D.

Professor of Medicine, University of Colorado School of Medicine; Head, Medical Oncology, University of Colorado Health Sciences Center, Denver

Charles H. Scoggin, M.D.

Associate Professor of Medicine, University of Colorado School of Medicine; Senior Fellow, Eleanor Roosevelt Institute for Cancer Research, Denver

John S. Simon, M.D.

Assistant Clinical Professor of Surgery, University of Colorado School of Medicine; Attending Surgeon, Rose Medical Center, Denver

Marc J. Sorkin, M.D.

Clinical Instructor in Dermatology, University of Colorado School of Medicine; Attending Physician and Head, Dermatology Section, St. Joseph's Hospital, Denver

Robert E. Wall, M.D.

Assistant Clinical Professor, Department of Obstetrics and Gynecology, University of Colorado School of Medicine; Coordinator of Resident Education, Department of Obstetrics and Gynecology, Rose Medical Center, Denver

Paul Wexler, M.D.

Clinical Professor of Obstetrics and Gynecology, University of Colorado School of Medicine; Chairman, Department of Obstetrics and Gynecology, Rose Medical Center, Denver

Phillip S. Wolf, M.D.

Clinical Professor of Medicine, University of Colorado School of Medicine; Attending Physician, Rose Medical Center, Denver

MEDICAL CARE OF THE PREGNANT PATIENT

Truth telling to patients is often debated as though the only issue is whether physicians are obligated to tell what they know.
Far more consequential are these questions:
Does the physician always know the truth?
Is there an art to truth telling . . . ?
What is the effect of truth on the patient?
—Norman Cousins
Human Options

1. BIOETHICAL CONSIDERATIONS FOR HIGH-RISK PREGNANCY
Fredrick R. Abrams

"Anything worth doing well . . . is worth doing poorly."* This witty and rueful aphorism acknowledges that the results of our efforts are sometimes less than perfect. We persevere in idealistic pursuits, trusting that overall we will improve the human condition even when we cannot make it perfect.

CLINICAL APPLICATION OF THE DISCIPLINE OF BIOETHICS

Humans are set apart from the lower animals by (1) a self-conscious use of the intellect and (2) an appreciation that we live in a time continuum (i.e., there is a future affected by our present actions). The use of this intellect "to convince rather than coerce" is the epitome of human behavior. Ethical theories are the distillate of scholars over many centuries of human thought and of diverse origins, struggling to determine the universal behavioral guidelines to enable humans to live in harmony. As used in this chapter, bioethics has two applications; it serves first as the basis of a code of behavior in medical practice and second as a guide for decision making at the bedside.

Many medical decisions are easy. When we empirically observe "a good result" from a "medical action" that places our patient at little or no risk, there is little call for in-depth analysis. Volumes have been written questioning the meaning of *good.* The meaning of *medical action* is also controversial [1]. The terms as used in this chapter should be taken to mean that which is generally accepted by physicians in medical practice. When we are confronted with a problem in which our

*H. Tristram Engelhardt, Jr., M.D., Ph.D., Professor, Center for Ethics, Medicine, and Public Issues, Baylor College of Medicine.

choices lie not between good versus bad, but rather between good and better, or bad and worse, then we must pause for reflection. When there is a decision to be made, when something of value must be sacrificed, we turn to ethics, sometimes called the logic of tragedy.

Ethics is a method of analysis enabling us, as temporary intruders on human agonies, to play our critical role in such a way as to make our intervention appropriate and our behavior consistent. The world does not always operate on this highly intellectual level. We can ask of ourselves that we keep our heads in the clouds of idealism, but our feet must be solidly on the ground of actual (and often emotionally governed) human interaction. Not all medical behavior is involved with critical decision making. Much is concerned with patient and physician relationships, and the rights and obligations assumed in the interactions. Is the relationship contractual? Is it fiduciary? Is it some other model? Bioethics helps us to derive the duties of our profession based on general ethical principles, particularized to the medical model.

TWO UNIQUE ASPECTS OF DECISIONS IN PREGNANCY

The most obvious aspect is the presence of two patients, the mother and the fetus. Most dilemmas arise when their interests are conflicting. Courts have tended to vest increasing rights in the fetus as term approaches. *Roe v. Wade* (93 S.Ct. 705 [1973]) gave no rights to the first-trimester fetus if the mother and physician felt abortion was indicated. At the other end of the spectrum is a recent Colorado court decision (Civil Action #79JN83) in which a mother was ordered to undergo cesarean delivery, for fetal distress, which she had refused while in labor. (She agreed after the court, hastily convened in the hospital, made its ruling.) The court held the infant, still in utero, to have a right to be wellborn that superseded the hazard of surgery for the mother [2].

Such a case in Georgia reached the Supreme Court of that state. A woman refused to have a cesarean delivery for a placenta previa on religious grounds. The court ordered the necessary laboratory tests repeated, against the patient's will, in the interest of the unborn child. Also, the court ruled that a cesarean delivery would have to be done if a placenta previa were proved. The case resulted in a vaginal delivery at term, as the placenta previa was found not to be present late in the third trimester. The decision invested the unborn near-term baby with rights not accorded the first-trimester fetus [3].

With the advent of in utero fetal surgery, we will face additional dilemmas in balancing fetal and maternal rights, if the state finds the interest of the unborn in conflict with maternal interest and desire [4,5]. Should a law be passed investing the conceptus with all the legal rights of a "person," the consequences would be revolutionary upon medicine as it is now practiced. Not only would abortion be illegal, but certain methods of contraception such as the IUD and techniques for in vitro fertilization could become "homicidal" as well. Amniocentesis, if it led to inadvertent spontaneous abortion, could become grounds for parental and/or doctor indictment for manslaughter. For the conceptus there is a maze of manifold crippling or lethal potentialities, before being launched down the birth canal into the sea of visible independent human interaction. I believe it is as foolish to designate a newly joined egg and sperm with the metaphysical title of "person" as it is to place your hammock between two newly planted sequoia seeds with the expectation of resting soon in their shade. Zygotes are not people, seeds are not trees, and neither can be counted on to grow to maturity, even when carefully nurtured. The determination of when human life begins is necessarily a retrospective one. We can look at an adult and safely say his life, as a unique combination of chromosomes, began at conception. (The components of his genetic structure, however, have been alive and human for eons.) But when the fertilization occurred, the initial conceptus could have become two or more individuals, or even a genetic mosaic. The initial conceptus also differentiates into embryo and placenta with membranes. The latter are also alive and human cells but are not "human life." The entity of "blighted ovum" in which only the membranes and placenta continue to develop to eight to ten weeks of gestation often results in spontaneous abortion. To accord that early conceptus full legal equivalence to a mother reduces one to the absurd position of unknowingly defending an adult against a placenta. Fifteen to twenty percent of conceptions fail to develop and are aborted spontaneously by the third month. To call a zygote a person will not make it behave like one. Adult persons have developed a wide variety of reactions to a conceptus, and a law will not change their conventional wisdom.

A second problem is "medicalization" of the birth process. Pregnancy is not an illness. Some complications (such as mild toxemia or hypertension) are not immediately apparent to the mother, in that she may be symptom free. There are cultural biases, folklore, religious and social implications, and widely diverse attitudes about pregnancy and the birth processes of which medical personnel must be cognizant if a satisfactory relationship and outcome are to be achieved. In many aspects of pregnancy the experienced mother may have more knowledge than the physician. Many decisions are social, not medical, and the physician may have no special knowledge to advise alterations in life-style. Think back only a few years to the taboo on vaginal exam in labor, the "essential" perineal shave, and the routine enema. Recent resurgence in interest in home delivery illustrates how important the lay person feels about the personal character of this paramount family experience, which medical personnel may mistakenly mark as "just another delivery." Great care must be taken to maintain appropriate empathy so that the psychological impact of the experience is not trivialized.

It is important to assure the patient of a working relationship with medical care programs, so that complicated pregnancies will not be lost to appropriate follow-up. Otherwise, a patient may perceive a message incorrectly: that she must either leave the medical system or relinquish control to medical personnel. She may then opt for a medically unsound but emotionally more acceptable experience. That message must be clearly repudiated and a cooperative venture planned instead.

With these special considerations in mind, general ethical theories can be applied to medical problems in pregnancy in a manner similar to that used in other disciplines.

BASIC ETHICAL THEORIES

There are two principal themes that pervade all ethical theory. Actions are ethical if they are well motivated. Or, actions are ethical if their consequences are good. The former theories are grouped together as deontological (*deon* = duty), the latter as utilitarian.

Kant, an eighteenth-century philosopher, sought to ground morality on an unconditional duty—an action not based on desire or intuition—so that all rational persons would recognize their duty given the same circumstances. One version of his unconditional duty (or categorical imperative) was stated, "Act only according to that maxim by which you can at the same time will it become universal law" [6]. His was a classic example of a (deontological) theory based on obligation, indicating that an action is moral if, and only if, it fulfills certain conditions, regardless of consequences. He contrasted this with utilitarian ethics and felt that it was superior because one cannot predict the outcome of all actions. Therefore, acting in hope of achieving a good result "could not be" an adequate basis for action.

Mill, an admirer of the earlier philosopher Bentham, presented his theory, utilitarianism, in the nineteenth century. Its principle was that "actions are right in proportion as they tend to promote happiness, wrong as they tend to produce the reverse of happiness" [7]. This is a theory alternatively called teleologic (*telos* = end) or consequentialist, since an action's "rightness" depends on its consequence—its contribution to some happy end.

Good arguments have been raised both to support and to refute these approaches, and most current writers point out they are not necessarily theories in contradiction. Often the same conclusions are reached by different pathways. A simple example: A utilitarian may agree in a given circumstance that lying would be an unethical action, for if people could not be trusted to tell the truth, much unhappiness would result. A deontologist would also feel that lying was unethical because one could not wish lying to become a universal law. Social discourse and function would be impossible were truth not implicit in conversation.

Beauchamp and Childress espouse four primary principles for ethical behavior [8]. They are prima facie principles—trumps by themselves—unless one overrides another. The authors do not rank the principles, thus leaving the dilemma of any pluralistic system. How are issues decided when principles are in conflict? This task requires the decision makers' personal involvement because values must be ranked in order to be consistent in action decisions.

It may be that this is a strength rather than a weakness. The ability to reorder the principles gives the flexibility necessary to adapt to differing needs in cases that at first glance seem identical. For example, consider the decision on the vigor of resuscitative measures for two 750-g premature infants. What factors might make a difference? One of the infants was the product of a pregnancy by parents after five years of infertility, which followed three spontaneous abortions. They urge resuscitation after discussing and accepting the possibility of future neurologic handicap. The other infant was delivered from a 14-year-old retarded child, pregnant by her stepfather, now nowhere to be found. Are the differences in the human situation morally relevant, and do they enter into the action decision?

I would offer the caveat of Stephen Toulmin:

Practical reasoning in ethics, as elsewhere, is a matter of judgment, of weighing different considerations against one another, never a matter of formal theoretical deduction from strict or self evident axioms. . . . We must remain on guard against the moral enthusiasts. In their determination to nail their principles to the mast, they succeed only in blinding themselves to the equities embodied in real life situations and problems [9].

Toulmin pointed out that wherever relations had to continue after an issue had been settled, negotiations and arbitration were chosen as the best decision-making device (e.g., union-management interaction). If arguments rested on principles alone and equity were not considered, there could be nothing but an adversarial relationship, with no hope of resolution.

FOUR ETHICAL PRINCIPLES

For guidance then, as boundaries within which to work freely rather than pathways leading directly to answers, I will attempt to present briefly several principles about which volumes have been written. The reader may wish to consider these principles more fully in the literature cited. The principles are autonomy, nonmaleficence, beneficence, and justice.

The Principle of Autonomy

Autonomy, most simply stated, is self-rule. In medicine it often means that the patient has the final decision as to what to do with his or her body. Kant further expressed that autonomous decisions were not whimsical or arbitrary, but based on consistent, self-imposed principles (which one could wish to become universal law). Thus, one must regard other persons' judgments as valid even when in disagreement with one's own, and not impede the actions those persons undertake in accordance with their principles. To do so would violate their autonomy (which would then mean one's own autonomy is at risk). Mill also felt that the individual must have freedom of action up to the point where it might impose upon another's freedom. This conforms to the principle of utility in that unimpeded persons would be most creative and able to maximize the "happiness" of society.

Commonsense limits on behavior are necessary because some persons are not autonomous. For example, prisoners, the retarded, the ignorant or uninformed may not be capable of autonomous decisions. Seriously ill or obtunded persons, many children and elderly, those under the influence of drugs often cannot act autonomously.

But the physician is constrained to honor a patient's autonomous decisions even if they do not appear to promote health. *The patient may have values to which life and health are subordinate.* The patient, if competent and well informed, should be allowed to make even tragic decisions. Issues of autonomy in medical situations might arise in the right to refuse treatment (even lifesaving treatment), attempted suicide, informed consent, the right to know diagnosis and prognosis, and nontherapeutic experimentation.

The issue of truth telling may be derived from this principle. Without having all the information available—all the truths—about their situation, patients cannot act autonomously. Therefore, those who derive the duty of veracity from the principle of autonomy (rather than feeling that truth telling is an inviolable freestanding principle) would base it on the duty to support, foster, and respect the autonomous strivings of the individual.

The Principle of Nonmaleficence

All physicians are familiar with *Primum non nocere*: "First and foremost, do no harm." Certainly there can be no argument about avoiding intentional harm. Failure to guard against risk, or to exercise sufficient care, or to be as knowledgeable as one is reasonably expected to be, or purports to be, is also physician failure of this duty. Courts have held applicable a legal version of this physician responsibility in cases of wrongful birth or wrongful life, when a parent was not advised of genetic hazards because of a physician's lack of knowledge or failure to disclose information before the birth of a damaged infant. Excellent summaries of ethical aspects of genetic screening and antenatal diagnosis have been published by Fletcher [10]. Sarto has included legal considerations that have been capably updated by Wright and Shaw [11,12]. Always acting to ensure that one will do no harm may paradoxically be a violation of duty. Many modalities of therapy offering great

promise for patients also have hazards or inevitably harmful side effects. A fair exposition of risk-benefit ratios followed by obtaining an autonomous patient's consent would clear one of a violation of the duty of nonmaleficence.

A problem arises, particularly in obstetrics and neonatology, when the issue of competence to make a decision is raised. The useful principle of autonomy shifts to that of nonmaleficence under such a circumstance. For example, take the birth of a Down's syndrome child with coincident bowel obstruction. The question of corrective surgery arises. If nothing is done, the infant will expire from starvation. If the infant survives the surgery, it will live the life of a retarded person. Is the fact of retardation morally relevant to the decision, and to the principle of nonmaleficence? Regardless of the decision, it may be viewed as a poor one by different parties [13]. In Maryland, the family, the physician, and the nursery personnel agreed not to intervene and the infant expired [14]. In New Jersey and Colorado, nursery personnel reported to the judiciary, who declared the newborn a ward of the court, which then ordered surgery performed. Cases in which the parents consent to surgery initially, of course, have no reason to become public knowledge. They remain quiet, personal tragedies or triumphs of a different nature.

The question of surgery on infants with meningomyelocele, hydrocephalus, or other major defects raises the issue of quality of life. Consideration must be given to whether enabling or prolonging a life of physical or emotional suffering adheres better to the principle of nonmaleficence than doing nothing at all. It may be that well-intentioned but short-sighted intervention only momentarily solves problems, later to create new ones.

Rosalyn Darling, in the *Hastings Center Report* [15], pointed out that, cure oriented, physicians were more likely to define a severely handicapped life as intolerable than were the parents of the afflicted child, concluding:

Those who have lived with the handicapped seem to reject any necessary incompatibility between being handicapped and leading a worthwhile life, a conclusion that ought to be taken into account by those charged with making decisions about the "right to life" of infants with birth defects.

I have no doubt that Darling's *"retrospective consensus"* is a true expression of many parents' current feelings about their handicapped children. Fortunately, people, especially parents, are very adaptable and can make their situations bearable by positive thinking. There are those who would *prospectively* choose to have no child, rather than a severely handicapped one. Many would prefer to try again for a healthy pregnancy outcome if there were a way to avoid a life substantially devoted to raising a handicapped child. In a letter to the *New York Times* magazine section editor, April 4, 1982, in response to an article on potential in utero treatment of the hydrocephalic infant, a parent wrote the following:

As the parent of a hydrocephalic, severely retarded two-year-old, I want to address . . . those cases in which the baby is neither cured nor dies, but sustains a severe handicap. . . .

Many of us caught in the heartbreaking process of watching our children not grow up, are seeing up close the extreme limitations of their lives, believe parents deserve to have a realistic picture of what they might be gambling on. Jargon about "developmental delays" and "special children" sadly masks the horror of what severe mental retardation means in terms of the quality of a child's life and what it is like for a family to live in a continuing context of hospitals and emergency situations.

. . . It is important to remember that doctors go home to dinner, but it is the parents and child who bear the life-affecting, long term consequences of these medical decisions.

The dimensions of the ongoing tragedy can be illustrated by the case cited by John Freeman, in which a child with an untreated meningomyelocele, at T-12, was transferred to a state institution after 5½ months. A shunt was placed. Over the next seven years, the child suffered a large number of orthopedic procedures for fractures, dislocated hip, and tendon surgery. He was found to be blind. When hydronephrosis was diagnosed, an ileal pouch was formed. A spinal fusion to allow him to sit and further revision of the ileal stoma were being planned. His mental age had not progressed beyond infancy [16].

The basic conflict revolves around two worthy goals. One is the prevention of suffering; the other is the preservation of life. The dilemma lies in how much abnormality makes life not worth living. A newly afflicted adult may decide for himself, and the criteria may be extremely diverse for different people. How much more difficult to decide for a second party, such as a severely compromised newborn! An argument in favor of passive euthanasia has been that a neonate will not suffer emotionally because a newborn is not conscious of its own existence. No one, of course, denies its capability to suffer physically. There is no way to measure a rapid demise against the life of the infant described [17]. Does one consider only the infant patient, or must the effects on its social constella-tion—parents and sibs—be considered as well? The concept of a specific fetal advocate was presented in an article on in utero fetal surgery. In the discussion the authors stated:

Finally, any proposed fetal treatment really involves two patients: the fetus and the mother. Whereas parents may consent to allow the fetus to be treated through the mother's body, who can give consent for the fetus? We believe that it is appropriately the parents themselves who bear this responsibility, but we also believe that it is best if a separate advocate can be identified for the fetus. This person not only seeks the best treatment for the fetus but also protects it from unwarranted or unnecessary assaults. Being separate from the fetus and the parents, the advocate can more objectively view the entire situation and the potential interventions. In some cases, the advocate may recommend no intervention and thus relieve potential parental guilt. Finally, since the advocate stands between the fetus and the physicians who are called on to render potential treatment, he or she can give an unbiased informed consent [34].

I must disagree with the notion of a fetal advocate. Such one-on-one advocacy gives far too much weight to a conceptual person vis-à-vis the actual parents and their clearly definable interests. An advocate for the fetus conjures up nightmarish visions of an adversary proceeding in which an unborn potential person is pitted against its parents. Should this acquire legal status, who will drag the unassenting mother to the operating room to undergo a surgical assault in the interest of a neurologically compromised fetus? How can anyone be a proxy for the tabula rasa of a fetus? The theologian and neonatologist chosen as fetal advocates in the above cited article [34] can only react culturally as clergy and physician. The incomprehensible and uncomprehending hydrocephalic fetus is neither self-conscious nor capable of emotional suffering. In a milieu of seductive technology, parental guilt, and wishful thinking, truly and meticulously informed maternal consent with alternative choices must always remain a primary and incontestable prerequisite to fetal surgery.

Lorber made a notable attempt to list criteria for treatment of infants with spina bifida [18]. He argued that those selected for surgery would have a reasonable quality of life. Nevertheless, many infants not selected would also survive. If physicians were able to prognosticate perfectly, the decision would be easier. This is obviously not the circumstance. Robert Reid suggests:

Supposing that a change in ethical attitudes was such that euthanasia was introduced in specifically defined cases of spina bifida. Is it reasonable to assume that, automatically, it will be part of a doctor's charitable duty to carry out the act of euthanasia? Currently it is no more than realistic to acknowledge that euthanasia applied to newborn infants is daily, widely, though secretly, practiced by doctors and others who believe that the patient, the infant, would be better off dead. Should all doctors, therefore, be expected to participate in the act of ending life, in the way that it is expected they will fulfill their other functions? Clearly not. There are many doctors to whom the very idea of ending the life of a child merely because it is deformed is both inadmissible and repugnant. But some doctors find abortion repugnant. And yet the abortion of a deformed fetus after prenatal diagnosis is now widely and easily acceptable in non-Catholic western countries.

There can be no doubt that the act itself will be no more or less repellent than the legal action of abortion in later stages of pregnancy, when the fetus, to all outward appearances, is a child. If euthanasia were morally or legally acceptable, most doctors would not find it outside the scope of their capabilities [19].

An additional sphere in which the principle of nonmaleficence arises is that of obligatory versus nonobligatory treatment [20]. "To stimulate the moral imagination,"* five ethical guidelines are listed upon which the Optimum Care Committee of the Massachusetts General Hospital based its protocol for dealing with this dilemma.

1. Life is not the absolute or ultimate good nor death the absolute evil.
2. Clinical decisions to stop "heroics" apply only to patients who are irreversibly moribund.
3. The will of the patient, not the health of the patient, should be supreme law.
4. Treatments that cannot reverse illness in a moribund patient are not necessary (they may be justifiable, but not necessary) and, when they will cause more suffering than benefit, are contraindicated.
5. Stopping treatment is ethically no different from never starting it.

Thus, the principle of nonmaleficence is seen in issues of prolongation of dying; killing versus letting die; quality versus equality of life (often stated as quality of life versus sanctity of life) [22]; the moral relevance of mental defects or physical handicaps; failure to advise or failure to disclose information critical for exercising the option of abortion for potential genetic defects; and substituted judgment for incompetent patients. One can

see that the choice of decision makers is often of paramount importance and that family, physician, consultants, committees, and courts may all be involved in the need to protect the patient's interests.

The Principle of Beneficence
In medicine it is a duty of practitioners to confer benefit because this characteristic is generally assumed to be essential to their chosen societal role. (Beneficence as a principle must be distinguished from the praiseworthy, but not duty-bound, activities more accurately described as benevolent.) The benefit may sometimes be accompanied by ill effect but should overall produce a positive result for the patient. Surgical procedures might result in such a trade. For example, a surgical procedure might eliminate a valued function such as fertility to achieve greater value by removing a life-threatening tumor (provided both the patient and the doctor rank their values in the same manner).

Beneficence, as a duty, also arises in an individual's relationship to society at large. One must give to society because one takes from society. Thus, there may be a moral basis for expecting a subject to participate in a nontherapeutic medical experiment, if little risk is involved, because that subject has benefited or may benefit from another's participation in the past. Where duty ceases and simple charity begins may be difficult to determine. Society's view of health care providers imposes a more personal obligation because of what they profess to do and to be (see Pellegrino [23] on the act of profession) and possibly because of society's contribution to the process by which they acquire their skills. Whereas passersby may not be duty-bound to aid an accident victim, professionals morally (usually not legally) could be expected to have a duty, imposed by their chosen role, to help.

The principle of beneficence may conflict with that of autonomy. Clinicians must be certain that they have set their own subjective needs aside before they act to deprive a patient of autonomous choice or withhold deserved information because they presume that they can make better choices than the patient. In the last analysis, most people know what is best for their own needs. Paternalism, better expressed in our gender-conscious society as "parentalism," is a mode of behavior arrogantly assumed by a practitioner who "knows what is best." Often the behavior arises, not from arrogance, but rather from a clinician's considered interpretation that the patient lacks true autonomy or is temporarily incompetent because of the stress of illness or other external factors.

*This phrase originated with Callahan and Bok [21], who listed and explained five goals for the study of ethics: (1) stimulating the moral imagination, (2) recognizing ethical issues, (3) eliciting a sense of moral obligation, (4) developing analytic skills, and (5) tolerating and reducing disagreements and ambiguity.

The patient's idea of health may not coincide with the physician's idea of health. Unless there is a violation of the clinician's principles serious enough to prohibit continued participation in the patient's care, a truly empathic effort must be made to comply with the patient's conception of optimum health goals. However, there is nothing wrong with a patient's delegating some decisions to a trusted medical expert, presumed to have a fiduciary relationship, in the same spirit we delegate some of our autonomous power to other social functionaries and institutions. There are situations in which the technical complexity is best evaluated by the physician. Even the most ardent autonomist must value years of training and experience. This judgment presupposes familiarity and sufficient communication so that the physician can apply expert judgment on how best to achieve the patient's goals, *yet not usurp the patient's right to decide what these goals should be.*

"Therapeutic privilege" is a principle invoked in defense of some parentalistic actions. Grounded in beneficence, it is the withholding of information that is felt to carry a significant harm, in and of itself, simply by its revelation. There are few legitimate occasions for this type of action with the sophisticated and curious lay public we now encounter. There may be justification for temporary parentalistic behavior to gather evidence that the patient is competent, if otherwise significant risk would be entailed for the patient by permitting a hasty (autonomous) action.

The Principle of Justice
The common and elementary principle found in justice theory is stated *formally:* Equals should be treated equally, and unequals treated unequally. When applied, it must be refined by a morally relevant delineation of what constitutes equals and unequals. Such defining characteristics would be referred to as *material principles* of justice. If isolettes were to be allotted in an intensive care unit, prematurity would clearly be a morally relevant material principle, and race or sex would not. Society has supported the closely allied principle of fairness, and in particular fairness of opportunity, pointing out that it is unjust to deny benefits based on characteristics for which an individual has no responsibility.

In the interest of justice, what is society's responsibility to rectify inequities in the "natural lottery," the inherent physical and mental capabilities with which we were born? Is there a different obligation to rectify untoward life events in which we must carefully distinguish the unfortunate (e.g., some crippling illnesses) from the unfair (e.g., de-

liberate radiation exposure and illness suffered without consent by a military draftee)?

Another issue is that of allocation of resources. Decisions are easier when there are no scarcities, but physicians may be forced to make choices. I believe society expects the individual physician to act as if no scarcity exists in dealing with the individual patient. Patient trust, which is a sine qua non in the therapeutic relationship, must not be imperiled by doubts as to whether the doctor is acting exclusively in the patient's interest. In the abstract, a physician's opinion may favor societal policies and rules that will, in the future, exclude certain individuals from care. In any specific case, it is not reasonable to expect the physician to act for society, in a utilitarian manner, rather than on behalf of his patient, unless definite social prohibitions (i.e., rules or laws) have been widely circulated and are publicly known in advance.

A CODE FOR PHYSICIANS
Is there a suitable guide for the physician involved in day-to-day care of nonhypothetical patients? We have long historical precedent for a code to guide the profession. The oaths of antiquity, like the toga, were suitable for the climate and society in which they originated, but they no longer cover the contemporary body politic or sociomedical climate. The affirmation (Table 1-1) is suitable for a physician dealing with a patient in a society with a pluralistic moral legacy. This affirmation is elucidated in accordance with the principles in the following paragraphs.

The basis for a moral relationship is *respect* for an autonomous person. The *trust* is that of a fiduciary relationship. The physician is characterized as a *professional* with self-imposed standards and a defined objective that he professes.

The dual aspect of medicine as both *art* and *science* must be appreciated. The argument of autonomy versus parentalism may be encountered [25], since the debate over how best to *benefit* the patient raises the issue of truth telling. First and foremost the actions of the physician must be directed to benefit the patient (not the practitioner), in keeping with the principle of beneficence.

The risk-benefit ratio and *full disclosure* necessary for intelligent autonomous choice are stressed, but the physician does not abdicate responsibility for the patient's choice. The doctor's role, as a *guide,* may be used to warn of obstacles, or to show shortcuts, through territory with which the physician is thoroughly familiar but through which the patient, despite all native capability, has

Table 1-1. A physician's affirmation

In order to be worthy of self respect, I pledge to respect others who place their trust in me as a professional in the healing arts. Therefore:

I will practice my art and my science to benefit my patients.

I will disclose to my patients that which I know of their disease, and any hazards of the remedies I might suggest, that I may guide them to choose the course that suits them best.

I will offer care and comfort when they are ill, and when death becomes inevitable, I will ease their way as best I can in keeping with their expressed plan.

I will recognize their right to self determination, and if conflicts should arise with my own ethical constraints, make them aware without judging wherein we differ, that they should consider seeking help elsewhere for their complaints.

I will intercede on their behalf within the scope of my authority if I perceive they are being treated without regard for their humanity.

I will hold in confidence that which is seen or heard in my role as physician.

I will ever be a student to sharpen my skills and further my knowledge that I may be a better clinician.

If I act in this way I may aspire to join the men and women who through the ages, have approached the loftiest ideals of the healing mission, for I will have earned the faith and trust which is the strongest tie in the bond between patient and physician.

Source: From Abrams [24]

never traveled. The principles of nonmaleficence and of beneficence are underscored.

The doctor must go beyond a simple contractual relationship to offer *care* and *comfort.* When confronting the prospect of a patient's death, the physician must remember that there is much more that can be done *for* the patient, if the patient wishes, despite the fact that there is nothing more to be done *against* the disease. Again, the principle of beneficence is advanced.

Patient and physician autonomy is an important theme emphasizing the physician's duty to inform the patient of *ethical differences* and to withdraw, if withdrawal is indicated, rather than to impose those differences on the patient.

A positive duty is to be a patient advocate, recognizing the importance of *individual human dignity.*

The time-honored concept of confidentiality is upheld, derived from the principle of autonomy.

A professional, in a rapidly expanding technical field, has the duty of continued study. In the absence of such study, the implied promise (i.e., offering the highest skill one has) is violated, breaching the concept of fidelity and the principle of nonmaleficence.

What is to be gained by the physician's following these principles? Certainly, we cannot measure a physician's success with a marketplace yardstick. Although all ethics should be the same, sly little phrases, such as "Business is business," and timeworn acknowledgments, such as "Caveat emptor," reveal acceptable scotomas in commercial dealings. Professional pride, the example of respected forebears, individual conscience, and the respect of colleagues elicit more reliable performance than contracts under the laws.

Dr. Eric Cassell [26], in a review of a book by sociologist Charles A. Bosk [27], states:

There is no way to regulate medicine or surgery on the basis of catching every error or making rules for every step; it simply will not work. The only way to cope with the problems raised by inadequate knowledge and uncertainty is to build, in each physician, a specifically medical conscience. Such moral training is one of the functions of internships and residencies. . . . When the training has been well done, even a 50-year-old doctor will get back out of bed at night to do what he has let lapse, because he can still hear the voice of the great chief resident in the sky. . . . Too much regulation may have a negative effect. It begins to undermine the moral rules, the conscience by which physicians regulate themselves. . . . Constant litigation and over-regulation can supersede the conscience, making it seem unnecessary. . . . The moral constraints on the profession will continue to be at least as powerful as legal ones in governing doctors' behavior, and moral constraints are more trustworthy. Policymakers should take care that in strengthening the one they don't weaken the other [26].

I would only add that medicine is a profession in which the spirit and the letter of the law may be as far apart as life and death.

CLINICAL DECISION MAKING

With this background the task becomes one of honing the skills of analysis and synthesis so as to apply broad principles and values to specific problems (Table 1-2).

Objective 1. Determine whose decision it is. This is least complex when there is an informed autonomous patient. Complexities arise when family, for example, wishes information withheld, or if there is a question of competence. If there is incompetence and a question of substituted judgment arises, the physician should feel that the best interests of the patient are being served—an especially difficult problem with the abnormal newborn. For further emphasis on the importance of this step for final action decisions, see objective 3.

Objective 2. Gather all medical data. This should be the area most familiar for the physician. Sometimes complete data resolve ethical dilemmas.

Table 1-2. Objectives: solving bioethical problems

Objective 1. Determine whose decision it is.

Objective 2. Gather all medical data.

Objective 3. Gather all value data from involved parties.

Objective 4. Determine conflicts and try to set priorities.

Objective 5. Using ethical principles, try to arrive at a rational resolution.

Objective 6. Discuss resolution with involved parties.

Objective 7. Synthesize physician's ethical resolution and involved parties' desires and needs.

Knowing that a newborn has anomalies incompatible with life as a neonate eliminates the need to consider surgical correction of malformations. The more statistical and prognostic information that is available, the better we are able to weigh risk-benefit decisions. One of the difficult facts of medical action that is frequently confronted is the need to act on incomplete data, despite our desires for more information.

Objective 3. Gather all value data from involved parties. It is important that communication be open to all interested parties. Being aware of diversity of feeling can alert the doctor to inform and to discuss, so that consensus can be reached without rancor [21]. This step may be at the heart of the matter. Be aware that some values held by concerned parties may be irreconcilable, but they are rationally held by people of good will. If *relief of suffering*, for example, were held the highest value by a family whose latest member was a hopelessly deformed infant (but one nevertheless having sufficient faculties to survive with special care), the family's decision might be to permit the infant to expire by withholding such care. Another family might hold it obligatory to *preserve life,* however limited and remote from normal, and therefore wish to provide all care at all costs. Can opposite decisions be made in similar cases and both be ethical? Indeed they can! When actual situations are encountered, persons involved can have equally compelling values upon which they base their decisions. Neither is wrong. Both are ethical. Thus, the values of the decision maker would be paramount in the action or inaction to be taken [13].

Objective 4. Determine conflicts and try to set priorities. The more involved an individual is with the patient, the more weight will be given to a person's value. Conflicts unresolvable within the hospital setting may sometimes move to the courts. To clarify your own thinking, define conflicts. Is society's value (principle of beneficence) of preserving life conflicting with a parent's value (non-maleficence) to relieve suffering? Is a patient's value (principle of autonomy) of consent to transfusion conflicting with a doctor's value (principle of beneficence) to preserve life?

Objective 5. Using ethical principles, try to arrive at a rational resolution. Remember Toulmin's caveat: "We must remain on guard against the moral enthusiasts. In their determination to nail their principles to the mast, they succeed only in blinding themselves to the equities embodied in real life situations and problems" [9]. Rational objectivity must be sought by the physician, but not to the exclusion of the equities. Consultation with social workers, clergy, nursing staff, and other experts can be very helpful in arriving at conclusions from as broad an information base as possible. Other professionals may help to reveal your biases to you. Keep in mind that ethical principles were evolved by people concerned with a just and rational way of life. They are ideals, and if everyone were to follow them to their paramount end, we would be living in a much different world. Since they are not followed by all (and never even thought about by many), we as clinicians involved in real and pragmatic decisions must accede to the facts of our situations. We must not lose sight of the ideal but must act in a world that is less than that.

Objective 6. Discuss resolution with involved parties. This does not mean you have solved the problem and are providing the answer. Instead, it is a presentation of the problem in a systematic and coherent way to the decision maker(s), getting feedback and clarifying issues by elucidating facts and responding to questions preparing for:

Objective 7. Synthesize physician's ethical resolution and involved parties' desires and needs.

All of these objectives may be intermingled in an ongoing clinical situation, but it is well to step out of the action for a time of reflection on objective 5 (using ethical principles, try to arrive at a rational solution) and to clarify your own thoughts. This will better prepare you to present objective 6 (Discuss resolution with involved parties) and fit the various segments into a cohesive whole. Objectives 6 and 7 could be rapidly sequential.

CASE PRESENTATION AND DECISION-MAKING ANALYSIS

A 19-year-old juvenile diabetic, already the parent of an 18-month-old child with possible developmental delay, was delivered of a viable male infant, at 37 weeks' gestation, by repeat cesarean section, after sporadic prenatal care. She had failed to keep many appointments and her diabetes was under poor control. The infant was holoprosencephalic with an unusually large facial defect, cleft lip and palate, and hydrocephaly. He cried spontaneously and needed no resuscitation.

The pediatrician in attendance was the same pediatrician who had "raised" the mother and cared for her throughout her years of juvenile diabetes. He hastily took the baby to the nursery before the mother could see it.

In the nursery it was apparent that the infant had sufficient midbrain function to survive, given ordinary care (i.e., feeding). Computed axial tomography and transillumination confirmed the virtual absence of cortex. The pediatrician requested cessation of the glucose and oxygen that had been started routinely on the infant of a diabetic. When the infant began to cry with hunger, several of the nurses fed him, using a special nipple adapted for cleft palate. The child became a very disturbing influence in the nursery, with nursery personnel in favor of maintenance care and the attending pediatrician firmly resolved against feeding. The entire nursery routine was disrupted and efficiency impaired.

After four days, a meeting was held with the nursery staff, attending pediatrician, other doctors, nurses, and paramedical personnel. The parents were not in attendance. The father had seen the baby shortly after birth. The mother did not see him until the third day, when, with the encouragement of nursery staff, she visited him. The pediatrician had discouraged the visit, feeling that the absence of facial features, replaced by a gaping cavity with open nares and a grotesquely enlarged head, would be too shocking a sight. He had not involved the parents in the decision to withhold feeding. He had discussed this tactic with them as the way the case would be managed. He explained at the meeting that he wished to spare the parents any guilt involved in shortening the life of the infant. A few days after the mother's first visit to the nursery, she learned to feed the infant.

As in many events with multiple observers, one finds a bare skeleton of facts. The events described by different observers show how a body of knowledge can be subject to widely varying interpretation. One observer states that the mother, with increasing confidence, accepted her nurturing role with the encouragement of staff. Another source maintained that the maternal role was imposed upon the mother by innuendo of being a bad person if she did not undertake to hold and feed the infant. It had been made clear from the beginning that the cortical damage of the infant was so great

that no intellectual capacity could ever be expected and life expectancy would be brief.

The pediatrician did not wish the infant to be discharged with the parents. After the social worker and other personnel became involved and discussed the situation with the parents and pediatrician, the infant went home with the mother. Two weeks later the infant was admitted to another institution and died of progressive apnea, despite active therapy, on the 28th day of life.

Analysis

Objective 1. Determine whose decision it is. The decision belongs to the patient. The patient is the infant, who is unable to make a decision. Who can speak for this patient? The pediatrician clearly was a parent advocate. The AMA Judicial Counsel opinion states: "Whether to treat a severely defective infant and exert maximal efforts to sustain life should be the choice of the parents" [28]. Although one could argue that feeding is neither treatment nor maximal effort, the implication of parent participation in treatment decisions is clear.

It is not difficult to understand the pediatrician's parentalistic involvement. He was virtually in loco parentis for the mother, having guided her through the maze of juvenile diabetes for over a decade. Many juvenile diabetics exercise denial. It is possible that the patient's denial of her diabetes and failure to comply with a rigid prenatal regimen resulted in an abnormal metabolic milieu that played some role in the actual anomaly encountered. One could argue that the mother was not an autonomous person by virtue of the disease process, which led to an unrealistic appraisal of her life situation. Nevertheless, only with great trepidation should autonomy as a principle be overridden by the parentalism derived from beneficence. Denial of the parents' participation in the decision not to feed the infant was a well-intended but overly subjective dismissal of their responsibility and right to share in the fate of their offspring. Their exclusion tended to foster the prominent mechanism of denial.

Objective 2. Gather all medical data. The significant medical data were simple and complete. The infant had absence of cortical function with no hope of help from medical or surgical therapy. The prognosis for intelligence was nil, and the probability of death, within months, was great. The infant was a sentient being, however, feeling pangs of hunger and distress allayed by feeding.

Objective 3. Gather all value data from involved parties. Optimally the parents should have been consulted, but since they were not, there were no data available. They might have been for or against feeding.

Nursery personnel were involved in the same way soldiers are given orders. Some may choose to follow those orders and absolve themselves of responsibility. Others may choose to assume responsibility. Some of the nurses did assume responsibility and chose to protest.

Clearly, had the parents chosen to allow feeding, the pediatrician would have had no basis for withholding it. I do not believe anyone would argue that the decision to feed would be a violation of the principle of justice, with the allocation of precious resources to an infant with no hope for meaningful life. Were the brain damage less, the performance of corrective surgery, both cerebral and facial, resulting in a still severely compromised infant, would raise the question of allocation of resources making it an issue unto itself. Nonmaleficence would be raised when considering the issue of the quality of life versus the fact of nonexistence.

Had the parents chosen not to feed the infant, the decision would have been met with the same protest. A conference such as was held, including the parents, might have sufficed. However, if the parents had held to their decision, the courts would probably have become involved [29].

What if no one had protested the order not to feed? The infant would have died sooner, but with more immediate suffering from starvation. Suffering would have been imposed upon it by other people, whose professed motives were to accomplish just the opposite: relief of suffering. The issue would have revolved around *whose* suffering was to be avoided.

Objective 4. Determine conflicts and try to set priorities. In this case, the initial conflict was between parentalistic beneficence (the pediatrician's desire to spare the parents the anguish of seeing the grotesque appearance of the infant, the decision to hasten its death and to avoid the possibility of bonding and the inevitable loss) and autonomous and realistic involvement in a tragedy (notwithstanding the possibility of maturation and emotional growth which experience may sometimes provide). It is true that these young parents may simply not have had the intellectual or emotional capacity to participate fully, but the alternatives should have been explored in the interest of promoting autonomy, however painful and fruitless the pediatrician believed this would be [30].

The true conflict was encountered between the beneficent motivation of the pediatrician toward the parents and the nonmaleficent principle of some of the nursery staff, who could neither participate in nor passively tolerate starving the infant to death. It suffered, to all appearances, when hungry. It appeared not to suffer when fed.

Objective 5. Using ethical principles, try to arrive at a rational resolution. A meeting with additional members of the Ethics Committee, including professional, administrative, and secretarial hospital personnel, was held in the spirit of Fost's recommendation for the "ideal ethical observer" [31]. The pain of the infant, reflected in the anguish of the nurses, was expressed. Without formal decision or formal actions, the pediatrician finally involved the parents, who visited the nursery, learned to feed the infant, and eventually took him home. The principle most cogent was that of nonmaleficence. In the very delicate balance of suffering, it appeared that the physical pain of the hungry infant outweighed the parents' mental anguish.

Objective 6. Discuss resolution with involved parties. The pain of the nursery staff was not ignored. A practical bonus was the restoration of a smoothly functioning intensive care nursery. The pediatrician still felt that the parents suffered unnecessarily, yet he acceded to the solution. He pointed out how difficult the situation had been at home and how useless it had been to prolong life, until the inevitable readmission and death. Others did not agree that it had been useless but felt that it was valuable for the parents' grieving process and in assuaging their assumed guilt for bearing an imperfect child.

An argument could be made, at this point, for active rather than passive euthanasia. The prognosis for any meaningful life was nil [32]. Death, when it came, was associated with pain and suffering that appeared to be meaningless. This type of existence, especially if a painful demise was to be encountered, is a cogent argument for active euthanasia [33]. A moral claim to a quick and painless death could be made by analogy to a person inextricably trapped in a burning wreck with more pain and suffering to come. It is possible to stipulate very specific conditions under which active euthanasia might not subject anguished parents or their sympathetic physicians to prosecution. A complete discussion of euthanasia, however, is beyond the scope of this book.

In this case, objectives 5, 6, and 7 were contemporaneous. After the infant's demise, efforts were made to include the parents in a small hospital support group with other parents who had suffered the death of a child.

A physician's task is always to be supportive of the involved people, aware that many problems have no happy solutions. Whether we cure or comfort (or fail to do either), we should be able to review our thought processes and conclude that our action (or inaction) was (at least) appropriate and consistent.

REFERENCES

1. Illich I. Medical nemesis. New York: Pantheon Books, 1976.
2. *People of the State of Colorado in the Interest of Unborn Baby ———, Civil Action #79JN83,* Juvenile Court, City and County of Denver (1979).
3. *Jefferson v. Griffin Spalding County Hospital Authority,* 247 Ga. 86, 274 S.E.2d 457 (1981).
4. Harrison MR, Golbus MS, Filly RA. Management of the fetus with a correctable congenital defect. JAMA. 1981; 246:774–7.
5. Fletcher JC. The fetus as patient: ethical issues. JAMA. 1981; 246:772–3. editorial.
6. Kant Immanuel. Foundations of the metaphysics of morals. tr. Beck LW. Indianapolis: Bobbs-Merrill, 1959.
7. Mill JS. Utilitarianism. ed. Gorovitz S. Indianapolis: Bobbs-Merrill, 1971.
8. Beauchamp TL, Childress JF. Principles of biomedical ethics. New York: Oxford University Press, 1979.
9. Toulmin S. The tyranny of principles. Hastings Cent Rep. 1981; 11:31–9.
10. Fletcher JC. Ethical issues in genetic screening and antenatal diagnosis. Clin Obstet Gynecol. 1981; 24:1151–68.
11. Sarto GE. Ethical and legal considerations of antenatal diagnosis. Clin Obstet Gynaecol. 1980; 7:135–41.
12. Wright EE, Shaw MW. Legal liability in genetic screening, genetic counseling, and prenatal diagnosis. Clin Obstet Gynecol. 1981; 24:1133–49.
13. Taub S. Withholding treatment from defective newborns. Law Med Health Care. 1982; 10:4–10.
14. Gustafson JF. Mongolism, parental desires, and the right to life. Perspect Biol Med. 1973; 16:529–57.
15. Darling RB. Parents, physicians, and spina bifida. Hastings Cent Rep. 1977; 7:10–4.
16. Freeman JM. The shortsighted treatment of myelomeningocele. Pediatrics. 1974; 53:311–3.
17. Furrow BR. The causes of "wrongful life" suits.

Ruminations on the diffusion of medical technologies. Law Med Health Care. 1982; 10:11–4.
18. Lorber J. Early results of selective treatment of spina bifida cystica. Br Med J. 1973; 4:201–4.
19. Reid R. My children, my children. New York: Harcourt Brace Jovanovich, 1977.
20. Cassem N. When illness is judged irreversible: imperative and elective treatments. Man Med. 1980; 5:154–66.
21. Callahan D, Bok S., eds. Ethics teaching in higher education. New York: Plenum, 1980.
22. McCormick RA. The quality of life, the sanctity of life. Hastings Cent Rep. 1978; 8:30–6.
23. Pellegrino ED. Toward a reconstruction of medical morality: the primacy of the act of profession and the fact of illness. J Med Philos. 1979; 4:32–56.
24. Abrams FR. Social needs and the physician's duties: a physician's affirmation. People Policy. 1979; 1:18–21.
25. Veatch RM. Professional ethics: new principles for physicians? Hastings Cent Rep. 1980; 10:16–9.
26. Cassell E. The great chief resident in the sky. Wall Street Journal. Vol. 193, No. 91:1979.
27. Bosk C. Forgive & remember. Chicago: Univ. of Chicago Press, 1979.
28. Quality of life. In: Current opinions of the judicial council of the American Medical Association. Chicago: AMA, 1981:8–9.
29. Robertson JA. Involuntary euthanasia of defective newborns: a legal analysis. Stanford Law Rev. 1975; 17:213–69.
30. Pauli RM, Cassell EJ. Nurturing a defective newborn. Hastings Cent Rep. 1978; 8:13–4.
31. Fost N. Counseling families who have a child with a severe congenital anomaly. Pediatrics. 1981; 67:321–4.
32. Fletcher J. Indicators of humanhood: a tentative profile of man. Hastings Cent Rep. 1972; 2:1–4.
33. Leake HC III, Rachels J, Foot P. Active euthanasia with parental consent. Hastings Cent Rep. 1979; 9:19–21.
34. Clewell WH, Johnson ML, Meier PR, et al. A surgical approach to the treatment of fetal hydrocephalus. N Engl J Med. 1982; 306:1320–25.

With us always has been the question of
when the life of the individual begins and
when society begins to protect this life because
it has gained the dignity of a human being.
Eggs and sperm die separately without any
pangs of conscience.
—Eugene Stead

2. LEGAL CONSIDERATIONS FOR HIGH-RISK PREGNANCY

George D. Dikeou and Gerald A. Niederman

Legal principles concerning a physician's treatment of the high-risk pregnancy have undergone substantial change in the recent past. Indeed, if this book were being written 20 years ago, a section on legal considerations would scarcely touch upon a central theme of the present chapter: the rights of the unborn fetus and the ramifications flowing from recognition of such rights. Amidst rapid legal evolution, it is clear that the focus of medical treatment in this area has shifted from an almost exclusive concern for the mother's well-being to a shared concern for the well-being of both the mother-to-be and the fetus. In fact, if present trends continue, the scope of physician responsibilities may well extend even farther to encompass the father-to-be, siblings, and other close kin.

This chapter discusses some of the legal developments that may affect the rights and obligations of a physician in the treatment of a high-risk pregnancy. At the outset, however, the authors feel obliged to state several lawyer-like disclaimers concerning this work. First, no effort has been made to discuss all applicable law in an exhaustive way. The limited focus of the chapter does not permit a comprehensive description of this evolving area of law. In addition to reviewing the cited court decisions themselves, the interested reader is urged to consult some of the excellent articles noted for further treatment of relevant legal issues [1–6].

Various jurisdictions may differ with respect to the legal principles actually applied. This chapter is not a substitute for personal legal advice rendered by a skilled local attorney. It is hoped that, by becoming more sensitive to possible legal issues related to high-risk pregnancy, the responsible physician will more readily consult legal counsel as a particular occasion warrants.

THE GENERAL LAW OF PHYSICIAN ACCOUNTABILITY

The general law of physician accountability to patients may be summarized quite simply. A lawsuit alleging medical malpractice may be framed upon different legal theories such as negligence, breach of contract, battery, lack of informed consent, or some combination of these legal concepts. Regardless of how the action is nominally titled, the issues before a court are generally similar.

To begin with, the physician must owe a duty to the patient. This duty can arise by express or implied contract, by mere implication based on a physician's conduct, or by statute, as under so-called Good Samaritan statutes applicable in certain states. More typically, however, it arises because the parties embark on a physician-patient relationship wherein the patient entrusts her well-being to a specific physician or team of physicians.

However established, a physician's duty is to conduct himself or herself in a manner commensurate with that which a reasonably prudent physician would assume under a similar set of circumstances. This standard of care, universally recognized, is the standard which must be understood and adhered to by any practicing physician dealing in the arena of high-risk pregnancy. To the extent that physicians hold themselves out to the public as specialists (e.g., in Ob-Gyn), they will further be held to a higher standard of a specialist's expertise.

If a physician's conduct falls below the applicable standard of care, and if the substandard treatment is viewed as the legal cause of injury to a patient, the physician will be held accountable to the patient and damages will be assessed to compensate for the injury suffered.

These principles of physician accountability, as

well as the entire notion of "medical malpractice," may seem inflexible and intimidating on the surface. In reality, however, the standard of responsibility is nothing more than what is expected of professionals generally, whether physicians, attorneys, accountants, or architects. One is expected to be as well read, to know as much concerning the availability of diagnostic techniques, and to be as capable of rendering the level of care necessary to protect a patient's rights and interests as are other physicians in that field. As with all professional conduct, the practicing physician should recognize personal limitations when dealing with the high-risk pregnancy and seek the assistance of particular specialists when necessary.

One element of the general law of physician accountability merits special emphasis because of its importance to the treatment of high-risk pregnancies. This is the requirement of informed consent. Simply put, a physician must obtain a patient's informed consent to diagnostic procedures, to medical and surgical treatment, and, conversely, to the decision to forego such procedures and treatment.

What is informed consent by a patient will, of course, vary with individual circumstances. Perhaps the most common definition is the objective "reasonable patient" standard: A patient must be provided with that amount and type of information regarding risks and alternatives which a reasonable patient would need to make a decision regarding her course of treatment [7]. A minority of courts have gone even farther and applied a "subjective" patient standard in determining the adequacy of informed consent. The subjective standard would require full disclosure of all information regarding the particular patient's decision whether or not to undergo treatment, irrespective of the reasonable patient's hypothetical needs [8].

Whether the measure be objective or subjective, it is clear that a physician must intelligibly communicate to a patient enough relevant facts concerning circumstances and risks so that the patient can make an informed decision whether to proceed with treatment or to forgo it. This is especially important in connection with the high-risk pregnancy. As discussed subsequently, much of the litigation involving physician accountability revolves around the patient's exercise of her option to abort or to carry a fetus to term, and the related issue of whether that option has legitimately been made available to her. However well-intentioned, paternalistic decision making for a patient is anathema to the physician concerned with maintaining proper standards of legal accountability. This must be contrasted, of course, with the counseling role necessarily played by a diligent physi-

cian in the overall treatment of a patient; from a legal standpoint, this honorable activity by a physician retains its legitimacy, provided that ultimate decisions are made by the patient after proper disclosure of all relevant matters.

APPLICATION OF LEGAL PRINCIPLES TO HIGH-RISK PREGNANCY
Central Themes in an Era of Change

Over the last 10 to 20 years, two primary developments—one legal and one medical—have combined to force reshaping of legal principles governing physician accountability for treatment of the high-risk pregnancy. The result has been to require a shift in physician outlook from an almost exclusive concern for maternal well-being to a broader concern for the overall well-being of mother-to-be, fetus, and other affected family members.

The main legal impetus for change was the landmark abortion rights decision by the United States Supreme Court in *Roe v. Wade* [9]. As many readers will recall, the Supreme Court held in *Roe v. Wade* that a woman has an absolute right—primarily deriving from her constitutional right of privacy—to seek and secure an abortion during the first trimester of pregnancy without state limitation or interference. Indeed, the Court extended this absolute constitutional right to encompass second-trimester abortions as well. However, in recognition of the higher risk associated with second-trimester abortions, the Court permitted the states some latitude to prescribe certain regulations governing performance of second-trimester abortions in order to protect the woman's health and well-being. The Supreme Court further held that once a fetus became viable—viability being defined as occurring in the third trimester of pregnancy—the states were free to prohibit abortions altogether except where demonstrably necessary to preserve a woman's life or health.

Apart from all of its other implications—religious, political, legal, or medical—the decision in *Roe v. Wade* carries with it two specific consequences of concern to treatment of the high-risk pregnancy. First, the right of states to prohibit third-trimester abortion subsumes the fact that a third-trimester fetus is capable of life and hence is a valid object of legal protection in which legal rights may vest. A physician's obligation is thereby extended to encompass another patient—the fetus—apart from his initial responsibility to the mother-to-be as patient.

Second, the Supreme Court established a maternal option for termination of pregnancy that did not generally exist prior to the decision in *Roe v. Wade.* While a first- or second-trimester abortion may now be obtained for any reason or for no reason, the right to choose abortion means that abortion may also be chosen for a reason of great relevance to the treatment of high-risk pregnancy: that is, the possibility (or probability) that a fetus, if carried to term, might be born with "defects" of greater or lesser severity. A new constitutionally protected option has thereby been created for the pregnant woman. The availability of the option to abort a defective fetus has inevitably imposed a whole new set of diagnostic and treatment responsibilities on the physician in the sound discharge of his or her duty, under the general principles of accountability discussed above.

No ethical or moral prescriptions are intended by the foregoing statements concerning abortion. The wide-ranging, often heated debate concerning the propriety of the Court's holding in *Roe v. Wade* continues at a fast pace, and there are few physicians, attorneys, or lay citizens who have not considered the issues and arrived at a personal resolution thereof.

However, the operative legal fact is that first- or second-trimester abortion is now a woman's constitutionally protected right. As such, it is clearly within the realm of information that must be provided to and considered by a patient in order to obtain true informed consent to diagnostic or treatment procedures. Reconciling the abortion option with a particular physician's moral or social beliefs might be problematic in a given case, but recognition of the option and communication of it are essential to the sound discharge of professional responsibilities.

Complementing the emergence of a woman's right to abort, the second great change in the treatment of high-risk pregnancies has come about through changes in the practice of medicine itself. With the advent of genetic screening and diagnostic tests such as amniocentesis and ultrasound, the physician treating a high-risk pregnancy now has available tools that permit a woman to exercise her option to abort in a much more informed manner than was previously possible. In addition, the development of alternatives to childbearing—particularly the effective, widespread sterilization of men and women—further expands the scope of endeavors in which treating physicians must discharge their duty of care for patients' well-being.

It is within the context of such developments that the courts have begun to apply (and expand) traditional rules of physician accountability to diverse situations relating to the treatment of high-risk pregnancies.

The Emerging Case Law

The following discussion highlights some recent court decisions addressing physician responsibilities pertaining to treatment of the high-risk pregnancy. As noted above, no effort has been made to exhaustively cite all, or even most, cases affecting this area of law. Rather, the authors have selected a fairly arbitrary number of decisions deemed important both because of the specific points involved and because they illustrate more general principles of physician responsibility.

Litigation involving issues of physician accountability has spawned its own terminology to characterize the different types of claims asserted. Unfortunately, the labels so developed have not been applied with total consistency by courts and commentators [10]. In this chapter, the phrase *wrongful life* will be used to denote a lawsuit brought on behalf of an aggrieved child, usually against the parents' physicians. In such a suit it is generally claimed that the child should be compensated because he or she was born with defects rather than being aborted. The phrase *wrongful birth* will be used to describe a suit brought by the aggrieved parents themselves against their physician, regardless of whether their offspring was born healthy but was merely unplanned or was born with a defect or ailment that the parents claim was preventable or was at least susceptible to prenatal diagnosis.

A substantial number of courts have held that a physician who negligently performs a sterilization procedure is liable for certain damages flowing from the subsequent birth of an unintended child, whether healthy or not. The validity of such a claim, brought by an aggrieved parent, is fairly well established, and the main area of legal dispute is with respect to the damages properly recoverable in this type of lawsuit.

In *Speck v. Finegold* [11] the plaintiff father suffered from neurofibromatosis, which had been transmitted to his first two offspring. To prevent the possibility of conceiving more children with this malady, plaintiff engaged the defendant physician to perform a vasectomy. The sterilization procedure was performed negligently, however, and the plaintiff mother became pregnant. Remarkably, a subsequent abortion was also performed negligently by the same physician, and the plaintiff mother gave birth to a third child afflicted with the inherited disease. While denying the afflicted infant the right to sue in her own name for wrongful life, the Pennsylvania court upheld the parents' claim against the physician, analyzing it as a traditional medical malpractice suit. Upon presentation of satisfactory proof of their allegations, plaintiff parents could recover their pecuniary expenses incurred and to be incurred in the care and treatment of their diseased child, as well as damages for their mental distress and physical inconvenience attributable to the child's birth.

Similarly, in *Stribling v. DeQuevedo* [12] the parents of a child born with dextrocardia (and complications therefrom) after a tubal ligation was negligently performed on the mother were held to state a valid claim for relief against the physicians involved in the unsuccessful surgery. Recoverable damages included compensation for the mother's lost earnings, for the physical pain, suffering, and emotional distress incident to the negligent surgery, for the costs of delivery, and for the costs associated with treatment of the child's ailments.

Cockrum v. Baumgartner [13] involved two separate suits brought by the parents of healthy children born, respectively, after negligently performed sterilization procedures and a negligent misdiagnosis of pregnancy. In each instance, the Illinois Appellate Court held the aggrieved parents entitled to recover the full expenses of raising and educating the unplanned child as an element of damage flowing from the defendant physician's negligence. The court expressly rejected the so-called benefits rule to offset the parents' damages, whereby the presumed emotional rewards of parenthood would be applied in mitigation of the financial costs of raising the child. The court further refused to follow prior Illinois case law, which had limited parents' damages in a "wrongful conception" case to pregnancy- and birth-related costs only, stating that "public policy considerations [cannot] properly be used to deny recovery to parents of an unplanned child of the full measure of all damages proximately caused by a physician's negligence" [14]. On subsequent appeal, however, the Illinois Supreme Court held that the costs of raising a normal and healthy child in such circumstances could not be recovered as damages to the parents.

Similarly, several other courts have recognized claims by parents for negligent sterilization procedures but have limited the recoverable damages to the medical expenses of the unwanted pregnancy, the cost of the ineffective sterilization operation, the pain and suffering connected with the unanticipated pregnancy, the loss of the mother's wages, and the father's loss of his wife's consortium and services arising from the conception [15–21]. Perhaps the strongest statement of this narrower approach to compensable damages in the case of a healthy child born after negligent sterilization was made by the Florida Court of Appeals in *Public Health Trust v. Brown* [22]. In re-

versing that portion of a jury verdict awarding the plaintiff mother the reasonable cost of raising such a child to the age of 18, the court said:

It is a matter of universally-shared emotion that the intangible but all-important, incalculable but invaluable "benefits" of parenthood far outweigh any of the mere monetary burdens involved. . . . Speaking legally, this may be deemed conclusively presumed by the fact that a prospective parent does not abort or subsequently place the unwanted child for adoption [23].

With all due respect for the Florida tribunal, the foregoing cases suggest that there are few, if any, "universally" shared sentiments concerning the extent of physician accountability for unplanned human life [24]. What is abundantly clear, however, is that such liability will be imposed, to a greater or lesser extent, when a physician fails to effectively perform procedures designed to limit family size.

Apart from liability for failing to effectively render medical services to implement a family's decision not to have children, it appears that a physician will also be held liable for failing to diagnose a maternal disease that results in the birth of a defective child, thereby depriving the mother-to-be of her option to abort. *Robak v. United States* [25] was a suit brought by an enlisted man in the United States Army and his wife, who gave birth to a rubella syndrome child. The United States Court of Appeals for the Seventh Circuit, applying the state law of Alabama (where plaintiffs had been stationed at the relevant time), upheld a substantial judgment by a Chicago court against the defendants based on the following negligence by physicians at the Fort Rucker Ob-Gyn Clinic:

Mrs. Robak . . . was then approximately one month pregnant [and] had developed a rash and a fever. She was examined by [the physician], who performed a pregnancy test and a blood test for rubella [German measles]. [The physician] informed Mrs. Robak that she was pregnant and that the test for rubella was negative. Mrs. Robak took a second test for rubella a few days later at the clinic and this test returned positive. She returned to the clinic regularly for routine examinations during her pregnancy. Neither [the physician] nor anyone else at the hospital, however, ever informed Mrs. Robak that she had contracted rubella. She was also never advised of the serious consequences that the rubella virus could have upon her unborn fetus [26].

The plaintiff's daughter was born with serious speech, hearing, vision, and learning disabilities, requiring extensive care, supervision, and surgical treatment during her lifetime. Given that a woman has a constitutional right to decide whether to obtain a first-trimester abortion, the Court of Appeals held that:

the staff at the Ob-Gyn clinic . . . deprived Mrs. Robak of the opportunity to make an informed decision when they failed to tell her of the rubella and of the potential consequences on her fetus. Because of this negligence, the Robaks are faced with large expenses for Jennifer's care and special treatment . . . the defendant must bear the burden for injuries resulting from its own negligence. Any other ruling would in effect immunize from liability those in the medical field providing inadequate guidance to persons who would choose to exercise their constitutional right to abort fetuses, which, if born, would suffer from genetic [or other] defects [27].

The award of $900,000 in damages was affirmed.

The importance of providing the patient with timely and sufficient information so that she may knowingly decide whether to abort or to carry a fetus to term was underscored in *Comras v. Lewin* [28]. In *Comras,* the New Jersey appellate court upheld the validity of a woman's claim for relief against a physician for failing to diagnose plaintiff's pregnancy during the first trimester. The court reasoned that the physician's failure to diagnose the pregnancy until the second trimester deprived plaintiff of her option to have aborted the fetus during the first trimester even though she chose not to abort during the second trimester for health and emotional reasons. A jury was empowered to award damages based on this deprivation of a woman's rights [29].

Becker v. Schwartz [30] involved two cases consolidated for appellate review. In the first case, a 37-year-old woman gave birth to a Down's syndrome child, allegedly without being advised of the increased risk of mongolism in children born to women over age 35 and of the availability of amniocentesis as a diagnostic tool. In the second, companion case, parents whose first child suffered from polycystic kidney disease were allegedly not informed that the disease could be hereditary and conceived a second child born with the same affliction. The New York Court of Appeals declined to recognize a claim on behalf of the afflicted infants for wrongful life but upheld the respective parents' claims for wrongful birth based on the physicians' alleged failure to diagnose and inform. However, recoverable damages were limited to pecuniary expenses incurred or to be incurred for the care and treatment of the afflicted children; the court specifically rejected the parents' claim to damages for emotional injuries suffered by them as a result of their children's conditions.

It is also becoming clear that a physician will be held liable for failing to provide appropriate genetic counseling or testing, or for performing appropriate tests in a less than satisfactory manner. In *Gildiner v. Thomas Jefferson University Hospital* [31] the federal district court applied Pennsylvania law to sustain plaintiff parents' cause of action for negligent genetic testing. When Mrs. Gildiner became pregnant, she and her husband were given a Tay-Sachs test at the defendant hospital; it established that both husband and wife were carriers of Tay-Sachs disease. Plaintiffs subsequently returned for further testing to determine whether their child would be afflicted with Tay-Sachs disease and advised their physician that they would not go through with the pregnancy unless they were assured that their child would not be afflicted with the disease. At their doctor's recommendation, amniocentesis was performed, with the representation that results of the test "would categorically determine whether or not the fetus would have Tay-Sachs disease" [32]. Unfortunately, the test was improperly performed or interpreted. Defendant physicians informed plaintiffs that the results of the amniocentesis eliminated any possibility that the fetus would be born with Tay-Sachs disease. The plaintiffs elected to proceed with the pregnancy, and Mrs. Gildiner subsequently gave birth to a child afflicted with Tay-Sachs disease.

As have a majority of courts considering the issue, the court in *Gildiner* refused to recognize a separate claim for wrongful life brought by the afflicted infant himself, based on the consequences of being born with the disease instead of having been aborted. However, the court upheld the parents' right to recover damages caused by the negligently performed amniocentesis. Such damages would include, at a minimum, the cost of medical treatment for the afflicted child. For procedural reasons, the full scope of cognizable damages (e.g., emotional pain and suffering) was deferred for a later ruling by the court.

In *Berman v. Allan* [33] plaintiff parents gave birth to a Down's syndrome child. They had not been informed of the availability of amniocentesis by their treating physician and alleged that they would have aborted had they known of the likely result of the pregnancy but that they were deprived of this option by the physician's negligence. While denying wrongful-life recovery to the afflicted child because the court perceived that it would be impossible to measure appropriate damages, the New Jersey Supreme Court upheld the parents' right to recover compensation for the emotional injuries sustained as a result of the failure to perform appropriate genetic testing. See also *Phillips v. United States* [34], in which a federal district court applied South Carolina law in upholding the right of the parents of a Down's syndrome child to sue their physician for negligently failing to provide genetic counseling or testing.

In *Naccash v. Burger* [35] the Virginia Supreme Court affirmed most elements of a jury verdict against the defendant physicians. The defendants negligently failed to diagnose plaintiff parents as carriers of Tay-Sachs disease by mishandling the father's blood sample in a Tay-Sachs test; their child was born with the ailment and died after a period of suffering. The parents were awarded as damages the cost of care and treatment of the child during his lifetime, as well as compensation for their own emotional distress.

Another line of cases also indicates that a physician may owe a duty to parents of the child he treats or to any siblings to properly diagnose the child and inform the parents of genetic infirmities in their existing children so that they may make informed choices about the conception of future offspring. In *Turpin v. Sortini* [36] the defendant was a "licensed professional specializing in the diagnosis and treatment of speech and hearing defects," who negligently examined plaintiff parents' first child and failed to diagnose that she was totally deaf because of a hereditary ailment. Not knowing of their first child's hereditary condition, the plaintiffs conceived another child, who was also deaf. The California Supreme Court upheld the validity of claims filed by both the parents and the afflicted second child. Recoverable compensation did not include so-called general damages for depriving the second child of the right to be born as a "whole, functional human being." However, damages to plaintiffs did properly include the cost of specialized teaching, training, and hearing equipment needed by the second child throughout her lifetime as a result of the hearing impediment. (See also *Becker v. Schwartz* [30], in which a physician was held liable for failing to diagnose a prior child's condition as being hereditary, thereby allegedly *causing* the parents to conceive a second child born with the same affliction.)

A physician's duty to a pregnant woman was similarly expanded in *Schroeder v. Perkel* [37]. In *Schroeder* the defendant physician had treated plaintiff parents' first child for four years and had failed to diagnose the child as suffering from cystic fibrosis. The parents conceived another child and were not informed until the eighth month of the second pregnancy, too late to abort, that they were carriers of cystic fibrosis; their second child was also born suffering from the disease. The New Jersey Supreme Court upheld the parents' suit, holding that the physician had a duty to the parents to diagnose and disclose the first child's disease so that the plaintiffs could make an informed decision about further childbearing. The damages that might properly be assessed against the physician included the extraordinary medical expenses of raising the second afflicted child (i.e., the medical, hospital, and pharmaceutical expenses that would necessarily be incurred by the parents for the child's survival). The court reasoned that "If it is proved at trial that the defendant physicians deprived Mr. and Mrs. Schroeder of their right to choose whether or not to give birth to a child afflicted with cystic fibrosis, defendants should be liable for the incremental medical costs of a child born with that affliction" [38].

Yet another evolving area pertaining to physician accountability merits special attention. Given traditional principles of professional responsibility, it is clear that a physician cannot properly render treatment to a fetus that poses a risk of harm to the mother-to-be, at least in the absence of genuinely informed consent by the mother. The flip side of the coin is somewhat more controversial: When might a physician be deemed liable to a child who brings suit after birth for injuries sustained because of treatment provided to the mother prior to the birth?

The modern trend of the law generally permits a child, upon birth, to sue for injuries sustained during gestation, at least where the injury occurred at a time when the fetus was viable [39–42]. Apart from such liability for so-called prenatal torts, several courts have further held that a fetus born alive may maintain suit for injuries caused to it prior to conception. Thus, in *Bergstreser v. Mitchell* [43] an infant was alleged to have suffered a period of hypoxia or anoxia because of delivery by an emergency, cesarean delivery. The need for the emergency delivery was alleged to have resulted from defendant physicians' negligent performance of a prior cesarean delivery to the plaintiff's mother, damaging her uterus, which fact was never disclosed to the infant's mother prior to the second conception and birth. Under Missouri law, the afflicted infant was held to state a valid claim for relief against the physicians. See also *Jorgensen v. Meade Johnson Laboratories, Inc.* [44], and *Renslow v. Mennonite Hospital* [45] for other holdings affirming a child's right to sue for injuries resulting from a preconception tort.

A related area of controversy is currently posed by the issue of whether (and when) a fetus might be permitted to sue for deprivation of federally secured rights under color of state law. The issue of a child's right to sue as a "person" under the civil rights laws is particularly significant for physicians working in the public sector, against whom such liability might be assessed. Compare *Poole v. Endsley* [46] (in which the court held that a fetus is not a protected person within the meaning of federal civil rights laws) with *Douglas v. Town of Hartford* [47] (in which a 5½-month-old fetus was held to be a person capable of maintaining suit under civil rights laws for prenatal injuries).

On the surface, at least, the divergent holdings of some of these cases seem difficult to reconcile. The resulting niceties of legal doctrine obviously reflect the rapid state of flux attending this area of professional responsibility. For the physician, however, clearly a decision to treat a pregnant woman (or to forgo treatment) that results in injury to an unborn (or possibly not yet conceived) child may well subject the practitioner to later liability in a suit by a subsequently born child who has been injured thereby.

While the courts have obviously not considered all possible situations involving the high-risk pregnancy, the foregoing cases make apparent the general judicial willingness to apply and expand traditional principles of physician accountability to such situations as they emerge. The scope of possible damages may vary according to the particular jurisdiction, but obviously the governing standard of care that a physician must achieve and maintain includes successfully diagnosing and testing for genetic abnormalities, prior to and during pregnancy, as well as after the birth itself, and properly performing all procedures designed to limit conception. Above all, it is a physician's legal duty to apprise his patient of enough relevant facts so that the patient may make appropriate decisions concerning conception, abortion, and birth.

MEETING PROFESSIONAL RESPONSIBILITIES OF HIGH-RISK PREGNANCY

As this brief discussion indicates, the extent and scope of a physician's legal responsibilities are expanding at a rapid pace. No longer can the prudent, skillful physician focus solely on protecting maternal well-being, for he or she will increasingly be held accountable for the well-being of a second patient—the fetus—as well. Thus, decisions such as whether to conceive, to abort, to prescribe drugs potentially dangerous to the fetus must all be evaluated from a broader perspective than traditionally employed.

In the authors' opinion, the developments should be viewed, not with paranoia or distaste for the legal system, but as a challenge to practicing physicians to recognize and meet their increased professional responsibility, in the best tradition of the medical profession. Sensitivity and continued education regarding the remarkable medical advances of our era are essential to the practicing physician, both to maintain the quality of care rendered and to minimize potential legal exposure to an aggrieved patient or her family.

In the ideal situation, the physician with the best place in the arena of high-risk pregnancy (and the legal problems incident thereto) would consult with potential parents before conception to discuss their concerns about a future pregnancy. In such a case, the skilled physician could provide to the parents a full range of consultation and advice that would aid them in the initial decision of whether or not to conceive. For example, prospective parents might ask their physician for a determination of whether or not they will have a Tay-Sachs child. The responsible physician could then secure appropriate genetic screening and, with some degree of certainty, advise the parents of the probabilities of having such an afflicted child.

Unfortunately, the physician is rarely confronted with the ideal situation. The physician's first contact with the high-risk pregnancy patient often comes after conception. At that point the physician may be faced with potentially conflicting interests as between the protection of the mother and the protection of the fetus. Obviously, there is a continuing responsibility to meet the standard of care relative to treating the mother-to-be. The physician must always be cognizant of her well-being. Furthermore, it is the doctor's obligation not only to protect her health but also to provide her with adequate information so that she can intelligently decide whether to exercise her right to abort. However, to the extent that a fetus is viable, or if a maternal decision is made to carry a previable fetus to term, all reasonable steps must also be taken to preserve fetal well-being.

In any event, the responsible practicing physician might well develop a standard checklist or questionnaire to be used with either prospective parents or newly pregnant patients. The questionnaire might ask relevant questions about family histories, parental health, existing family genetic patterns, and other phenomena that would help the physician determine the need for genetic counseling, explanation of risks of pregnancy, and other appropriate medical consultation and advice. Such a procedure, regularly followed, properly interpreted, and duly implemented, would go far toward meeting a physician's standard of care in any litigation seeking to hold him or her personally responsible for alleged malpractice.

Other practical steps to follow in this area are similar to those ordinarily pursued in the general practice of medicine. Good rapport and communication between physician and patients are essential, as is a demonstrated sensitivity and concern by the physician for the patient's well-being. Apart from defusing possible legal problems before they emerge, such qualities also assist a physician, albeit in intangible ways, in establishing the propriety of professional conduct if later challenged in court. It should also be remembered that there are few substitutes for good, accurate documentation of a physician's efforts on the patient's behalf. This is especially important in the arena of high-risk pregnancy, where the sufficiency of a patient's informed consent is often the difference between vindication and liability in judicial proceedings.

FUTURE MEDICOLEGAL DEVELOPMENTS

Given the difficulty in stating the exact current status of the law in many specific instances, it is a perilous activity to predict future trends with any precision. It is, nonetheless, likely that physicians' accountability will continue to expand as does medical practice itself.

Thus, as the possibility of fetal treatment for particular disorders improves (e.g., through microsurgical or recombinant DNA techniques), a physician's duty of care will probably include both recognizing the availability of such techniques and performing them in a proper manner [48].

Similarly, the physician's duty may well expand to encompass other relatives of the patient. Comparable to the traditional duty to report certain contagious diseases, an obligation may arise to inform a pregnant woman's siblings that a particular genetic defect may be carried by other family members [36]. Reconciling such an obligation with the one-on-one confidentiality inherent in the traditional physician-patient relationship is well beyond the scope of this chapter. However, it seems to be a fertile area for future litigation to which increased sensitivity is suggested.

Another future development may be the redefinition of fetal viability to an earlier point than the third trimester, as more and more remarkable gains are made in neonatology. It remains to be seen whether the abortion standards set forth by the United States Supreme Court in *Roe v. Wade* will be revised accordingly in the foreseeable future. Such a revision would correspondingly alter the current balance in a physician's obligations as between mother-to-be and fetus.

In a related vein, the issue may well arise (as in other areas of medicine) as to who will bear the sometimes staggering costs of providing the best available diagnostic and treatment techniques. It is possible, for example, that a standard health insurance policy might require a pregnant woman to undergo genetic screening or other medical diagnostic procedures as a condition precedent to full coverage of newly born children.

Rather than reacting impulsively to the specter of our "brave new world," the legal system is likely to respond in traditional ways by applying evolved notions of physician responsibility grounded on established precedent. To the physician aware of professional responsibilities and devoted to improving his or her art, the future treatment of the high-risk pregnancy poses a challenge and an opportunity to better apply medical learning and professional dedication in the overall service of the patient.

REFERENCES

1. Note. Father and mother know best: defining the liability of physicians for inadequate genetic counseling. Yale L J. 1978; 87:1488–1515.
2. Comment. Wrongful life: the right not to be born. Tul L Rev. 1980; 54:480–99.
3. Capron AM. Tort liability and genetic counseling. Colum L Rev. 1979; 79:618–84.
4. Friedman JM. Legal implications of amniocentesis. U Pa L Rev. 1974; 123:93–156.
5. Comment. Live birth: a condition precedent to recognition of rights. Hofstra L Rev. 1976; 4:805–36.
6. King P. The juridical status of the fetus: a proposal for legal protection of the unborn. Mich L Rev. 1979; 77:1647–87.
7. *Canterbury v. Spence,* 464 F.2d 772 (D.C. Cir. Ct.), *cert. denied,* 409 U.S. 1064 (1972).
8. *Scott v. Bradford,* 606 P.2d 554 (Okla. 1979).
9. *Roe v. Wade,* 410 U.S. 113, 93 S.Ct. 705, 35 L.Ed.2d 147 (1973).
10. Compare *Phillips v. United States,* 508 F.Supp. 544, 545, N. 1 (D.S.C. 1981), with *Turpin v. Sortini,* 182 Cal.Rptr. 337, 340, N.4 (Cal. 1982).
11. *Speck v. Finegold,* 439 A.2d 110 (Pa. 1981).
12. *Stribling v. DeQuevedo,* 422 A.2d 505 (Pa. Super. Ct. 1980).
13. *Cockrum v. Baumgartner,* 425 N.E.2d 968 (Ill. App. 1981; __ N.E. 2d __, No. 55733 Ill. Feb. 2, 1983).
14. *Cockrum v. Baumgartner* at 970. *Compare, Ochs v. Borrelli,* 445 A.2d 883 (Conn. 1982), where the court upheld the award of child-rearing expenses to the parents of a child born after a negligent tubal ligation, but allowed the jury to offset the damages by the value of benefit conferred on the parents by the unplanned birth.
15. See *Kingsbury v. Smith,* 442 A.2d 1003 (N.H. 1982).
16. *White v. United States,* 510 F.Supp. 146 (D.Kan. 1981) (applying Georgia law).
17. *Sorkin v. Lee,* 434 N.Y.S.2d 300, 78 A.D.2d 180 (1980).
18. *Bushman v. Burns Clinic Medical Center,* 268 N.W.2d 683 (Mich. App. 1978).
19. *Hickman v. Myers,* 632 S.W.2d 869 (Tex. Civ.App. 1982).

20. *Wilbur v. Kerr,* 628 S.W.2d 568 (Ark. 1982).
21. *Boone v. Mullendore,* 416 So.2d 718 (Ala. 1982).
22. *Public Health Trust v. Brown,* 388 So.2d 1084 (Fla. App. 1980).
23. *Public Health Trust v. Brown* at 1085-6 (citations omitted).
24. *See, e.g., Wilbur v. Kerr* at 571-3 (Dudley, J., dissenting).
25. *Robak v. United States,* 658 F.2d 471 (7th Cir. Ct. 1981).
26. *Robak v. United States* at 473 (footnote omitted).
27. *Robak v. United States* at 476 (footnote omitted).
28. *Comras v. Lewin,* 443 A.2d 229 (N.J. App. 1982).
29. *Comras v. Lewin* at 230.
30. *Becker v. Schwartz,* 386 N.E.2d 807 (N.Y. 1978).
31. *Gildiner v. Thomas Jefferson University Hospital,* 451 F.Supp. 692 (E.D.Pa. 1978).
32. *Gildiner v. Thomas Jefferson University Hospital* at 694.
33. *Berman v. Allan,* 404 A.2d 8 (N.J. 1979).
34. *Phillips v. United States,* 508 F.Supp. 537 and 508, F.Supp. 544 (D.S.C. 1980).
35. *Naccash v. Burger,* 290 S.E.2d 825 (Va. 1982).
36. *Turpin v. Sortini,* 182 Cal.Rptr. 337 (Cal. 1982).
37. *Shroeder v. Perkel,* 432 A.2d 834 (N.J. 1981).
38. *Shroeder v. Perkel* at 842.
39. See, e.g., *Edresz v. Friedberg,* 248 N.E.2d 901 (N.Y. 1969).
40. *Seattle First National Bank v. Rankin,* 367 P.2d 835 (Wash. 1962).
41. *Libby v. Conway,* 192 Cal.App.2d 865, 13 Cal.Rptr. 830 (1961).
42. *Rodriquez v. Patti,* 415 Ill. 496, 114 N.E.2d 721 (1953).
43. *Bergstreser v. Mitchell,* 448 F.Supp. 10 (E.D.Mo.), *affirmed,* 577 F.2d 22 (8th Cir. Ct. 1978).
44. *Jorgensen v. Meade Johnson Laboratories, Inc.,* 483 F.2d 237 (10th Cir. Ct. 1973) (applying Oklahoma law).
45. *Renslow v. Mennonite Hospital,* 367 N.E.2d 1250 (Ill. 1977).
46. *Poole v. Endsley,* 371 F.Supp. 1379 (N.D.Fla. 1974).
47. *Douglas v. Town of Hartford,* 542 F.Supp. 1267 (D.Conn. 1982).
48. *Phillips v. United States,* 508 F.Supp. 537, 543, N.4 (D.S.C. 1980).

That they bred in and in, as might be shown,
marrying their cousins—nay, their aunts,
and nieces,
which always spoils the breed, if it increases.
—Lord Byron
Don Juan

3. PRENATAL GENETICS

Paul Wexler and James J. Nora

With the growing awareness of the risk of environmental agents, including intentionally ingested substances, the question as to why these agents affect some individuals, but not all, and why they affect some individuals to a greater or lesser extent than others, focuses attention on variation and the inherent constitution of the individual. The chapters on pharmacology (Chap. 6) and teratology (Chap. 7) consider the evidence of how endogenous or exogenous agents influence structure or function of the individual. Genetics must also be considered in an effort to understand how an individual responds to specific influences.

The complexity of genetic principles and the explosion in the technology of genetic study threaten the young student of basic genetics and completely repel the more senior clinician who had little or no foundation in the field. Yet a desire to provide a family with all the information possible about its risks and choices of conceiving and begetting a normal child requires that the clinician have a basic understanding of patterns of inheritance. It is also necessary that there be an awareness of the value of and indications for antenatal diagnosis and an openness about limitations in one's knowledge that may require another expert opinion.

A meticulous history eliciting information about family disease and addressing specific heritable conditions is as appropriate for the pregnant woman as for the general medical patient. Maternal and paternal drug exposure prior and subsequent to conception may offer little information that is helpful to a specific pregnancy but can allow a compilation of data that might be of value in the future. Isolated cases of problematic fetal outcomes may help to unmask the evidence required to create concern about specific influences. The pregnant woman is alert to environmental risks, and documentation of medication or disease in pregnancy is improving. Still, the interaction of heredity and environment will continue to cloud the appropriate allocation of responsibility to each of these factors.

Except for those individuals at special risk, most obstetric outcomes produce intact newborns. The availability of improved diagnostic techniques now provides the means to investigate gestation more carefully. It is clear that invasive methods for fetal assessment will not become standard care for all pregnant women. Noninvasive technology (e.g., ultrasound, serum alpha-fetoprotein, echocardiography) and changes in societal behavior (e.g., limitation of family size and delayed parenthood) may make prenatal diagnosis more attractive, even to the low-risk patient. As with most of medicine, the balance between indicated procedures and available knowledge and technology is delicate and dynamic. The patient, planning her family, will expect her physician to be knowledgeable in the applications of new medical advances to her situation. The information presented should serve as a substantial foundation upon which to build a working knowledge of the field, as it is today.

BASIC GENETIC PRINCIPLES

Although Charles Darwin attempted to address heritability in considering the factors responsible for evolution, and Gregor Mendel set forth many of the principles that helped to explain the end results of inherited characteristics, their work was not incorporated into the general body of medical knowledge. It is not surprising that the application of genetic principles to clinical medicine was delayed when one realizes that for more than 30 years prior to 1956 the teaching was that the human cell possessed 48 chromosomes. In 1956 Tijo and Levan, using improved techniques of preparation, correctly described the 46 chromosomes found in normal human diploid cells (22 pairs of autosomes and 2 sex chromosomes) [1]. Beginning in 1970, the introduction of new staining methods allowed chromosomes to be further characterized [2]. Prior to this time, the size of the chromosomes and the location of the centromere were the only methods employed for classifying chromosomes.

COMMON CHROMOSOME-STAINING METHODS

Quinacrine Mustard (Q Banding)
When chromosomes are stained with quinacrine mustard, bright and dull bands can be observed with the fluorescent microscope. The specific patterns can be used to separate different chromosomes from one another and to match homologous pairs (Fig. 3-1).

Giemsa Stain (G Banding)
If chromosomes are stained with Giemsa following trypsin treatment to denature protein, dark and light staining bands (G bands) are observed. The dark bands are the same as the bright bands seen with Q banding (Fig. 3-2).

It is possible to prepare chromosomes with reverse banding techniques (R banding), which reverse the light and dark bands seen with G banding. Centromeric banding (C banding) can identify small changes in the area of the centromere such as inversions or deletions. Stains are also available for studying limited areas of specific chromosomes (e.g., nucleolar organizing regions—NOR stain) or small contributions in satellited chromosomes (G

11 banding). If chromosomes are fixed, stained, and photographed just prior to metaphase when they are less contracted, they can be further characterized. In this way, small differences between chromosomes can be seen. This method of chromosome preparation (high-resolution chromosomes) may help to identify specific changes found in pathologic states. Most clinical studies are performed by means of G banding. The other methods of cell preparation are used when diagnosis is uncertain.

CLASSIFICATION OF GENETIC DISORDERS
The major genetic disorders are due to chromosomal abnormalities or single gene defects or may conform to the mode of multifactorial inheritance. Chromosomal abnormalities may occur with either an excess or a deficiency of all or part of one or more chromosomes. Being the most common cause of spontaneous abortions (more than 50%), they also account for a significant number of abnormal newborns (approximately 5 per 1,000 births) [3,4].

Single gene defects are due to mutations at a specific site on a chromosome. If the evidence of a gene is manifested by its presence when on only

Fig. 3-1. Human karyotype stained with fluorescent quinacrine mustard (QFQ banding). (Photograph courtesy of the Cytogenetics Laboratory, Rose Medical Center.)

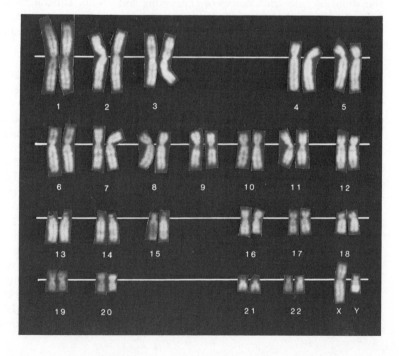

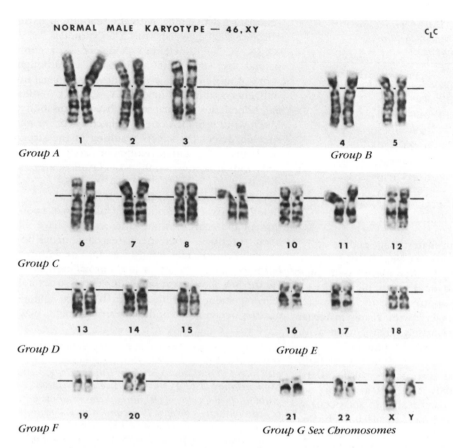

Fig. 3-2. Human karyotype stained with Giemsa following trypsin treatment (GTG banding). (Photograph courtesy of the Cytogenetics Laboratory, Rose Medical Center.)

one of a homologous pair of chromosomes (single dose), it is said to be dominant. If a mutant gene is seen (expressed) only when present on both chromosomes, it is called recessive.

A mutant gene can also be present on a sex chromosome. In a male with one X and one Y sex chromosome, in addition to 22 pairs of autosomes, a mutant gene on the X chromosome is likely to be expressed (X-linked disease—e.g. hemophilia A, Duchenne muscular dystrophy). Females (XX) possessing one normal and one mutant gene are "carriers" and are, usually, unaffected themselves. Only one Y-linked disorder is known ("hairy pinnae syndrome").

Multifactorial inheritance is responsible for most cases of the common birth defects, such as congenital heart anomalies, neural tube defects, cleft lip and palate, and clubfoot, and results from the interaction of several genes with the environment.

Chromosomal Abnormalities

Chromosomal defects may be divided into disor-ders of number (aneuploidy) and disorders of structure.

Aneuploidy

Abnormal chromosome numbers may be found in as many as 7 to 8% of all conceptions. Total absence of an autosome is usually incompatible with life. Absence of a sex chromosome is not, however, due to a biologic process in which only one X chromosome is required to carry the major genetic information. Duplication of an autosome or an extra sex chromosome often results in abortion, but pregnancies may continue to term. Approximately 1 in 200 newborns will demonstrate an abnormal chromosome number, abnormal numbers of sex chromosomes being slightly more frequent than abnormal autosome numbers. As many as 7% of stillborns will demonstrate aneuploidy [7]. Polyploidy (e.g., 69 or 92 chromosomes), a multiple of the haploid number of chromosomes (23 chromosomes) other than diploid (46 chromosomes), may be seen in abortions and tissue culture.

Down syndrome (trisomy 21), the disorder with which we are most familiar, occurs in approximately 1 in 800 births [4]. The incidence in-

Table 3-1. Approximate risk of chromosomal anomalies (including Down's syndrome) with advancing maternal age

Maternal age (yr)	Approximate risk (%)
<20	0.05– 0.08
20–24	0.08– 0.10
25–29	0.08– 0.15
30–34	0.12– 0.20
35–39	0.30– 0.80
40–42	0.90– 1.50
43–45	1.50– 3.00
46–49	2.00–10.00

creases with increasing maternal age and, possibly, if the paternal age is greater than 55 years [5,6]. Males conceiving a child after age 55 years may also have an increased incidence of mutant genes. Table 3-1 shows the approximate incidence of a chromosomal abnormality with rising maternal age. At present, approximately 20% of infants with Down's syndrome are born to women older than 35 years. The age-specific incidence is for both numerical and structural chromosomal disorders. Trisomy 18 and trisomy 13 result in a more severely affected child than trisomy 21 and occur in approximately 1 in 5,000 to 10,000 births. Trisomy 8 mosaicism (the existence of more than one cell line in the same individual) may be more common than was formerly realized and produces children with floppy ears, variable mental retardation, marked skeletal abnormalities, hands with deep palmar creases, and characteristic facies.

Excessive numbers of sex chromosomes also produce significant disease, the severity of mental retardation worsening with the amount of extra chromosomal material. Thus XO (Turner's), XXX, XXXX, XXY (Klinefelter), XYY are all accompanied by significant abnormalities. Although some of these disorders may allow for normal intelligence and functioning (XXY, 45,X; XYY) they are, nonetheless, the cause of substantial disability. Much work is being done to help characterize the specific defect or defects resulting in the structural, metabolic, and developmental abnormalities seen with abnormal numbers of chromosomes.

Structural Chromosomal Defects

Deletion (loss), duplication, and insertion of a portion of one chromosome into another have all been described. Unbalanced rearrangements between chromosomes (translocations) or within a chromosome can result in an abnormal individual. Figure 3-3 shows several examples of structural rearrangements. Rarely, other structural abnormalities occur. Some of these rearrangements may

Fig. 3-3. Examples of deletion, reciprocal translocation, and Robertsonian translocation. Idiograms modeled after International System for Human Cytogenetic Nomenclature (ISCN) (1981). A. Deletion: (a) Idiogram of chromosome 4; (b) normal chromosome 4; (c) chromosome 4 deleted. B. Reciprocal translocation: (a) Idiogram of chromosome 4; (b) normal chromosome 4; (c) chromosome 4, deleted; (d) idiogram of chromosome 21; (e) normal chromosome 21; (f) chromosome 21 with translocated portion of chromosome 4. C. Robertsonian translocation within chromosome group D (13, 14, 15): (a) Normal chromosome 13; (b) translocation between chromosomes 13 and 14; (c) normal chromosome 14; (d) normal chromosome 15. (Photograph courtesy of the Cytogenetics Laboratory, Rose Medical Center.)

Structural Chromosomal Rearrangements

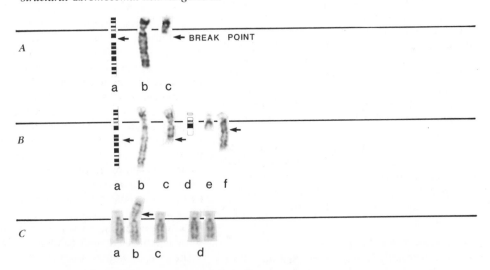

be unstable and fail to undergo normal cell division. Many result in substantial gain or loss of chromosomal material causing abnormal development.

Most translocations are between groups D and G (Fig. 3-2) and usually involve chromosome 21. Chromosome 14 is more commonly involved from group D (approximately 60%) although chromosomes 13 and 15 may be involved (approximately 20% for each). Translocations may be balanced (reciprocal—parts of two chromosomes are exchanged) or unbalanced (a portion of genetic material is lost). In a robertsonian translocation the breaks occur at the centromeres of two chromosomes, and entire chromosome arms are exchanged (Fig. 3-3).

Single Gene Defects
Autosomal Dominant
If a gene is manifested when it is present on only one of a pair of autosomes, it is called a dominant gene. If the gene is abnormal, a disease may result. More than 1,400 such diseases are known. It is characteristic of dominant inheritance that the trait will be transmitted to 50% of all offspring (Fig. 3-4). As a general rule, defects in structural protein are inherited as dominant disorders whereas enzymatic defects are usually transmitted in a recessive fashion. Since some autosomal dominant disorders are not expressed immediately, there may be a delay in diagnosis. Huntington's chorea, a disease in which there is mental deterioration and abnormal (choreic) movements, has a

Fig. 3-4. Autosomal dominant inheritance pattern (theoretical). □ = *normal male;* ■ = *affected male;* ○ = *normal female;* ● = *affected female.*

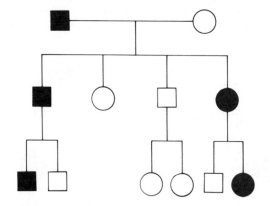

Males, females affected equally
50% of children inherit gene
50% of children are normal
All individuals with gene have the disease (severity may vary with expression of the gene)

variable age onset; by age 39 approximately 50% of individuals possessing the gene will have manifested the disease. Even at age 49 approximately 18% of individuals possessing the gene will not have demonstrated any symptoms. When the expression of a gene or trait is less than 100%, it is said to demonstrate reduced penetrance.

Autosomal Recessive
Most biochemical disorders demonstrate an autosomal recessive mode of inheritance (more than 1,100 diseases are known). Since expression of the disease requires the abnormal gene to be present on both of a homologous pair of autosomes, recognition of the carrier state often follows the birth of an affected child. The more rare an autosomal recessive disease, the lower the carrier state in the general population and the greater the probability of consanguinity. Conversely, cystic fibrosis, the most common autosomal recessive disease in whites, has a carrier frequency of about 1 in 20. Because the gene is so common in the general population, the occurrence of the disease in one child does not necessarily suggest consanguinity. The disease may affect as many as one child in every 1,600 births.

Included in the category of autosomal recessive diseases are many inborn errors of metabolism. Approximately 100 disorders that can be inherited in an autosomal recessive manner are accessible to antenatal diagnosis. Many more have yet to be diagnosed prenatally. Specific determination of the autosomal recessive mode of inheritance in any specific clinical case may elude proof. Twenty-five percent of children conceived to carrier couples will be affected, 25% will be unaffected and not possess the gene, and 50% will be unaffected but be carriers (Fig. 3-5).

Sex-Linked Disorders
As mentioned earlier, there is only one known Y-linked disorder (hairy pinnae syndrome). The inheritance of this disorder is not totally clear and may be due to some interaction between the X and Y chromosomes.

Females possess two X chromosomes, one of which is genetically active. One X chromosome is inactivated in each cell and can be identified as a Barr body, a dark-staining circular mass of chromatin seen in the perimeter of the nucleus of the cell. The inactivation of one X chromosome occurs randomly, and either the paternal or the maternal X chromosome is active in any one cell. As a result, women carrying a mutant gene on an X chromosome will be less seriously affected by the presence of a defective gene than a male because they

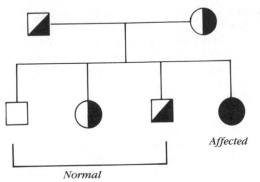

Affected

Normal

Males, females affected equally

Parents are carriers

50% of children carry abnormal gene and are
not affected (single dose)

25% of children affected with disease (double
dose)

25% of children are normal

67% of unaffected offspring are carriers of the
abnormal gene

*Fig. 3-5. Autosomal recessive inheritance pattern
(theoretical). □ = normal male; ▨ = carrier male;
● = affected female; ◐ = carrier female.*

usually have adequate primary gene product from the normal gene. An example is the lowered value of factor VIII (antihemophilic globulin) seen in mothers of a hemophiliac male child. The child's X chromosome must come from the mother since the Y originates from the father. Although the mother carries the mutant gene (obligate carrier), the disease is usually not clinically manifest in her.

X-linked disease may be dominant or recessive. If recessive, it will be expressed in all males with the abnormal gene (half of the male offspring) and one-half of the females will be carriers. X-linked dominant disorders are rare. Vitamin D–resistant

rickets (hypophosphatemia) is an example. There-fore, most sex-linked diseases are due to mutant genes on an X chromosome, are recessively inher-ited, and affect males. Transmission of X-linked dominant disease is from an affected mother to half of her daughters and half of her sons and from an affected male to all of his daughters and none of his sons (Fig. 3-6).

X-linked recessive disorders are usually severe and often fatal. Approximately 200 diseases with this mode of inheritance have been described. If the disorder is highly lethal in males, new cases will be caused, to a significant degree, by new mu-tations. Transmission is from a carrier female to 50% of all progeny. Of the 50% of the children re-ceiving the abnormal gene, all sons will be affected and all daughters will be carriers. There is no father-to-son transmission, and all daughters of an affected father are obligate carriers; that is, the in-herited paternal X will possess the mutant gene (Fig. 3-7).

Hemophilia A (AHG or factor VIII deficiency), hemophilia B, and Duchenne muscular dystrophy are examples of this mode of inheritance. X-linked hydrocephalus, secondary to aqueductal stenosis, gained international attention subsequent to the first report of transuterine placement of a func-tioning ventricular shunt [8].

It has also been suggested that X-linked mental retardation may be a common form of mental defi-ciency in males [9]. Some of these patients may demonstrate a secondary constriction or break at the distal end of the long arm of the X chromo-

*Fig. 3-6. Sex-linked dominant inheritance pattern
(theoretical). A. Male affected. B. Female affected.
□ = normal male; ■ = affected male; ○ = normal
female; ● = affected female.*

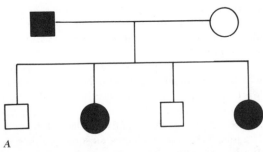

A

Anyone possessing gene is affected with disease

Males transmit abnormal gene to all daughters and
no sons

All daughters are affected with disease

All sons are normal

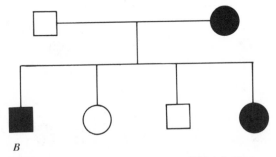

B

Women transmit abnormal gene to 50% of all sons
and daughters

50% of all children, regardless of sex, will have the
disease

50% of all children will be normal

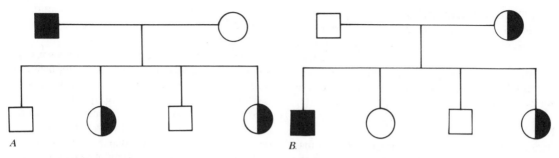

A

Male transmits abnormal gene to all daughters
No father to son transmission
Daughters with the abnormal gene are carriers

B.

Female transmits abnormal gene to 50% of daughters
 and 50% of sons
Sons inheriting the gene have the disease
Daughters inheriting the gene are carriers

Fig. 3-7. Sex-linked recessive inheritance pattern (theoretical). A. Male affected with disease. B. Female carrier. □ = normal male; ■ = affected male; ○ = normal female; ◑ = carrier female.

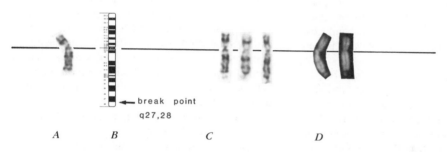

A   B   C   D

Fig. 3-8. Marker X. (A) Normal X chromosome. (B) Idiogram of X chromosome modeled after ISCN. (C) Marker-X (GTG banding). (D) Marker X (QFQ banding). (Photograph courtesy of the Cytogenetics Laboratory, Rose Medical Center.)

some (marker-X or fragile-X) when it is cultured in media 199, which is low in folic acid and thiamine (Fig. 3-8).

Multifactorial Inheritance

Multifactorial inheritance assumes an interaction between a genetic predisposition (usually polygenic) and an environmental trigger. It is felt that inheritance of traits, such as intelligence or height, is the result of the interaction between many genes and the environment; however, a major gene or a small number of genes may be visualized as having a required interaction with an environmental trigger. The appearance of a defect (e.g., heart or neural tube) may be explained as a specific inherited susceptibility within the individual and a specific threshold. The predictable and significant risk of phocomelia produced coincident with the ingestion of thalidomide failed to cause these defects in all exposed individuals and

demonstrates the relationship between susceptibility, threshold, and attack rates.

The recurrence risk of this mode of inheritance is related to a number of factors: the frequency of the defect in the population, the sex of the patient, even the season of the year. For example, the recurrence risk for pyloric stenosis in subsequent siblings is greater if the affected individual is female. This phenomenon may be due to the fact that the threshold for females is higher, implying that a greater genetic predisposition is needed for a female to get the disease. Also, the risk of recurrence in a family is greater when more than one family member is affected. Monozygotic twins are more often both affected than dizygotic twins, but frequently only one is affected. The risk of recurrence in a sibling of a disorder inherited in a multifactorial manner, if there is only one index case in the family, is approximately 1 to 5%.

Neural tube defects can often be diagnosed antenatally and conform to the mode of multifactorial inheritance. Congenital heart defects, cleft lip and palate, susceptibility to cancer, stroke, and heart attack are additional examples of diseases that recur in families in a multifactorial inheritance pattern.

ANTEPARTUM DIAGNOSIS

In addition to the methods described in Chapter 5 for assessing fetal well-being, antenatal testing methods can be applied to intrauterine diagnosis of abnormalities of the fetus and of the fetal-placental unit. Some of these methods are described below.

Ultrasound

Beginning very early in gestation, ultrasound may help to distinguish intrauterine versus extrauterine gestation and to follow the growth and development of the gestational sac and fetus. Although the cost-effectiveness of routine ultrasound screening for all pregnancies is questionable, it can be extremely valuable in problem pregnancies. Nonviable pregnancy (including hydatidiform mole) and multiple gestation can be reliably diagnosed with realtime ultrasound. Crown–rump measurements early in pregnancy and biparietal measurements later in pregnancy can help to answer the issue of uncertain gestational dates, that occurs in at least 25% of patients [10].

With realtime ultrasound screening, fixed B-scan ultrasound employing gray scale, and selective use of sector scanning, delineation of fetal organs and development has been remarkably enhanced. When combined with amniotic fluid alpha-fetoprotein, more than 90% of open neural tube defects are liable to diagnosis. Amniotic fluid acetylcholinesterase can help to further delineate the borderline cases. Routine testing for serum alpha-fetoprotein in pregnancy has been controversial in the United States because of a significant incidence of false positive results (approximately 3%) and a relatively low incidence of the disorder (3 per 1,000) [11]. In Great Britain, Ireland, and Wales, an incidence figure for neural tube defects approximating 1% has encouraged routine serum screening. Anencephaly can be detected by 13 to 14 weeks of gestation by the absence of the regular outline of the fetal skull. Amniocentesis is rarely necessary to confirm the diagnosis.

Diagnosis of hydrocephaly is based on the early detection of increasing ventricular size to head size ratios. The ratio should be below 0.5 after approximately 17 weeks of gestation. Later in pregnancy, a thinning of the cerebral mantle to below 1 cm may be indicative of a poor fetal prognosis [12]. Since the time when a ventricular shunt is placed can significantly affect the infant's prognosis, ultrasound may provide clinical information to help decide when to deliver an infant. If a transuterine placement of a ventricular shunt proves to be in the best interest of the fetus, ultrasound can direct the timing as well as the actual performance of the procedure [8].

Noninvasive detection of major fetal vascular and cardiac defects may soon be accomplished by utilization of advanced techniques in ultrasound, including fetal echocardiography [13–15]. Any cardiac defect that can be demonstrated with the maternal-fetal circulation intact might be liable to diagnosis (e.g., interventricular or interarterial defects, or malpositions of the great vessels).

The fetal stomach, intestine, liver, kidney, and urinary bladder can often be visualized during routine ultrasound examination. Fetal bowel obstruction (e.g., duodenal atresia, imperforate anus) as well as omphalocele, diaphragmatic hernia (often with coexisting lung atresia), ascites, and fetal pleural effusions have all been detected antenatally.

Fetal urethral obstruction, polycystic renal disease, and renal agenesis (Potter syndrome—renal agenesis or hypoplasia with characteristic facies and skeletal abnormalities) can also be diagnosed. If neither fetal bladder nor fetal kidneys can be seen after one or two hours of observation, intravenous administration of 20 to 40 mg furosemide to the mother, followed by repeat scan in 30 minutes, may demonstrate a previously undetected functioning renal system.

Careful measurement of limb growth can detect many cases of short-limb dysplasia, especially if it involves the long bones. Pathologic fractures occurring in patients at risk for some types of osteogenesis imperfecta may also be seen.

Amniocentesis

The incidence of chromosomal disorders is approximately 1 in 200 live-born infants [16]. As discussed earlier, some couples are at increased risk (e.g., increased maternal age, translocation carriers), and antenatal diagnosis can offer the family assurance of a chromosomally normal child, in most instances.

Amniocentesis is a method for acquiring viable fetal cells that are suspended in the amniotic liquor. The cells can be cultured, and after approximately two to three weeks enough cells are present to allow karyotyping. Detection of biochemical abnormalities may require three to five weeks or longer from the time of amniocentesis. Many tests can be performed by only one or very few laboratories in the country.

Occasionally, a careful genetic history will reveal one or more additional specific disorders that can be detected by amniocentesis. Therefore, most cytogenetics laboratories strongly encourage careful evaluation of the patient for amniocentesis prior to performing the procedure.

The incidence of immediate complications from amniocentesis (e.g., leakage of fluid or bleeding) is 1 to 2%. Approximately 3% of women will experience fetal loss, but the incidence is similar for women at risk who do not have amniocentesis [17]. It is likely, however, that injury to the fetus or disruption of the placenta will result in an occasional fetal loss that otherwise would not have occurred. The direct risk of fetal loss secondary to amniocentesis is unknown but should be less than 1 in 200 to 500 procedures. Cutaneous scarring of the fetus from superficial needle puncture can occur. Serious complications involving the fetus, yet not resulting in fetal loss, have been infrequent [18–22].

Amniocentesis is best performed at 15 to 17 weeks' gestation, when the volume of fluid is adequate (approximately 125–400 mL) [23]. Unfortunately, current methods do not allow detection of most chromosomal and biochemical disorders in the first trimester.

Although the risk of fetal loss was statistically no different for patients requiring one or two needle insertions, there was an increased incidence with repeated insertions (2.9%, 4.3%, and 8.1% for one, two, or three insertions respectively) as reported in the 1976 NICHD study [17]. Fetal loss decreased with the experience of the operator from 3.7% for clinicians who had performed fewer than 10 needle punctures to 0.3% when clinicians had gained experience by performing more than 50 punctures [18]. The benefits derived from preamniocentesis ultrasound are uncertain. It does allow fetal assessment, assurance of fetal viability, placental localization, and an opportunity for site selection. With realtime ultrasound, loops of umbilical cord can be identified and some attempt made to minimize the fetal hazard from the procedure.

Since amniocentesis requires careful evaluation of the patient for appropriate indications, consideration for special testing, and a working knowledge of ultrasound or an ultrasonographer, most physicians will choose to refer their patients to a diagnostic center. If referral is not feasible, consideration should be given to the advisability of pooling community expertise and resources so that amniotic fluid can be obtained safely and delivered to an appropriate laboratory facility. Although many laboratories will provide the physician with transport kits, a slight decrease in the likelihood of receiving a diagnosis should be expected due to the handling of viable cell preparations.

Identification of normal DNA sequences isolated from fetal fibroblasts obtained by amniocentesis, which represents the gene that codes for specific globin polypeptide chains, have enabled the diagnosis of some of the thalassemias, sickle cell anemia, and other major hemoglobinopathies to be made prenatally. Pooled placental blood aspiration or fetoscopy performed for the acquisition of fetal blood samples, under direct vision, has also been used for prenatal detection of some hemoglobinopathies. Details of fetoscopy and methods for acquiring fetal tissues or blood are discussed in a subsequent section. When the procedure is performed on fibroblasts obtained by conventional amniocentesis, the risks are no different from those of amniocentesis for chromosomal diagnosis.

Other Methods for Prenatal Diagnosis
Recombinant DNA Molecular
Hybridization
Conditions for which severe sequelae are probable—for example, sickle cell disease (HbSS), homozygous beta-thalassemia (Cooley anemia), and homozygous alpha-thalassemia—may make it appropriate to consider prenatal diagnosis. Cultured fibroblasts demonstrate only a fraction of the human genome. The method for detection of mutant genes is called molecular hybridization. It depends on the incubation of radiolabeled messenger RNA specific for the gene with denatured (single-stranded) DNA from normal or mutant cells. The DNA will merge with the messenger RNA to form a messenger RNA-DNA hybrid. An estimation of normal hybridization that will occur is made from incubation of labeled messenger RNA with known normal single-stranded DNA. If deletion of a gene has occurred, no hybridization will take place. The presence of less hybrid than might be expected is a sign of partial deletion of the gene. The method has been improved upon by means of hybrid techniques using copying DNA prepared from the purified gene-specific messenger RNA. Individuals carrying no copies of the gene (homozygous alpha-thalassemia), one copy (HbH disease), two copies (heterozygous alpha-thalassemia), three copies (alpha-thalassemia carrier), and four copies (normal) have now been identified [24–27].

Restriction Endonucleases
Another prenatal diagnostic method, which can also be applied to amniotic fluid fetal fibroblasts, employs commercially available restriction enzymes that cleave certain proteins (in this case

DNA) in specific sites. These bacterial endonu-cleases recognize specific nucleotide sequences. After cleavage, autoradiography is used to identify the specific fragments and compare them to a map of known globin chains treated with the same en-zymes. In sickle cell disease (HbSS) a change in the DNA sequence is found (GAGGAG is changed to GTGGAG). Recently an enzyme has been isolated that can cleave the DNA sequence, GAGG. There-fore, a normal individual would demonstrate this fragment whereas a patient with SS hemoglobin would not. Kan, using a different restriction en-donuclease, has been able to identify fetuses with HbS (fragments contain 13 kilobases and 7 kilobases) whereas normal individuals produce only 7 kilobase fragments [24]. Future applications to the hemoglobinopathies as well as utilization of these methods to further elucidate the activity of specific genes or regions of the genome should be forthcoming. For a more complete discussion of the methodology, the reader is referred to refer-ences 27 to 30.

Fetoscopy
Aspiration of placental blood guided by placental localization with ultrasound and immediately analyzed by a particle-size analyzer will identify the larger fetal red blood cell. Fetal blood aspira-tion can then be carried out. The fetus can be di-rectly visualized and fetal skin or fetal blood sam-ples obtained that are less contaminated by mater-nal blood or amniotic fluid using a fetoscope [30–36].

A 1.7-mm needlescope is placed in the amniotic sac, and a 26- or 27-gauge needle is used for fetal blood sampling. Skin biopsy is possible under di-rect vision, and limited vision of the fetus is often possible. Intravenous sedation administered to the mother before or during the procedure will re-duce the activity of the fetus. Candidates for this procedure include fetuses at risk for sex-linked disorders (hemophilia A or B) in which karyotyp-ing will allow detection only of the fetal sex (i.e., 50% of males will be affected), the hemo-globinopathies, some cases of neural tube defects in which laboratory results are inconclusive or in disagreement with one another, and some cases of limb dysplasias (e.g., Ellis-van Creveld, certain cases of dwarfism). Also, fetoscopy is useful with fetal cutaneous changes (epidermolysis bullosa letalis) in which coincident occurrence of other major constitutional problems in the fetus might justify prenatal diagnosis [36,37]. Diagnosis of X-linked Duchenne muscular dystrophy was de-scribed by Mahoney et al. in 1977, using assay of fetal plasma creatinine phosphokinase levels [38].

The assay has not proved to be as valuable as was originally believed because of false negative re-sults [39,40].

Fetal loss is variably reported as between 3 and 10% following fetoscopy. Antibiotics and tocolytic drugs have been used by some investigators. Am-nionitis, fetal death in utero, and preterm labor explain most of the losses.

Although the technique can provide informa-tion that may not be obtainable in any other way, the incidence of unsuccessful fetal outcomes fol-lowing its performance will keep fetoscopy lim-ited to patients requiring the information and in the hands of those expert in its performance.

Genetic Linkage
Genetic linkage analysis is based on the specific re-lationship between genes. Because of a close placement to one another on a chromosome, some genes tend to remain together, after cell multipli-cation, more often than might be explained by chance alone. Testing for linkage analysis is based on the presence or absence of an identifiable (rec-ognizable) marker that is found in conjunction with a specific disease. Autosomal dominant dis-eases in which no specific enzyme defect has been defined are likely candidates for study [41]. Edgell et al. used known linkage between the G6PD locus and the locus for hemophilia A [42]. Diagnosis by linkage analysis will always be liable to error, how-ever small, because recombination can occur even among closely linked loci.

If cells are incubated with and without a sus-pected deficient substance (e.g., enzyme provided either exogenously or by incubation with normal cells, which do produce the enzyme), it may be possible to distinguish normal from diseased cells. Demonstration of this distinction can allow for prenatal confirmation of a suspected defect and may even allow detection of an affected fetus, where the specific defect is unknown if character-istics between normal and diseased cells are differ-ent. Xeroderma pigmentosum, in which a defect in a thymine-splitting endonuclease is known, results in different susceptibility to environmental ma-nipulations, such as heat, pH, or ultraviolet light, than is found in normal cells.

Fetal Cells in the Maternal Circulation
Finally, Schröder and others described the trans-placental passage and appearance of fetal lympho-cytes in maternal blood that traverse the placenta in the first trimester [43–45]. Herzenberg, Sweet, and Herzenberg used a fluorescence-activated cell sorter for this purpose [46]. Approximately 1 in every 2,000 to 5,000 maternal white blood cells is of fetal origin. Occasional maternal samples will

show as many as 1% of the lymphocytes to be fetal. The fetal cells are refractive to mitogens, and karyotype analysis was not possible [44]. Even if this difficulty could be overcome, the presence of an XX karyotype would require differentiation from the maternal karyotype, and cells demonstrating an XY karyotype have been returned during a current pregnancy when a female infant was delivered. This event is presumed to be due to persistence of viable XY cells from a prior pregnancy. Much attention will be directed to this method in the next several years in the search for safe, noninvasive fetal diagnostic approaches.

INDICATIONS FOR PRENATAL DIAGNOSIS

In the preceding pages we have discussed basic principles in genetics and described various methods employed for prenatal diagnosis. It remains only to describe the selection of patients to be considered for prenatal diagnosis. Stephenson and Weaver compiled a list of almost 200 disorders that have been diagnosed antenatally [47]. History of recurrent familial disorders or abnormal progeny should lead to counseling from someone learned in patterns of inheritance. Conventional indications and possible indications for prenatal diagnosis are listed in Table 3-2. Many of the conditions listed under possible indications are found

Table 3-2. Candidates for prenatal diagnosis

Conventional indications
  Maternal age at delivery >35 years
  Previous child with known chromosomal defect
  Either parent a carrier of known chromosomal
    defect
  Previous child with neural tube defect
  Parents carriers of a diagnosable inborn error of
    metabolism
  Determination of sex-linked recessive disease
    (see Table 3-3)
Possible indications
  Parental metabolic derangements—e.g., diabetes,
    autoimmune thyroiditis, alpha₁-antitrypsin
    deficiency [50–53]
  X-ray exposure (see Chap. 8)
  Advanced paternal age [5, 6]
  Habitual abortion, especially if with known chromo-
    somal abnormality [48, 49, 54, 55]
  Induced ovulation [56, 57]
  Delayed fertilization (?)
  Artificial insemination (?)
  Parental chromosomal variants (?)
  Maternal age at delivery 30–34 years with any other
    risk factor

in patients in whom the difficulty of having achieved a pregnancy at all would make the small risk of prenatal diagnostic testing unacceptable.

Autosomal Dominant Inheritance
In many of the autosomal dominant disorders it falls to the genetic counselor to inform the patients of their statistical risks. Occasionally the disorder can be diagnosed prenatally by ultrasonography or linkage analysis. In couples in whom the father is a known or potential carrier of a defective gene, the couple may choose artificial insemination. Although the circumstances surrounding the issue and the legality of surrogate motherhood make this option less than optimum, some couples will choose it for circumstances in which the female is at risk. Disorders included in this category are Huntington chorea, Marfan syndrome, acute intermittent porphyria, achondroplasia, some types of polycystic kidney disease, dyslexia, and neurofibromatosis.

Autosomal Recessive Inheritance
The approximately 100 autosomal recessively inherited diseases that can be diagnosed antenatally make up the largest single category of diseases for consideration for prenatal diagnosis. Most are due to inborn errors of metabolism and they include some of the better-known disorders (Tay-Sachs, Sandhoff, Sanfilippo, Hurler, most glycogen storage diseases, such as Gaucher, Niemann-Pick, and Krabbe, disorders of amino acid metabolism, and other disorders usually characterized by an enzyme deficiency).

Sex-Linked Recessive Inheritance
Some X-linked recessive diseases are listed in Table 3-3. Except for Lesch-Nyhan, Fabry, G6PD deficiency, X-linked hydrocephalus, and possibly the hemophilias and Duchenne muscular dystrophy, diagnosis is by karyotype analysis of cultured amniotic fluid fibroblasts, with 50% of males being at risk for the disease. Further work will be necessary to distinguish normal from affected males.

Multifactorial Inheritance
Some of the disorders and possible methods for diagnosis are tabulated in Table 3-4.

Prenatal diagnosis should have the goal of recognition of disorders and correction of the defect. Except for isolated disorders (e.g., X-linked aqueductal stenosis, gastroschisis, and some neural tube defects), recognition does not result in intervention and correction. In many instances, the

Table 3-3. Some sex-linked recessive disorders

Disease	Deficiency	Prenatal diagnostic test
Hemophilia A	Factor VIII	Fetal sex (karyotype)
Hemophilia B	Factor IX	Fetal blood sampling Linkage analysis
Duchenne muscular dystrophy	Creatine phosphokinase	Fetal blood sampling (false negatives)
Hydrocephalus aqueductal stenosis		Fetal sex (karyotype) Ultrasound
Testicular feminization	Cytosol receptor protein (in most cases)	Fetal sex (karyotype)
Mental retardation (X-linked, recessive)		Karyotype (media-199 for marker-X)
Inborn Errors of Metabolism		
Lesch-Nyhan disease	Hypoxanthine-guanine phospho-ribosyl trans-ferase (HGPT)	Fetal sex (karyotype) Enzyme assay
Fabry disease	Ceramide trihexo-side galactosidase	Fetal sex (karyotype) Enzyme assay
G6PD deficiency	G6PD	Fetal sex (karyotype) Enzyme assay
Hunter syndrome	Sulfioduronide sulfatase	Fetal sex (karyotype)
Glycogen storage disease (type VIII)	Phosphorylase kinase	Fetal sex (karyotype)
Hyperammonemia I	Ornithine transcarbamylase	Fetal sex (karyotype)

Table 3-4. Some multifactorial diseases

Disease	Prenatal diagnostic test
Neural tube defects	Ultrasound, serum and amniotic fluid alpha-fetoprotein
Congenital heart disease	Ultrasound Echocardiography
Cleft lip and palate	Ultrasound Fetoscopy
Gastrointestinal anomalies	Ultrasound Fetography
Renal anomalies	Ultrasound
Skeletal anomalies	Ultrasound Fetography

correction, if undertaken, is less than optimum (see Chap. 1).

Advances in diagnosis often precede the introduction of therapeutic modalities, but progress in therapy will come slowly. At present, prenatal genetics serves to identify some families at risk and to diagnose the presence or absence of some disorders. Knowing the risks, the family, with the physician, can arrive at a reasonable decision. It remains for the perinatal investigators to expand the diagnostic capabilities in the antepartum period and to introduce those therapeutic approaches that can correct a problem, once recognized.

Abortions, Stillbirths, Neonatal and Early Childhood Deaths

It is essential that the details surrounding an intrauterine, neonatal, or early childhood loss of an infant be carefully researched to determine whether the family is at an increased risk of recurrence and whether a test for carrier status or prenatal detection of the disease exists. In recurrent abortion, consideration should be given to chromosome analysis of fetal tissue, if found. Careful pathologic examination should be done with all stillbirths and neonatal deaths looking for evidence of a pattern that might predictably repeat in subsequent pregnancies [48,49]. In children with multiple anomalies or in cases of neonatal death of unknown cause, chromosome analysis can be done. Tissue obtained from missed abortions or stillbirths will often fail to grow in culture. In the absence of comparative fluorescent studies or polymorphism with maternal blood lymphocytes, only the growth of XY cells in culture ensures the presence of fetal cells (see exception under Fetal Cells in the Maternal Circulation).

Indications and methods for antenatal fetal diagnosis will continue to expand. Although correction of detected fetal problems will offer hope to some families, the major emphasis for the next decade will be on the recognition of the family at risk and the early detection of fetal disease. With this as a foundation, correction, and possibly prevention, may follow.

REFERENCES

1. Tijo JH, Levan A. The chromosome number of man. Hereditas. 1956; 42:1–6.
2. Caspersson T, Zech L, eds. Chromosome identification. 23rd Nobel Symposium. New York: Academic Press, 1973.
3. Boué J, Boué A, Lazar P. Retrospective and prospective epidemiological studies of 1500 karyotyped spontaneous human abortions. Teratology. 1975; 12:11–26.
4. Simpson JL. Diagnosing fetal chromosomal abnormalities. In: Queenan JT, ed. Management of high-risk pregnancy. Oradell, NJ: Medical Economics, 1980:35–45.
5. Matsunaga E, Tonomura A, Oishi H, Kikuchi Y. Reexamination of paternal age effect in Down's syndrome. Hum Genet. 1978; 40:259–68.
6. Stene J, Fischer G, Stene E, Mikkelsen M, Petersen E. Paternal age effect in Down's syndrome. Ann Hum Genet. 1977; 40:299–306.
7. Bauld, R, Sutherland GR, Bain AD. Chromosome studies in investigation of stillbirths and neonatal deaths. Arch Dis Child. 1974; 49:782–8.
8. Clewell WH, Johnson ML, Meier PR, et al. A surgical approach to the treatment of fetal hydrocephalus. N Engl J Med. 1982; 306:1320–5.
9. Turner G, Brookwell R, Daniel A, Selikowitz M, Zilibowitz M. Heterozygous expression of X-linked mental retardation and X-chromosome marker fra (X) (q27). N Engl J Med. 1980; 303:662–4.
10. Grennert L, Persson PH, Gennser G. Benefits of ultrasonic screening of a pregnant population. Acta Obstet Gynecol Scand [Suppl]. 1978; 78:5–14.
11. Queenan JT. Maternal serum α-fetoprotein screening. In: Queenan JT, ed. Management of high-risk pregnancy. Oradell NJ: Medical Economics, 1980:67–70.
12. Hobbins JC, Grannum PA, Berkowitz RL, Silverman R, Mahoney MJ. Ultrasound in the diagnosis of congenital anomalies. Am J Obstet Gynecol. 1979; 134:331–45.
13. Roczen, RS. Fetal echocardiography: present and future applications. JCU. 1981; 9:223–9.
14. Winsberg F. Echocardiography of the fetal and newborn heart. Invest Radiol. 1972; 7:152–8.
15. Kleinman CS, Hobbins JC, Jaffe CC, Lynch DC, Talner NS. Echocardiographic studies of the human fetus: prenatal diagnosis of congenital heart disease and cardiac dysrhythmias. Pediatrics. 1980; 65:1059–67.
16. Lubs HA, Ruddle FH. Chromosomal abnormalities in the human population: estimation of rates based on New Haven newborn study. Science. 1970; 169:495–7.
17. The NICHD National Registry for Amniocentesis Study Group. Midtrimester amniocentesis for prenatal diagnosis. JAMA. 1976; 236:1471–6.
18. Karp LE, Hayden PW. Fetal puncture during midtrimester amniocentesis. Obstet Gynecol. 1977; 49:115–7.
19. Lamb MP. Gangrene of a fetal limb due to amniocentesis. Br J Obstet Gynaecol. 1975; 82:829–30.
20. Rickwood AM. A case of ileal atresia and ileocutaneous fistula caused by amniocentesis. J Pediatr. 1977; 91:312.
21. Young PE, Matson MR, Jones OW. Fetal exsanguination and other vascular injuries from midtrimester genetic amniocentesis. Am J Obstet Gynecol. 1977; 129:21–4.
22. Verjaal M, Leschart NJ. Risk of amniocentesis and laboratory findings in a series of 1500 prenatal diagnoses. Prenatal Diagnosis I. 1978:173–81.
23. Queenan JT, Thompson W, Whitfield CR, Shah SI. Amniotic fluid volumes in normal pregnancies. Am J Obstet Gynecol. 1972; 114:34–8.
24. Kan YW, Golbus MS, Dozy AM. Prenatal diagnosis of α-thalassemia. Clinical application of molecular hybridization. N Engl J Med. 1976; 295:1165–7.
25. Koenig HM, Vedvick TS, Dozy AM, Golbus MS, Kan YW. Prenatal diagnosis of hemoglobin H disease. J Pediatr. 1978; 92:278–81.
26. Wong V, Ma HK, Todd D, Golbus MS, Dozy AM, Kan YW. Diagnosis of homozygous α-thalassemia in cultured amniotic-fluid fibroblasts. N Engl J Med. 1978; 298:669–70.
27. Seale TW, Rennert OM. Prenatal prognosis of thalassemias and hemoglobinopathies. Ann Clin Lab Sci. 1980; 10:383–94.
28. Boyer SH, Boyer ML, Noyes AN, Belding PK. Immunologic basis for detecting sickle cell hemoglobin phenotypes in amniotic fluid erythrocytes. Ann NY Acad Sci. 1974; 241:699–713.
29. Chang H, Modell CB, Alter BP, et al. Expression of the beta-thalassemia gene in the first trimester fetus. Proc Natl Acad Sci USA. 1975; 72:3633–7.
30. Hobbins JC, Mahoney MJ. In utero diagnosis of hemoglobinopathies—technique for obtaining fetal blood. N Engl J Med. 1974; 290:1065–7.
31. Rodeck CH, Campbell S. Sampling pure fetal blood by fetoscopy in second trimester of pregnancy. Br Med J. 1978; 2:728–30.
32. Benzie RJ, Malone RM, Miskin M. Rudd NL, Schofield PA. Prenatal diagnosis by fetoscopy with subsequent normal delivery: report of a case. Am J Obstet Gynecol. 1976;126:287–8.

33. Rodeck CH, Campbell S. Early prenatal diagnosis of neural-tube defects by ultrasound-guided fetoscopy. Lancet. 1978; 1:1128–9.

34. Rodeck CH, Campbell S. Umbilical-cord insertion as source of pure fetal blood for prenatal diagnosis. Lancet. 1979; 1:1244–5.

35. Hobbins JC. Diagnosing with the fetoscope. Contemp Ob Gyn. 1979; 13:143–52.

36. Rodeck CH. Fetoscopy guided by real-time ultrasound for pure fetal blood samples, fetal skin samples, and examination of the fetus in utero. Br J Obstet Gynaecol. 1980; 87:449–56.

37. Rodeck CH, Eady RA, Godden CM. Prenatal diagnosis of epidermolysis bullosa letalis. Lancet. 1980; 1:949–52.

38. Mahoney MJ, Haseltine FP, Hobbins JC, Banher BQ, Caskey CT, Golbus MS. Prenatal diagnosis of Duchenne's muscular dystrophy. N Engl J Med. 1977; 297:968–73.

39. Golbus MS, Stephens JD, Mahoney MJ, et al. Failure of fetal creatine phosphokinase as a diagnostic indicator of Duchenne muscular dystrophy. N Engl J Med. 1979; 300:860–1.

40. Emery AE. Duchenne muscular dystrophy. Genetic aspects, carrier detection and antenatal diagnosis. Br Med Bull. 1980; 36:117–22.

41. Simpson JL. Antenatal monitoring of genetic disorders. Clin Obstet Gynaecol. 1979; 61:259–93.

42. Edgell CJ, Kirkman HN, Clemons E, Buchanan PD, Miller CH. Prenatal diagnosis by linkage: hemophilia A and polymorphic glucose-6-phosphate dehydrogenase. Am J Hum Genet. 1978; 30:80–4.

43. Schröder J. Transplacental passage of blood cells. J Med Genet. 1975; 12:230–42.

44. Schröder J, Schröder E, Cann HM. Fetal cells in the maternal blood. Lack of response of fetal cells in maternal blood to mitogens and mixed leukocyte culture. Hum Genet. 1977; 38:91–7.

45. Walknkowska J, Conte FA, Grumbach MM. Practical and theoretical implications of fetal maternal lymphocyte transfer. Lancet. 1969; 1:1119–22.

46. Herzenberg LA, Sweet RG, Herzenberg LA. Fluorescence-activated cell sorting. Sci Am. 1976; 234:108–17.

47. Stephenson SR, Weaver DD. Prenatal diagnosis—a compilation of diagnosed conditions. Am J Obstet Gynecol. 1981; 141:319–43.

48. Nordenson I. Increased frequencies of chromosomal abnormalities in families with a history of fetal wastage. Clin Genet. 1981; 19:168–73.

49. Hassold TJ. A cytogenetic study of repeated spontaneous abortions. Am J Hum Genet. 1980; 32:723–30.

50. Milunsky A. Glucose intolerance in the parents of children with Down's syndrome. Am J Ment Defic. 1970; 74:475–8.

51. Fialkow PJ. Thyroid antibodies, Down's syndrome, and maternal age. Nature. 1967; 214:1253–4.

52. Kueppers F, O'Brien P, Passarge E, Rudiger H. Alpha 1-antitrypsin phenotypes in sex chromosome mosaicism. Med Genet. 1975; 12:263–4.

53. Fineman RM, Kidd KK, Johnson AM, Breg WR. Increased frequency of heterozygotes for α-1 antitrypsin variants in individuals with either sex chromosome mosaicism or trisomy 21. Nature. 1976; 260:320–1.

54. Nordenson I. Increased frequencies of chromosomal abnormalities in families with a history of fetal wastage. Clin Genet. 1981; 19:168–73.

55. Mennuti MT, Jingeleski S, Schwarz RH, Mellman WJ. An evaluation of cytogenetic analysis as a primary tool in the assessment of recurrent pregnancy wastage. Obstet Gynecol. 1978; 52:308–13.

56. Boué JG, Boué A. Increased frequency of chromosomal anomalies in abortions after induced ovulation. Lancet. 1973; 1:679–80.

57. Oakley GP, Flynt JW. Increased prevalence of Down's syndrome (mongolism) among the offspring of women treated with ovulation-inducing agents. Teratology. 1972; 5:264.

Sir, she came in, great with child, and
Longing for . . . stew'd prunes.
—William Shakespeare
Measure for Measure

4. NUTRITIONAL PROBLEMS DURING PREGNANCY
Robert E. Wall

Historically, interest and knowledge in nutrition have been neglected by most medical educators and practitioners [1,2]. The impact of poor nutrition on the developing fetus was minimized in the belief that the fetoplacental unit represented a true parasite capable of extracting all the nutritional needs from its mother, regardless of any deficient or surplus caloric, protein, or nutrient consumption.

During the last decade, the nutritional relationship between the mother and her fetus has been more thoroughly investigated and reviewed [3–7]. The following discussion presents an overview of gestational nutrition and considers some societal influences on nutritional patterns.

NUTRITIONAL REQUIREMENTS DURING PREGNANCY
Energy/Calories

Changes in maternal tissues, growth of the fetus and the placenta, and the general increase in maternal metabolic activity during pregnancy increase the energy requirements for the pregnant woman. The estimated total caloric need for a term pregnancy is an additional 80,000 kilocalories (kcal), or an increase of 15% over the nonpregnant state. Very little additional energy is necessary until the end of the first trimester, when a dramatic rise occurs and remains nearly constant until delivery. The World Health Organization recommends an additional 150 kcal per day through the first trimester. During the second and third trimesters, an increase of 350 kcal per day is preferred [8]. During the second trimester, the additional energy intake is used primarily for the expansion of the maternal blood volume, for the increase in uterine and breast size, and for the accumulation of fat stores in the mother. The increased caloric needs in the third trimester are for fetal and placental growth [9].

In order to avoid suboptimal protein utilization, total caloric intake for the pregnant woman should not fall below 36 kcal per kilogram per day during pregnancy [10].

Protein and Amino Acids

Dietary protein requirements for the pregnant woman are difficult to assess. Most authors suggest estimates of minimal protein requirement based on nitrogen balance studies, which probably overestimate actual fetal-maternal needs. The recommended additional allowance of dietary protein is 30 g per day. Baseline protein requirements vary with age (1.3–1.7 g/kg/day). Because baseline protein requirements of women under 19 years of age are higher, the daily protein consumption by a pregnant teenager must be significantly greater to ensure optimal fetal growth and development (Table 4-1). Protein metabolism and utilization are dependent on caloric intake. Below 36 kcal/kg/day, protein utilization in the adult becomes suboptimal since protein must be used as a primary energy source [10].

Serum protein concentration decreases during pregnancy to approximately 70% of prepregnancy level by the beginning of the third trimester. Albumin levels fall rapidly in the first trimester. Changes in the amount of protein ingested have little influence on this normal physiologic alteration. Because of the marked decrease in albumin, the albumin-globulin ratio falls. Globulin concentrations are also altered during pregnancy. The direction of the change varies with the globulin being considered (Table 4-2).

Most of the serum proteins, particularly albumin, are transported across the placenta by simple diffusion. Transfer of IgG immunoglobulin is through both passive diffusion and a selectively operable carrier system that allows the fetus to maintain relatively stable IgG levels even during times when the maternal levels are, transiently, low [12]. This facilitated transfer of IgG is most efficient during the last half of pregnancy.

Maternal serum amino acid levels fall in normal pregnancy. The fetus demonstrates higher serum

Table 4-1. Total daily dietary protein requirements during pregnancy

Adult	1.3 g/kg/day
Ages 15–18	1.4 g/kg/day
Ages 11–14	1.7 g/kg/day

Source: National Research Council [11].

Table 4-2. Alteration of maternal serum protein levels during pregnancy

Proteins	Changes during pregnancy
Total proteins	Decreased
Albumin	Decreased
Albumin-globulin ratio	Decreased
α_1-Globulins	Increased
α_1-Lipoprotein	Unchanged
α_1-Antitrypsin	Increased
α_1-Glycoprotein (easily precipitable)	Increased
Gc globulin	Increased
α_2-Globulins	Increased
Haptoglobulin	Unchanged
Ceruloplasmin	Increased
α_2-Macroglobulin	Unchanged
β-Globulins	Increased
Transferrin	Increased
Thermopexin	Unchanged
Fibrinogen	Increased
β_1-Lipoprotein	Unchanged
β_1-AC($C'3$)	Unchanged
γ-Globulin	Decreased
Specific proteins	
α_1-Fetoprotein	Marked increase
Pregnancy zone protein (α_2)	Appearance and marked increase

Source: From Moghissi [12].

Table 4-3. Elemental iron content of supplements

Preparation	Iron (%)
Ferrous gluconate	11
Ferrous sulfate	20–30
Ferrous fumarate	32.5

300 to 400 mg is needed to supply fetal erythropoietic needs [14]. Thus, almost 1 g of elemental iron must be absorbed to supply the maternal-fetal unit during a term pregnancy. The usual American diet provides approximately 15 mg of elemental iron daily, of which only 10% is absorbed in healthy individuals. Even if iron absorption improves during pregnancy, as has been suggested, dietary iron alone is inadequate to meet the requirements of the pregnant woman [3]. Balanced meals, including meat and high levels of ascorbic acid, appear to maximize iron absorption [15,16]. Maternal stores are unlikely to be able to meet the increased demand. Interestingly, the fetus appears to act as a true parasite with respect to iron metabolism and its own erythropoiesis. Despite marked maternal iron deficiency, the developing fetus is able to extract needed iron and produce normal red cell volumes although fetal iron stores remain reduced.

The current recommendation during pregnancy is for oral supplementation of 30 to 60 mg of ferrous iron per day [11]. Table 4-3 lists the percentage of elemental iron supplied by some of the commonly used oral iron preparations.

Continuation of iron supplementation for two to three months after delivery is suggested to maximize maternal iron stores following the demands of a term pregnancy and delivery. In rare instances of inadequate absorption or poor patient compliance, parenteral iron supplementation may prove worthwhile during or following pregnancy.

Folic Acid

Folic acid (pteroylglutamic acid or folate) deficiency is the most common vitamin deficiency in pregnant women. Estimates by the World Health Organization suggest that one-third to one-half of all pregnant women demonstrate a relative deficiency of this water-soluble vitamin during pregnancy [17]. Folic acid is essential for DNA synthesis, and increased amounts are, therefore, necessary for rapidly dividing cells, including those in the maternal bone marrow and the feto-placental unit. Humans cannot synthesize folic acid. Major dietary sources of folates include green leafy vegetables, meats, liver, peanuts, citrus fruits,

levels than its mother secondary to the active transport of amino acids across the placenta [13]. Contributions to the fetal amino acid pool are also made through fetal swallowing of amniotic fluid proteins and their degradation and subsequent absorption into the fetal circulation.

Iron

The role of iron in maternal nutrition deserves special attention. Augmented maternal erythropoiesis and initiation of fetal erythropoiesis must occur despite relatively meager maternal iron stores. Maternal red cell volume in pregnancy increases by approximately 20%, with most of the increase occurring in the last two trimesters. Elemental iron in the amount of 500 to 600 mg is required to meet the maternal demand alone. An additional

Table 4-4. Nutritional allowances in normal pregnancy

Requirement*	Amount (per day)	Comments
Energy	300 additional kcal	Energy requirement is minimally altered during early gestation, increases sharply at end of first trimester, and remains constant until term
Iron	18 mg	Most diets do not supply adequate iron; supplementation with 30–60 mg of ferrous iron is necessary
Folic acid	800 μg	Normal diets are frequently inadequate for folic acid; supplement can be given routinely
Vitamin A	1,000 retinol equivalents (4,000–5,000 IU)	Blood levels increase during normal pregnancy
Vitamin D	400–600 IU	Requirement increases to facilitate greater calcium absorption
Vitamin E	10 mg	Requirement increases because of increased caloric intake
Ascorbic acid	80 mg	Maternal blood levels of most water-soluble vitamins fall during gestation, and fetal blood levels exceed maternal by 50–100%
Pyridoxine	2.6 mg	Requirement increases to provide for increased maternal protein ingestion and fetal transfer
Thiamin	1.4 mg	Requirement increases early in gestation; attainable in balanced diet
Riboflavin	1.5 mg	Requirement increases during pregnancy; deficiency manifested by cheilosis, dermatitis, or glossitis
Niacin	15 mg	Increased energy requirements necessitate 15% increase
Vitamin B_{12}	4 μg	Requirement increases because of considerable fetal accumulation
Calcium	1,200 mg	RDA exceeds fetal needs; however, maternal absorption is incomplete
Magnesium	450 mg	—
Zinc	20 mg	Deficiency in experimental animals produces an increased rate of fetal malformations
Iodide	175 μg	Requirement increases because of fetal transfer and increased maternal loss.

Requirement is defined as the minimum amount needed to prevent deficiency, whereas *allowance* is generally placed at a higher level to account for individual variability and to provide a margin of safety.
Source: Data from National Research Council [11].

and yeast. Because it is rapidly destroyed by heat, folic acid is inactivated by prolonged cooking.

Manifestations of folate deficiency may develop if intake is inadequate for four months or more [11]. Mild folic acid deficiency has been incriminated in a variety of pregnancy complications (e.g., abruptio placenta, fetal loss). The correlation between mild deficiency and untoward maternal or fetal outcome is tenuous, however. Severe deficiencies of the vitamin may lead to megaloblastic anemia. Although the subject is somewhat controversial, the author agrees with the recommendation for folate supplementation during normal pregnancy [18]. The current recommended dietary allowance (RDA) is double the nonpregnant requirements with levels approaching 1 mg/day during gestation (see Table 4-4). Pregnancies complicated by excessive bleeding, anemia, chronic hemolysis, upper bowel disease, intestinal bypass, or twins all require daily folate supplementation. Where phenytoin or the diuretic triamterene has been used on a chronic basis, the reduced form of folate (folinic acid) may be needed to overcome the drug-induced deficiency of folate [17].

Calcium

The total calcium requirement during pregnancy is 30 g. Most is utilized for calcification of the fetal skeleton during the third trimester. The current RDA is an additional 400 mg per day for a total of 1,200 mg/day during gestation. This requirement can be met by ingesting a liter of milk daily. Women who restrict their intake of milk and milk products or who cannot tolerate ingestion of large amounts of lactose should be offered calcium supplementation.

Maternal serum levels of calcium normally decrease during pregnancy because of the physiologic fall in albumin. Calcium ions are actively transported across the placenta, producing elevated fetal calcium and calcitonin levels and reduced fetal parathyroid hormone levels. Thus an optimal environment is provided for the mineralization of the fetal skeleton matrix during the latter half of pregnancy [3,19].

Sodium

Recommendations for sodium intake during pregnancy have changed greatly in recent years. Previously, the ingestion of sodium was implicated in the development of toxemia and the pathologic edema that accompanies it [20]. More recently, pregnancy has been recognized as a salt-wasting state with glomerular filtration of an additional 5,000 to 10,000 mEq of sodium per day. Progesterone promotes further naturesis. Physiologic compensation for the sodium loss results in increased activity of the renin-angiotensin-aldosterone system. Specifically, the adrenal cortex is stimulated by elevated levels of angiotensin to release aldosterone, promoting the tubular reabsorption of sodium and attenuating the otherwise marked sodium loss.

Despite a net loss of total body sodium during pregnancy, normal maternal dietary ingestion of sodium provides adequate replacement. Salt supplementation is unnecessary [20]. Treatment of toxemia or the edema of normal pregnancy with salt-wasting diuretics or salt restriction is contraindicated [3,21].

Fat-Soluble Vitamins
Vitamin A

Vitamin A (retinol) is necessary, in the human, for normal visual function and maintenance of mucous membranes. It is absorbed, from the normal diet, as retinol or as any number of provitamins, beta-carotene being the most prevalent. Mild deficiency of vitamin A, in the nonpregnant state, results in impaired adaptation to the dark and subsequently may lead to ocular damage [11]. Although vitamin A activity has been expressed in international units (IU) in the past, more recently it has been reported as an equivalent weight of retinol or "retinol equivalents" [11]. Because of elevated serum lipid levels during pregnancy, maternal serum vitamin A levels increase during gestation. In mothers with adequate prenatal nutrition, the amounts of vitamin A that may be re-

quired over several months can be stored in the liver. The fetus sequesters significant amounts of vitamin A, necessitating a 25% increase in the maternal intake to 1,000 retinol equivalents per day (4,000–5,000 IU).

Vitamin D

The regulation of calcium and phosphate metabolism requires the presence of adequate amounts of vitamin D. Exposure to sunlight with formation of cholecalciferol and ingestion of plant or animal foods containing natural or supplementary vitamin D are the usual sources of vitamin D. Like all fat-soluble vitamins, vitamin D traverses the placenta by simple diffusion [19]. As fetal skeletal growth is completed, requirements for vitamin D fall. In pregnant women past the age of 22 the RDA is 10 μg (400 IU), double that of nonpregnant women. For pregnant teenagers the RDA is increased another 25 to 50% to allow for the mother's own skeletal growth. One liter of "fortified" milk contains 10 μg vitamin D, although other excellent dietary sources of the vitamin are fish, liver, eggs, and butter [11]. Exposure to sunlight is usually adequate to meet the requirements for the nonpregnant adult.

Vitamin E

Clinical evidence of vitamin E deficiency, in humans, has been observed in patients with long-standing fat malabsorption [11]. Vitamin E activity is derived from a variety of plant compounds. Alpha-tocopherol is the most common and potent. Vitamin E nutritional requirements increase with the amount of polyunsaturated fats consumed. Fortunately, foods highest in polyunsaturated fats (vegetable oils and margarine) also contain the largest amounts of vitamin E. Because of the additional vitamin E requirement for the developing fetus, the RDA should be increased 25% to 10 mg alpha-tocopherol equivalents (15 IU). Increased caloric intake with balanced dietary sources should supply adequate levels of vitamin E for the needs of the pregnant woman and her fetus throughout gestation.

Vitamin K

Vitamin K is necessary for the synthesis of a number of proteins found in the liver, bone, and kidney. Among these are the vitamin K–dependent clotting factors, including prothrombin (factor II) [22]. In addition to the vitamin K found in large amounts in green leafy vegetables (phylloquinone), half of the vitamin K found in the human liver is vitamin K_2 (menaquinone), synthesized by endogenous bowel flora [23]. Vitamin K deficiency

Table 4-5. Common dietary sources of vitamins

Vitamins	Source
Vitamin A	Carrots, liver, spinach, cantaloupe
Vitamin D	Milk, fresh liver oils, egg yolk
Vitamin E	Vegetable oil, dark green leafy vegetables
Vitamin K	Turnip greens, broccoli, green tea
Ascorbic acid	Citrus fruits and juices, broccoli, turnip greens, brussels sprouts
Folic acid	Brewer's yeast, liver, green leafy vegetables, beets
Thiamin	Brewer's yeast, whole grain cereals
Riboflavin	Liver, milk, yogurt, cottage cheese
Niacin	Liver, nuts, chicken, salmon
Pyridoxine	Liver, meat, fish, chicken, whole grain bread
Vitamin B_{12}	Meat, eggs, shellfish, liver

is therefore uncommon except in severe malabsorption. There is no specific RDA for the nonpregnant or pregnant female since the contribution by normal intestinal bacteria should be adequate. The normal adult requirement for vitamin K is approximately 2 μg per kilogram per day [24]. If parenteral vitamin K is necessary, phylloquinone preparations (vitamin K_1) are preferred. Some of the common dietary sources of fat-soluble vitamins are given in Table 4-5.

Water-Soluble Vitamins

Unlike the fat-soluble vitamin group, serum levels of water-soluble vitamins decrease during pregnancy [9]. This fall probably represents a normal physiologic adjustment favoring fetal growth at the expense of maternal well-being [9,25]. Although pharmacologic supplementation of these vitamins may normalize serum levels, present allowances suggest the need for only modest increases during pregnancy. These vitamins are carried by active transport across the placenta. Levels in the fetal serum may exceed those in the maternal circulation by 50 to 100% [9,19].

Ascorbic Acid

Ascorbic acid (vitamin C) is necessary for the proper formation of collagen. Because humans cannot synthesize ascorbic acid, prolonged dietary deficiency results in a disease characterized by poor collagen integrity and capillary fragility. In developed countries pregnancy is rarely complicated by vitamin C deficiency since high levels are found in many fruits, particularly citrus. Because of the enhanced transfer of vitamin C to the fetal circulation, the RDA during pregnancy increases 33% to 80 mg per day.

Thiamin

Thiamin (vitamin B_1) requirements during pregnancy increase early in gestation. The RDA increases from approximately 1.0 to 1.4 mg per day. Dietary deficiencies of vitamin B_1 may be seen in countries where unenriched white rice or white flour are the mainstays of the diet. Alcoholism (with its associated poor nutrition) and long-term dialysis may result in thiamin deficiency [11]. Clinical vitamin B_1 deficiency (beriberi) affects the nervous and cardiovascular systems primarily.

Riboflavin

Vitamin B_2 (riboflavin) is necessary for optimal protein metabolism. The RDA in pregnancy is an additional 0.3 mg. Deficiency of this nutrient is most frequently evidenced by cheilosis, dermatitis, or glossitis.

Niacin

Niacin (nicotinic acid or vitamin B_5) is an important component of human coenzymes. Clinical deficiency (pellagra) results in dermatitis and, ultimately, dementia. Dietary tryptophan is converted to niacin. The increased caloric intake and energy requirements during pregnancy require an increase of approximately 15% or 2 niacin equivalents, when compared to the nonpregnant RDA.

Pyridoxine

Vitamin B_6 (pyridoxine and its related pyridines) is a necessary coenzyme for amino acid metabolism. The requirement for vitamin B_6 intake varies directly with dietary protein ingestion. During pregnancy a 25% increase is recommended, to a level of 2.6 mg/day. In addition, elevated estrogen levels in pregnancy increase tryptophan oxygenase activity, resulting in an increased requirement for pyridoxine in pregnancy [26]. Balanced dietary intake is adequate to supply the vitamin B_6 requirement in pregnancy. Earlier reports that pyridoxine supplementation lowers the incidence of preeclampsia have been refuted [27–29]. Supplements to the normal diet do not appear to be necessary nor advantageous.

Vitamin B_{12}

Vitamin B_{12} (cobalamin) is necessary for appropriate amino acid, fatty acid, and nucleic acid metabolism. Absorption from the gastrointestinal tract occurs in the ileum and requires "intrinsic factor" secreted by gastric mucosal cells. Because of an efficient reutilization of vitamin B_{12} via the enterohepatic circulation, clinically significant vitamin B_{12} deficiency may take several years to develop. Vitamin B_{12} requirements increase during pregnancy. The RDA is 4 µg per day as compared with approximately 3 µg per day for nonpregnant adults. Mothers on pure vegetarian diets may develop significant vitamin B_{12} deficiency accompanied by megaloblastic anemia and neurologic dysfunction. Some of the common dietary sources of water-soluble vitamins are given in Table 4-5.

Trace Minerals
A number of minerals, in addition to calcium and iron, are required for a variety of metabolic processes in humans. Magnesium is plentiful in the environment. The RDA for magnesium is increased 50% in pregnancy. Iodide, zinc, copper, manganese, cobalt, molybdenum, selenium, chromium, and tin are also essential for many human enzyme systems [30]. Only iodide and zinc have been studied extensively and have a daily allowance recommended. Substantial increases of these minerals (17 and 33%, respectively) are suggested during pregnancy. Several reviews detail the present knowledge regarding some trace elements and their implications during pregnancy [30–32]. Some of the common dietary sources of minerals are given in Table 4-6.

MATERNAL WEIGHT GAIN AND FETAL WELL-BEING
Maternal weight gain is a crude indicator of gestational nutrition. The average woman can be expected to gain 10 to 12 kg during a term pregnancy, with younger women tending toward greater weight gain than older women [3]. Maternal and neonatal morbidity is lowest if weight gain re-

Table 4-6. Common dietary sources of minerals

Minerals	Source
Sodium	Table salt, cheese, milk (present in virtually all processed foods)
Potassium	Fresh fruits, dried fruits (apricots, raisins, dates), milk, meat, salt substitute (KCl)
Chloride	Table salt or salt substitute
Molybdenum	Meat, grains, legumes, nuts
Chromium	Brewer's yeast, meat, cheese, whole grains
Fluoride	Sardines, tea, fluoridated water
Copper	Oysters, nuts, liver, corn oil margarine
Manganese	Nuts, grains, vegetables, fruits
Selenium	Seafood, meat, egg yolk
Iodide	Table salt (iodized), white bread, seafood
Zinc	Meat, shellfish, eggs, liver, poultry, nuts
Iron	Meat, poultry, fish, dried fruits
Calcium	Milk, cheese, yogurt, sardines
Phosphorus	Liver, turkey, cheese, milk, dried beans
Magnesium	Dried beans, dark green leafy vegetables

mains within this range. The pattern of weight gain is also important. A small weight gain (1–2 kg) during the first trimester is to be expected. After 9 to 10 weeks' gestation, the average increase in weight should be approximately 0.35 to 0.4 kg/ week until term (Fig. 4-1) [9].

Excessive Weight Gain
Excessive weight gain has been implicated in a variety of obstetric complications, including pre-

Fig. 4-1. Pattern and components of average maternal weight gain during pregnancy. (From Pitkin [3].)

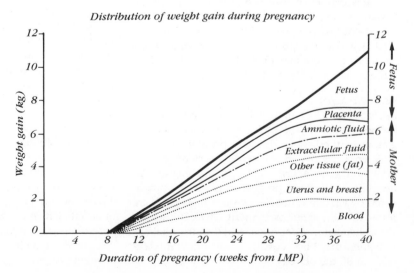

Distribution of weight gain during pregnancy

Duration of pregnancy (weeks from LMP)

· eclampsia. In the past marked caloric restrictions were imposed to limit weight gain to 7 kg in pregnancy hoping to reduce the risk of toxemia. Although excessive weight gain in pregnancy probably contributes to the number of patients troubled by obesity later in life, it does not result in an increase in either the incidence or the types of obstetric complications seen in the mother or infant. The problems of the obese pregnant patient are discussed later in this chapter.

Inadequate Weight Gain

Insufficient weight gain during pregnancy is defined as a weight gain of 1 kg or less per month [6]. Since inadequate weight gain is associated with decreased birth weight and increased neonatal and maternal morbidity, the patient's diet should be evaluated and nutritional counseling undertaken. Taylor has recently commented: "There has been too much attention given to weight control during pregnancy and not enough to weight gain and a proper daily diet" [2].

Birth Weight

Infant birth weight is a crude measure of intrauterine nutrition but an accurate predictor of neonatal morbidity and mortality [6,9]. Fetal growth retardation, in some instances, may be caused by poor maternal nutrition or, more precisely, fetal malnutrition. Infants who have been malnourished in utero are typically long and thin with minimal subcutaneous fat deposition. They have a smaller number of total body cells, lower organ weights, limited cranial volumes, and reduced RNA, DNA, protein, cholesterol, and phospholipid in the brain [6,12]. Psychomotor development is also slowed [33].

Aside from the length of gestation, maternal weight gain during normal pregnancy is the primary determinant of birth weight. Prepregnancy maternal weight is also directly related to birth weight [6,9]. The relationship between prepregnancy height and birth weight have been disputed. It has been suggested that maternal height may be an index of genetic influences on the developing fetus [32].

VEGETARIAN AND RESTRICTED DIETS DURING PREGNANCY
Vegetarian Diets

In assessing the nutritional impact of vegetarian diets during pregnancy, it is necessary to define the type of diet consumed. Lacto-ovovegetarians include eggs and dairy products in their diet in addition to plant substances. Those who consume dairy products and plant food, while omitting eggs, are termed lactovegetarians. Strict vegetarians, called "vegans," omit eggs and dairy products, consuming only plant substances.

Women whose dietary intake is dominated by plant substances may have difficulty ingesting an adequate volume of food to meet the increased caloric requirements of pregnancy. The problem is accentuated later in pregnancy, when gastric capacity decreases. The pregnant adolescent vegetarian is at greater risk since her basic caloric requirement is increased by an additional 100 to 300 kcal per day over that of her adult counterpart [11]. During chronic caloric deprivation, utilization of protein as a primary energy source may interfere with protein anabolism.

Of the 20 amino acids required for the body to make proteins, humans are unable to synthesize eight: leucine, isoleucine, phenylalanine, valine, lysine, methionine, threonine, and tryptophan. Because some plant proteins contain only a few of the essential amino acids, a variety of plant proteins must be ingested in order to supply adequate amounts of all of these amino acids. Since eggs and dairy products are complete proteins which supply all the essential amino acids, the problem is peculiar to the vegan. Vegetarian diets that contain both grain protein and proteins derived from legumes will provide adequate amounts of methionine and lysine, the most difficult amino acids to acquire in the strict vegetarian diet [34]. Lappe has developed a practical guide to assist the vegan in developing a more complete diet [35]. Because reduced digestibility lowers the net protein utilization of vegetable protein, protein requirements for vegans are higher than those for pregnant women on a normal diet [11]. Since calculation of the nutritional benefit of a vegan diet may be difficult, the services of a skilled nutritionist are usually required.

Vitamin B_{12} deficiency in the strict vegetarian can be severe. Since there are *no* vegetable sources of vitamin B_{12}, supplementation or vitamin B_{12}–fortified soy milk must be used to avoid the sequelae of vitamin B_{12} deficiency, particularly the neurologic changes, which may not be reversible.

Absorbable iron appears to be less available from vegetable sources than from meat. However, even strict vegetarians do not seem to be more likely to develop iron deficiency than their omnivorous counterparts [36]. Dietary zinc is primarily found in meat. Vegetable sources of zinc include wheat germ, nuts, and yeast. The absorption of zinc and iron is decreased by the presence of phytates, found in whole grains and cereals [16,34].

Without milk and other dairy products, vegetarians must consume larger amounts of green leafy vegetables, including broccoli, cabbage, and the greens of turnips, mustard, collards, and kale. Tofu, fortified soy milk, sesame seeds, and almonds are also good sources of dietary calcium. Because of the rapidity with which nutritional difficulties may develop in strict vegetarians during pregnancy, professional nutritional counseling is advised. Most vegans are able to fulfill the necessary nutritional requirements to ensure normal fetal and maternal growth and development during pregnancy if they follow the nutritional guidance that is available [34,35,37].

Zen Macrobiotic Diets

The Zen macrobiotic diet is a series of ten dietary regimens that become increasingly more restrictive at the "higher levels." Developed in Japan by George Ohsawa in 1971, it is increasing in popularity and can produce nutritional problems in pregnancy [38]. It requires the avoidance of all animal products, refined or processed foods, seasonings and spices, stimulant food or drinks, and tropical or semitropical fruits. Fluids are restricted. The macrobiotic life-style encourages the use of whole grain cereals as the major or only element in the diet [34,39]. Deficiency states are common, particularly in the higher level diets. Calcium, iron, riboflavin, and vitamin B_{12} deficiencies may occur [34]. The caloric demands of pregnancy can be met only by frequent feedings. In general, adherence to macrobiotic diets during pregnancy should be condemned. Brown and Bergan recommend careful selection of varied, acceptable macrobiotic foodstuffs for those who insist on this dietary approach [40]. Safety of this approach during pregnancy has not been demonstrated.

Pediatric Implications of Restricted Diets

Physicians are frequently unable to drastically alter the nutritional philosophies of pregnant women who have chosen restricted diets. These women require extensive nutritional support and counseling, close observation of infant growth and development, and occasionally court-ordered intervention. Children of vegan mothers who are either breast-fed or placed on vegetarian diets early in life are at risk [41–44]. Vyhmeister et al. recommend a number of vegetarian alternatives to ensure adequate nutrition in these children [45].

Severely restrictive diets may place the child at risk for starvation or vitamin deficiency [46–48]. In these circumstances, the physician's responsibility cannot end with delivery of the infant; appropriate social surveillance must be initiated to protect the neonate [48].

FETAL AND NEONATAL EFFECTS OF INADEQUATE OR EXCESSIVE NUTRIENTS

Investigations into the effects of inadequate or excessive nutrient ingestion on the developing fetus began with the report of Hale in 1933, which described congenital malformations in pigs following deficient vitamin A intake in pregnancy [49]. Most of the studies have been performed on experimental animals; however, several reports have specifically considered human development. An extensive review of all the possible effects is beyond the scope of this discussion. Relationships that are reasonably well substantiated or strongly suspected in the human species are considered in Table 4-7.

Overt Malnutrition

Severe dietary restriction during pregnancy is believed to increase the risk of fetal growth retardation, neonatal mortality, and abnormalities in infant and child development [50–52]. Severe nutritional deprivation in the third trimester dramatically reduces birth weight, particularly in women with inadequate nutritional reserves at the onset of pregnancy [25].

Maternal starvation has been incriminated in the development of a variety of structural and functional abnormalities of the fetal central nervous system. The exact role of maternal ketosis is undefined. Nevertheless, maternal ketosis should be prevented by adequate caloric intake and hydration. Although balanced dietary supplementation is recommended to rectify overt malnutrition, any caloric supplements, including those utilizing only carbohydrate sources, can dramatically reduce the incidence of low-birth-weight babies [12,53,54].

Excessive caloric intake does not increase the risk of toxemia. In the absence of hyperglycemia, direct deleterious effects on the developing infant have not been observed. Nevertheless, the correlation between excessive calories consumed during pregnancy and subsequent maternal obesity is well known. Caloric restraint, not restriction, should be encouraged during pregnancy, except in the underweight patient.

Protein and Amino Acids

Optimal growth and development requires adequate simultaneous supplies of all of the eight essential amino acids. Few studies have isolated the effects of protein versus calorie restriction. Con-

Table 4-7. Possible fetal/neonatal effects of inadequate or excessive administration of nutrients during human pregnancy

Nutrient	Effects of deficiency state	Effects of excessive administration
Calories	Low birth weight Increased neonatal mortality Suboptimal somatic growth and development Suboptimal mental growth and development	?
Protein	Low birth weight	Preterm birth Increased neonatal mortality
Phenylalanine	?	Low birth weight Mental retardation Microcephaly
Carbohydrate	Low birth weight Increased neonatal mortality Suboptimal somatic growth and development Suboptimal mental growth and development	?
Galactose	?	Mental retardation Cataracts
Vitamin A	?	Urologic anomalies Neural tube defects Hydrocephalus
Vitamin D	Neonatal hypocalcemia Neonatal tetany Neonatal rickets Enamel hypoplasia Increased dental caries	Neonatal hypercalcemia Neonatal hypoparathyroidism Craniofacial anomalies Supravalvular aortic and pulmonic stenosis Multiple organ calcification Mental retardation Neurologic dysfunction Kidney failure
Vitamin E	Neonatal hemoglobinopathy	"Reproductive failure"
Vitamin K	Lowered neonatal prothrombin levels	Increased neonatal bilirubin levels (synthetic analog administration)
Ascorbic acid	Increased risk of abortion	Conditioned neonatal scurvy
Thiamin	Congenital beriberi Congestive heart failure Increased neonatal mortality	?
Pyridoxine	Neurologic dysfunction Lowered neonatal immunocompetence	?
Folic acid	Increased risk of abortion Craniofacial anomalies Skeletal anomalies Miscellaneous organ anomalies Megaloblastic anemia	?
Vitamin B_{12}	Megaloblastic anemia Neurologic dysfunction	?
Calcium	Suboptimal fetal skeletal ossification Neonatal hypocalcemia Neonatal tetany	?
Zinc	Low birth weight Preterm birth Increased neonatal mortality Neural tube defects Hydrocephalus Craniofacial anomalies Skeletal anomalies Heart and lung abnormalities	?
Copper	Neural tube defects	Increased risk of abortion
Iodide	Cretinism	Congenital goiter Neonatal hypothyroidism

Refer to text for specific references.

trolled experiments in laboratory animals, as well as observations in protein-restricted humans, confirms a decrease in the birth weight of the offspring of mothers with inadequate protein intake [55]. In the Guatemalan Food Supplementation Study, increases in nonprotein calories appeared to ameliorate some of the fetal growth retardation, despite continued dietary protein inadequacy [56]. In a randomized controlled trial in New York City, high-protein supplements were administered to pregnant women with otherwise inadequate diets. Surprisingly, an excess of preterm births and higher infant mortality were observed in the protein-supplemented group [57].

Deficiencies of specific amino acids have not been noted to produce detrimental effects on the developing human fetus. Animal data suggest that the omission of some essential amino acids (e.g., methionine) may not only decrease birth weight but also be overtly teratogenic [55]. Strict vegetarians must ingest varied and large amounts of plant protein to protect against specific amino acid deficiencies.

A number of animal studies have confirmed the deleterious effects of excessive amounts of some amino acids when used in pharmacologic amounts. The multisystem effects of phenylketonuria in humans document the teratogenic risks of increased phenylalanine. Similar effects have been demonstrated in other mammalian species [55].

Carbohydrates

Carbohydrate deprivation has been discussed previously. Without adequate carbohydrate intake, protein is consumed as a primary energy source and is unavailable for fetal growth and development.

No apparent ill effects have been observed from general carbohydrate excess. However, high blood levels of galactose during pregnancy appear to have harmful effects on the developing fetus in a number of mammalian species [55].

Lipids

Essential fatty acids (e.g., linoleic acids) are required for normal growth and development, both before and after birth. No congenital anomalies have been reported as a result of dietary lipid deficiency. The effects of dietary excess of cholesterol and other lipids remain undefined at the present time [55].

Vitamin A

The well-known teratogenic risks of high doses of vitamin A supplementation in animals appear to apply to the human fetus as well. Congenital urologic abnormalities have been observed in women ingesting more than 35,000 IU daily during pregnancy [58]. Neural tube defects and hydrocephalus in humans—and laboratory animals—ingesting pharmacologic doses of vitamin A have also been reported [32,59]. No obvious neonatal risks have been noted that were due to vitamin A deficiency during pregnancy.

Vitamin D

Hypervitaminosis D is detrimental to adults and children. If vitamin D is ingested in excessive amounts during pregnancy, neonatal hypercalcemia and hypoparathyroidism with craniofacial anomalies may result. Supravalvular aortic and pulmonic stenosis, brain and kidney calcification, mental retardation, generalized neurologic dysfunction, and kidney failure have also been reported [29,58,59]. However, pregnant women with hypoparathyroidism, given large doses of vitamin D, delivered normal infants [55]. Unlike inadequate vitamin A intake, deficiency of vitamin D during pregnancy can affect the neonate. Neonatal hypocalcemia and tetany may appear soon after birth. Skeletal evidence of neonatal rickets has been noted. Finally, enamel hypoplasia and increased dental caries are also found more frequently in offspring of vitamin D–deficient pregnant women [3,29,58].

Vitamin E

Because of the ubiquitous nature of vitamin E, deficiencies are uncommon. Newborn hemoglobinopathies have been attributed to vitamin E deficiency [6,30]. Specific detrimental fetal effects of excessive vitamin E ingestion during human pregnancy have not been demonstrated. Caution should be observed, however, because of the risks demonstrated with excess ingestion of other fat-soluble vitamins. Roberts has commented: "Megadoses of vitamin E should be used with restraint. This includes sophisticated health-conscious pregnant women" [60].

Vitamin K

Although vitamin K deficiency is rare in adults, neonatal hypoprothrombinemia can result if inadequate amounts of this vitamin are available to the pregnant women [6,30]. Administration of large doses of synthetic vitamin K analogs during labor have been associated with neonatal hyperbilirubinemia [61].

Vitamin C

Vitamin C deficiency is rare in developed nations. Inadequate vitamin C intake during pregnancy has been correlated with an increased risk of spontaneous abortion [58]. Large doses of vitamin C during gestation may condition the developing fetus to high ascorbic acid requirements, with resultant scurvy in the neonatal period [58,61].

Thiamin

Significant deficiencies of thiamin during pregnancy may be asymptomatic in the mother. Infants may demonstrate acute congestive heart failure, typical of beriberi, which can lead to neonatal death. Early or immediate perinatal administration of thiamin may prevent this life-threatening complication [62]. No detrimental effects have been reported secondary to excessive thiamin intake.

Pyridoxine

Deficient pyridoxine intake may lower neonatal immunocompetence [63]. Neonatal seizure activity and pyridoxine-responsive anemia in the newborn have also been reported [64]. Excesses of vitamin B_6 do not appear to be detrimental to the fetus.

Folic Acid

Administration of aminopterin, a folic acid antagonist, during human pregnancy has resulted in increased rates of abortion and fetal malformations, including those of the trunk, skeleton, brain, heart, and kidneys [18,55,58]. Alcohol and phenytoin also interfere with folate absorption and metabolism in humans and may cause congenital anomalies [18]. Retrospective studies on mothers giving birth to malformed children have suggested a high incidence of folate deficiency. There is, at present, no conclusive evidence linking teratogenesis with dietary folate deficiency. Laurence et al. demonstrated a decrease in the recurrence risk for neural tube defects by dietary counseling or folate supplementation in pregnant women with inadequate diet in the prior pregnancies [65,66]. Neonatal megaloblastic anemia has also been reported with folate deficiency during pregnancy [30].

Vitamin B_{12}

Vitamin B_{12} deficiency during pregnancy is rare except in the strict vegetarian not taking B_{12} supplementation. In this case neurologic deficits and megaloblastic anemia may be demonstrated in the newborn as well [6,44].

As yet, no deleterious effects to the neonate have been reported after maternal supplementation with large amounts of vitamin B_{12}.

Calcium

Decreased maternal calcium ingestion has been correlated with the development of neonatal hypocalcemia and tetany [3,58]. Optimal ossification of the fetal skeleton requires adequate dietary intake of calcium, although the maternal skeleton has a small reservoir of calcium that can be used during minor deficiency states [32,55]. Teratogenesis has not been reported with excessive calcium intake.

Zinc

The importance of the trace element zinc is just being realized. Although few controlled trials in humans have been conducted, it appears that maternal zinc deficiency may increase the risk of intrauterine and neonatal growth retardation, preterm delivery, and neonatal mortality [67–70]. Neural tube defects have been reported to be more common in populations known to have diets deficient in zinc [32,68]. Increased urinary loss of zinc following maternal alcohol ingestion may play a role in the development of fetal alcohol syndrome [58]. Other congenital anomalies that have been attributed to zinc deficiency include craniofacial abnormalities, spine and foot deformities, and anomalous development of heart and lungs [30].

Other Minerals

Deficiency in dietary copper intake has been implicated in an increased incidence of neural tube defects [68]. Women with marked increases in total body copper, secondary to untreated Wilson's disease, have a higher rate of spontaneous miscarriage [32].

Maternal iodide deficiency during pregnancy is a major factor in the development of endemic cretinism. Ingestion or absorption of large quantities of iodide during pregnancy contributes to the development of fetal goiter and neonatal hypothyroidism [71,72].

Although many of the effects of nutrient deficiency or excess during pregnancy are unproved, the possibility of significant detrimental neonatal effects must constantly be considered. Studies in laboratory animals cannot be directly extrapolated to humans; however, human investigations are currently in progress. A nutritional approach based on moderation and caution should be followed by the pregnant woman and her physician in order to avoid any deleterious influences that are as yet unrecognized.

PREGNANCY IN THE UNDERWEIGHT PATIENT

Underweight may be defined as 90% or less of an individual's standard weight for height (Table 4-8)

[3]. Underweight gravidas are at increased risk for delivery of growth-retarded infants. As pregravid weights decrease, the risk of growth retardation in the fetus increases [74]. In one study, when poor maternal weight gain was superimposed on a low pregravid weight, the incidence of growth-retarded infants was greater than 40%. This compared with a 2% incidence of growth-retarded infants in mothers of standard weight with adequate weight gain during pregnancy [75]. It has been suggested that the underweight woman contributes involuntarily to her own body mass during pregnancy at the expense of her infant's growth [74]. Dietary counseling and food supplementation in underweight patients increase birth weight in these patients [3]. The incidence of toxemia, antepartum hemorrhage, prematurity, and anemia is increased in women who enter pregnancy at less than 90% of their standard weight [76,77].

Convincing the underweight woman that she needs to gain weight may be difficult. Protein and caloric supplementation has been suggested to attempt to achieve an appropriate weight for the patient, in addition to the 11 kg necessary for optimal infant development [58,74,78]. Goals for adequate weight gain can more easily be achieved if the gain is carried out over the entire gestation. Anderson has recommended initial supplementation, in the form of eggs and dairy products, as available sources of protein and energy [74]. Consultation with professional nutritionists may be necessary if simple dietary alterations do not show signs of ameliorating the condition.

MANAGEMENT OF OBESITY DURING PREGNANCY

Obesity is the most common nutritional disorder in the United States today [79]. Obesity may be defined as 20% above standard weight for height (Table 4-8). Forty percent of the women in the United States and Canada over 40 years of age are obese [79,80]. Increased maternal age and multiparity correlate closely with obesity. Obesity usually results from the ingestion of excessive amounts of calories. The foods are often of high caloric content yet low nutritive value. Thus, the obese patient may, paradoxically, also be malnourished [74].

The fetus of the obese pregnant woman has the same nutritional requirements as the developing infant whose mother is of ideal body weight. The caloric intake should not be markedly restricted. There is not complete agreement on optimal weight gain for obese pregnant patients. A consensus does exist that excess weight gain should be avoided by encouraging some caloric restraint. If given appropriate nutritional counseling, many obese patients will gain less than the average (11 kg) during pregnancy. A number of authors have suggested that a weight gain of 8 to 9 kg may correlate with an improved perinatal outcome [74,78,80].

Marked restriction of caloric intake for weight control or weight reduction in pregnancy is contraindicated. The development of maternal ketosis has been correlated in some studies with decreased intelligence in the offspring [81–83]. In addition to the utilization of amino acids as a primary energy source, severe caloric restriction may foster the development of vitamin and mineral deficiencies. Following pregnancy and lactation, a careful program for weight reduction should be undertaken.

Obese patients are at an increased risk for developing chronic hypertension, toxemia, diabetes mellitus, and thromboembolic complications [80,84]. Some authors have recommended low-dose subcutaneous heparin post partum or postoperatively to minimize the risk of thromboembolic phenomena in morbidly obese patients [85,86].

The exact relationship between maternal obesity and obstetric complications is unclear. Obese mothers have a higher rate of growth-retarded and macrosomic infants [84,87]. Although the incidence of cesarean birth is not increased, the relationship between dysfunctional or prolonged labor and maternal obesity is controversial [84,88].

The risk of surgery in obese patients is undoubtedly increased. Cardiovascular, respiratory, and anesthetic complications are more frequent [79]. Wound infections occur more often. Suction drainage of the subcutaneous space or secondary wound closure is recommended to decrease the incidence of such infections [85,89,90]. Because of the possible increased incidence of wound dehiscence and incisional hernia, internal retention sutures of the Smead-Jones type should be routine [85,91].

Following intestinal bypass surgery for obesity, vitamins K and B_{12}, folate, iron, and calcium deficiencies can occur [18,92,93]. Parenteral administration of some nutrients may be necessary. Despite an increased incidence of growth-retarded infants [94,95], if pregnancy occurs two years or more after surgery, a good pregnancy outcome may be anticipated. In one series, a higher, though statistically insignificant, incidence of congenital malformations was reported [96].

Table 4-8. Ideal and deviations of pregravid weights for height

Height	Ideal Weight*	Underweight (%)					Normal range											Overweight (%)											
		−30	−25	−20	−15	−10	+10	+15	+20	+25	+30	+35	+40	+45	+50	+55	+60	+65	+70	+75	+80	+85	+90	+95	+100	+105	+110	+115	+120
4'9"	104	73	78	83	88	94	114	120	125	130	135	140	146	151	156	161	166	172	177	182	187	192	198	203	208	213	218	224	229
4'10"	107	75	80	86	91	96	118	123	128	134	139	144	150	155	161	166	171	177	182	187	193	198	203	209	214	219	225	230	235
4'11"	110	77	83	88	94	99	121	127	132	138	143	149	154	160	165	171	176	182	187	193	198	204	209	215	220	226	231	237	242
5'0"	113	79	85	90	96	102	124	130	136	141	147	153	158	164	170	175	181	186	192	198	203	209	215	220	226	232	237	243	249
5'1"	116	81	87	93	99	104	128	133	139	145	151	157	162	168	174	180	186	191	197	203	209	215	220	226	232	238	244	249	255
5'2"	118	83	89	94	100	106	130	136	142	148	153	159	165	171	177	183	189	195	201	207	212	218	224	230	236	242	248	254	260
5'3"	123	86	92	98	105	111	136	141	148	154	160	166	172	178	185	191	197	203	209	215	221	228	234	240	246	252	258	264	271
5'4"	128	90	96	102	108	115	141	147	154	160	166	173	179	186	192	198	205	211	218	224	230	237	243	250	256	262	269	275	282
5'5"	132	92	99	106	112	119	145	152	158	165	172	178	185	191	198	205	211	218	224	231	238	244	251	257	264	271	277	284	290
5'6"	136	95	102	109	116	122	150	156	163	170	177	184	190	197	204	211	218	224	231	238	245	252	258	265	271	279	286	293	299
5'7"	140	98	105	112	119	126	154	161	168	175	182	189	196	203	210	217	224	231	238	245	252	259	266	273	280	287	294	301	308
5'8"	144	101	108	115	122	130	158	166	173	180	187	194	202	209	216	223	230	238	245	252	259	266	274	281	288	295	302	310	317
5'9"	148	104	111	118	126	133	163	170	178	185	192	200	207	215	222	229	237	244	252	259	266	274	281	289	296	303	311	318	326
5'10"	152	106	114	122	129	137	167	175	182	190	198	205	213	220	228	236	243	251	258	266	274	281	289	296	304	312	319	327	334

*Ideal weights for heights from Metropolitan Life Insurance Company, New York City.

Source: Luke [73].

NUTRITION AND THE PREGNANT ADOLESCENT

In the United States, one million teenagers become pregnant annually. Thirty thousand are less than 15 years of age. More than half of these pregnant women elect to continue their pregnancy, and 25% will experience another unwanted pregnancy within one year [97].

The prognosis for pregnancy in the adolescent female appears to be more closely related to the degree of physical maturity than to the patient's chronologic age [97–99]. The major obstetric risks for the young mother is the development of toxemia or the delivery of a low-birth-weight infant [100]. Inadequate nutrition may be an important risk factor in the adolescent who has yet to reach physiologic maturity [7].

The most rapid rate of skeletal and muscle growth occurs *prior* to the onset of menses. Within two to three years following menarche, most body growth is completed and physiologic adulthood commences. Women with late menarche are close to completing their somatic growth by the time ovulation begins. If menarche occurs at an early age, the young woman may still experience significant somatic growth during this fertile period. These differences must be considered when one calculates the nutritional requirements of the pregnant adolescent. If a pregnancy occurs within two years of menarche, particularly if menses began at an early chronologic age, there is an increased risk to the mother and fetus [101]. When pregnancy ensues more than two years after a normal menarche, the risk in that pregnancy is no greater than in the adult woman [97] (Fig. 4-2).

Once she becomes pregnant, the adolescent should be offered nutritional counseling. She may demonstrate poor eating habits and may attempt to reduce her food intake in an attempt to maintain her figure. An adequate morning meal is a necessity. Repeated assurances that a trim physique may once again be achieved following pregnancy and lactation are helpful. If caloric restriction has been self-imposed prior to her growth spurt, skeletal developmental abnormalities may already be present [7]. Caloric deprivation following peak adolescent growth may leave the pregnant teenager nutritionally deficient.

Adolescent pregnant women often restrict carbohydrates and fats to maintain an optimal body image. Protein intake is, usually, adequate. However, failure to consume enough carbohydrate calories may result in protein utilization as a primary energy source. Because of the likelihood of low iron stores and inadequate intake, oral iron supplementation of 30 to 60 mg of elemental iron per day is essential [102].

Calcium stores are usually adequate. In order to avoid depleting calcium reserves and to ensure optimal mineralization of the fetal skeleton, the RDA for calcium in this age group increases from 1.2 to 1.6 g per day. For women likely to undergo significant growth during and following pregnancy, additional dietary calcium may prove beneficial.

Recommended allowances for vitamin A, folic acid, pyridoxine, and zinc may not be met by the teenager's diet [103–105]. Dietary counseling and supplemental folic acid should remedy these deficiencies. Zinc supplementation through in-

Fig. 4-2. Growth rates around the mean age of menarche and incidence of pregnancies by age. Menarche is normalized at 12.5 years of age. The curves may be displaced horizontally for populations with different ages of menarche. (From Beal [97].)

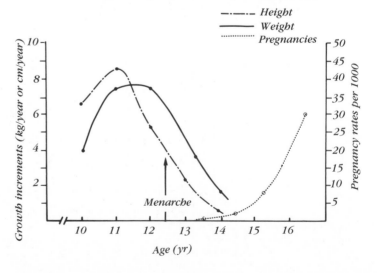

creased amounts of eggs, meat, liver or seafood is recommended, since sexual maturation and growth requires additional amounts of zinc [67,103].

CRAVINGS, AVERSIONS, AND PICA

Food aversions and cravings during pregnancy are reported in up to two-thirds of women. Aversions appear to occur as commonly as cravings [106].

Cravings and aversions can develop at any time during pregnancy, although the majority seem to begin early in pregnancy and disappear by 20 weeks' gestation [106]. Only in rare instances do these perversions persist into the puerperium.

Cravings for fruits, especially apples, are common [106]. A variety of other foods have also been reported. Aversions for high-protein foods are more common than cravings for these items. Aversions for coffee, tea, fried foods, and tobacco also occur.

Although reports of cravings for sweet foods are common, Dippel and Elias noted a marked decrease in the desire for sweets during all trimesters of pregnancy [106,107]. This confirmed previous observations in laboratory animals. The authors attributed this phenomenon to high progesterone levels in pregnancy, which decreases the sensitivity of estrogen-dependent taste mechanisms.

Pregnant women frequently demonstrate cravings and aversions for multiple substances. As many as five aversions in combination with three cravings have been reported in one patient [106].

In 24 patients with malignant neoplasms, Brewin reported food cravings or aversions that were identical to those they had experienced during earlier pregnancies [108]. He proposed that a similar host immunotolerance to tumors and to the fetus might be related to the development of these taste disorders.

Although pica was first recognized in the sixth century, the etiology remains obscure. Pica is defined as compulsive ingestion, usually of nonnutritive substances. The more common cravings include ice, starch, clay, and chalk. Various causes have been proposed, including iron deficiency, hunger, superstition, social acceptance, and mental illness [109].

Cultural and social pressures to practice pica appear to be important. A review of pica in Georgia by O'Rourke et al. showed a higher than usual incidence in low-income older rural blacks [110]. The sale of white clay, as a delicacy, was commonplace. A follow-up of the same population published seven years later showed a significant decrease in the incidence of pica with routine iron administra-

tion and intensive education efforts [111]. Edwards et al. described the ingestion of a number of nonnutritive substances as a treatment for various ills of pregnancy and to promote the health of the unborn child [112].

For years it was believed that inadequate nutrition led to the iron deficiency anemia observed in a large proportion of patients practicing pica. Minnich et al. demonstrated that clays ingested by Turkish women had the ability, through cation exchange, to irreversibly bind ingested iron into nonabsorbable compounds [110,113,114]. Talkington and colleagues, however, found no significant impairment of iron absorption by starch or clay in Texas [115]. Several authors have reported that expeditious correction of pica can be expected by oral or parenteral administration of iron [116–118]. Even in patients without overt anemia, pica could be effectively treated with iron supplementation. In a double-blind study, Coltman showed an immediate cessation in pica with iron supplementation [119]. Crosby believes that pica is a common complication of iron deficiency. He regarded cravings for iron-poor foodstuffs as a symptom of iron deficiency that often could be corrected by iron administration [109].

In addition to the nutritional deficiencies that accompany pica, dysfunctional labor, bowel obstruction and even death have occasionally been reported [120–122].

ANOREXIA NERVOSA AND BULIMIA DURING PREGNANCY

Anorexia nervosa is a psychiatric disorder characterized by a delusional denial of thinness, hyperactivity, a constant striving for perfection, and a distorted attitude toward eating that overrides hunger, warnings, and threats. It is most common in females during the second and third decades of life. Usually the disorder is associated with amenorrhea. Nevertheless, a few patients with anorexia nervosa have been reported during pregnancy [126–128]. In three of these cases ovulation was induced with gonadotropins [127]. These patients may suffer hypokalemia, ketosis, hypochloremic alkalosis due to vomiting, as well as weight loss. The exact risk to the fetus is unknown. However, severe dietary restriction during pregnancy is believed to have particularly severe consequences for fetal growth and development [50–52].

A variant of anorexia nervosa, bulimia is characterized by episodes of gorging followed by self-induced emesis. This problem may be difficult to distinguish from hyperemesis gravidarum. In one reported case it was necessary to maintain adequate nutrition with the use of an oral-gastric feeding tube. In this case the authors felt that the cessation of vomiting during continuous feeding helped distinguish bulimia from hyperemesis, since vomiting would likely not have ceased had the patient suffered from hyperemesis [128].

Therapy for each of these disorders is both nutritional and psychiatric. Hospitalization is desirable for restoration of fluid and electrolyte balance. In some cases malnutrition may be so advanced that parenteral alimentation is required [124].

ASSESSMENT OF NUTRITIONAL STATUS AND IDENTIFICATION OF PATIENTS AT RISK

Approximately 20 to 30% of pregnant women require special nutritional counseling during pregnancy [74]. Although some patients can be easily identified, a significant number require a careful history and physical examination and close prenatal care to detect a nutritional disorder (Table 4-9).

The underweight pregnant patient, particularly if she delays antepartum care until late in pregnancy, may not be easily identified. The obese patient may feel that the increased caloric demands of pregnancy will enable her to achieve weight control or reduction. Although subject to significant error, weight versus height charts can provide the physician with a baseline estimate (Table 4-8). Wrist circumference measurements have been suggested to more accurately determine body frame size and optimal prepregnancy weight [74].

A thorough medical and obstetric history may help identify patients at high nutritional risk. A previous history of systemic disease, large or growth-retarded infants, or preterm births requires careful evaluation and close observation of maternal weight gain during pregnancy. A history of successive pregnancies within a limited time period can indicate inadequate maternal nutrient stores. Similar problems can affect pregnancies occurring during or shortly following lactation. Numerous investigations of the nutritional effects of oral contraceptive use have been reported in the literature [3]. Pyridoxine and folic acid deficiency can occur; only folic acid deficiency appears to be of clinical concern during pregnancy. Folate supplementation should be considered for patients who conceive shortly after the discontinuation of birth control pills [123].

Patients who have a history of anemia or glucose intolerance require periodic laboratory evaluation during gestation. Chronic systemic disease, especially if it calls for dietary restriction, may necessi-

Table 4-9. Factors in identifying pregnant patients at nutritional risk

I. Past obstetric history
   A. Repetitive conceptions at brief intervals
   B. Recent discontinuation of lactation
   C. Previous growth-retarded infant
   D. Previous preterm delivery
   E. Previous macrosomic infant
   F. Previous stillbirth
   G. History of gestational glucose intolerance
   H. History of gestational anemia

II. Past medical history
   A. History of chronic systemic disease
   B. History of glucose intolerance
   C. History of anemia
   D. Recent discontinuation of oral contraceptives
   E. History of drug ingestion interfering with nutrient absorption or utilization

III. Social history
   A. Teenager, particularly if close to early menarche
   B. Unwanted pregnancy
   C. Substance abuser
   D. Low socioeconomic status
   E. Ingesting fad or restricted diets

IV. Physical examination
   A. Prepregnancy weight 10% less than optimal weight for height
   B. Prepregnancy weight 20% greater than optimal weight for height
   C. Systemic evidence of nutritional deficiency (e.g., glossitis, gingivitis, cheilosis, dental caries, dermatitis)

V. Laboratory assessment
   A. Decreased hematocrit
   B. Abnormal red cell or white cell morphology on peripheral smear
   C. Presence of sugar, protein, or ketones in routine urinary screen

VI. Course of pregnancy
   A. Severe nausea and vomiting
   B. Multiple gestation
   C. Total weight gain during first half of pregnancy <4 kg
   D. Significant vaginal bleeding
   E. Weight gain <1 kg per month after 20 weeks
   F. Weight gain of >1 kg per week
   G. Development of significant edema

tate careful dietary review and adjustments when needed. Some medications interfere with normal nutrient metabolism, increasing requirements during pregnancy.

Teenage pregnant patients must receive close attention, especially if they have conceived shortly after menarche and have not achieved their full growth potential. If the pregnancy is unwanted, much support will be required to ensure adequate motivation for attention to nutritive needs.

Patients with severe nausea and vomiting during early pregnancy must be observed for nutritional deficiency. Restrained use of antiemetic medications may be necessary if dietary approaches such as frequent carbohydrate feedings are unsuccessful. In the most severe cases, total parenteral nutrition must be considered [124].

Patients from low socioeconomic backgrounds are likely to be nutritionally deprived. Food supplementation may be necessary and will result in increased birth weights and decreased perinatal mortality [54].

Pregnant women who are substance abusers are often nutritionally deprived. These patients must be encouraged to improve dietary habits, while being supported in their attempts to curb their abuse.

The presence of multiple gestation or significant blood loss during pregnancy necessitates additional nutrient intake.

Adherence to fad or nutritionally restrictive diets may be an indication for supplementation of the pregnant woman (e.g., the vegan who needs varied vegetable proteins as well as B_{12} supplementation).

Weight gain of <1 kg per month after 20 weeks of pregnancy may be seen with suboptimal nutrition and poor fetal growth. Total weight gain during the first half of pregnancy of less than 4 kg warrants careful investigation and therapy. Excessive weight gain, particularly toward the end of pregnancy, may be an indication of glucose intolerance and fat deposition or of marked accumulation of extracellular fluid associated with toxemia.

Measurement of urinary glucose, protein, and ketones should be performed at each prenatal visit during pregnancy. Serial measurements of hematocrit should be obtained, particularly in patients at high risk for developing iron deficiency during pregnancy. The normal alterations in laboratory studies during pregnancy must be considered when interpreting these results [125]. No single test is a reliable marker of general nutritional status.

Despite their inherent inaccuracies, diet diaries for patients at nutritional risk, if not for all pregnant women, may provide enough information to make adjustments in protein and caloric intake possible. If adequate amounts of such "perfect" foods as dairy products and eggs are not being included, appropriate substitutions can be introduced. Consultation with nutritional counselors is recommended for complex problems, such as vegans, women with malabsorption syndromes, diabetics, or patients who have recently had intestinal bypass surgery.

REFERENCES

1. Pitkin RM, Kaminetzky HA, Newton M, Pritchard JA. Maternal nutrition. A selective review of clinical topics. Obstet Gynecol. 1972; 40:773–85.
2. Taylor ES. Editorial. Obstet Gynecol Surv. 1982; 37:229–31.
3. Pitkin RM. Nutritional support in obstetrics and gynecology. Clin Obstet Gynecol. 1976; 19:489–513.
4. Leader A. Maternal nutrition in pregnancy. Current Prob Obstet Gynecol. 1983; 6:1–47.
5. Luke B. Maternal nutrition. Boston: Little, Brown, 1979.
6. Leader A, Wong KH, Deitel M. Maternal nutrition in pregnancy. Part I: a review. Can Med Assoc J. 1981; 125:545–9.
7. Worthington-Roberts BS, Vermeersch J, Williams SR. Nutrition in pregnancy and lactation. 2nd ed. St. Louis: Mosby, 1981.
8. Joint FAO/WHO Ad Hoc Expert Committee on Energy and Protein Requirements. Energy and protein requirements. Rome: Food and Agriculture Organization of the United Nations, 1973.
9. Pitkin RM. Assessment of nutritional status of mother, fetus, and newborn. Am J Clin Nutr. 1981; 34:658–68.
10. Oldham H, Sheft BB. Effect of caloric intake on nitrogen utilization during pregnancy. J Am Diet Assoc. 1951; 27:847–54.
11. National Research Council. Committee on Dietary Allowances. Recommended dietary allowances. 9th rev. ed. Washington, D.C.: National Academy of Sciences, 1980.
12. Moghissi KS. Maternal nutrition in pregnancy. Clin Obstet Gynecol. 1978; 21:297–310.
13. Ghadimi H, Pecora P. Free amino acids of cord plasma as compared with maternal plasma during pregnancy. Pediatrics. 1964; 33:500–6.
14. McFee JG. Iron metabolism and iron deficiency during pregnancy. Clin Obstet Gynecol. 1979; 22:799–808.
15. Munro HN. Nutrient requirements during pregnancy—II. Am J Clin Nutr. 1981; 34:679–84.
16. Finch CA, Huebers H. Perspectives in iron metabolism. N Engl J Med. 1982; 306:1520–8.
17. Uses of folic acid in pregnancy and in clinical disorders. Med Lett Drugs Ther. 1972; 14:50–2.

18. Kitay DZ. Folic acid and reproduction. Clin Obstet Gynecol. 1979; 22:809–17.

19. Robertson WVB. Maternal-infant nutrition. In: Quilligan EJ, Kretchmer N, eds. Fetal and maternal medicine. New York: Wiley, 1980:123–40.

20. Lindheimer MD, Katz AI. Sodium and diuretics in pregnancy. N Engl J Med. 1973; 288:891–4.

21. Hytten FE. Weight gain in pregnancy—30 years of research. S Afr Med J. 1981; 60:15–9.

22. Olson RE, Suttie JW. Vitamin K and gamma-carboxyglutamate biosynthesis. Vitam Horm. 1977; 35:59–108.

23. Rietz P, Gloor U, Wiss O. Menadione aus menschlicher leber und faulschlamm. Int Z Vitam Ernahrungsforsch [Beih]. 1970; 40:351–62.

24. Olson RE. Vitamin K. In: Goodhart RS, Shils ME, eds. Modern nutrition in health and disease. 5th ed. Philadelphia: Lea & Febiger, 1973:166–74.

25. Hytten FE. Nutrition in pregnancy. Postgrad Med J. 1979; 55:295–302.

26. Rose DP. Oral contraceptives and vitamin B_6. In: Human vitamin B_6 requirements. Washington, D.C.: National Academy of Sciences, 1978:193–201.

27. Sprince H, Lowy RS, Folsome CE, Behrman JS. Studies on urinary excretion of "xanthurenic acid" during normal and abnormal pregnancy: survey of excretion of "xanthurenic acid" in normal nonpregnant, normal pregnant, pre-eclamptic and eclamptic women. Am J Obstet Gynecol. 1951; 62:84–92.

28. Klieger JA, Evrard JR, Pierce R. Abnormal pyridoxine metabolism in toxemia of pregnancy. Am J Obstet Gynecol. 1966; 94:316–21.

29. Hillman LS, Haddad JG. Human perinatal vitamin D metabolism. I. 25-Hydroxyvitamin D in maternal and cord blood. J Pediatr. 1974; 84:742–9.

30. Kaminetzky HA, Baker H. Micronutrients in pregnancy. Clin Obstet Gynecol. 1977; 20:363–80.

31. Hurley LS. Developmental nutrition. Englewood Cliffs, N.J.: Prentice-Hall, 1980.

32. Moghissi KS. Risks and benefits of nutritional supplements during pregnancy. Obstet Gynecol. 1981; 58:68S–78S.

33. Osofsky HJ. Antenatal malnutrition: its relationship to subsequent infant and child development. Am J Obstet Gynecol. 1969; 105:1150–9.

34. Cohn SD. Vegetarian nutrition: an overview. Issues Health Care Women. 1978; 1:1–4.

35. Lappe FM. Diet for a small planet. New York: Ballantine, 1971.

36. Ellis FR, Mumford P. The nutritional status of vegans and vegetarians. Proc Nutr Soc. 1967; 26:205–12.

37. Williams ER. Making vegetarian diets nutritious. Am J Nurs. 1975; 75:2168–73.

38. Ohsawa G. Macrobiotics: an invitation to health and happiness. Oroville, Calif.: George Ohsawa Macrobiotic Foundation, 1971.

39. Tauraso NM. Recommendations for healthful living—an holistic approach. Frederick, Md: Hidden Valley Press, 1981.

40. Brown PT, Bergan JG. The dietary status of "new" vegetarians. J Am Diet Assoc. 1975; 67:455–9.

41. Robson JR. Food faddism. Pediatr Clin North Am. 1977; 24:189–201.

42. American Academy of Pediatrics. Committee on Nutrition. Nutritional aspects of vegetarianism, health foods, and fad diets. Pediatrics. 1977; 59:460–4.

43. Shull MW, Reed RB, Valadian I, Palombo R, Thorne H, Dwyer, JT. Velocities of growth in vegetarian preschool children. Pediatrics. 1977; 60:410–7.

44. Higginbottom MC, Sweetman L, Nyhan WL. A syndrome of methylmalonic aciduria, homocystinuria, megaloblastic anemia and neurologic abnormalities in a vitamin B_{12}-deficient breast-fed infant of a strict vegetarian. N Engl J Med. 1978; 299:317–23.

45. Vyhmeister IB, Register UD, Sonenberg LM. Safe vegetarian diets for children. Pediatr Clin North Am. 1977; 24:203–10.

46. Robson JR, Konlande JE, Larkin FA, et al. Zen macrobiotic dietary problems in infancy. Pediatrics. 1974; 53:326–9.

47. Berkelhamer JE, Thorp FK, Cobbs S. Kwashiorkor in Chicago. Am J Dis Child. 1975; 129:1240.

48. Roberts IF, West RJ, Ogilvie D, Dillon MJ. Malnutrition in infants receiving cult diets: a form of child abuse. Br Med J. 1979; 1:296–8.

49. Hale F. Pigs born without eye balls. J Hered. 1933; 24:105–6.

50. Osofsky HJ. Relationships between nutrition during pregnancy and subsequent infant and child development. Obstet Gynecol Surv. 1975; 30:227–41.

51. Philips C. Johnson NE. The impact of quality of diet and other factors on birth weight of infants. Am J Clin Nutr. 1977; 30:215–25.

52. Falkner F. Maternal nutrition and fetal growth. Am J Clin Nutr. 1981; 34:769–74.

53. Stein Z, Susser M, Rush D. Prenatal nutrition and birth weight: experiments and quasi-experiments in the past decade. J Reprod Med. 1978; 21:287–99.

54. Susser M. Prenatal nutrition, birthweight, and psychological development: an overview of experiments, quasi-experiments, and natural experiments in the past decade. Am J Clin Nutr. 1981; 34:784–803.

55. Hurley LS. Nutritional deficiencies and excesses. In: Wilson JG, Fraser FC, eds. Handbook of teratology. Vol. I. New York: Plenum, 1977:261–308.

56. Lechtig A, Habicht JP, Delgado H, et al. Effect of food supplementation during pregnancy on birthweight. Pediatrics. 1975; 56:508–20.

57. Rush D, Stein Z, Susser M. A randomized controlled trial of prenatal nutritional supplementation in New York City. Pediatrics. 1980; 65:683–97.

58. Rosso P. Nutrition and abnormal fetal growth. In: Queenan JT, ed. Management of high-risk pregnancy. Oradell, NJ: Medical Economics, 1980:7–13.

59. Nutrition in pregnancy. Med Lett Drugs Ther. 1978; 20:65–6.

60. Roberts HJ. Perspective on vitamin E as therapy. JAMA 1981; 246:129–31.

61. Cochrane WA. Overnutrition in prenatal and neonatal life: a problem? Can Med Assoc J. 1965; 93:893–9.

62. Rosso P. Nutrition and maternal-fetal exchange. Am J Clin Nutr. 1981; 34:744–55.

63. Vitamin B_6 deficiency and immune responses. Nutr Rev. 1976; 34:188–9.

64. Requirement of vitamin B_6 during pregnancy. Nutr Rev. 1976; 34:15–6.

65. Laurence KM, James N, Miller M, Campbell M. Increased risk of recurrence of pregnancies complicated by fetal neural tube defects in mothers receiving poor diets and possible benefit of dietary counseling. Br Med J. 1980; 281:1592–4.

66. Laurence KM, James N, Miller MH, Tennant GB, Campbell H. Double-blind randomised controlled trial of folate treatment before conception to prevent recurrence of neural-tube defects. Br Med J. 1981; 282:1509–11.

67. Butrimovitz GP, Purdy WC. Zinc nutrition and growth in a childhood population. Am J Clin Nutr. 1978; 31:1409–12.

68. Hurley LS. Teratogenic aspects of manganese, zinc, and copper nutrition. Physiol Rev. 1981; 61:249–95.

69. Meadows NJ, Ruse W, Smith MF, et al. Zinc and small babies. Lancet. 1981; 2:1135–7.

70. Patrick J, Dervish G, Gillieson M. Zinc and small babies. Lancet. 1982; 1:169–70.

71. Carswell F, Kerr MM, Hutchison JH. Congenital goitre and hypothyroidism produced by maternal ingestion of iodides. Lancet. 1970; 1:1241–3.

72. Vorherr H, Vorherr UF, Mehta P, Ulrich JA, Messer RH. Vaginal absorption of povidone-iodine. JAMA. 1980; 244:2628–9.

73. Luke B. A nutritional assessment of the expectant mother: how and why. Keeping Abreast J. 1977; 2:280–91.

74. Anderson GD. Nutrition in pregnancy—1978. South Med J. 1979; 72:1304–14.

75. Rosso P, Luke B. The influence of maternal weight gain on the incidence of fetal growth retardation. Am J Clin Nutr. 1978; 31:696. abstract.

76. Pitkin RM. Nutritional influences during pregnancy. Med Clin North Am. 1977; 61:3–15.

77. Edwards LE, Alton IR, Barrada MI, Hakanson EY. Pregnancy in the underweight woman: course, outcome and growth patterns of the infant. Am J Obstet Gynecol. 1979; 135:297–302.

78. Naeye RL. Weight gain and the outcome of pregnancy. Am J Obstet Gynecol. 1979; 135:3–9.

79. Strauss RJ, Wise L. Operative risks of obesity. Surg Gynecol Obstet. 1978; 146:286–91.

80. Gould SF, Makowski EL. Obesity in pregnancy. Perinatol Neonatol. 1981; 5:49–59.

81. Churchill JA, Berendes HW, Nemore J. Neuropsychological deficits in children of diabetic mothers. Am J Obstet Gynecol. 1969; 105:257–68.

82. Dr. Atkins' diet revolution. Med Lett Drugs Ther. 1973; 15:41–2.

83. Stehbens JA, Baker GL, Kitchell M. Outcome at ages 1, 3, and 5 years of children born to diabetic women. Am J Obstet Gynecol. 1977; 127:408–13.

84. Calandra C, Abell DA, Beischer NA. Maternal obesity in pregnancy. Obstet Gynecol. 1981; 57:8–12.

85. Morrow CP, Hernandez WL, Townsend DE, Disaia PJ. Pelvic celiotomy in the obese patient. Am J Obstet Gynecol. 1977; 127:335–9.

86. Laros RK, Alger LS. Thromboembolism and pregnancy. Clin Obstet Gynecol. 1979; 22:871–8.

87. Harrison GG, Udall JN, Morrow G. Maternal obesity, weight gain in pregnancy, and infant birth weight. Am J Obstet Gynecol. 1980; 136:411–2.

88. Gross T, Sokol RJ, King KC. Obesity in pregnancy: risks and outcome. Obstet Gynecol. 1980; 56:446–50.

89. McIlrath DC, van Heerden JA, Edis AJ, Dozois RR. Closure of abdominal incisions with subcutaneous catheters. Surgery. 1976; 80:411–6.

90. Ahern JK, Goodlin RC. Cesarean section in the massively obese. Obstet Gynecol. 1978; 51:509–10.

91. Wallace D, Hernandez W, Schlaerth JB, Malick RN, Morrow CP. Prevention of abdominal wound disruption utilizing the Smead-Jones closure technique. Obstet Gynecol. 1980; 56:226–30.

92. Wills CE. Obstetrical delivery after jejuno-ileostomy for obesity. J Med Assoc Ga. 1971; 60:39–42.

93. Wong KH, Leader A, Deitel M. Maternal nutrition in pregnancy. Part II: the implications of previous gastrointestinal operations and bowel disorders. Can Med Assoc J. 1981; 125:550–2.

94. Taylor JL, O'Leary JP. Pregnancy following jejunoileal bypass. Effects on fetal outcome. Obstet Gynecol. 1976; 48:425–7.

95. Ingardia CJ, Fischer JR. Pregnancy after jejunoileal bypass and the SGA infant. Obstet Gynecol. 1978; 52:215–8.

96. Savel LE, Simon SR, Maxon WS. Pregnancy after jejunoileal bypass. A review and report of one case. Obstet Gynecol. 1978; 52:58S–60S.

97. Beal VA. Assessment of nutritional status in pregnancy—II. Am J Clin Nutr. 1981; 34:691–6.

98. Grant JA, Heald FP. Complications of adolescent pregnancy. Survey of the literature on fetal outcome in adolescence. Clin Pediatr. 1972; 11:567–70.

99. Carruth BR. Adolescent pregnancy and nutrition. J Med Soc NJ. 1981; 78:217–8.

100. Committee on Adolescence, American Academy of Pediatrics. Statement on teenage pregnancy. Pediatrics. 1979; 63:795–7.

101. Zlatnik FJ, Burmeister LF. Low "gynecologic age": an obstetric risk factor. Am J Obstet Gynecol. 1977; 128:183–6.

102. Elsborg L, Rosenquist A, Helms P. Iron intake by teenage girls and by pregnant women. Int J Vitam Nutr Res. 1979; 49:210–4.

103. Greger JL, Higgins MM, Abernathy RP, Kirksey A, DeCorso MB, Baligar P. Nutritional status of adolescent girls in regard to zinc, copper, and iron. Am J Clin Nutr. 1978; 31:269–75.

104. Kirksey A, Keaton K, Abernathy RP, Greger, JL. Vitamin B$_6$ nutritional status of a group of female adolescents. Am J Clin Nutr. 1978; 31:946–54.

105. Tyrer LB, Mazlen RG, Bradshaw LE. Meeting the special needs of pregnant teenagers. Clin Obstet Gynecol. 1978; 21:1199–213.

106. Trethowan WH, Dickens G. Cravings, aversions and pica of pregnancy. In: Howells JG, ed. Modern perspectives in psycho-obstetrics. New York: Brunner/Mazel, 1972:251–68.

107. Dippel RL, Elias JW. Preferences for sweet in relationship to use of oral contraceptives and pregnancy. Horm Behav. 1980; 14:1–6.

108. Brewin TB. Can a tumour cause the same appetite perversion or taste change as a pregnancy? Lancet. 1980; 2:907–8.

109. Crosby WH. Pica. JAMA. 1976; 235:2765.

110. O'Rourke DE, Quinn JG, Nicholson JO, Gibson HH. Geophagia during pregnancy. Obstet Gynecol. 1967; 29:581–4.

111. Bronstein ES, Dollar J. Pica in pregnancy. J Med Assoc Ga. 1974; 63:332–5.

112. Edwards CH, McDonald S, Mitchell JR, et al. Clay- and cornstarch-eating women. J Am Diet Assoc. 1959; 35:810–5.

113. Minnich V, Okuoglu A, Tarcon Y, et al. Pica in Turkey: II. Effect of clay upon iron absorption. Am J Clin Nutr. 1968; 21:78–86.

114. Blum M, Orton CG, Rose L. Effect of starch ingestion on excessive iron absorption. Ann Intern Med. 1968; 68:1165. abstract.

115. Talkington KM, Gant NF, Scott DE, Pritchard JA. Effect of ingestion of starch and some clays on iron absorption. Am J Obstet Gynecol. 1970; 108:262–7.

116. Lanzkowsky P. Investigation into the aetiology and treatment of pica. Arch Dis Child. 1959; 34:140–8.

117. McDonald R, Marshall SR. The value of iron therapy in pica. Pediatrics. 1964; 34:558–62.

118. Reynolds RD, Binder HJ, Miller MB, et al. Pagophagia and iron-deficiency anemia. Ann Intern Med. 1968; 69:435–40.

119. Coltman CA. Pagophagia and iron lack. JAMA. 1969; 207:513–6.

120. Holt WA, Hendricks CH. Dysfunctional labor due to fecal impaction. Obstet Gynecol. 1969; 34:502–5.

121. Gusdon JP, Tunca C. Pica mimicking abruptio placenta. A case report. Obstet Gynecol. 1974; 43:197–9.

122. Key TC, Horger EO, Miller JM. Geophagia as a cause of maternal death. Obstet Gynecol. 1982; 60:525–6.

123. Streiff RR. Folate deficiency and oral contraceptives. JAMA. 1970; 214:105–8.

124. Hew LR, Deitel M. Total parenteral nutrition in gynecology and obstetrics. Obstet Gynecol. 1980; 55:464–8.

125. National Research Council. Committee on Nutrition of the Mother and Preschool Child. Laboratory indices of nutritional status in pregnancy. Washington, D.C.: National Academy of Sciences, 1978.

126. Lakoff KM, Feldman JD. Anorexia nervosa associated with pregnancy. Obstet Gynecol 1972; 39:699–701.

127. Hart T, Kase N, Kimball CP. Induction of ovulation and pregnancy in patients with anorexia nervosa. Am J Obstet Gynecol 1970; 108:580–4.

128. Weinfeld RH, Dubay M, Burchell RC, Millerick JD, Kennedy AT. Pregnancy associated with anorexia and starvation. Am J Obstet Gynecol 1977; 129:698–99.

5. ANTENATAL FETAL ASSESSMENT
Robert E. Wall

Auscultation of the fetal heart as an indicator of fetal well-being was first proposed in 1821 by Kergaradec, a French nobleman who never practiced obstetrics [1]. Since that time, obstetricians have searched for subtle changes in fetal heart rate before and during labor that might accurately reflect the intrauterine health of the fetus.

Despite earlier biochemical attempts to find an optimal marker for antenatal fetal assessment, the introduction of the oxytocin challenge test into clinical practice, by Ray and Freeman in 1972, began a new era in antenatal fetal testing [2]. Current utilization of antepartum monitoring of spontaneous fetal heart rate (nonstress test) or antepartum monitoring of the fetal heart rate following uterine contractions (contraction stress test) has provided clinicians with a reliable system for documenting fetal well-being in high-risk pregnancies, including those complicated by medical illness. Although the perfect biochemical or biophysical test has yet to be defined, the nonstress test is currently the mainstay of antenatal fetal assessment in most perinatal centers in this country.

The exact role of antenatal testing in low-risk pregnancies is unclear. Although some physicians have advocated nonstress testing for all pregnancies, maternal assessment of fetal activity is the only test of fetal well-being widely utilized at present in low-risk pregnancies [3].

The following discussion is intended to familiarize practitioners with the basic clinical principles of the most valuable antenatal tests of fetal well-being in use today.

BIOPHYSICAL TESTING—FETAL MOVEMENT

For many years obstetricians considered the subjective assessment of fetal movement by the pregnant woman an indirect confirmation of pregnancy. Not until 1958 did Smyth and Farrow suggest that decreased fetal movements could be clinically useful in diagnosing impending fetal asphyxia or death [1].

Sadovsky and colleagues have contributed greatly to our knowledge of normal and pathologic fetal movement. In 1973 they proposed that the subjective maternal assessment of fetal activity was a clinically useful method of monitoring the unborn child [4]. At present, assessment of fetal movement is included by most perinatal centers for monitoring both low- and high-risk pregnancies.

Fetal movement (quickening) is usually perceived by pregnant women as "a flutter" between the fifteenth and the twentieth gestational weeks. Such recognition is often influenced by the mother's personality, cooperation, and occupation, as well as by the condition of the fetus [5]. Using objective discernment of fetal movements by ultrasound as a standard, most women are able to accurately perceive 80 to 90% of all fetal movements [6].

In the opinion of most investigators, the frequency of fetal movement appears to increase with gestational age, peaking at 32 weeks. Thereafter, fetal activity slowly declines, with the postmature fetus demonstrating little activity (Fig. 5-1). Several authors have attributed the normal decrease in fetal movement in the last weeks of pregnancy to decreased amniotic fluid or increased fetal sleep periods with central nervous system maturation [6].

The average number of fetal movements per day, perceived by the mother, in the third trimester is highly variable. *Except in cases of absent or very few movements, the absolute number of fetal movements is not clinically significant.* In 127 pregnant women with normal pregnancy outcomes, the average daily number of fetal movements at 32 weeks' gestation was 575 (range 50–956). As few as four to ten movements per day

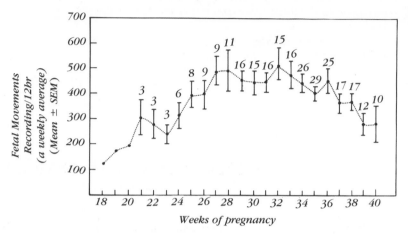

Fig. 5-1. Mean values of daily fetal movement recording in normal pregnancy. (From Sadovsky et al. [7].)

were reported without poor results [6]. Maternal lateral recumbency, the rapid eye movement stage of sleep, exposure to ultrasound, and increased blood sugar appear to increase fetal movements in most instances. Cigarette smoking and some pharmacologic depressants, in addition to fetal hypoxia and poor fetal condition, may reduce fetal activity [1,5,6].

Whether a normal diurnal variation in fetal movements exists is controversial. Most authors believe that the period of least fetal movement occurs in the morning, with a relative increase during the evening hours. Marked variations in fetal activity occur throughout the day. Independently of maternal sleep-wake cycles, the normal fetus demonstrates rest periods, with little or no movement, varying in length up to 120 minutes [8,9]. Sadovsky has suggested that reduction in fetal activity to three movements in 24 hours or cessation of all activity for 12 hours is a "movement alarm signal (MAS)." He believes this may indicate a fetus in severe distress secondary to chronic uteroplacental insufficiency [6]. Unfortunately, intrauterine demise secondary to abruptio placentae or cord complications are rarely preceded by decreased fetal activity. A marked increase in sudden strong vigorous fetal movements followed by abrupt cessation of all activity may occur with cord complications, acute fetal distress, and fetal death [5].

Leader et al. prospectively studied fetal movement in 262 high-risk pregnancies [10]. They considered fetal movement abnormal when (1) a day passed with no fetal movement or (2) the number of movements fell below ten per day on two consecutive days. Poor fetal outcome occurred in the normal movement group in 1% of cases while almost half of the abnormal movement group demonstrated significant fetal morbidity, including

stillbirth in 38%. There were no stillbirths in the 223 patients with normal fetal movement.

Harper et al. prospectively monitored 91, mostly high-risk, pregnancies with weekly fetal heart rate testing, biweekly serum unconjugated estriol determinations, and daily fetal movement recording [11]. Only 1 of 87 women without cessation of fetal activity demonstrated an abnormal fetal heart rate pattern. In three of four women with no fetal movement, abnormal fetal heart rate patterns were noted, with one subsequent neonatal death.

In clinical practice, both low- and high-risk patients should be instructed about the value of fetal movement as an indicator of fetal well-being. In the last trimester, each encounter with the patient should include questions regarding fetal activity. Thus the patient will realize the importance of fetal activity and its prognostic significance. She should include subjective assessment of daily fetal activity as an integral part of her antepartum care. In high-risk pregnancies, objective recording of the number of fetal movements during multiple distinct periods of observation is preferred. Three or four half-hour periods should be set aside throughout the day to evaluate the number of movements. Observation periods must be extended in patients who feel little or no movement during recording sessions. Patients who note less than ten movements per day, despite constant prolonged observation, or those who note a marked decrease in fetal activity, particularly with diminished strength of movements, should be evaluated further to confirm fetal well-being. Patients who note less than four movements per day or who feel no movement in 12 hours are at extreme risk for impending fetal demise. Immediate evaluation is mandatory.

Daily maternal assessment of fetal movement is a reliable, safe, inexpensive indicator of fetal well-being that should be applied to all pregnancies. In all instances, the clinical situation and other parameters of fetal well-being must be considered in order to properly evaluate the patient and her fetus.

ANTEPARTUM FETAL HEART RATE TESTING

Contraction Stress Test

The early contributions of Hon and associates, as well as those of Caldeyro-Barcia and his colleagues, provided a foundation for antepartum fetal heart monitoring in high-risk pregnancies [12–14]. Although European investigators first described the antenatal induction of uterine contractions by means of exogenous oxytocin in high-risk patients, the definitive description of the "stress test" in this country came from Ray and associates in 1972 [2]. They proposed that a compromised fetus could be identified on an external fetal heart rate monitor by the occurrence of repetitive "late decelerations" in response to regular uterine contractions stimulated by oxytocin. The absence of decelerations was felt to be evidence of fetal well-being. This "oxytocin challenge test" (contraction stress test) was quickly included in the screening protocols of most high-risk obstetric centers. The contraction stress test (CST) still remains an accurate evaluator of fetal well-being.

The contraction stress test is indicated in those pregnancies at risk for uteroplacental insufficiency. Postmaturity, intrauterine growth retardation, pregnancy-induced or chronic hypertension,

and diabetes mellitus make up the majority of such indications. Relative contraindications to the CST include placenta previa, ruptured membranes, premature labor, premature cervical dilatation, previous classical cesarean delivery, and overdistended uterus (e.g., multiple gestation or polyhydramnios).

The patient is placed in semi-Fowler's position, and baseline vital signs are recorded. An external fetal heart rate transducer and tocodynamometer are positioned carefully to optimize the recording of the fetal heart rate. After a ten-minute baseline tracing is obtained, a dilute intravenous infusion of oxytocin is begun and slowly increased until firm uterine contractions have reached a frequency of every two to three minutes, lasting 40 to 60 seconds. When three contractions have occurred within a ten-minute period, the stimulation is withdrawn and the fetal heart rate tracing reviewed.

A few centers have recently employed nipple stimulation to avoid oxytocin infusion. Either hand-held breast pump or digital twisting and traction to the nipple by the patient will induce adequate uterine contractions to evaluate the fetal heart rate in 50 to 80% of cases. As yet, few published reports are available in the literature regarding this procedural variation [15].

The appearance of late decelerations associated with the majority of contractions recorded is interpreted as a *positive* test (Fig. 5-2). If no late decelerations are noted, the test is *negative* and repeated in seven days. When occasional late decelerations are noted, the test is *equivocal* or *suspicious* and repeated within 24 hours (Table 5-1).

A negative contraction stress test virtually rules out the possibility of imminent intrauterine demise on the basis of poor uteroplacental function [16,17]. Impending stillbirth, secondary to cord accident or abruptio placentae, cannot be predicted with the CST. Using these definitions,

Fig. 5-2. Representative drawing of recurrent late decelerations, by Sarah Gustafson, Media Center, Rose Medical Center. FHR = fetal heart rate; UC = uterine contractions.

Positive contraction stress test

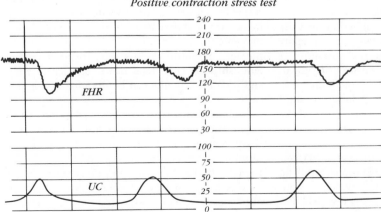

Table 5-1. Classical interpretation of the CST

Interpretation	Description
Negative	No late deceleration(s) present on tracing with uterine activity that is adequate
Positive	Late decelerations present with most (more than half) of the uterine contractions (unless hyperstimulation present), even if uterine activity is less than adequate
Suspicious	Adequate uterine activity with some late deceleration(s), but does not meet criteria for a positive test
Hyperstimulation	Late deceleration(s) present with or following excessive uterine activity
Unsatisfactory	Quality of tracing inadequate for accurate interpretation, or adequate uterine activity cannot be achieved

Source: Huddleston and Freeman [16].

Huddleston et al. found only one fetal death in over 1,000 patients evaluated by the contraction stress test [18]. Alteration in the fetal milieu (e.g., hypertensive crisis or deterioration of diabetic control) necessitates retesting more frequently than at the usual weekly intervals. Likewise, more frequent stress testing may be desirable in patients with complex medical or obstetric problems.

The contraction stress test carries a high false positive rate. As many as 50% of babies with a positive test show no further evidence of fetal distress or poor outcome if subjected to a trial of labor [19]. Some authors have proposed that fetal heart rate accelerations with fetal movement during a positive contraction stress test may help to identify many of the "healthy" infants with false positive tests [18,20]. With a positive contraction stress test, other parameters of fetal well-being and maturity should be assessed. The fetal and maternal risks of delivery must be weighed against the reliability of fetal well-being assessments. In many instances, the gravity of the maternal condition or the absence of other signs of fetal well-being will dictate delivery. Determination of fetal lung maturity, by amniocentesis and amniotic fluid phospholipid analysis, may be of value, particularly when the various tests of fetal well-being are contradictory.

Because of the high rate of equivocal tests demonstrating occasional late decelerations, Schifrin, in 1977, proposed the "ten-minute window" concept to define the contraction stress test [21]. If a ten-minute window is identified containing three firm uterine contractions, each with late decelerations, the test is termed positive. Further fetal assessment is recommended. If a ten-minute window is identified with no late decelerations after any of the three contractions, the test is termed negative, demonstrating fetal well-being. A negative test is routinely repeated within seven days. If no positive or negative ten-minute window can be identified, the test is called equivocal and must be repeated within 24 hours. The rate of equivocal tests is markedly reduced if these window definitions are used. However, the rate of false negative evaluations appears to increase, since the stillbirth rate rises to 7 per 1,000 [22].

Nonstress Test
Initial observations regarding baseline fetal heart rate parameters and fetal well-being were made in Europe in the 1960s. The earliest publication in the United States correlating fetal heart rate accelerations (reactivity) with fetal well-being was by Lee et al. in 1975 [23]. Shortly thereafter, Trierweiler et al. and Rochard and colleagues independently confirmed this association, and the nonstress test (NST) quickly assumed a significant role in screening high-risk pregnancies [24,25]. It is currently the primary surveillance tool for evaluating high-risk pregnancies.

The indications for nonstress testing are identical to those listed above for the CST. The evaluation is intended to indirectly assess uteroplacental function and will not predict intrauterine catastrophes such as abruptio placentae or cord accident. A significant advantage to nonstress testing is the absence of contraindications. Because no oxytocin is utilized, it is without risk, regardless of the clinical situation or the obstetric complication being evaluated.

To perform the nonstress test, the patient is placed in semi-Fowler's position and vital signs are recorded initially and at periodic intervals. An external fetal heart rate transducer and tocodynamometer are attached, and the patient records fetal movements by depressing the marker button of the fetal monitor. In this way, the temporal relationship between fetal heart rate accelerations and fetal movements can be documented graphically.

Various protocols have been proposed to describe the reactive nonstress test. There is some disagreement about the number, amplitude, and duration of fetal heart rate accelerations as well as the time period in which they must occur. Nevertheless, no statistical difference exists between the published protocols and their ability to document

Table 5-2. Predictive reliability of the reactive nonstress test

Author	Year	Total NSTs	Total patients	Definition of reactive			Corrected PNM*/reactive tests	Predictive reliability
				Acceleration	Time period	Amplitude		
Nochimson et al. [26]	1978	812	421	4	20 min	15 bpm × 15 sec	0/407	100.0%
Evertson et al. [27]	1979	2,422	1,169	5	20 min	15 bpm × ? sec	5/493	99.0%
Lee and Drukker [28]	1979	722	471	2	?	10 bpm × ? sec	0/462	100.0%
Schifrin et al. [3]	1979	4,517	2,003	2	10 min	15 bpm × 15 sec	2/1,876	99.9%
Pratt et al. [29]	1979	1,000	362	2	30 min	15 bpm × 30 sec	1/271	99.6%
Mendenhall et al. [30]	1980	1,005	367	1	30 min	10 bpm × ? sec	0/302	100.0%
Keegan and Paul [31]	1980	1,877	895	2	20 min	15 bpm × 15 sec	3/572	99.5%
DeVoe [32]	1980	961	441	3	30 min	15 bpm × 15 sec	1/349	99.7%
Weingold et al. [33]	1980	1,281	509	5	20 min	15 bpm × 15 sec	3/444	99.3%
Ingardia et al. [34]	1980	2,592	862	5	20 min	15 bpm × 15 sec	3/733	99.6%
Phelan [35]	1981	3,000	1,452	4	20 min	15 bpm × ? sec	4/1,001	99.6%
Keane et al. [36]	1981	1,328	566	2	20 min	15 bpm × ? sec	2/459	99.6%
Barrett et al. [37]	1981	2,510	1,000	2	10 min	15 bpm × 15 sec	4/661	99.4%
Brown and Patrick [38]	1981	1,101	333	5	20 min	15 bpm × 15 sec	0/326	100.0%

*Corrected PNM = perinatal mortality with abruptio placentae and congenital anomalies incompatible with life excluded, if reported.

fetal well-being (Table 5-2). Our current protocol requires that a reactive tracing have at least two accelerations of fetal heart rate within a ten-minute period, each associated with fetal movement. The accelerations must last 15 seconds and reach a maximum level of at least 15 beats per minute above the baseline fetal heart rate. After a reactive test, the NST may be repeated weekly unless the maternal condition worsens or the fetus is at extreme risk.

If the criteria for reactivity are not met during a 40-minute observation period, despite external uterine manipulation of the fetus, the test is termed *nonreactive* and the fetus is evaluated, the same day, by contraction stress testing.

The corrected perinatal mortality within seven days of a reactive nonstress test is approximately 5 per 1,000. Table 5-2 reviews 14 publications between 1978 and 1981 that analyzed the clinical outcomes after 25,000 NSTs in more than 10,000 patients. The corrected perinatal mortality within seven days of a reactive NST in this combined series is 3 per 1,000.

Freeman et al. have recently reported a prospective, nonrandomized multi-institutional study of primary surveillance with the contraction stress test in 4,626 high-risk patients compared to assessment with the nonstress test in 1,542 patients. The corrected perinatal mortality within 7 days of a reactive NST was 7 per 1,000. This compared to a corrected perinatal mortality within seven days of a negative CST of 3.5 per 1,000 [39].

Between 5 and 20% of nonstress tests are interpreted as nonreactive. When nonreactive NSTs are followed by a contraction stress test, the majority of CSTs will be negative, indicating fetal well-being despite the nonstress test result. However, most authors still believe that the fetus with a nonreactive nonstress test is at a higher risk despite negative contraction stress testing [31,34,40]. Physicians should consider this fact when devising a management plan in any high-risk pregnancy being evaluated by nonstress testing.

The meaning of *variable* decelerations during nonstress testing has yet to be clearly defined. Variable decelerations of the fetal heart rate are those that have a sharp descending and ascending slope while varying in shape from one another [13]. The pathogenesis is believed to be umbilical cord compression. In 1979 Lee and Drukker divided variable decelerations into three categories [28]. *Mild* variable decelerations were of short duration and small amplitude and had abrupt onset and return to the baseline. These were present in 15% of reactive nonstress tests and were associated with no increase in fetal or neonatal risk. More prolonged decelerations, *stressed* variables, were associated with a normal outcome if more frequent nonstress testing was utilized to detect deterioration in fetal condition. In a small number of cases, a *distressed* variable pattern with smoothly curved deceleration and recovery angles was seen. This was associated with intrauterine fetal compromise necessitating immediate intervention.

In 1980 Keegan and Paul reported marked variable decelerations with fundal or suprapubic pressure in 3 of 657 reactive nonstress tests that they reviewed [31]. In two cases these decelerations were noted in patients who were postterm (>42 weeks' gestation) with clinical oligohydramnios. Subsequent induction of labor produced severe repetitive variable decelerations necessitating cesarean delivery for fetal distress. A third case unassociated with either postdatism or oligohydramnios delivered vaginally without problems.

In reviewing 469 NSTs, O'Leary et al. reported 34 patients with reactive NSTs and more than three variable decelerations of more than ten beats per minute, each lasting at least ten seconds [41]. In 94% of these patients, spontaneous labor within seven days of the test was accompanied by significant fetal heart rate variable decelerations or cord complications during labor and delivery. Twenty-four percent required cesarean delivery. No intrauterine demise occurred within seven days of the reactive nonstress test despite the presence of significant variable decelerations.

Phelan and Lewis reviewed 2,000 nonstress tests and found that 110 tests in 94 pregnancies

exhibited variable decelerations in response to fetal activity [42]. During labor, 60% had variable decelerations, 55% demonstrated abnormal cord position, and 8% required cesarean delivery for fetal distress. Of the 94 pregnancies, three patients had an intrauterine fetal demise secondary to cord accidents. The authors suggested ultrasound evaluation of cord position and amniotic fluid volume as well as contraction stress testing (regardless of the NST results) in all cases of variable decelerations in response to fetal movement or uterine contractions.

In postterm pregnancies, Miyazaki and Miyazaki reported two cases in which reactive NSTs with variable decelerations were followed by abnormal contraction stress tests [43]. Both patients were delivered by cesarean delivery for fetal distress during induction of labor.

Six percent of more than 1,000 reactive NSTs reviewed by Brown and Patrick in 1981 exhibited one to three variable decelerations of at least 15 beats per minute for at least 15 seconds [38]. The authors found no perinatal morbidity or mortality in this group.

It is evident that more data are needed regarding the prognosis for patients with variable decelerations during nonstress testing. Despite the inconsistencies in the information reported, the data suggest that patients with variable decelerations during antepartum fetal heart rate testing are at increased risk for fetal morbidity and mortality. The presence of significant variable decelerations with fetal movement, particularly when frequent, prolonged, severe, *stressed* or *distressed,* requires a contraction stress test, a realtime ultrasound evaluation to detect oligohydramnios or abnormal cord position, and more frequent nonstress testing.

In summary, the nonstress test is a convenient, inexpensive, and accurate evaluator of fetal well-being that can be used in all pregnancies. The risk of an intrauterine fetal demise, within seven days of a reactive nonstress test, is extremely low—approximately 5 per 1,000. The literature is unclear as to which definition of a reactive nonstress test is the most reliable. Although the majority of nonreactive nonstress tests will be followed by a negative contraction stress test, these patients are probably at higher risk for fetal morbidity and mortality than those with a reactive nonstress test. Weekly nonstress tests may *not* be frequent enough to adequately evaluate the rapidly changing fetal-maternal unit in the highest-risk pregnancies complicated by disorders such as diabetes, postdatism, or intrauterine growth retardation.

BIOCHEMICAL TESTS
Estriol

In the normal female, estriol is the least active of all the estrogens, representing the major peripheral metabolite of the more potent estradiol and estrone produced in the ovary.

During pregnancy, the major C-21 estrogen precursor, 5-pregnenolone, is converted by the fetal adrenal gland into dehydroepiandrosterone sulfate, a C-19 androgenic steroid. Once estriol is released into the maternal circulation, more than 90% is conjugated in the maternal liver at the 16-carbon position. Bile excretion of more than half of these conjugates into the gastrointestinal tract is followed by hydrolysis by gut flora and absorption into the maternal blood as free estriol. Conjugated estriol is ultimately excreted via the maternal kidney [44] (Fig. 5-3).

As pregnancy progresses, increasing quantities of estriol and its conjugates are produced and can be found in the maternal serum and urine. Excretion and production of estriol are increased by a factor of 1,000 during pregnancy. Because of both the placental and the fetal contributions to its formation, increasing estriol production, during pregnancy, has been used as a reflection of fetal-placental well-being in high-risk pregnancies.

Spielman and associates first described the fall in blood estrogens associated with intrauterine demise in 1933 [46]. Smith and Smith in 1941 were the first investigators to propose falling blood and urinary estrogen levels as a predictor of placental insufficiency [47]. These early observations required expensive and complicated biologic assays to measure estrogen activity. Clinical application was severely limited. With the advent of biochemical determination of estrogen in the mid-1950s, the clinical usefulness of estriol determination in monitoring placental function was confirmed [48].

Greene and Touchstone published a report of the first large series of high-risk pregnancies monitored by maternal urinary estriol excretion [49]. They established a normal range for estriol excretion and demonstrated a strong correlation between normal daily urinary estriol excretion and fetal well-being. Plasma estriol determination and rapid radioimmunoassay techniques contributed to the clinical usefulness and to the popularity of estriol determinations during the 1970s [50,51]. With the introduction of nonstress testing in the late 1970s, maternal estriol determinations have been less commonly employed as a primary tool for assessment of fetal well-being in high-risk pregnancies.

Twenty-four-hour total urinary estriol assays have proved to be an inconvenient and expensive tool fraught with many sources of error and delay in obtaining clinically useful results. Measurement of plasma estriol is complicated by a wide diurnal variation [52,53]. Investigators have attempted to refine the usefulness of plasma estriol by measuring only the unconjugated fraction. Wide temporal variation still exists, and plasma estriol determinations must be performed frequently [52,53]. A significant fall in estriol does not herald fetal jeopardy in most cases [54,55]. Because of this high false positive rate, other tests of fetal well-being must be performed as soon as a significant fall in estriol is discovered. Antepartum fetal heart rate testing should help to identify patients whose fetuses are not in immediate danger [54,55]. However, in the presence of documented fetal lung maturity, particularly in the diabetic patient, delivery of the infant must be considered [55].

Estriol determinations still have clinical relevance in the management of the pregnant diabetic. Whittle et al. found unconjugated daily plasma es-

Fig. 5-3. The androgen compounds utilized for estrogen synthesis in human pregnancy are derived from the maternal bloodstream, in the early months of gestation. By the twentieth week of pregnancy, the vast majority of estrogen excreted in the maternal urine is derived from fetal androgens. (From Speroff et al. [45].)

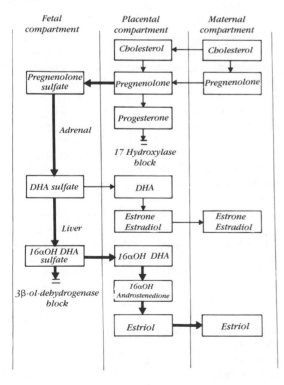

triol determinations to be a useful screening tool in diabetic pregnancies [54]. In the absence of a 40% fall, diabetic pregnancies were allowed to continue to maturity with no increase in perinatal mortality. Jorge and associates used a combination of biophysical and biochemical surveillance techniques [55]. They found that falling plasma unconjugated estriol is an accurate early indicator of fetal compromise when used in conjunction with nonstress and contraction stress testing. They encouraged its continued use in diabetic pregnancies.

Estriol screening requires a dedicated biochemical laboratory, accurate and frequent determination of plasma or urinary estriol, and timely results. These requirements are difficult to achieve. Likewise, antepartum fetal heart rate testing should be available to ensure that a normal pregnancy is not interrupted by a spurious estriol value.

Human Placental Lactogen

Human placental lactogen (HPL) is a polypeptide secreted by the placental syncytiotrophoblast that is similar in structure to growth hormone. Intimately involved in maternal carbohydrate metabolism during pregnancy, little hormone crosses the placenta to the fetal circulation. Its major role appears to be the amelioration of maternal starvation effects by its mobilization of stored lipids to free fatty acids.

Fukushima isolated HPL in 1961 [56]. Since that time, its value as a test for fetal well-being has been debated. Most studies have shown a low sensitivity and specificity [57]. Spellacy et al., in a prospective study, demonstrated a significant reduction in perinatal mortality when serum HPL was used as a routine screen in high-risk pregnancies [58]. With the availability and extensive experience accumulated with other tests of fetal well-being, HPL has assumed a limited role, if any, in assessing the integrity of placental function in high-risk pregnancies.

ULTRASOUND EVALUATION
Serial B-Scan

The application of high-frequency sound waves (B-scan ultrasound) to the field of obstetrics by Donald et al. in 1958 was a major advance in the safe and accurate antenatal assessment of fetal well-being [59]. Although some investigators have advocated the routine antenatal use of ultrasound in all pregnancies, the majority of opinion is that "ultrasound should be used judiciously and only when indicated" [60,61]. Ultrasound is particularly valuable for following pregnancies complicated by systemic disease.

The optimal management of pregnancy requires an accurate assessment of gestational age. In gestations complicated by maternal medical illness, the correct gestational age is essential for determination of the optimal time for intervention, if required.

Intrauterine gestation can be documented by ultrasound as early as five to six weeks from the last menstrual period. By six weeks, the standard gestational sac diameter measures 2 cm, subsequently increasing approximately 7 mm each week. By ten weeks, the sac has reached a diameter of nearly 5 cm. The accuracy of this mode of gestational age determination is approximately ± seven days [62].

Eight weeks from the last menstrual period, the active fetus can be consistently demonstrated within the amniotic sac and the crown–rump length can be determined. Robinson has studied this mode of gestational dating and reports an accuracy of ± three to four days, using crown–rump length calculations [63,64]. Standard crown–rump length at eight weeks is 1.5 cm. The growth thereafter equals approximately 1 cm weekly. Most clinicians have found the use of realtime dynamic image ultrasound scanning optimal for determination of crown–rump length.

Fetal biparietal diameter measurement is the accepted method of gestational age determination in the second trimester of pregnancy. The fetal skull can be identified, beginning at 12 weeks' gestation. A variety of tables relating gestational age to biparietal diameter are available and reflect variations in study populations, ultrasonic equipment, and methodology of measurement. Because of the decreasing rate of growth of the fetal skull, the accuracy of biparietal dating decreases with advancing gestational age. In general, the earlier in gestation a biparietal diameter is measured, the more accurate the gestational age determination. Evaluations made by 16 weeks' gestation are accurate to within seven days. In contrast, scans after 28 weeks' gestation are acccurate only to within 21 days.

O'Brien and Queenan have recently assessed gestational age, during the second trimester, using femur length estimates determined by realtime ultrasonography [65]. The accuracy of the assessment was shown to be ± seven days. Femur length at this time should be used to confirm dates obtained with biparietal diameter measurements. When the position of the fetal vertex does not allow accurate dating, femur length is an excellent alternative.

With recent improvements in dynamic image ultrasonographic transducers, antenatal diagnosis of many congenital anomalies can be confirmed (see Chap. 3) [66–68]. In pregnancies at high risk for fetal malformations secondary to systemic disease (e.g., diabetes mellitus), or because of the treatment of such disease during organogenesis, serial screening during the first and second trimesters should be considered.

Some major abnormalities may be diagnosed in the first trimester. Absence of fetal heart motion or disorganized or absent fetal parts, by nine weeks' gestation, indicates fetal demise. Accurate assessment of gestational age is essential in these cases. If any doubt exists, a follow-up scan in 10 to 14 days will confirm the diagnosis. During the second trimester, precise imaging of the central nervous system may allow detection of anomalous development. The application of intrauterine neurosurgical techniques may allow corrective attempts in selected cases of central nervous system abnormality, particularly later in pregnancy when termination may not be an alternative [69].

Genitourinary anomalies may be diagnosed antenatally with ultrasound scanning. Abnormalities incompatible with life (e.g., renal agenesis) are amenable to ultrasonic diagnosis and early termination. Bladder dilatation secondary to urethral stenosis is potentially correctable in utero, allowing for normal anterior somite growth and development.

Cardiac, gastrointestinal, soft tissue, and skeletal abnormalities are also being recognized with increasing frequency prior to delivery. The knowledge that a fetus has an abnormality allows the physician to prepare the family emotionally and to optimize the mode of delivery and available neonatal care. In situations incompatible with fetal survival, the safest method of delivery for the mother may be chosen.

Fetal Breathing

It was not until 1970 that investigators demonstrated the existence of intrauterine fetal breathing in mammalian species [70]. Using A-scan ultrasound evaluation, Boddy and Robinson clearly demonstrated human fetal breathing in utero soon thereafter [71]. With the introduction of dynamic image realtime ultrasound, the evaluation of fetal breathing, through the direct observation of fetal chest wall movement, has become accurate and markedly simplified [72,73].

Periodic episodes of fetal breathing movements are present in the normal fetus during the third trimester. Continuous, regular respiratory movements at a rate of 30 to 90 breaths per minute, lasting up to 10 minutes, can be observed. Total apnea for 30 minutes has been associated with increased

fetal morbidity and mortality but has also been noted in the normal fetus [72,73]. The presence of slow, high-amplitude "gasping" fetal breathing appears to have a high correlation with impending fetal distress [74]. Hypoxemia, hypoglycemia, infection, smoking, maternal exercise, and normal labor may result in decreased fetal breathing movements [72–75]. In 1978 Platt et al. evaluated 125 high-risk pregnancies, recording the percentage of time that fetal breathing movement was observed during a 30-minute period [73]. Although fetal breathing movements were noted between 0 and 90% of the 30-minute period, infants in whom fetal breathing was present demonstrated a significantly higher one- and five-minute Apgar scores than infants in whom no fetal breathing movement had been observed. Fetuses with absent breathing were more likely to have cesarean deliveries for fetal distress. Also, these infants more frequently had significant growth retardation as compared to infants with fetal breathing.

Manning et al. utilized fetal breathing movement as one of five variables evaluated in constructing a "biophysical profile" of fetal well-being [76,77]. Although fetal breathing was present in the vast majority of high-risk patients evaluated, this parameter was more frequently falsely abnormal than any of the other four variables evaluated.

Observation of fetal breathing movement can be a worthwhile *adjunct* in the documentation of fetal well-being in high-risk pregnancies. The evaluation protocol most useful in clinical practice has yet to be established. The *presence* of normal fetal breathing movement does correlate closely with good perinatal outcome.

FETAL LUNG MATURITY

Determination of fetal lung maturity prior to delivery has proved to be invaluable in managing pregnancies with medical or obstetric complications. Evaluation of amniotic fluid creatinine, bilirubin, and osmolality, as well as examination of desquamated fetal cells from amniotic fluid stained with Nile blue sulfate, provided some assistance during the 1960s and early 1970s [78]. The description of the amniotic fluid lecithin/sphingomyelin ratio in the mature fetus by Gluck and associates in 1971 enabled clinicians to confidently deliver infants when the L/S ratio reached 2 or greater [79,80]. Most recently, the presence of a specific acidic phospholipid, phosphatidylglycerol, in amniotic fluid, has virtually guaranteed fetal lung maturity, even in pregnancies complicated by diabetes mellitus and erythroblastosis fetalis [81,82]. The determination of the specific phospholipid content of

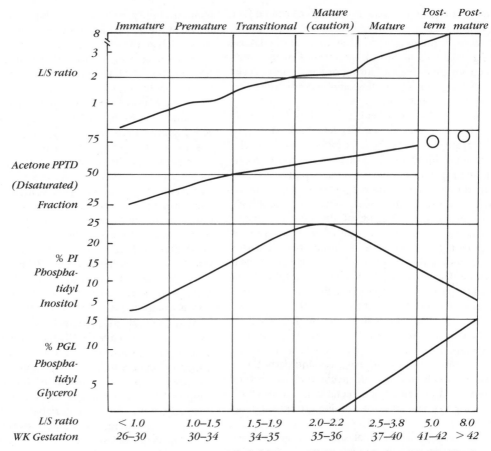

Fig. 5-4. Form used to report the lung profile. The four determinations are plotted on the ordinate and the weeks of gestation on the abscissa (as well as the L/S ratio as an "internal standard"). When these are plotted, they fall into a given grid that identifies the stage of development of the lung as shown in the upper part of the form. The designation "mature (caution)" refers to the patients, other than those with diabetes, who can be delivered with safety when the values fall in the "mature" grid, as decribed elsewhere. (From Kulovich et al. [82].)

amniotic fluid, the "lung profile," has become the optimal method of documenting fetal lung maturity (Fig. 5-4). With realtime ultrasonic guidance and careful selection of cases, the risks of amniocentesis at term can be minimized, though not entirely eliminated [83]. Rupture of membranes, premature labor, fetal injury, and, rarely, fetal death must all be weighed against the benefits of fetal lung maturity determination.

In 1979 Grannum et al. described a system for evaluating placental characteristics determined by ultrasonography that correlated closely with fetal lung maturation [84]. In a small series, they reported that 100% of patients with grade III placental changes had fetal pulmonary maturity as determined by the L/S ratio (Fig. 5-5 and Table 5-3). This study requires further confirmation as anecdotal cases of grade III placental changes associated with neonatal respiratory distress syndrome have been reported [85]. Ultrasonic inspection of the placenta may prove valuable, particularly in instances where safe amniocentesis is not feasible.

Tests for evaluation of the fetal condition can offer the clinician significant information about the intrauterine environment. With major advances in treating the intrauterine fetus or critically ill neonate, it is now possible to weigh the risks of extrauterine life against those of a hostile intrauterine environment. The exact combination of antenatal tests that will best predict fetal outcome has not been determined. Intelligent utilization of one or more of the tests described above will minimize the risks to both mother and fetus. Still, none of these tests alone will replace the judgment of a skilled and experienced clinician, using all the available tools.

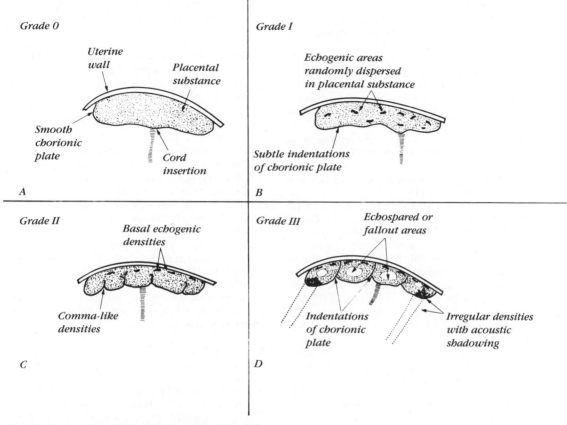

Fig. 5-5. Evaluation of placental characteristics. (A)
The ultrasonic appearance of a grade 0 placenta. (B)
Grade I placenta. (C) Grade II placenta. (D) Grade III
placenta. (From Grannum et al. [84].)

Table 5-3. Summary of placental grading

Section of placenta	Grade 0	Grade I	Grade II	Grade III
Chorionic plate	Straight and well defined	Subtle undulations	Indentations extending into placenta but not to basal layer	Indentations communicating with basal layer
Placental substance	Homogeneous	Few scattered EGAs*	Linear echogenic densities (comma-like densities)	Circular densities with echo-spared areas in center; large, irregular densities that cast acoustic shadows
Basal layer	No densities	No densities	Linear arrangement of small EGAs (basal stippling)	Large and somewhat confluent basal EGAs; can create acoustic shadows

*Echogenic areas
Source: Adapted from Grannum et al. [84].

REFERENCES

1. Goodlin RC. History of fetal monitoring. Am J Obstet Gynecol. 1979; 133:323–52.
2. Ray M, Freeman R, Pine S, Hesselgesser R. Clinical experience with the oxytocin challenge test. Am J Obstet Gynecol. 1972; 114:1–9.
3. Schifrin BS, Foye G, Amato J, Kates R, MacKenna J. Routine fetal heart rate monitoring in the antepartum period. Obstet Gynecol. 1979; 54:21–5.
4. Sadovsky E, Yaffe H. Daily fetal movement recording and fetal prognosis. Obstet Gynecol. 1973; 41:845–50.
5. Sadovsky E, Polishuk WZ. Fetal movements in utero: nature, assessment, prognostic value, timing of delivery. Obstet Gynecol. 1977; 50:49–55.
6. Sadovsky E. Fetal movements and fetal health. Semin Perinatol. 1981; 5:131–43.
7. Sadovsky E, Evron S, Weinstein D. Daily fetal movement recording in normal pregnancy. Riv Obstet Ginecol Pract Med Perinatol. 1979; 59:395–403.
8. Hoppenbrouwers T, Ugartechea JC, Combs D, Hodgman JE, Harper RM, Sterman MB. Studies of maternal-fetal interaction during the last trimester of pregnancy: ontogenesis of the basic rest-activity cycle. Exp Neurol. 1978; 61:136–53.
9. Granat M, Lavie P, Adar D, Sharf M. Short-term cycles in human fetal activity. Am J Obstet Gynécol. 1979; 134:696–701.
10. Leader LR, Baillie P, Van Schalkwyk DJ. Fetal movements and fetal outcome: a prospective study. Obstet Gynecol. 1981; 57:431–6.
11. Harper RG, Greenberg M, Farahani G, Glassman I, Kierney CM. Fetal movement, biochemical and biophysical parameters, and the outcome of pregnancy. Am J Obstet Gynecol. 1981; 141:39–42.
12. Hon EH. The electronic evaluation of the fetal heart rate; preliminary report. Am J Obstet Gynecol. 1958; 75:1215–30.
13. Hon EH, Quilligan EJ. The classification of fetal heart rate. II. A revised working classification. Conn Med. 1967; 31:779–84.
14. Caldeyro-Barcia R, Mendez-Bauer C, Poseiro JJ, et al. Control of human fetal heart rate during labor. In: Cassels DE, ed. The heart and circulation in the newborn and infant. New York: Grune & Stratton, 1966.
15. Resnik R. Symposium. NST or CST? What's best for spotting the high-risk fetus? Contemp Ob Gyn. 1982; 19:92–127.
16. Huddleston JF, Freeman RK. Assessment of fetal well-being by antepartum fetal heart rate testing. In: Bolognese RJ, Schwarz RH, Schneider J, eds. Perinatal medicine: Management of the high-risk fetus and neonate. 2nd ed. Baltimore: Williams & Wilkins, 1982.
17. Jarrell SE, Sokol RJ. Clinical use of stressed and nonstressed monitoring techniques. Clin Obstet Gynecol. 1979; 22:617–32.
18. Huddleston JF, Sutliff G, Carney FE, Flowers CE. Oxytocin challenge test for antepartum fetal assessment. Am J Obstet Gynecol. 1979; 135:609–14.
19. Paul RH, Miller FC. Antepartum fetal heart rate monitoring. Clin Obstet Gynecol. 1978; 21:375–84.
20. Braly P, Freeman RK. The significance of fetal heart rate reactivity with a positive oxytocin challenge test. Obstet Gynecol. 1977; 50:689–93.
21. Schifrin BS. Antepartum fetal heart rate monitoring. In: Gluck L, ed. Intrauterine asphyxia and the developing fetal brain. Chicago: Year Book, 1977:205–24.
22. Evertson LR, Paul RH. Antepartum fetal heart rate testing: the nonstress test. Am J Obstet Gynecol. 1978; 132:895–900.
23. Lee CY, Di Loreto PC, O'Lane JM. A study of fetal heart rate acceleration patterns. Obstet Gynecol. 1975; 45:142–6.
24. Trierweiler MW, Freeman RK, James J. Baseline fetal heart rate characteristics as an indicator of fetal status during the antepartum period. Am J Obstet Gynecol. 1976; 125:618–23.
25. Rochard F, Schifrin BS, Goupil F, LeGrand H, Blottiere J, Sureau C. Nonstressed fetal heart rate monitoring in the antepartum period. Am J Obstet Gynecol. 1976; 126:699–706.
26. Nochimson DJ, Turbeville JS, Terry JE, Petrie RH, Lundy LE. The nonstress test. Obstet Gynecol. 1978; 51:419–21.
27. Evertson LR, Gauthier RJ, Schifrin BS, Paul RH. Antepartum fetal heart rate testing. I. Evolution of the nonstress test. Am J Obstet Gynecol. 1979; 133:29–33.
28. Lee CY, Drukker B. The nonstress test for the antepartum assessment of fetal reserve. Am J Obstet Gynecol. 1979; 134:460–70.
29. Pratt D, Diamond F, Yen H, Bieniarz J, Burd L. Fetal stress and nonstress tests: an analysis and comparison of their ability to identify fetal outcome. Obstet Gynecol. 1979; 54:419–23.
30. Mendenhall HW, O'Leary JA, Phillips KO. The nonstress test: the value of a single acceleration in evaluating the fetus at risk. Am J Obstet Gynecol. 1980; 136:87–91.
31. Keegan KA Jr, Paul RH. Antepartum fetal heart rate testing. IV. The nonstress test as a primary approach. Am J Obstet Gynecol. 1980; 136:75–80.
32. Devoe LD. Clinical implications of prospective antepartum fetal heart rate testing. Am J Obstet Gynecol. 1980; 137:983–90.
33. Weingold AB, Yonekura ML, O'Kieffe J. Nonstress testing. Am J Obstet Gynecol. 1980; 138:195–202.
34. Ingardia CJ, Cetrulo CL, Knuppel RA, et al. Prognostic components of the nonreactive nonstress test. Obstet Gynecol. 1980; 56:305–10.
35. Phelan JP. The nonstress test: a review of 3,000 tests. Am J Obstet Gynecol. 1981; 139:7–10.
36. Keane MW, Horger EO III, Vice L. Comparative study of stressed and nonstressed antepartum fetal heart rate testing. Obstet Gynecol. 1981; 57:320–4.
37. Barrett JM, Salyer SL, Boehm FH. The nonstress test: an evaluation of 1,000 patients. Am J Obstet Gynecol. 1981; 141:153–7.
38. Brown R, Patrick J. The nonstress test: how long is enough? Am J Obstet Gynecol. 1981; 141:646–51.

39. Freeman RK, Anderson G, Dorchester W. A prospective multi-institutional study of antepartum fetal heart rate monitoring. II. Contraction stress test versus nonstress test for primary surveillance. Am J Obstet Gynecol. 1982; 143:778–81.

40. Druzin ML, Gratacos J, Paul RH. Antepartum fetal heart rate testing. VI. Predictive reliability of "normal" tests in the prevention of antepartum death. Am J Obstet Gynecol. 1980; 137:746–7.

41. O'Leary JA, Andrinopoulos GC, Giordano PC. Variable decelerations and the nonstress test: an indication of cord compromise. Am J Obstet Gynecol. 1980; 137:704–6.

42. Phelan JP, Lewis PE Jr. Fetal heart rate decelerations during a nonstress test. Obstet Gynecol. 1981; 57:228–32.

43. Miyazaki FS, Miyazaki BA. False reactive nonstress tests in post term pregnancies. Am J Obstet Gynecol. 1981; 140:269–76.

44. Gabbe SG, Hagerman DD. Clinical application of estriol analysis. Clin Obstet Gynecol. 1978; 21:353–62.

45. Speroff L, Glass RH, Kase NG. Clinical gynecologic endocrinology and infertility. 3rd ed. Baltimore: Williams & Wilkins, 1983:276.

46. Spielman F, Goldberger MA, Frank, RT. Hormone diagnosis of viability of pregnancy. JAMA. 1933; 101:266–8.

47. Smith GV, Smith OW. Estrogen and progestin metabolism in pregnancy. Clin Endocrinol. 1941; 1:470–6.

48. Brown JB. A chemical method for determination of oestriol, oestrone and oestradiol in human urine. Biochem J. 1955; 60:185–93.

49. Greene JW, Touchstone JC. Urinary estriol as an index of placental function. Am J Obstet Gynecol. 1963; 85:1–9.

50. Nachtigall L, Bassett M, Hogsander U, Levitz M. Plasma estriol levels in normal and abnormal pregnancies: an index of fetal welfare. Am J Obstet Gynecol. 1968; 101:638–48.

51. Taylor ES, Hagerman DD, Betz G, Williams KL, Grey PA. Estriol concentrations in blood during pregnancy. Am J Obstet Gynecol. 1970; 108:868–75.

52. Katagiri H, Distler W, Freeman RK, Goebelsmann, U. Estriol in pregnancy. IV. Normal concentrations, diurnal and/or episodic variations, and day-to-day changes of unconjugated and total estriol in late pregnancy plasma. Am J Obstet Gynecol. 1976; 124:272–80.

53. Distler W, Gabbe SG, Freeman RK, Mestman JH, Goebelsmann, U. Estriol in pregnancy. V. Unconjugated and total plasma estriol in the management of pregnant diabetic patients. Am J Obstet Gynecol. 1978; 130:424–31.

54. Whittle MJ, Anderson D, Lowensohn RI, Mestman JH, Paul RH, Goebelsmann U. Estriol in pregnancy. VI. Experience with unconjugated plasma estriol assays and antepartum fetal heart rate testing in diabetic pregnancies. Am J Obstet Gynecol. 1979; 135:764–72.

55. Jorge CS, Artal R, Paul RH, et al. Antepartum fetal surveillance in diabetic pregnant patients. Am J Obstet Gynecol. 1981; 141:641–5.

56. Fukushima M. Studies on somatotropic hormone secretion in gynecology and obstetrics. Tohoku J Exp Med. 1961; 74:161–74.

57. Hobbins JC, Berkowitz RL. Current status of human placental lactogen. Clin Obstet Gynecol. 1978; 21:363–73.

58. Spellacy WN, Buhi WC, Birk SA. The effectiveness of human placental lactogen measurements as an adjunct in decreasing perinatal deaths. Am J Obstet Gynecol. 1975; 121:835–44.

59. Donald I, MacVicar J, Brown TG. Investigation of abdominal masses by pulsed ultrasound. Lancet. 1958; 1:1188–95.

60. Committee on Technical Bulletins of The American College of Obstetricians and Gynecologists. Diagnostic ultrasound in obstetrics and gynecology. ACOG Tech Bull. 1981; 63:1–5.

61. Marsden DE, ed. Use of ultrasound. In: Collected letters of the International Correspondence Society of Obstetricians Gynecologists. 1982; 23:25–32.

62. Hellman LM, Kobayashi M, Fillisti L, Lavenhar M, Cromb E. Growth and development of the human fetus prior to the twentieth week of gestation. Am J Obstet Gynecol. 1969; 103:789–800.

63. Robinson HP. Sonar measurement of fetal crown–rump length as means of assessing maturity in first trimester pregnancy. Br Med J. 1973; 4:28–31.

64. Robinson HP, Fleming JEE. A critical evaluation of sonar "crown–rump length" measurements. Br J Obstet Gynaecol. 1975; 82:702–10.

65. O'Brien GD, Queenan JT. Growth of the ultrasound fetal femur length during normal pregnancy. Part I. Am J Obstet Gynecol. 1981; 141:833–7.

66. Hobbins JC, Grannum PA, Berkowitz RL, Silverman R, Mahoney MJ. Ultrasound in the diagnosis of congenital anomalies. Am J Obstet Gynecol. 1979; 134:331–45.

67. Deter RL, Hadlock FP, Carpenter RJ, Klima TF, Kim HS, Park SK. Use of dynamic image (real-time) ultrasonography in the detection of fetal anomalies. Perinatol Neonatol. 1982; 6:35–46.

68. Sabbagha RE, Tamura RK, Dal Campo S. Obstetric ultrasonography in perspective. Perinatol Neonatol. 1982; 6:53–62.

69. Clewell WH, Johnson ML, Meier PR, et al. A surgical approach to the treatment of fetal hydrocephalus. N Engl J Med. 1982; 306:1320–5.

70. Dawes GS, Fox HE, Leduc BM, et al. Respiratory movements and paradoxical sleep in the foetal lamb. J. Physiol (London). 1970; 210:47P–48P.

71. Boddy K, Robinson JS. External method for detection of fetal breathing in utero. Lancet. 1971; 2:1231–3.

72. Manning FA. Fetal breathing movements as a reflection of fetal status. Postgrad Med. 1977; 61:116–22.

73. Platt LD, Manning FA, Lemay M, Sipos L. Human fetal breathing: relationship to fetal condition. Am J Obstet Gynecol. 1978; 132:514–8.

74. Boddy K. Fetal breathing: its physiologic and clinical implications. Hosp Pract. 1979; 14:89–96.

75. Boylan P, Lewis PJ. Fetal breathing in labor. Obstet Gynecol. 1980; 56:35–8.

76. Manning FA, Platt LD, Sipos L. Antepartum fetal evaluation: development of a fetal biophysical profile. Am J Obstet Gynecol. 1980; 136:787–95.

77. Manning FA, Baskett TF, Morrison I, Lange I. Fetal biophysical profile scoring: a prospective study of 1,184 high-risk patients. Am J Obstet Gynecol. 1981; 140:289–94.

78. Perkins RP. Antenatal assessment of fetal maturity. Obstet Gynecol Surv. 1974; 29:369–84.

79. Gluck L, Kulovich MV, Borer RC, Brenner PH, Anderson GG, Spellacy WN. Diagnosis of the respiratory distress syndrome by amniocentesis. Am J Obstet Gynecol. 1971; 109:440–5.

80. Gluck L, Kulovich MV. Lecithin-sphingomyelin ratios in amniotic fluid in normal and abnormal pregnancy. Am J Obstet Gynecol. 1973; 115:539–46.

81. Hallman M, Kulovich M, Kirkpatrick E, Sugarman RG, Gluck L. Phosphatidylinositol and phosphatidylglycerol in amniotic fluid: indices of lung maturity. Am J Obstet Gynecol. 1976; 125:613–7.

82. Kulovich MV, Hallman MB, Gluck L. The lung profile. I. Normal pregnancy. Am J Obstet Gynecol. 1979; 135:57–63.

83. Platt LD, Manning FA, Lemay M. Real-time B-scan-directed amniocentesis. Am J Obstet Gynecol. 1978; 130:700–3.

84. Grannum PA, Berkowitz RL, Hobbins JC. The ultrasonic changes in the maturing placenta and their relation to fetal pulmonic maturity. Am J Obstet Gynecol. 1979; 133:915–22.

85. Quinlan RW, Cruz AC. Ultrasonic placental grading and fetal pulmonary maturity. Am J Obstet Gynecol. 1982; 142:110–1.

When you have a doctor, a patient, and a drug,
there is room for misunderstanding.
—Eugene Stead

6. PHARMACOLOGIC PRINCIPLES
David K. Manchester

Physicians caring for women of childbearing age confront a major dilemma: Treatment of serious medical disorders frequently requires the use of drugs potentially harmful to offspring. While it is a fact that most drugs do not harm developing offspring, clearly some do. Because drug effects on human reproduction may not be predictable from our current data base, some decisions involving drug treatment must be made on the basis of very little information. Several blanket responses seem unwise, however, including wholesale admonitions against having a family, discontinuation of needed medications, and unnecessary abortion. Equally unwise would be the unthinking use of medication without clear indication or the adoption of careless attitudes based on the fact that human reproduction usually produces healthy infants despite hostile environments. Some understanding of the reproductive effects of drugs must be sought. This chapter briefly highlights what is known and not known about drug therapy and human reproduction. Based on this review, some general guidelines for drug therapy are advanced. Questions regarding specific drugs and therapy of specific disorders will be discussed by other authors in separate chapters. Whenever possible, the reader will be referred to books and published reviews that will provide further understanding of basic principles.

It is important for physicians to understand that the public's apparent preoccupation with the potential adverse effects of drugs on reproductive function and outcome is not a fad. Although most children are born healthy and vigorous, reproduction is not as successful as we think, and fear of possible tragedy is based in common human experience. Congenital abnormalities, in fact, occur frequently. Miscarriages are even more common. While relatively few abnormal infants deliver compared to the numbers of conceptuses that are lost early in pregnancy, 10–11% of the population is affected in one way or another by congenital abnormalities [1].

Given the central role of reproduction in biology, it is not surprising to find emotional and physiologic functions upset by reproductive disorders and losses. Since ancient times, explanations for reproductive problems in congenital abnormalities have included environmental factors [2]. Thalidomide confirmed our worst fears, and the reaction to the increased understanding of the toxic effects of the chemical environment was predictable. People are frightened by the fact that reproduction occasionally ends in tragedy, and the inclusion of poorly understood synthetic chemicals, such as drugs, increases anxieties. Patients' questions regarding the effects of drugs on offspring should be taken very seriously. Reasons for use or avoidance of drugs need to be carefully considered and communicated.

DRUG ACTION IN DEVELOPING ORGANISMS
Receptor Interactions
The central proposition of pharmacology holds that drug effects are dose dependent. In the confusion stemming from concern over birth defects, this dose-response relationship has been frequently neglected. Because birth defects are threshold phenomena—that is, they are either present or absent—there has been a tendency to regard drugs as having either an adverse effect on developing offspring or no effect at all. Birth defects are the morphologic result of interactions between developmental, genetic, and environmental factors. Drugs interact through dose-dependent effects on cell function; they do not cause abnormalities directly. The dose dependency of drug contributions to congenital abnormalities has been repeatedly demonstrated in animal systems. The number of fetuses in a litter of mice affected with cleft palate, for example, is a predictable function of the dose of corticosteroid given at a critical period of development [3].

Reproducible dose-response curves imply the presence of drug receptors. Embryonic and fetal responses to drugs are mechanistically the same as those of adults. Drug receptor interactions and drug effects on cellular function are probably quite similar in developing and adult tissues. The differences are in the physiologic effects that pharmacologically altered cell function produces in developing, as opposed to adult, organisms. Because we lack understanding of physiology early in gestation, we are unable to predict drug effects during this period. Our knowledge of physiology improves, however, in later gestation, when the effects of drugs become more predictable. In all cases, concentration-dependent drug receptor interactions are the rule.

Drug receptors can now be studied in vitro by binding studies. This technique has supported an explosion of investigations confirming the presence of drug receptors in developing tissues. The studies describe a fascinating spectrum of patterns of development and interactions between receptor systems. Few, if any, "fetal" receptors, however, have been identified. When present, receptors in fetal tissues bind drugs with affinities that are predictable from adult data [4]. These findings underscore the continuity of pharmacologic response at the molecular level and again point to the need to understand embryonic and fetal physiology. In practical terms, this means that dose-dependent drug effects during development ought eventually to be predictable.

Metabolic Activation

Some adverse effects of drugs in adults are idiosyncratic. The same is probably true during development. Many idiosyncratic reactions in adults involve metabolism of drugs to more active, or toxic compounds. Hepatotoxicity of drugs, for example, frequently involves their metabolism [5] and may result from genetically determined imbalances in detoxification pathways [5–7]. While cytotoxicity produced by metabolites in adults may or may not produce illness, it is likely to be devastating during development. Cell death is one of the more common mechanisms of teratogenesis, and metabolism of drugs to toxic products can result in cell death [8]. Recent evidence indicates that metabolism of thalidomide to a toxic metabolite in certain species including humans causes cell death and could explain its ability to produce birth defects in some animals and not in others [10]. Although drug metabolism by human fetal tissues is generally immature relative to that in adults, it is important to point out that it develops to a significantly greater extent during human gestation than during the gestation of laboratory animals [9].

Human embryopathies have occasionally been associated with other drugs that are capable of being metabolized to active or toxic compounds. The number of drugs potentially toxic through metabolic activation is unknown, but agents felt to be likely candidates are compounds like phenytoin, which has been associated with birth defects [11] and with metabolism-dependent hepatotoxicity in adults [7]. Carcinogens are often toxic because of metabolic activation, and many are also teratogenic [12]. Our current understanding of chemical toxicity resulting from metabolic activation in humans is limited, but metabolic activation is certainly involved in chemical carcinogenesis and teratogenesis in animals [13,14].

Available Data

At this time, we do not have access to enough physiologic and pharmacologic data to predict many drug effects on offspring early in pregnancy. The practicing physician must therefore respect this ignorance and carefully consider indications for drug use. In order to assess risks, he or she often must consult tabulations of animal studies and human case reports. These sources of information can be helpful if put into proper perspective. First, it should be recognized that the value of animal studies lies mainly in their ability to delineate teratogenic mechanisms. Many are therefore designed using high doses—doses that will reproducibly cause birth defects. Mechanisms identified by such studies need, then, to be put into human contexts. For example, Longo has elegantly worked out the effects of carbon monoxide on oxygenation in fetal sheep [15]. This understanding of the effects of carbon monoxide in animals provides a sound basis for discussion of risks in humans, given known exposures. The data predict significant toxicity above 20 mg/dL carboxyhemoglobin contents but few serious effects at lower levels.

Human case reports are also important, but the information they provide is limited. Reports of congenital abnormalities associated with a drug exposure must be considered against a background of commonly occurring sporadic birth defects. Since drug exposures also occur commonly, apparent associations are likely. Although few such associations actually result from cause and effect relationships, these observations have nonetheless been of considerable value. They raise questions and present possibilities. They are valuable because they suggest mechanisms that can be investigated in animals. They also provide the impetus for prospective studies assessing risks in humans. While such tedious consideration of case reports is a very inefficient approach, it has, in fact, identified every known human drug-related embryopathy [16]. The piecing together of the story of human fetal toxicity associated with high-level ethanol exposures is a good example of this process [17].

The practitioner must be cautious in interpreting the literature. A case report, or a series of case reports, neither proves cause and effect nor establishes risks. It simply says that two things may be related. Risks are ratios; they require a denominator that can be supplied only by prospective studies or retrospective investigations of entire populations at risk. Such studies are exceedingly difficult, and the physician is often forced to deal with incomplete information. This frustrating situation stems largely from the fact that many aspects of human reproduction are unique, and human populations are heterogeneous. Case reports should be communicated to patients and to the public as limited observations.

Fetal Therapy

To this point, the discussion of drug effects on offspring has focused solely on adverse outcomes. It should be emphasized that increased understanding of fetal physiology and drug-receptor interactions may provide new opportunities to treat the fetus as a patient. Successful examples of fetal pharmacology to date include transplacental induction of surfactant synthesis by corticosteroids and other agents, and treatment of in utero heart failure with digoxin [18,19]. The same principles of drug action apply to both fetal therapy and toxicity.

Placental Transport of Drugs

In order to directly affect developing humans, drugs must traverse the placenta. An understanding of this organ's development and function is therefore important. Placentation and placentas are impressively diverse among mammalian species, a fact that must be remembered when interpreting animal studies [20]. Human placentation is relatively unique. The process of implantation begins approximately three days after conception and is completed by day 13. Human placentation precedes organogenesis. Trophoblastic tissue invades the endometrium and grows over maternal blood vessels. These vessels atrophy, and maternal blood begins to percolate through lacunae (hollow areas) surrounded by trophoblast. Villi form as projections into these spaces and later become vascularized from the fetal side. Maternal blood actually leaves the maternal circulation and flows through intervillous spaces entirely surrounded by "fetal" tissue. This type of placentation is called hemomonochorionic, which means that only a single cell layer, derived from the chorion, separates maternal from fetal circulations [21]. Figure 6-1 illustrates this relationship as it appears near term. Note the proximity of the fetal capillary to the intervillous space.

The single cell layer constituting the "placental barrier" in humans is called syncytiotrophoblast. From the standpoint of drug passage, two characteristics of this cell type need to be considered: (1) its permeability and (2) its capacity for metabolism. Syncytiotrophoblastic cells are not much different from other cells in the body. Their membranes exclude very large, polar charged, or highly water-soluble molecules. The properties of drugs that allow them to be absorbed and to distribute across maternal cell membranes will also allow them to traverse placental cells. Thus, there is no placental barrier for most drugs. Drugs passively diffuse across the placenta; they move down concentration gradients, and their rates of transfer are determined by their chemistry and that of the syncytiotrophoblast. The question, therefore, should be not whether a drug crosses the placenta but rather what concentration it achieves in the fetus and with what fetal receptors it interacts.

The placenta is a very active metabolic tissue. At term, syncytiotrophoblast produces gram quantities of peptide hormones, metabolizes and synthesizes steroids, allows pinocytosis of macromolecules, and actively transports selected compounds against concentration gradients. Although it also possesses many components of drug detoxification systems (e.g., cytochrome P-450, glucuronyl transferase, epoxide hydrolase, and glutathione S-transferase), the placenta is not a major organ of drug metabolism. Rather, the systems present seem geared to metabolism of other xenobiotics such as aromatic hydrocarbons [22]. Most drugs therefore gain essentially free access to the fetus.

Pharmacokinetics

Drug concentrations are determined by dose and the kinetic processes of absorption, distribution, and metabolism. It is convenient to consider various components of the body as pharmacokinetic compartments and to describe the disposition of drugs in terms of rates of change of concentrations in each compartment. The fetus (here meaning the fetus, placenta, and amniotic fluid) behaves as a "deep" compartment. A somewhat oversimplified, but nonetheless conceptually useful, construct for describing disposition of drugs during pregnancy is a two-compartment model (Fig. 6-2). In this model, drug is directly injected or absorbed into the central (maternal) compartment and then diffuses into and back out of the peripheral (fetal) compartment. Drug is finally eliminated from the central compartment. Kinetic constants for the rates of transfer into or out of each compartment can be described. These constants reflect the permeability of the membranes involved, as well as rates of metabolism and absorption. Knowing or

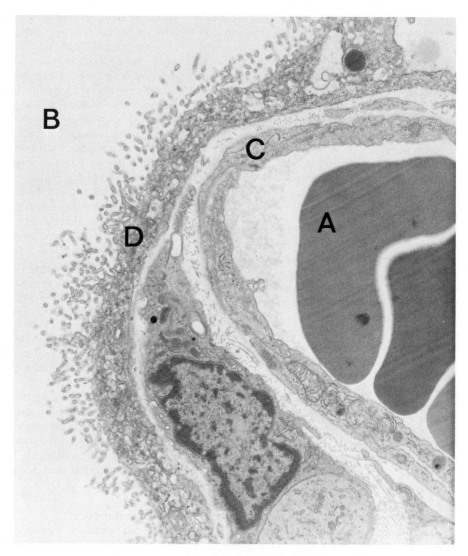

Fig. 6-1. Electron micrograph (× 4,800) of a human placenta at term. Fetal red blood cells (A) and plasma are separated from the maternal circulation (B) by capillary endothelium (C) and syncytiotrophoblast (D). The distance between the two circulations progressively decreases during gestation. (Photograph courtesy William Clewell, M.D., Department of Obstetrics, University of Colorado School of Medicine.)

estimating the constants, we can predict changes in drug levels over time. Two additional kinetic parameters can also be described: the volume of distribution (the apparent size of a body compartment into which the drug must spread in order to result in a given concentration) and clearance (the amount of a body fluid from which a drug is removed over a given period of time). The latter entity has the greatest biologic significance. It can be broken down into the kinetic constant describing the rate of elimination from the central compartment (Ke1) and the volume of distribution.

Determinants of drug disposition affect fetal levels differently when drugs are administered as a single dose than when they are given chronically and levels reach a steady state. At steady state, the amount of drug absorbed over a given period is equal to the amount eliminated; the drug has completely distributed through all compartments, and its level in each remains constant. Following single doses, the level of drug in any compartment may be influenced as much by factors determining the rate of distribution as by factors responsible for its elimination. Differences between steady-state and single-dose kinetics are important when considering drug levels in peripheral compartments.

At steady state, the rates of transfer of drugs

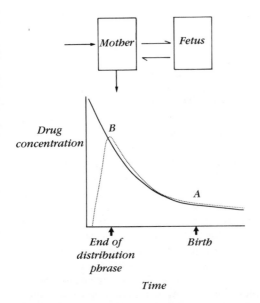

Fig. 6-2. Simplified kinetic consideration of the fetal-maternal unit as a two-compartment open model. A single dose of drug B is assumed to have been administered intravenously into mother. The solid line (–) depicts drug concentration in maternal plasma. The dotted line (.....) represents drug concentration in fetal plasma.

across cell membranes such as those of the placenta have little impact, and the ratio of drug concentrations between fetal and maternal plasma tends toward unity. Differences in steady-state levels of total drug reflect factors such as ionization and protein binding. Differences in protein or tissue binding, however, do not lead to different levels of free drug. Differences in pH between maternal (pH 7.35–7.40) and fetal (pH 7.20–7.25) blood can lead to unequal levels of total drugs when the pKa approaches the physiologic range. For example, the pKa of most local anesthetics falls between pH 8 and pH 9. At physiologic pH 5, up to 20% of the drug is un-ionized and can cross the placenta. The percentage of drug ionized is greater in fetal blood with its lower pH since these compounds are weak bases. Ionization traps drugs on the fetal side, and total drug appears to accumulate. The ratio of levels of un-ionized drug at steady state in the two compartments remains constant, however. Lowering fetal pH, as with asphyxia, leads to more trapping and greater accumulation of total drug.

Many drugs given in pregnancy, especially those administered during labor, do not achieve steady state. Under these circumstances, factors affecting rate of distribution become very important. Concentrations of drugs in maternal and fetal compartments change over time roughly in the manner depicted in Figure 6-2. Ionization and protein binding slow diffusion from both sides of the placenta. The result is often an apparent lag in clearance of drug from the fetal compartment. Drug levels in cord blood at point A in Figure 6-2 are higher than those in mother. Such observations should not be taken to indicate active transport nor do they necessarily mean that drug concentrates on the fetal side. Questions regarding placental contributions to transport should be approached only at steady state.

The pattern of distribution after intravenous administration of a single dose as shown in Figure 6-2 illustrates another important point with respect to drug distribution after administration of single doses. At point B, distribution is complete, and the drug in fetal plasma has reached its peak. From this point, elimination from the fetal and maternal compartments tends to be parallel, but the rates reflect primarily maternal excretion processes. The peak height at point B is directly proportional to the level of drug at the start of the distribution phase in maternal plasma [23]. This means that the peak level of drug in the fetal compartment can be affected by the route of administration of maternal drug. With intravenous administration, a bolus effect creates a greater gradient than with either intramuscular or oral administration. Thus, the rapid intravenous administration of a narcotic drug for pain during labor is associated with higher levels in fetal plasma and may be an important determinant of respiratory depression at the time of delivery. On the other hand, intravenous administration of a drug to a mother may be useful if it is desirable to achieve a high fetal drug level. In most cases of fetal therapy, however, the best approach to maintaining a therapeutic level in the fetus is to achieve and maintain a therapeutic steady-state level in the mother.

Although the above discussion is an oversimplification, the principles presented are of practical use. The discussion assumes, however, that little, if any, metabolism takes place in fetal tissues. This assumption is valid for the majority of drugs. Human fetal liver contains enzymes capable of drug metabolism. Although the capacity for metabolism is greater in human than in animal fetuses, the rates of metabolism are so slow relative to those of the mother that fetal metabolism has little effect on distribution of maternally administered drug. These slow rates of metabolism continue for variable periods of time postnatally, meaning that infants delivered with significant levels of drug transferred from mother may maintain those levels for extended lengths of time postnatally [9]. Thus, the effect of a drug, like propranolol, on a fetus may be relatively short lived, whereas the same drug may produce a significantly more prolonged effect if the infant is delivered soon after administration [24].

Maternal Drug Effects

Maternal adaptations to pregnancy include changes in nearly every physiologic system in the body. It is likely, therefore, that pregnancy affects the action and disposition of drugs. Little information, however, is available describing pregnancy's influences on pharmacodynamics and pharmacokinetics.

Drug disposition will be influenced by changes in renal and hepatic function as well as by changes in body composition. Drug absorption may also be affected. In practical terms, the pharmacokinetic consequences of these changes translate into drug concentrations that are greater or less than expected after a single dose, and drug clearances that exceed or fall below those of nonpregnant women. A few examples of altered drug disposition have been described during pregnancy including decreased clearance of caffeine [20] and lower than expected levels of phenytoin. The latter result from poor absorption, increased clearance, or both [25].

The effects of pregnancy on drug action need more study. Few, if any, investigations have documented physiologic responses to drugs administered in expectant women. Nonetheless, women recount a wide variety of alterations in perceptions and reactions to foreign compounds. For example, many women report aversion to alcohol, tobacco smoke, and foods that are not necessarily linked to morning sickness [26]. Understanding the changes in maternal response to drugs during gestation may both provide insight into specific physiologic adaptations and identify the need to modify therapeutic approaches.

Critical Periods

The cellular actions of drugs will affect an organism differently at different stages of development. Observations of adverse effects of drugs on morphogenesis have given rise to the concept of critical periods of development—intervals during which specific cellular interactions irreversibly affect the structure or function of a developing organ. From the discussion of drug action above, however, it is obvious that drugs are pharmacologically active throughout development. The tendency has been to consider drug effects on development as important only during organogenesis. This is emphatically not the case. The following section briefly reviews some examples of how

drugs may produce effects throughout reproduction.

Preconception

Drug exposures affect gametogenesis and fertility. Ovulation can be pharmacologically prevented and stimulated. The first meiotic division in human females occurs in utero. Mutagenic effects of maternally administered drugs could become manifest, therefore, in subsequent generations [27].

Recently, attention has been directed to several aspects of drug effects on reproductive function in men [28]. Drugs can affect both sperm counts and motility. It may also be expected that many drugs will diffuse into semen, and the list of compounds that have been detected in ejaculates is growing. Their effects, however, are unknown. Most concern has been directed toward the effects of cytotoxic agents on spermatogenesis. Several studies have demonstrated decreased sperm counts and infertility during treatments with cancer chemotherapeutic agents. Nevertheless, drug effects on spermatogenesis may be transient, since new spermatocytes are produced every 78 days. Evidence indicates varying sensitivities of developing sperm at different stages of maturation. Stem cells appear to be relatively insensitive, at least to the effects of cytotoxic agents [27,28]. Several reports of the return of fertility following cancer chemotherapy have appeared. These studies may indicate considerable potential for recovery of spermatogenesis following treatment with cytotoxic agents.

Concern is growing over the effects of drug exposures in utero on reproductive function in adults. Although the effects of diethylstilbestrol were initially believed to be only cervical abnormalities, vaginal adenosis, and an increased risk for vaginal cancer, pregnancy outcome also appears to be affected, with a threefold increase in prematurity [29]. Equally disturbing are reports of reproductive effects of drugs like phenobarbital, which can influence testosterone levels and reproductive function in animals exposed in utero [30]. Animals exhibit imprinting of sex dependent metabolism and behavior to a much greater extent than do humans. These studies provide insight into mechanisms by which drugs may affect reproduction.

Preimplantation

Very little is known about drug effects on zygotes during the first two weeks following conception. This period of human gestation is spent in blastocyst formation and in implantation. It has been suggested that this period is relatively resistant to adverse drug effects. Observation reveals that there is little association between drug exposures during this time and congenital abnormalities. Three explanations are possible. The first is that drugs have little or no access to the zygote prior to completion of placentation. This is not likely to be the case since drugs diffuse widely throughout body compartments. Probably, however, levels of drugs encountered in the fallopian tube and uterine cavity are lower than those in plasma. A second possibility is that there are few drug receptors present at this stage of development. The pharmacology of cells in the early stages of development has been intensively studied in amphibians and is now approachable in mammalian systems through techniques of in vitro fertilization and zygote implantation. Therapeutic concentrations of drugs are active in organisms at this stage [31,32]. In vivo studies of haloperidol administered during implantation in rodents, for example, suggest that it can induce a prolongation of gestation (diapause)[33]. Drugs appear to be pharmacologically active at this stage of development.

A third interpretation of the apparent lack of association between abnormalities observed at birth and early drug exposures holds that any adverse effects produced at these early stages are likely to be devastating to the pregnancy and to result in its loss. A great deal of evidence now supports the fact that abnormal cellular function in early gestation leads to pregnancy loss. Spontaneous miscarriages occur in approximately 15% of diagnosed pregnancies, and many more losses occur than parents are aware of. The pathology of these losses yields a high percentage of chromosomal, structural, and other abnormalities [34]. Developmental abnormalities, therefore, most commonly result in pregnancy loss. Births of infants with congenital abnormalities represent only a fraction of the total fetal loss. The contributions of drug-induced abnormalities to this spectrum of pregnancy loss has not been quantified. Studies of mechanisms in animals indicate that drug-induced embryotoxicity is manifest primarily as pregnancy loss [8]. Nonetheless, early drug toxicity can be manifest at birth. It is, therefore, inappropriate to conclude that adverse effects of drug exposures occurring during the preimplantation period will necessarily result only in pregnancy loss. It may also be wrong to conclude that because a pregnancy has progressed beyond a certain point it has escaped any injurious effects of previously administered drugs. The tenuousness of development during implantation predicts immediate losses and lower risks for abnormalities in liveborns exposed to drugs during this period, but it does not preclude the possibility of adverse drug effects.

Organogenesis

The interval of organogenesis, roughly 2 to 12 weeks after conception, has received most attention as a critical period in human development. Adverse pharmacologic effects at this time can lead to irreversible malformations, many of which are compatible with continued growth and eventual live birth. Thalidomide represents the best known of the human teratogens operating in this period. The number of drugs proved to cause human abnormalities during organogenesis is actually rather small—less than a dozen compounds [35]. The number of drugs suspected of causing such problems, or associated with birth defects in case reports, however, is considerably larger.

The interplay between pharmacologic, genetic, and developmental factors is partially responsible for the discrepancy between retrospective associations and what can actually be shown to be cause and effect. It is also possible that the potential for drugs to cause birth defects is less than generally feared. Again, animal studies show that cytotoxicity, abnormalities of cellular growth and differentiation, and failure of cell migration are the major mechanisms producing birth defects [8]. Since the potential for drugs to be cytotoxic and to affect rates of cell growth and migration is substantial, concern over the possibility that drugs may induce malformations during organogenesis should remain high.

Fetal Development

Concern about adverse drug effects during fetal development, from roughly 12 weeks after conception to term, has tended to be less than for earlier periods of development. The fetal period is characterized by growth and functional maturation of the conceptus. This interval is relatively prolonged in human development and represents a period of significant growth and organization within the central nervous system (CNS). Adverse effects of drugs during this time can be expected to be manifest in abnormalities of fetal growth and brain function. Chronic drug exposures frequently affect postnatal growth, and it appears likely that many will affect intrauterine growth as well [36]. Few surveys of drug effects have included fetal size as an end point. Among the drugs suspected of altering fetal growth are propranolol, steroids, and a variety of CNS-active compounds, including anticonvulsants, sedatives, and tranquilizers. The fetal alcohol syndrome, characterized by abnormalities of brain and body growth, is largely a disorder of the fetal period. Cessation of drinking early in the fetal period, while having no effect on problems encountered during organogenesis, substantially improves brain growth and development [17].

The newly established field of behavioral teratology concentrates on drug effects during the fetal period and on brain function [37]. Although the magnitude of the problem of adverse effects of drugs on developing brain is unknown, the potential for significant problems is great [38]. Elucidation of the mechanisms involved will be more difficult since the end point to be measured will be largely behavioral. Functional maturation of liver, lung, gonads, and other organs may also be affected during fetal growth. The fetal period, then, is likely to turn out to be as critical, with respect to irreversible adverse effects, as any previous stage of development. Great caution should be exercised in using drugs throughout pregnancy, and use of drugs known to affect the central nervous system should be carefully considered before use during the fetal period.

Perinatal Period

Equally critical to pregnancy outcome is the immediate perinatal period—the interval of adjustment to extrauterine life beginning with preparation for labor, including delivery, and the first few weeks following. This is a period of increasing drug usage as perinatal medicine intensifies its efforts to affect pregnancy outcome. It should also be noted that abnormal adjustment to extrauterine life contributes significantly to mortality and is a leading cause of mental deficiency. The processes of birth and adjustment to extrauterine life are complex and involve both specialized and usual physiologic functions. Drugs, clearly, have a therapeutic role during this period, but they also possess considerable potential for harm [39].

All of the drugs used to prevent premature delivery can affect extrauterine adjustment responses. Prostaglandin synthetase inhibitors are effective tocolytics, for instance, but they may lead to in utero closure of the ductus arteriosus and have been associated with primary pulmonary hypertension in neonates born during treatment with these agents [40]. Certain effects of beta-sympathomimetic agents on postnatal cardiovascular and metabolic adjustments are predictable, and problems with hypotension, hypoglycemia, and decreased gastrointestinal motility have been reported [41]. Use of drugs that depress respirations pose obvious threats, but maternally administered drugs, present in significant levels in infants at birth, can affect other important functions such as infant arousal, temperature control, suckling behavior, and sleep.

Since the neonate, in general, clears drugs slowly, effects of maternally administered drugs may last for several hours or days after birth. During this period, the neonate not only must make cardiorespiratory adjustments but also must become metabolically independent. Many hepatic functions mature postnatally, among them the capacity to conjugate bilirubin. Since excessive amounts of free, unconjugated bilirubin are toxic to the central nervous system, the effects of drugs administered during labor on bilirubin metabolism and protein binding should be carefully considered. As with any other drug effect, the potential for maternally administered compounds to affect neonatal bilirubin disposition depends on the concentration of drug present. Few known cases of kernicterus, the neuropathologic correlate of bilirubin-induced brain damage, can be directly attributed to maternally administered drugs. On the other hand, significant fetal concentrations of drugs, like sulfonamides, which could interfere with bilirubin metabolism and protein binding, may be achieved after maternal administration [42]. A continued cautious approach is worthwhile.

Pharmacologic responses in the newborn exposed to drugs administered to the mother during labor need not preclude their use. In many instances, the potential benefits to mother and infant far outweigh the risks. Problems such as hypoglycemia and hypotension can be effectively treated in the neonate if they are anticipated and recognized. Maternal drug therapy may be an indication for pediatric consultation and pediatric presence at delivery. Good communication between physicians caring for mothers and infants is mandatory.

Drugs administered to women during the postpartum period can be expected to diffuse into breast milk. The composition of human breast milk is such that it will contain both lipid- and water-soluble compounds. Few drugs are actively excreted into breast milk. Most diffuse down concentration gradients determined by maternal plasma levels. Thus, the total amounts of most drugs ingested by infants through milk will be low and the physiologic effects minimal. A few potent compounds, such as antimetabolites, are best avoided [43]. Given decreased clearance of drugs by newborns, continuous administration of even low doses of certain drugs could lead to accumulation and effective levels. It may be more important to document levels of drug in fetal plasma after nursing than to measure drug levels in milk. Symptoms in infants that might be related to maternal drugs absorbed from breast milk should be investigated and documentation of the infant's blood levels sought. In general, concern over administration of drugs to nursing women centers more on the effects of the drugs on milk production than on infant responses [43].

In many cases, the event of birth also means the abrupt discontinuation of transplacentally acquired drugs. Although clearance of the drug may be delayed to some extent, the newborn infant must soon adjust to life without drugs. Withdrawal symptoms associated with narcotics, barbiturates, and other addictive drugs are well documented during the neonatal period [44]. The phenomenon may be more common than was previously realized. Withdrawal symptoms in neonates have also been associated with maternal administration of reserpine and antihistamines [45]. Metabolic and physiologic readjustments will occur in infants suddenly deprived of many drugs.

APPROACH TO DRUG THERAPY DURING PREGNANCY

The foregoing discussions have attempted to present general principles of developmental pharmacology. By themselves, these principles did not eliminate the dilemmas described in the introductory paragraphs. The following section outlines a practical approach to the potential problems of drug therapy during pregnancy based on the principles discussed.

Anticipatory Counseling

Both disease states themselves and the drugs used to treat them can affect reproductive outcome. Much of what follows in this book will be devoted to providing specific examples. All physicians caring for individuals of childbearing age, both men and women, should develop a specific sensitivity to reproductive issues and talk them over with their patients. Discussions of the prognosis and management of chronic disease should include consideration of adverse effects on reproduction. Whenever possible, specific answers to questions concerning risks should be sought. The chapters in this book and the literature cited may be helpful, but formal counseling may also be advantageous. Geneticists and genetic counselors can frequently provide much useful information. Perinatologists, neonatologists, obstetricians, and pediatricians may also be helpful. Choices about reproduction rightfully belong to individuals, but physicians have a responsibility to provide information that may be relevant to decision making.

The advantages of anticipatory counseling are obvious. Inheritance of disorders can be discussed and effects of pregnancy assessed. In some cases, specific modifications of treatment regimens may be possible, prior to conception.

Early Recognition of Pregnancy

Women requiring chronic medication who wish to have children should be encouraged to test for pregnancy as soon as they suspect it. Management of a pregnancy complicated by a serious medical problem often requires the coordinated efforts of several physicians. Keys to such management are accurate estimates of gestational age and, often, early therapeutic adjustments of medication. Perhaps the best indicator of fetal well-being is uterine growth. Early diagnosis of pregnancy and examination by a physician will establish this important data base.

Indications for Drug Therapy

Indications for use of all drugs should be reviewed during pregnancy. As mentioned above, good clinical practice includes such reviews prior to conception. Consideration of the natural history and physiologic ramifications of many diseases can be expected to support the use of drugs. The general contention that significant maternal disease, if left untreated, will adversely affect pregnancy outcome is well documented in the succeeding chapters in this book. This is not to say that drugs used in pregnancy will necessarily be safe. The information reviewed in the previous sections predicts that maternally administered drugs will be pharmacologically active in the conceptus. Adverse responses will occur, and some may produce irreversible effects.

Drugs that are indicated should be administered in effective doses and the pregnant patient monitored for the therapeutic effect, drug level, or both. If drug therapy is indicated in order to improve maternal physiologic function, and thereby protect the fetus from the effects of maternal disease, then it is important to use the drug as effectively as possible. Since, as discussed above, pregnancy may affect drug disposition and pharmacodynamics, careful monitoring is called for. The expense involved is justified by the fact that careful monitoring generally leads to use of the minimally effective dose of an agent, prevents toxicity due to accumulation of drug, and avoids addition of other drugs when levels are subtherapeutic. Monitoring also identifies noncompliance, a common problem in drug therapy that may actually place the conceptus at higher risk.

Whenever possible, drugs with which there has been some experience in pregnancy should be selected. This approach creates, to a certain extent, a new "therapeutic orphan"—the pregnant woman. Because maternal diseases have the potential for significant impact on the developing offspring, there is a great need for new and creative approaches to medical management. Use of new or unprecedented drugs during pregnancy should be recognized as experimental and informed consent obtained. In some cases, there may be little or no experience with the drug of choice for a specific problem. In such instances, the parents should be informed of this lack of experience. It is still possible, even when experience with a compound in pregnancy is limited, to present expectant parents with medical recommendations favoring the use of a drug.

Discussion of Risks

The use of any drug entails acceptance of risks. Use of a drug during pregnancy implies acceptance of additional risks and necessitates careful communication between physician and patient. The discussions mandated by this situation require a specific data base. First, the indications for the drug use must be discerned and the alternatives to its use considered. The potential effects of the drug on both mother and fetus need to be considered. Since the specific response of the conceptus will depend on genetic and developmental factors in addition to dose-dependent pharmacologic effects, information about genetic background and the progress of gestation should be included. Genetic background is particularly important. Risks for all drugs used in pregnancy should be discussed against a background of risks in the general population. Generally accepted estimates of pregnancy outcomes indicate that approximately 15% of diagnosed pregnancies spontaneously abort and 3 to 5% of infants are born with a congenital abnormality. Careful family histories may identify individuals who fall outside the general population. For instance, a family history of neural tube defects, congenital heart disease, or other birth defects would suggest that risks for use of a drug during the critical periods of organogenesis are theoretically higher than they would be for the general population. While this increase in risk may not be quantifiable, its theoretical presence may influence decisions, and both parties need to be aware that they are accepting risks potentially higher than in usual circumstances.

The progress of pregnancy also needs to be reviewed. Frequently, the malady for which a drug is being prescribed may already be affecting fetal well-being in addition to maternal health. Thus, in addition to monitoring maternal response to drug, fetal response can also be monitored depending on gestational age, by such objective criteria as rate of growth, heart rate, and perceived movement (see Chap. 5, Antenatal Fetal Assessment). Use of ultrasound promises to improve monitoring

of fetal responses to drugs, but at present this application of the technique is experimental.

The following format is useful in communicating complex information to concerned prospective parents. The approach involves three steps. First, what is known and not known about the disease, drug, and particular pregnancy is reviewed. Next, interactions between these elements are discussed and priorities established. Finally, a medical recommendation for a specific treatment plan is offered. Questions are continually addressed. This approach efficiently communicates information about risks and benefits and at the same time incorporates the patient in the decision process. The approach usually results in a reasonable recommendation that clearly identifies both interpretation and judgment.

Detecting Drug Effects

Since pregnancy can affect drug disposition, monitoring of maternal levels of chronically administered drugs is recommended. The use of specific drugs is considered in subsequent chapters. The goal, as always, is to achieve and maintain a therapeutic level.

Frequently, women taking medications will discontinue them after discovering that they are pregnant. They are then left wondering whether their fetus has been adversely affected. This question also arises when women continue to take medication during pregnancy. Although prenatal diagnosis has advanced considerably through use of genetic amniocentesis, radiography, and ultrasound, the specific role of these techniques in monitoring drug effects has yet to be established. Since few drugs produce chromosomal abnormalities, genetic amniocentesis is of no specific value in monitoring drug effects. Although ultrasound imaging has been improved by better resolution and more experience, the ability of ultrasound to screen for birth defects remains limited. Drug exposures alone do not currently constitute an indication for ultrasound examinations. Rather, ultrasound appears to be more informative when used for obstetric indications, abnormal uterine size or growth, or when genetic predispositions exist for specific identifiable anomalies. Few drugs are associated with abnormalities that can be detected by ultrasound, especially early in gestation.

Case reports have associated exposures to several drugs with neural tube defects. No cause and effect relationships have been established yet, but screening for such defects can be accomplished by measuring maternal serum alpha-fetoprotein. This test is not diagnostic, but rather a screening tool for defects in the neural tube. So far, no studies have determined its value in screening for drug-related exposures, but its potential may be worth discussing with patients who have had exposures during early organogenesis.

POSTNATAL FOLLOW-UP

Drug therapy in pregnant women is, in many ways, experimental. Given our inability to discern fetal pharmacologic effects in utero, careful examination after birth is essential.

Relatively few children exposed to drugs in utero have been followed from birth—unfortunately, since documentation of administration of drugs during pregnancy is tantamount to enrollment in a prospective study. The result of this lack of follow-up is well illustrated by the current dilemma presented by use of sodium warfarin (Coumadin) during pregnancy. During the 1960s, several studies reported that normal infants were delivered after maternal Coumadin therapy. Normality was based on nursery admission examinations. Later, cartilaginous deformities, extraosseous calcifications, and ocular abnormalities in a few infants were, retrospectively, linked to Coumadin exposures early in gestation. In light of these case reports, questions about the safety of using Coumadin during gestation have been raised. Because "prospectively" identified infants have been lost to follow-up, risks for such untoward effects cannot now be accurately estimated [46]. Since use of drugs in pregnancy often amounts to experimental medicine, all persons involved share the obligation to complete the experiment through documented follow-up. This challenge will be met only through careful communication and good medical practice.

REFERENCES

1. Murphy EA, Chase GA. Principles of genetic counseling. Chicago: Year Book, 1975.
2. Warkany J. Congenital malformations. Chicago: Year Book, 1971.
3. Biddle FG. Use of dose-response relationships to discriminate between the mechanisms of cleft-palate induction by different teratogens: an argument for discussion. Teratology. 1978; 18:247–52.
4. Boreus LO. Drug-receptor interactions and biologic maturation. In: Mirkin BL, ed. Clinical pharmacology and therapeutics: a pediatric perspective. Chicago: Year Book, 1978:3–22.
5. Zimmerman HJ. Hepatotoxicity: the adverse effects of drugs and other chemicals on the liver. New York: Appleton-Century-Crofts, 1978.
6. Mitchell JR, and Jollows DJ. Metabolic activation of drugs to toxic substances. Gastroenterology. 1975; 68:392–410.
7. Spielberg SP, Gordon GB, Blake DA, Goldstein DA, Herlong HF. Predisposition to phenytoin hepatotoxicity assessed in vitro. N Engl J Med. 1981; 305:722–7.
8. Wilson JG. Current status of teratology: general principles and mechanisms derived from animal studies. In: Wilson JG, Fraser FE, eds. Handbook of teratology. Vol. 1. New York: Plenum, 1977:47–74.
9. Neims AH, Warner M, Loughnan PM, Aranda JV. Developmental aspects of the hepatic cytochrome p. 450 monooxygenase system. Annu Rev Pharmacol Toxicol. 1976; 16:427–45.
10. Gordon GB, Spielberg SP, Blake DA, Balasubramanian V. Thalidomide teratogenesis: evidence for a toxic arene oxide metabolite. Proc Natl Acad Sci USA. 1981; 78:2545–8.
11. Hassell TM, Johnston MC, Dudley KH, eds. Phenytoin-induced teratology and gingival pathology. New York: Raven Press, 1980.
12. Harbison RD. Chemical-biological reactions common to teratogenesis and mutagenesis. Environ Health Perspect. 1978; 24:87–100.
13. Shum S, Jensen NM, Nebert DW. The murine Ah locus: in utero toxicity and teratogenesis associated with genetic differences in benzo(a)pyrene metabolism. Teratology. 1979; 20:365–76.
14. Nebert DW. Etiology of birth defects: potential importance of genetic differences in drug metabolism. In: Soyka LF, Redmond GP, eds. Drug metabolism in the immature human. New York: Raven Press, 1981:1–17.
15. Longo LD. The biological effects of carbon monoxide on the pregnant woman, fetus, and newborn infant. Am J Obstet Gynecol. 1977; 129:69–103.
16. Fraser FC. Prevention of birth defects: how are we doing? Teratology. 1978; 17:193–201.
17. Rosett HL. The effects of alcohol on the fetus and offspring. In: Kalant OJ, ed. Alcohol and drug problems in women. Vol. 5 of Research advances in alcohol and drug problems. New York: Plenum, 1980:595–652.
18. Avery ME. Pharmacological approaches to the acceleration of fetal lung maturation. Br Med Bull. 1975; 31:13–7.
19. Kleinman CS, Donnerstein RL, DeVore GR, et al. Fetal echocardiography for evaluation of in utero congestive heart failure. N Engl J Med. 1982; 306:568–75.
20. Christensen HD, Manion CV, Kling OR. Caffeine kinetics in late pregnancy. In: Soyka LF, Redmond GP, eds. Drug metabolism in the immature human. New York: Raven Press, 1981:163–82.
21. Fox H. Pathology of the placenta. London: Saunders, 1978:1–49.
22. Juchau MR. Enzymatic bioactivation and inactivation of chemical teratogens and transplacental carcinogens/mutagens. In: Juchan MR, ed. The biochemical basis of chemical teratogenesis. New York: Elsevier North Holland, 1981:63–94.
23. Gibaldi M, Perrier D. Pharmacokinetics. New York: Marcel Dekker, 1975:45–128.

24. Hill RM, Stern L. Drugs in pregnancy: effects on the fetus and newborn. Drugs. 1979; 17:182–97.

25. Hassell TM, Johnson MC, Dudley KH. Phenytoin induced teratology and gingival pathology. New York: Raven Press, 1980:1–236.

26. Hook EB. Changes in tobacco smoking and ingestion of alcohol and caffeinated beverages during early pregnancy. In: Kelley S, Hook EB, Janerich DT, Porter IH, eds. Birth defects: risks and consequences. New York: Academic Press, 1976:173–83.

27. Vogel F, Motulsky AG. Human Genetics: problems and approaches. New York: Springer-Verlag, 1979:18–81.

28. Lee IP, Dixon RL. Factors influencing reproduction and genetic toxic effects on male gonads. Environ Health Perspect. 1978; 24:117–27.

29. Herbst AL, Hubby MM, Azizi F, Makii MM. Reproductive and gynecologic surgical experience in diethylstilbestrol-exposed daughters. Am J Obstet Gynecol. 1981; 141:1019–28.

30. Gupta C, Yaffe SJ, Shapiro BH. Prenatal exposure to phenobarbital permanently decreases testosterone and causes reproductive dysfunction. Science. 1982; 216:640–2.

31. Bell E, ed. Molecular and cellular aspects of development. New York: Harper & Row, 1965.

32. Galloway SM, Perry PE, Meneses J, Nebert DW, Pedersen RA. Cultured mouse embryos metabolize benzo(a)pyrene during early gestation. Proc Natl Acad Sci USA. 1980; 77:3524–8.

33. Tuchmann-Duplessis H. Drug effects on the fetus. Sydney: ADIS Press, 1975:153–5.

34. Porter IH, Hook EB, eds. Human embryonic and fetal deaths. New York: Academic Press, 1980.

35. Wilson JG. Embryotoxicity of drugs in man. In: Wilson JG, Fraser FC, eds. Handbook of teratology. Vol. 1. New York: Plenum, 1977:309–55.

36. Redmond GP. Effects of drugs on intrauterine growth. Clin Perinatol. 1979; 6:5–19.

37. Rodier PM. Behavioral teratology. In: Wilson JG, Fraser FC, eds. Handbook of teratology. Vol. 4. New York: Plenum, 1978:397–428.

38. Prasad KN, Vernadakis A. Mechanisms of actions of neurotoxic substances. New York: Raven Press, 1982.

39. Manchester DK, Neims AH. The evaluation of pharmacologic approaches to perinatal asphyxia. In: Gluck L, ed. Intrauterine asphyxia and the developing fetal brain. Chicago: Year Book, 1977:334–48.

40. Manchester D, Margolis HS, Sheldon RE. Possible association between maternal indomethacin therapy and primary pulmonary hypertension of the newborn. Am J Obstet Gynecol. 1976; 126:467–9.

41. Niebyl JR. Drugs for inhibition of premature labor. Clin Perinatol. 1979; 6:53–63.

42. Brodersen R. Bilirubin transport in the newborn infant, reviewed with relation to kernicterus. J Pediatr. 1980; 96:349–56.

43. Bowes WA. The effects of medications on the lactating mother and her infant. Clin Obstet Gynecol. 1980; 23:1073–80.

44. Finnegan LP, Fehr KO. The effects of opiates, sedative-hypnotics, amphetamines, cannabis, and other psychoactive drugs on the fetus and newborn. In: Kalant OJ, ed. Alcohol and drug problems in women. Vol. 5 of Research advances in alcohol and drug problems. New York: Plenum, 1980:653–723.

45. Hill RM. Adverse effects of prenatal drug therapy. In: Mirkin BL, ed. Clinical pharmacology and therapeutics: a pediatric perspective. Chicago: Year Book, 1978:199–219.

46. Hall JG, Pauli RM, Wilson KM. Maternal and fetal sequelae of anticoagulation during pregnancy. Am J Med. 1980; 68:122–40.

There is therefore no deformity but in monstrosity, wherein notwithstanding there is a kind of beauty, Nature so ingeniously contriving those irregular parts, as they become sometimes more remarkable than the principall Fabrick.
—Sir Thomas Browne
Religio Medici

7. PRINCIPLES OF TERATOLOGY

James J. Nora, Audrey Hart Nora, and Paul Wexler

Only two decades ago the concept that the fetus was almost invulnerable within the maternal environment was widely accepted. The experience with rubella in Australia in 1941 seemed to be almost an aberrant episode [1]. Then came thalidomide—and it became clear that drugs as well as a rogue virus could malform the human fetus [2]. Yet it is only within the past decade that the broad dimensions of the problem of environmental teratogens have become apparent. In the first edition of a textbook of medical genetics published in 1974 only two teratogens were listed as being firmly established (rubella and thalidomide) and teratogenic exposure was not even on the list of the 25 most common reasons for referral to a genetics clinic. In the 1981 second edition of the same textbook only a rather arbitrary selection from among many teratogens could be accommodated within the limitations of space—and teratogenic exposures had become the sixth most common reason for genetic referral and the occasion for more "genetic" telephone consultations than all other reasons combined [3]. Thus, in the past decade, patients as well as physicians have become aware of the vulnerability of the fetus and profoundly concerned about protecting pregnancies from adverse environmental influences.

GENERAL CONSIDERATIONS

From the point of view of the practicing physician, the principles of teratology can be reduced to a very simple approach, can be highly complex, or can fall somewhere in between. In the simplest terms one may assume that any drug that is capable of pharmacologic activity can be a threat to the developing fetus. Therefore, the overview would be that the pregnant woman should avoid all chemicals and drugs that she can safely avoid during her pregnancy. This is not to say that drugs that are clearly indicated should be withheld, but that

the potential risks and benefits should be understood by the physician and the patient. The patient should be an informed participant in the decision to take a medication during pregnancy. The highly complex side of the issue of drugs in pregnancy is that for almost every study that raises an alarm about the potential hazards of a given drug another study essentially exonerates that drug. These are methodologic problems for epidemiologists to debate, but they are very real to the physician trying to decide which drugs might be safe to use in pregnancy. How drugs and chemicals produce maldevelopment has been largely a mystery, although clues to possible solutions are beginning to emerge. For example, a cellular basis for the teratogenicity of thalidomide, has recently been proposed [4].

Some investigators may argue that, because each step in causality from maternal exposure to a drug leading to a birth defect in a baby cannot be demonstrated for most drugs, we cannot be confident that a suspected drug is truly teratogenic. Most workers take a position that is somewhere between the simple and the complex. It is acknowledged that, while irrefutable data are hard to find, potent pharmacologic agents must be approached with caution because of their potential damage to the unborn, and the imperfect data we possess.

Within this framework, the requisites of a teratogenic exposure may be explored. There are three essentials and several corollaries. The essentials that will be developed in subsequent paragraphs are

1. Exposure at a vulnerable period of embryogenesis
2. Genetic predisposition to react adversely to the effects of a given teratogen
3. Genetic predisposition to one or more malformations

Among the corollaries to be mentioned now is a concept that must always be kept in mind: The developing embryo is not a little adult. What is required to construct an organ, such as the heart, in an embryo weighing only a few grams is quite different from what is required to maintain a heart in a 70-kg adult. Another corollary is that the dosage of a drug that will be teratogenic in experimental animals usually overlaps the dosage that will kill some embryos. This is not invariably the case, but a general concept is that a sublethal dose malforms the embryo. A further concept that is relevant in an age of polypharmacology is that combinations of drugs may interact and produce defects that would not be caused by a single drug alone.

Exposure at a Vulnerable Period of Embryogenesis

The failure to recognize this very straightforward principle plagues most epidemiologic studies of teratogens and leads to conflicting conclusions. If there is a drug exposure *after* a critical stage of embryogenesis (such as truncoconal septation of the heart), the drug exposure cannot be blamed. Conversely, if a study contains many cases in which the drug was used after the critical stage, the fact that a defect did not occur cannot be ascribed to the drug's not being able to produce the malformation. The drug was simply given too late to cause a problem.

From the point of view of a physician being consulted by a troubled patient exposed to an infection, a drug or chemical, or other potential teratogen, it is essential to know when in pregnancy the exposure occurred. For most developing structures (Table 7-1), the vulnerable period is from about two weeks after conception (four weeks' gestation) through about eight weeks' conceptional age (ten weeks' gestational age), the highest concentration of risk being in the first six weeks after conception.

What is treacherous about teratogenic insults is that the embryo is most vulnerable during the

Table 7-1. Period of conceptus vulnerability to teratogens

Fetal age	Gestational age (fetal age + 2 wk)	Teratogenic risk
0–2 wk	0–4 wk	Negligible
3–6 wk	5–8 wk	Highest
7–8 wk	9–10 wk	High
9–13 wk	11–15 wk	Decreasing
14–38 wk	16–40 wk	Low (with exceptions)

period when the mother may not be sure whether or not she is pregnant. Before implantation, and for about the first two weeks after conception, the fertilized egg is relatively invulnerable to insults that can malform a fetus. If the environmental trigger is highly potent, a spontaneous abortion will result rather than a birth defect. The next one-month is the period of highest risk (third through sixth weeks) for major malformations. Sometime during this highest-risk period, many women realize that they are pregnant and begin to make changes in their life-styles that are compatible with protecting the pregnancies. Unfortunately, they may start too late. A substantial number of women do not even begin to make protective changes until the highest-risk period has already passed. A recommendation that we make to sexually active women in the reproductive age is that they assume they are pregnant from the day their period is due until the period comes. The day the period is due (in reasonably regular cycles) is about the day the embryo becomes vulnerable to teratogens. This is the time to stop alcohol and unnecessary drug and other teratogenic exposures.

With some exceptions, the type of exposure that is most likely to cause structural birth defects is the short-term one. The experience with thalidomide was that in some cases only one dose was sufficient to do the damage. Long-term exposures are more likely to cause the death of an embryo or not produce damage at all—possibly on the basis of the lack of genetic predisposition to react adversely to the agent. Certainly some teratogens, such as alcohol, will have a continuing deleterious effect from long-term exposure during pregnancy. Although the developing heart is vulnerable to teratogens for only a short period during early pregnancy, the developing brain and physical growth are vulnerable throughout (and after) pregnancy to environmental insults. The concept here would appear to be that there are some long-term sublethal teratogenic influences that may not cause maldevelopment of heart or limb but may still adversely affect growth and brain development. The effect of maternal smoking throughout pregnancy on the birth weight of babies is another example.

A final point, also derived from the thalidomide experience, is that the exposure to many teratogens that will malform a developing organ occurs about five days to two weeks *before* the completion of that aspect of development. To cause transposition of the great arteries, for example, the teratogenic exposure is not at 34 days (when truncoconal septation is completed) but at about 28 days.

Genetic Predisposition to React Adversely to the Effects of a Given Teratogen

This topic is covered in detail in Chapter 6, Pharmacologic Principles. Here only a few observations will be reemphasized. Some individuals can tolerate (and have tolerated) exposures to agents as potent as thalidomide without the development of a birth defect. Other individuals can have minimal exposures to agents well tolerated by the great majority of the population and have adverse reactions. While it is not always the rule, some teratogens cause birth defects that are characteristic enough to suggest the etiology. Phocomelia and thalidomide, rubella and rubella syndrome, lithium and Epstein anomaly are in this category. In other situations, certain patterns of malformations are compatible with a given teratogenic exposure but not diagnostic. Finally, recent evidence has suggested that it is often not the drug itself that does the damage but a metabolite of the original chemical.

Genetic Predisposition to One or More Malformations

Just as some individuals and families are susceptible to the effects of a drug or chemical, there are individuals and families predisposed to birth defects of various types. In obtaining family histories, the clinical geneticist is struck by how certain diseases and malformations cluster in families. Some families are cancer prone, some are heart attack prone, and some seem to have more than their share of birth defects. As one looks carefully at these families, it frequently turns out that the type of birth defect found in a family is rather specific.

This point may be illustrated by looking at congenital heart disease, starting with animal models that we have investigated and showing how the

same pattern holds in human families. About 1% of C57BL/6 mice spontaneously have congenital heart defects (the same rate as humans), and the defect is almost always ventricular septal defect (VSD). If you expose the pregnant female on day 8 of gestation to a single large dose of dextroamphetamine, the rate of congenital defects, mostly VSD, goes up to 11% [5]. If the teratogen is antiheart antibody, the rate of heart defects climbs to 20%—the predominant defect is still VSD. If the A/J strain of mice is used, amphetamines cause a heart defect rate of 13%. The defect, however, is not VSD but mostly atrial septal defect (ASD), the defect that the A/J strain has spontaneously in about 1% of fetuses. In a continuation of the experiment with antiheart antibody the defect rate was increased to 22%, but again mostly ASD. The defect that these experimental models get from different teratogens is the defect running in the family.

So too in human populations: If one child in a family (or a parent) has a VSD, the most likely congenital heart defect to recur in the family is VSD. The same is found for ASD and the full gamut of congenital heart defects. A patient gets the defect running in the family.

This is not to say that only one defect is possible or only one defect can run in families. Some children (and mice) have several malformations. In these cases the basic predisposition to maldevelopment can encompass more than one organ system, and a profound teratogenic insult, as with thalidomide or rubella virus, can malform several simultaneously developing structures such as the heart, spine, limbs, eyes, kidneys, and ears. If the teratogen is given too late to malform the heart, it may malform structures that are still early enough in development to be vulnerable.

The hereditary predisposition to maldevelopment is often illustrated by curves and thresholds, as shown in Figure 7-1. The polygenic predisposi-

Fig. 7-1. The threshold of the genetic environmental interaction.

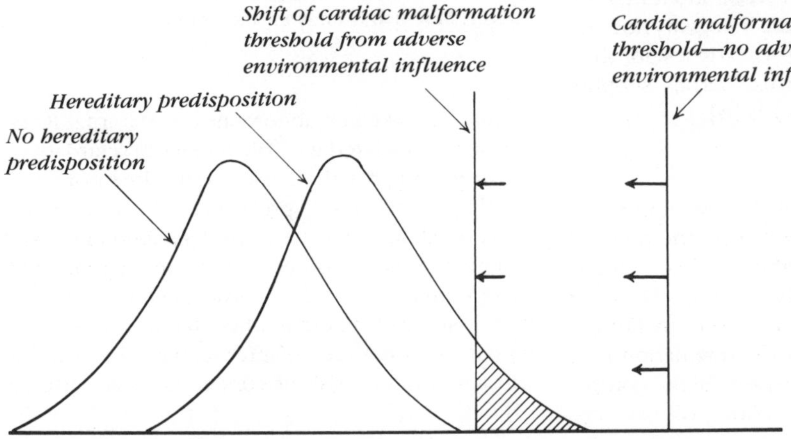

Shift of cardiac malformation threshold from adverse environmental influence

Hereditary predisposition

No hereditary predisposition

Cardiac malformation threshold—no adverse environmental influence

tion is suggested by the hypothetical curve and the enviromental influence by the vertical threshold line. Since the discussion up to now has used congenital heart disease as a specific example of maldevelopment, visualize that on the right side of the vertical threshold line lies VSD and on the left side, no heart defect. If the curve of predisposition is moved to the right, a defect occurs on the basis of increased genetic susceptibility. If the curve is to the left, genetic predisposition is minimal or absent, depending on how far to the left the curve of genetic predisposition is located with respect to the threshold. The corollary is that a teratogenic insult moves the threshold line to the left. The key is the relationship of the curves to the thresholds.

SELECTED TERATOGENS

Table 7-2 provides a partial list of teratogens that are of historical or present clinical interest. They may be subdivided into infections, maternal conditions, and drugs and radiation.

Infections

Rubella, while no longer a major threat to populations in which girls and women are immunized, must be discussed as the prototype of infectious teratogens. The original rubella syndrome, recognized in 1941, consisted of cataracts, deafness, and patent ductus arteriosus. The extended rubella syndrome was described during the 1964–1965 pandemic and greatly broadened the spectrum of anomalies [6]. Some lessons to be learned from this teratogen are that a characteristic pattern of anomalies may point to a specific teratogenic exposure. However, a single anomaly or a cluster of anomalies that do not conform to the original triad may also result from the same teratogenic insult. Several other infectious agents have been implicated in the cause of birth defects, and there are probably a large number still to be identified. Of fundamental importance is the necessity for the agent to cross the placenta. Clearly established teratogens are cytomegalovirus, herpes simplex virus, syphilis, and toxoplasmosis [6].

Maternal Conditions

The major content of this book deals with this subject matter. Of greatest interest from the point of view of teratology are diabetes, fever, lupus erythematosus, and phenylketonuria. Maternal diabetes carries with it an increase in malformation risk of two to five times the population risk, apparently depending on the quality of the control of the diabetes. The most common problems are

Table 7-2. Selected teratogens in humans

Teratogens	Approximate frequency of maldevelopment
Infections	
Rubella	35–70%
Cytomegalovirus	10%
Herpes simplex virus (HSV) as teratogen	?
Syphilis	Very high
Toxoplasmosis	15%
Coxsackie B virus	?
Maternal conditions	
Diabetes	5%
(for reversible cardiomegaly)	(30%)
Fever	?
Lupus erythematosus	20–40%
Phenylketonuria— untreated	Very high
Phenylketonuria— treated	Lower
Drugs and radiation	
Thalidomide	50–80%
Radiation	Dose dependent
Alcohol (chronic alcoholism)	20–30%
Amphetamines	5–10%
Anticoagulants, oral	5–10%
Anticonvulsants	
Hydantoin (phenytoin)	5–10%
Phenobarbital	?
Trimethadione	? 20%
Chemotherapeutic agents	High
Lithium	10%
Minor tranquilizers	
Diazepam	? (very low)
Meprobamate	? (very low)
Sex hormones	
Male	? low
Progestagen/estrogen	5%
Stilbestrol	?

Source: Modified from Nora and Fraser [3].

cardiac and skeletal abnormalities. Maternal fever has been associated with birth defects; retardation, seizures, and growth deficiency are the most commonly encountered problems [7]. Congenital heart block has recently been described in fetuses and newborns of mothers with systemic lupus and other connective tissue disorders and represents a high risk [8]. Maternal phenylketonuria carries with it a very high risk of microcephaly in offspring and a substantial risk of congenital heart disease [9].

Drugs and Radiation

In this section we briefly discuss some drugs of concern and mention radiation, which is taken up in Chapter 8. Lists of chemicals that may cause damage reflect the experience and interest of the compilers. With the exception of thalidomide, conclusions regarding drugs are subject to considerable discussion. One could also reasonably ask why drug A or chemical B is not included. Our answer is that there are many other potential teratogens awaiting more definitive evaluation. And we repeat that any drug that is capable of real and useful pharmacologic activity may also be capable of doing harm under the right conditions of genetic vulnerability and timing of exposure.

Thalidomide must be considered the prototype of drug teratogenicity, just as rubella virus is the prototype infectious teratogen, although neither agent is typical of the great majority of teratogens. Both rubella and thalidomide malform a much higher percentage of exposed fetuses and produce a much more characteristic syndrome than do other teratogens. Many of the lessons learned from thalidomide have been described earlier in this presentation. The most striking lesson, however, is that a drug that malformed 50 to 80% of fetuses exposed at a vulnerable period of development, and produced a very rare anomaly (phocomelia), still required four years before the data were convincing enough to necessitate withdrawal of the drug.

Alcohol is another drug that has only recently been widely accepted as being teratogenic. In retrospect it is now easy to go back to biblical times to find an injunction against drinking or to eighteenth-century England to find the Parliament expressing concern about the unhealthy offspring of mothers who, during pregnancy, consumed large quantities of the inexpensive gin that was available at the time. Yet as recently as the 1960s a sizable study in France associating birth defects with maternal alcoholism was largely ignored. Finally the description of the fetal alcohol syndrome provided the right combination of timing and clinical definition to bring the problem into focus [10]. The full fetal alcohol syndrome with physical and mental retardation, congenital heart disease, small palpebral fissures, and facial hypoplasia occurs in 20 to 30% of offspring of women who chronically consume four or more drinks per day, and in perhaps as many as 10% following two to four drinks per day.

Anticoagulants of the coumarin type have been associated with birth defects resembling those found in the autosomal recessive Conradi's syndrome. Stippled epiphyses, nasal hypoplasia, and occasionally optic atrophy and mental retardation have been found in as many as 5 to 10% of babies whose mothers required these anticoagulants [11]. The indications for the anticoagulants are most often intracardiac prosthetic valves and thrombophlebitis.

Anticonvulsants as a group of drugs illustrate some of the problems connected with implicating teratogens in human malformations. The first suspicion was raised in 1968, by Meadows, who reported an increased frequency of cleft lip and palate and congenital heart disease in the babies of mothers who used anticonvulsants [12]. Alert practitioner observations represent the starting point for the discovery of most human teratogens. A description of the fetal hydantoin syndrome that included the unusual findings of severe terminal digital hypoplasia rounded out the clinical description [13]. Follow-up observations from large-scale surveillance studies are often considered an important next step in producing definitive evidence. The large collaborative perinatal study in the United States, in an initial report, concluded that an increased frequency of congenital heart disease and cleft lip and palate was causally associated with maternal exposure to hydantoin (phenytoin). However, shortly after reaching this conclusion, the United States perinatal study group, in conjunction with a Finnish group, came to a conclusion differing from the one just published: It was not the phenytoin that caused the birth defects but the presence of epilepsy in either the mother or the father. Clinicians who are oriented toward thinking of biologic processes and syndromes are less likely to accept statistically significant conclusions that conflict too strikingly with clinical observations.

Chemotherapeutic agents, lithium, minor tranquilizers, and sex hormones illustrate problems and principles that have been covered in the previous discussion of other drug teratogens. The levels of risk appear in Table 7-2.

In 1979, the FDA established five categories to describe a drug's potential to cause birth defects (FDA Drug Bulletin 1982:13; No. 2). By 1984 most prescription drugs will have been classified. The descriptions are as follows:

A—Controlled studies in women fail to demonstrate a risk to the fetus in the first trimester. The possibility of fetal harm is remote.

B—Animal studies do not indicate a risk to the fetus and there are no controlled human studies, or animal studies do show an adverse effect on the fetus, but well-controlled studies in pregnant women have failed to demonstrate a risk to the fetus.

C—Studies have shown drug to have animal teratogenic or embryocidal effects, but there are no controlled studies in women, or no studies are available in either animals or women.

D—Positive evidence of human fetal risk exists, but benefits in certain situations (e.g., life-threatening situations or serious diseases for which safer drugs cannot be used or are ineffective) may make use of the drug acceptable despite its risks.

X—Studies in animals or humans have demonstrated fetal abnormalities, or there is evidence of fetal risk based on human experience, or both, and the risk clearly outweighs any possible benefit.

Street drugs clearly are important problems from the point of view of addiction, psychosocial adjustment, and financial considerations. However, reliable data are still not available with respect to their teratogenic potential. In theory, one can project how substances such as cocaine or marijuana could damage the fetus. There have also been some well-meaning and sensationalized reports based on inadequate information that appear to strongly implicate street drugs as teratogens. Certainly, one does not need this ammunition in addition to the other very compelling reasons for not using substances of abuse. The pregnant woman who uses one substance probably uses several substances and probably pays less attention to nutrition and many other aspects of her general health and hygiene. In general, there is little reason to challenge the concept that substances of abuse taken during pregnancy are potentially damaging to mother and fetus. However, the actual data on specific substances must still be gathered and sorted out.

Over-the-counter drugs represent another category of potential for damage that will require a great deal of investigation to implicate specific teratogens. Again, the data have yet to be obtained. For both street drugs and over-the-counter drugs, both the logistics of obtaining the data and problems of analysis are enormous. Nevertheless, the methodology is available. Precisely designed studies can find the answers.

Radiation is justifiably a cause of concern with regard to the genetic damage that it can cause. It is the prototype agent for producing gene mutations. It can also cause chromosomal breaks. However, the teratogenic effect of radiation, the damage to an embryo or a fetus, is a different problem and this occupies the next chapter.

In conclusion, the environment in industrialized societies contains a wealth of potential hazards to the pregnant woman and her unborn child. During the past decade many hazards have been recognized, but definitive studies on the great majority of potential teratogens have yet to be performed. Recent investigations of teratogens have pointed the way to more precise methodology in data collection and analysis. It should now be possible to identify many low-risk teratogens, with the goal of eliminating them from the environment of the pregnant woman, and to reduce substantially the number of birth defects in our population.

REFERENCES

1. Gregg NM. Congenital cataract following German measles in mother. Trans Ophthalmol Soc Aust (1941). 1942; 3:35–46.
2. Lenz W. Chemicals and malformations in man. In: Second international conference on congenital malformations. New York: International Medical Congress, 1964:263–76.
3. Nora JJ, Fraser FC. Medical genetics: principles and practice. 2nd ed. Philadelphia: Lea & Febiger, 1981.
4. Gordon GB, Spielberg SP, Blake DA, Balasubramanian V. Thalidomide teratogenesis: evidence for a toxic arene oxide metabolite. Proc Natl Acad Sci USA. 1981; 78:2545–8.
5. Nora JJ, Sommerville RJ, Fraser FC. Homologies for congenital heart diseases: murine models, influenced by dextroamphetamine. Teratology. 1968; 1:413–6.
6. Kurent JE, Sever JL. Infectious diseases. In: Wilson JG, Fraser FC, eds. Handbook of teratology. Vol. 1. New York: Plenum, 1977:225–59.
7. Smith DW, Clarren SK, Harvey MA. Hyperthermia as a possible teratogenic agent. J Pediatr. 1978; 92:878–83.
8. McCue CM, Mantakas ME, Tingelstad JB, Ruddy S. Congenital heart block in newborns of mothers with connective tissue disease. Circulation. 1977; 56:82–90.
9. Stevenson RE, Huntley CC. Congenital malformations in offspring of phenylketonuric mothers. Pediatrics. 1967; 40:33–45.
10. Clarren SK, Smith DW. The fetal alcohol syndrome. N Engl J Med. 1978; 298:1063–7.
11. Carson M, Reid M. Warfarin and fetal abnormality. Lancet. 1976; 1:1127.
12. Meadows SR. Anticonvulsant drugs and congenital abnormalities. Lancet. 1968; 2:1296.
13. Hanson JW, Myrianthopoulos NC, Harvey MA, et al. Risks to the offspring of women treated with hydantoin anticonvulsants, with emphasis on the fetal hydantoin syndrome. J Pediatr. 1976; 89:662–8.

8. RISKS OF RADIATION EXPOSURE

William C. Earley

There is an enormous body of technical literature concerning the effects and risks of exposure to low-dose ionizing radiation. Experts differ on the magnitude of those risks or even whether risks exist. The following discussion attempts to evaluate some of the research related to the fetal and maternal risks of irradiation during pregnancy.

DEFINITIONS

Recently, a new system of radiation units has been proposed to replace the conventional units. Both sets of units with conversion factors are given in Table 8-1 [1]. For this discussion the familiar units of rads, rems, and roentgens will be used.

A rad is a unit of measurement of the absorbed dose of ionizing radiation. One rad corresponds to the energy transfer of 100 ergs per gram of an absorbing material including human tissue. A rem refers to a quantity of ionizing radiation that has the same biologic effect as an equal number of rads of x-rays (rem = rad × relative biologic effectiveness).

A term that is not familiar to many readers is *relative biologic effectiveness* (RBE). One rad of energy delivered by x or gamma photons does not have nearly the biologic effect of one rad of energy delivered by neutrons. The RBE of the neutron beam may be up to ten times greater. *Linear energy transfer* (LET) refers to the number of ion pairs produced in tissue per unit length of travel. Alpha particles have the highest LET while gamma and x photons have the lowest.

A principle of radiation dosimetry and effect is that the amount of radiation delivered in one dose over minutes or hours causes more effect (damage) than the same amount of radiation delivered in small doses over months or years. Bond defines low-level radiation exposure as single exposures of 10 or 15 rads or less and high-level exposure as 25 to 100 rads delivered in minutes to a few hours. High dose rate is defined as 5 to 10 rads per minute while low dose rate is less than 5 rads per year [2]. This chapter deals primarily with x and gamma radiation of RBE 1, low LET, low-level radiation exposures, and low dose rates.

Two other terms are mentioned here since each appears in many articles: *stochastic* and *nonstochastic*. These terms describe the biologic effects of radiation. Stochastic effects are those in which the probability of the occurrence, but not the severity of the effect, is a function of dose. The effect is all or none. Examples include the induction of mutations or cancer by low-dose radiation.

In nonstochastic effects of radiation, the severity of the effect varies with the dose of radiation. These effects usually result from high-dose radiation and cause cell death. An example of a nonstochastic effect is bone marrow suppression following high total body radiation exposure to 200 rads. Both stochastic and nonstochastic radiation effects may manifest a critical threshold level.

MATERNAL GENETIC AND CANCER RISKS

Considerable controversy exists regarding the mutation and cancer risks from low-dose radiation. Lack of agreement can be due to biases, emotions, and politics. However, there are at least three other major reasons for it: (1) Much of the estimation of human risk from low-dose radiation is extrapolated from high-dose exposures of research animals and from high-dose exposures of humans (some pregnant) who survived the Nagasaki and Hiroshima atomic explosions. The disagreement is in the selection of the correct equation for the curve to evaluate the data [3]. (2) The estimation of doses of radiation to human casualties of Hiroshima and Nagasaki has been subject to review and revision [4]. (3) The number of mutations and cancers induced by low-dose radiation is simply too small to be detected in the background of naturally occurring mutation and cancer. In

Table 8-1. Radiation quantities and units

Quantity	Conventional unit	SI unit*	Conversion
Exposure	Roentgen (R)	Coulomb per kilogram (c/kg)	$1 \text{ R} = 2.58 \times 10^{-4}$ c/kg
Dose	Rad (100 ergs/g)	Gray (Gy)(joule/kg)	1 rad = 0.01 Gy
Dose equivalent	Rem (rad $\times$ RBE)	Sievert (Sv)(Gy $\times$ RBE)	1 rem = 0.01 Sv

*Système Internationale d'Unités
Source: Gibbs et al. [1].

electronic terms, the signal-to-noise ratio is too low [2]. Land has estimated that to accurately establish the increased risk of cancer of the breast from mammography it would be necessary to follow 60 million women from age 35 until death to accumulate adequate numbers of case studies and controls [5].

Genetic Risk
Despite the controversy described above, reasonable estimates of genetic risk from low-dose radiation can be established. Although no conclusive experimental human data have been compiled regarding radiation-induced transmitted genetic damage, there are data from people exposed in Hiroshima and Nagasaki [6,7]. Also, animal data are available. It is from these data that most of the estimates of genetic risk are derived.

In order to understand the genetic risks from low-dose radiation, it is necessary to know the risk of spontaneous genetic defects. The Committee on the Biological Effects of Ionizing Radiations III (BEIR III) estimated that of 1,000,000 live-born infants approximately 107,000 will have some discernible genetic defect. What is at issue is to discover the additional risk of genetic damage from exposure to low-dose radiation, and the specific dose of radiation that will increase the mutation rate. Table 8-2 shows estimates of the increase in the rate of various inherited disorders including chromosomal abnormalities, which may occur in the first postirradiation generation (F_1) or in many

generations in the future (genetic equilibrium) as a result of a one time population exposure to a given amount of radiation (1 rem per generation per million live births in table cited). Therefore, 1 rem of radiation per generation per million live births to a population would result in an additional 20 autosomal dominant and X-linked diseases in the first postirradiation generation and ultimately an additional 100 of these diseases at genetic equilibrium (UNSCEAR) [9]. BEIR III estimates are shown in the last two columns [8]. Similar estimates are given for other radiation-induced mutations.

The term *doubling dose* is defined as a dose of radiation required to double the spontaneous mutation rate. This dose has been estimated as 156 rems by Shull et al., as 50 to 250 rems by BEIR III, based on reanalysis of data from atomic bomb survivors, and as 100 rems by the United Nations Scientific Committee on the Effects of Atomic Radiation (UNSCEAR) [7,8,9]. It is from these estimates of doubling dose that the mutation risks of low-dose radiation have been calculated.

Somatic (Cancer) Risk
That high-dose radiation may cause cancer is well known. In England, patients with ankylosing spondylitis treated with therapeutic doses of radiation have been reported to have an increased incidence of leukemia [10]. In addition, an increased incidence of breast cancer has been reported in

Table 8-2. Genetic risk of radiation; estimated effect of average population dose equivalent of 0.01 sv (1 rem) per generation (per million live births)

Disease classification	Current incidence	UNSCEAR F_1	Equilibrium	BEIR III F_1	Equilibrium
Autosomal dominant and X-linked	10,000	20	100	5–65	40–200
Irregularly inherited	90,000	5	45		20–900
Recessive	1,100	Slight [a]		Few	[a]
Chromosomal aberrations	6,000	38	40	<10	[b]
Total	107,100	63	185	5–75	60–1,100
Percent of current incidence		0.06	0.17	0.005–0.07	0.06–1.0

[a]Very slow increase.
[b]Increases only slightly.
Source: Modified from Gibbs et al. [1].

Table 8-3. Equations relating increased cancer incidence to dose of radiation

Linear model	$(1) I = \alpha_0 + \alpha_1 D$
Quadratic model	$(2) I = \alpha_0 + \alpha_1 D^2$
Linear quadratic model	$(3) I = \alpha_0 + \alpha_1 D + \alpha_2 D^2$

I = cancer incidence; D = dose; α_0 = spontaneous cancer incidence; α_1, α_2 = constants.

Table 8-4. Annual risk rates in the United States population from various causes

Event	Chance of injury or death per year
Auto accident (disability)	1/100
Cancer (all types and causes)	1/700
Cancer (from smoking)	1/2,000
Auto death	1/4,000
Fire death	1/25,000
"Pill" death	1/25,000
Drowning	1/30,000
Electrocution	1/200,000
Airplane trip (from New York City to San Francisco and return)	1/1,000,000
Reactor emanation site boundary (5–10 millirems per year)	<1/1,000,000
Average for population within 50 miles of reactor	<1/10,000,000

Source: Modified from Bond [2].

women treated with therapeutic x-rays for post-partum mastitis [11]. There are many other examples of cancer caused by high-dose ionizing radiation [12,13].

The association between cancer and exposure to low-dose radiation is much more difficult to establish. Since the ratio of cancers caused by low-dose radiation to naturally occurring cancers is so small, very large populations are required for statistically accurate data. Gibbs cites a number of articles [14–18] that report a statistically significant association between diagnostic x-ray exposure and leukemia [1]. However, he also cites other articles [19,20] that failed to confirm any correlation. Furthermore, those retrospective studies that did show an association did not show cause and effect. In many instances, the x-ray exam may have been necessary because of underlying illness associated with undiagnosed leukemia. Also, as with all retrospective studies, the studies cited above were subject to sampling bias, and genetic predisposition probably plays a role (see Chap. 7).

Since human data from low-dose radiation exposure are inconclusive, it is necessary to extrapolate from high-dose data. The equations that must be used to facilitate the extrapolation evoke considerable disagreement. Three equations have been proposed to relate the increased incidence of cancer to dose of radiation (Table 8-3). Although arguments exist supporting or refuting each model, the BEIR III committee selected the linear quadratic model [8].

There appears to be general agreement that the cancer risk from low-dose radiation is quite small. Bond and UNSCEAR suggest that a maximum of eight additional cancers per 1,000,000 people (or 1 per 125,000) would occur as a result of exposures to 1 rad [2,9]. For interest and comparison, Table 8-4 shows the chance of serious injury or death per year to the United States population from various activities [2].

THE EMBRYO AND FETUS

Most of the preceding presentation has dealt with the risk of low-dose radiation to adult humans or animals. The risk to the developing embryo or fetus is another matter. There are several reasons why the embryo or fetus is more sensitive to radiation: (1) Rapidly dividing cells or rapidly growing tissue is more sensitive to radiation. (2) Damage to or death of a few cells in a developing embryo may produce a marked effect in the fetus, at term. (3) Radiation exposure to the fetus is, frequently, to the whole body.

Genetic Risk

The time, during gestation, when radiation exposure occurs is critical. The first trimester (during organogenesis) represents the greatest risk. Most of the available data have been extrapolated from animals to humans. Also, most of the animal radiation exposures were in the high-dose range of 50 to 200 rads [21]. Some human data, from high-dose exposure to the fetus at different times during gestation, do exist. These data were obtained from women who received radiation therapy for cancer or from women exposed to the atomic bomb blast in Japan during pregnancy [22–29].

There has been good correlation between animal and human data. Brent cites several reports of fetal exposure to 100 rads or more, in the first trimester [30]. The effects most commonly seen were microcephaly, eye anomalies, and intra-uterine growth retardation. Most of the micro-cephalic children were mentally retarded. Included with eye anomalies were microphthalmia, cataracts, strabismus, retinal degeneration, and

Table 8-5. A compilation of the effects of 10 rads or less
*acute radiation at various stages of gestation in rat and mouse**

	Stage of gestation (days)				
	Preimplantation	Implantation	Early organogenesis	Late organogenesis	Fetal stages
Mouse	0–4½	4½–6½	6½–8½	8½–12	12–18
Rat	0–5½	5½–8	8–10	10–13	13–22
Corresponding human gestation period	0–9	9–14	15–28	28–50	50–280
Lethality	+	−	−	−	−
Growth retardation at term	−	−	−	−	−
Growth retardation as adult	−	−	−	−	−
Gross malformations (aplasia, hyperplasia, absence of over-growth of organs or tissues)	±	−	−	−	−
Cell depletions, minimal but measurable tissue hypoplasia	−	−	−	−	−
Sterility	−	−	−	−	−
Significant increase in germ cell mutations	±	±	±	±	±
Cytogenic abnormalities	−	−	−	−	−
Neuropathology	−	−	−	−	−
Tumor induction	−	−	±	±	±
Behavior disorders	−	−	−	−	−
Reduction in life-span	−	−	−	−	−

*Dose fractionation or protraction effectively reduces the biologic result of all the pathologic effects reported in this table.
−, no observed effect; ±, questionable but reported or suggested effect; +, demonstrated effect.
Source: Brent [30].

optic atrophy. No visceral, limb, or other abnormalities were found unless the child exhibited intrauterine growth retardation, microcephaly, or readily apparent eye malformations. It is likely, therefore, that the isolated limb or visceral defect occurred independently of the radiation exposure, or that the increased risk of these isolated defects from high-dose radiation exposure is slight.

Several mechanisms have been postulated to explain radiation effects on the embryo. These mechanisms include cell death, mitotic delay, abnormalities of cell migration, and alteration in macromolecular structure. One or more mechanisms may be operative at different stages of embryo development. For example, prior to the blastocyst stage, when the embryo is a multicellular organism, cell death or death of the embryo is the major result with little or no growth retardation or teratogenic effects. During organogenesis the embryo is very sensitive to teratogenic effects or growth retardation but less likely to suffer cell or embryonic death. Tables 8-5 and 8-6 show the effects of 10 rads and 100 rads, respectively, on development at various stages of gestation in the rat and mouse (the corresponding human gestational period is included). On the basis of these data Brent maintains that the hazards of radiation exposure in the range of diagnostic roentgenology (0.02–5.0 rads) present an extremely low risk to the embryo when compared to spontaneous events.

Cancer Risk

Stewart et al. [31–34] and others [14,16,17] found that 1 to 2 rads of exposure, in utero, increased the risk of leukemia in the offspring by a factor of 1.5 to 2.0 over the natural incidence. However, Kato studied 1,300 people, who received in utero exposure to radiation from the atomic bomb. There was no increase in malignancy in 24 years of follow-up in this group [35].

Miller found the incidence of leukemia in non-radiation-exposed siblings of leukemic children to be 1 per 720 [36]. This incidence exceeds the 1 in 2,000 risk for leukemia following pelvimetry exposure and the 1 in 3,000 risk for leukemia in the

Table 8-6. A compilation of the effects of 100 rads acute radiation on embryonic development at various stages of gestation in rat and mouse*

	Stage of gestation (days)				
	Preimplan- tation	Implan- tation	Early organogenesis	Late organogenesis	Fetal stages
Mouse	0–4½	4½–6½	6½–8½	8½–12	12–18
Rat	0–5½	5½–8	8–10	10–13	13–22
Corresponding human gestation period	0–9	9–14	15–28	28–50	50–280
Lethality	+ + +	+	+ +	±	−
Growth retardation at term	−	+	+ + +	+ +	+
Growth retardation as adult	−	+	+ +	+ + +	+ +
Gross malformations (aplasia, hypoplasia, absence or over- growth of organs or tissues)	−	−	+ + +	+	−
Cell depletions, minimal but measurable tissue hypoplasia	−	−	±	+ +	+
Sterility	−	−	±	−	+ +
Significant increase in germ cell mutations	±	±	±	±	±
Cytogenic abnormalities	±			+	+
Cataracts	−	−	+	+	+
Neuropathology	−	−	+ + +	+ +	+
Tumor induction	−	−	±	±	±
Behavioral disorders	−	−	+	+	±
Reduction in life-span	−	−	−	−	−

*Dose fractionation or protraction effectively reduced the biologic result of all the pathologic effects reported in this table.
−, no observed effect; ±, questionable but reported or suggested effect; +, demonstrated effect, + +, readily appar-ent effect; + + +, occurs in high incidence.
Source: Brent [30].

general population of children. These data suggest that factors other than radiation exposure account for the high incidence of leukemia in siblings. Fur-thermore, animal studies show that exposure of pregnant mice, at varying times in gestation, to high doses (30–100 rads) of x-irradiation failed to produce an increased incidence of tumors in the offspring [30,37–39].

SOURCES OF LOW-DOSE RADIATION

The major sources of low-dose radiation exposure include standard diagnostic radiographic proce-dures, such as barium enemas, upper gastrointesti-nal and excretory urography series, CT scans, and diagnostic nuclear medicine procedures, such as lung, bone, and biliary scans. Table 8-7 lists the ap-proximate gonadal and fetal exposure from vari-ous diagnostic procedures [1]. This table does not include the radiation exposure from fluoroscopy.

Fluoroscopy, as part of a radiographic proce-dure, contributes a significant exposure to the maternal ovaries and fetus, particularly with pro-cedures such as hysterosalpingography and bar-ium enema. A reasonable estimate of fluoroscopy dose to fetus and ovaries can be made with the fol-lowing assumptions [45]: (1) fluoroscopy gener-ated by 80 to 90 kV, (2) fetus and maternal ovaries at an average depth of about 10 cm from skin sur-face, (3) skin dose about 1 rad per minute per mil-liampere, (4) dose to fetus–maternal ovaries ap-proximately 10 to 20% of skin dose. Thus, a hys-terosalpingogram using x photons generated by 80 kV, 2 milliamperes, and 1 minute fluoroscopy time would deliver approximately 0.2 to 0.4 rad to the fetus and maternal ovaries.

The calculation of dose to the fetus and maternal ovaries from the administration of radionuclides is complicated. Although the uterus containing the fetus is close to the maternal ovaries, the dose to each may differ, depending, in large part, on two factors: (1) Most of the radiopharmaceuticals ad-

*Table 8-7. Ovarian and embryonic
exposure from diagnostic radiology*

Examination	Number of films*	Dose in millirads (mrads)	
		Ovaries	Embryo
Chest	1.5	0.06	0.06
Skull	4.1	<0.01	<0.01
Cervical spine	3.7	<0.01	<0.01
Ribs	3.0	0.4	0.4
Shoulder	1.8	<0.01	<0.01
Thoracic spine	2.1	1.0	0.1
Cholecystogram	3.2	6.0	5.0
Lumbar spine	2.9	400	410
Upper GI	4.3	45	50
KUB	1.7	210	260
Barium enema	4.0	790	820
Lumbosacral spine	3.4	640	640
IVP	5.5	640	820
Pelvis	1.3	150	200
Hip	2.0	80	130
Mammography	2.0	<0.01	<0.01
Urethrocystogram		1,500†	NA
Hysterosalpingo-gram		590†	NA
Dental	1.0	0.01	NA
CT scan brain	5.0	7.0	NA
CT scan abdomen	5.0	40	NA

NA = data not available.
*Average number of films per study.
†Majority of dose from fluoroscopy.
Source: Gibbs et al. [1].

*Table 8-8. Thyroidal
radioiodine ^{131}I exposure of the fetus*

Gestation period	Fetal/maternal ratio (thyroid gland)	Dose to thyroid (fetus) (rad/μCi ^{131}I)
10–12 wk	—	0.001 (precursor)
12–13 wk	1.2	0.7
2nd trimester	1.8	6.0
3rd trimester	7.5	—
Birth imminent	—	8.0

Source: Kereiakes et al. [47].

ministered are partially eliminated from the body via the urinary tract. Since the urinary bladder is much nearer to the uterus than it is to the ovaries, the dose to the uterus and fetus is greater. (2) The human placenta transports different radionuclides variably. There are no human data for transport of radionuclides across the placenta early in pregnancy. Animal data, cited by Husak and Wiedermann, showed no placental passage early in pregnancy of ^{67}Ga citrate and the bone-scanning agents but there was passage of ^{99m}Tc pertechnetate [46]. Later in pregnancy, when the placenta is well formed, some radiopharmaceuticals will cross the placenta. Iodide crosses the placenta beginning at 12 to 13 weeks' gestation and is trapped by the fetal thyroid, with increasing efficiency. At term the radiation dose to the fetal thyroid can be eight times that to the maternal thyroid (Table 8-8) [47].

Winter et al. demonstrated radioactivity in the bladder of a 31-week human fetus after injection of 3 mCi of ^{99m}Tc pyridoxylideneglutamate, a biliary scanning agent, into the mother [48]. Gaulden and Datz (unpublished data) imaged the epiphyses of a 30-week fetus after the injection of 10 mCi of ^{99m}Tc MDP, a bone-scanning agent, into the mother [49]. The doses to the fetus shown in Table 8-9 were calculated on the assumption of no placental transfer [46,47].

RADIONUCLIDES IN BREAST MILK
Nursing mothers may need diagnostic nuclear medicine studies, such as lung, biliary, and bone scans. It is known that ^{99m}Tc and ^{131}I are secreted in human breast milk [50–54]. Wyburn accurately measured the quantities of these isotopes in breast milk over a period of 230 hours after administration of 200 μCi of ^{131}I-MAA (lung-scanning agent), 12 mCi ^{99m}Tc pertechnetate, and 10 mCi of ^{99m}Tc EDTA [55]. On the basis of his findings and recommendations from the International Commission on Radiological Protection (ICRP), he stated that in the case of the ^{131}I-MAA, breast-feeding should be interrupted for 10 to 12 days. Following ^{99m}Tc EDTA, 20 to 32 hours' interruption was sufficient [55,56]. Currently, in nuclear medicine, ^{131}I is used very little for imaging while ^{99m}Tc-labeled compounds are used almost exclusively. Although data concerning secretion in breast milk of all ^{99m}Tc-labeled pharmaceuticals are not available, it would seem reasonable to assume similar data for them and to advise interruption of breast-feeding for 48 hours. A breast pump can be used to maintain the flow of milk during this period. ^{67}Ga citrate, used for detecting infection and neoplasm, tends to concentrate in breast tissue, particularly

Table 8-9. Dose to ovaries and embryo from various nuclear medicine procedures

Radiopharmaceutical	Study	Dose to Ovaries (mrad/μCi)	Embryo
^{67}Ga citrate	Tumor and abscess imaging	0.26	0.25*
^{99m}Tc DPTA	Brain and renal imaging	0.027	0.035*
^{99m}Tc glucoheptonate	Brain and renal imaging	0.007	0.034*
^{99m}Tc albumin	Blood pool and cardiovascular imaging	0.015	
^{99m}Tc HIDA	Hepatobiliary imaging	0.050	
^{99m}Tc aggregate (microsphere and macroaggregated albumin)	Lung perfusion imaging	0.009	0.035
^{99m}Sodium pertechnetate	Brain and thyroid imaging	0.017	0.037
^{99m}Tc phosphates	Bone and myocardial infarct imaging	0.046	0.036
^{99m}Tc sulfur colloid	Liver, spleen, and bone marrow imaging	0.023	0.032
^{111}In DPTA	Cisternogram	0.07	
^{133}Xe gas	Ventilation lung scanning	0.26	
^{201}Tl chloride	Myocardial imaging	0.39	
^{131}I hippurate	Renogram renal imaging	0.30	
^{131}I sodium iodide	Thyroid uptake and imaging (15% uptake in mother)	0.25	0.100
^{123}I sodium iodide	Thyroid uptake and imaging (15% uptake in mother)	0.025	0.032

*From Kereiakes et al. [47].
From Husak and Weidermann [46].

in lactating women. Although no data are available, with this agent it would seem prudent to stop breast-feeding permanently, since gallium might be secreted in breast milk for as long as 30 to 40 days.

THERAPEUTIC RADIATION
Occasionally, the fetus is exposed to high-dose radiation from the treatment of pelvic or abdominal cancer during pregnancy. The dose to the fetus in these cases may be several hundred rads. Each case must be individually evaluated. Although therapeutic abortion is generally recommended, there are anecdotal cases reporting the birth of a normal infant. Normal outcome has been reported after irradiation dosage of 680 rads in pregnancy, with the irradiated fetus subsequently fathering a normal infant 24 years later [57].

COUNSELING FOR RADIATION EXPOSURE
A systematic approach is vital. Brent [30] recommends that the following information be obtained and documented:

1. Stage of pregnancy at time of exposure
2. Menstrual history
3. Previous pregnancy history
4. History of congenital malformations
5. Other potential environmental factors present during this pregnancy
6. Age of mother and father
7. Type of radiation study and dates and numbers of studies performed
8. Calculation of embryonic exposure by a medical physicist or radiologist
9. State of this pregnancy: wanted or unwanted
10. Evaluation of this information. Arriving at decision by both patient and counselor
11. Placing a summary of the information provided and a statement that the patient has been informed that something may go wrong with the pregnancy in the medical record; also, documenting that no one has guaranteed a normal outcome to the pregnancy
12. Use of amniocentesis and ultrasound to evaluate the fetus considered on a case-by-case basis

The overwhelming body of opinion is that an exposure of 5 rads or less to the fetus produces no significant increased risk of genetic or somatic damage and no significant increased risk of malignancy later in life. Most diagnostic studies result in fetal doses of less than 2 rads. Therefore, the pa-

Table 8-10. Dose to fetus and ovaries
in example case (approximated dose in mrad)

Study	Ovaries	Fetus
KUB	124	153
Cholecystogram	6	5
HIDA scan	400	500*
Barium enema	790	820
Fluoroscopy	300	300
Upper GI	40	50
Total mrads	1,660	1,828
Rads	1.66	1.83

*Estimated from the dose to the ovaries.

tient should be reassured and may continue the pregnancy if the exposure to the fetus is less than 5 rads. A hypothetical case is given to demonstrate estimation of radiation dose.

A 23-year-old married female with abdominal pain had a single supine film. This was followed by an oral cholecystogram, which showed slight opacification of the gallbladder, and no stones. A radionuclide scan of the biliary tract was done using 8 mCi of ^{99m}Tc HIDA. Because these studies were normal, a barium enema and a GI series were performed. Two minutes of fluoroscopy was required for the barium enema, with one minute of that time including the uterus and ovaries. Approximately 1½ minutes of fluoroscopy was required for the upper GI series. The ovaries and uterus were not in the field during any of that time.

Subsequently, the young woman was found to be pregnant and was estimated to have been in approximately the third week of gestation when the diagnostic studies were done. The radiation exposure to maternal ovaries and fetus are tabulated in Table 8-10. Despite the number of studies, the total exposure was less than 2 rads.

Animal and human data support the conclusion that no increase in abortion, intrauterine growth retardation, or gross congenital malformation results from radiation exposures below 5 rads [42, 58], and probably below 10 rads. Diagnostic roentgenographic and nuclear medicine studies can be done when there is a definite medical indication. Since the approximate incidence of spontaneous abortion is 10 to 15%, major congenital malformations at term 2.5 to 3.0%, intrauterine growth retardation 4%, and early- or late-onset genetic disease 10 to 11%, the added risk of diagnostic radiation exposure is small [30]. Nevertheless, minimizing radiation exposure during pregnancy is always prudent. Diagnostic studies should be postponed until a diagnosis of early pregnancy can be excluded, if at all possible. An attempt to choose an appropriate time in pregnancy to perform diagnostic radiologic studies is spurious since the effects can be undetected or significantly delayed, and patient susceptibility and threshold undoubtedly plays a role. The "safety" of the first ten days following a menstrual period also does not ensure that radiation will have no biologic effect [40].

Exposing a pregnant or potentially pregnant woman to radiation should always be done with careful thought. If, with equally satisfactory results, the risk of radiation exposure could be avoided by choosing a nonradiation procedure, the latter should be used. On the other hand, because of the low risk of diagnostic procedures to the developing embryo or fetus, this potentially valuable diagnostic tool should not be withheld because of irrational fears of fetal injury [41–44].

REFERENCES

1. Gibbs JS, et al. Radiation risks in medical practice, Dept of Radiology and Radiologic Sciences, Vanderbilt Univ. School of Medicine. Work in progress.
2. Bond VP. A basis for estimating the risks of low-level radiation. In: Fullerton GD, Kopp DT, Waggener RG, Webster EW, eds. Biological risks of medical irradiations. Medical Physics Monograph 5. New York: American Institute of Physics, 1980:21–32.
3. Webster EW. Estimates of cancer risks from low-level exposure to ionizing radiation: the BEIR report 1980. In: Fullerton GD, Kopp DT, Waggener RG, Webster EW, eds. Biological risks of medical irradiations. Medical Physics Monograph. New York: American Institute of Physics, 1980:55–77.
4. Loewe WE, Mendelsohn E. Revised dose estimates at Hiroshima and Nagasaki. Health Phys. 1981; 41:663–6.
5. Land CE. Estimating cancer risks from low doses of ionizing radiation. Science. 1980; 209:1197–1203.
6. Selby PB. Genetic effects of low-level irradiation. In: Fullerton GD, Kopp DT, Waggener RG, Webster EW, eds. Biological risks of medical irradiations. Medical Physics Monograph 5. New York: American Institute of Physics, 1980:1–20.
7. Schull WJ, Otake M, Neel JV. Genetic effects of the atomic bombs; a reappraisal. Science. 1981; 213:1220–7.
8. National Research Council. Committee on the Biological Effects of Ionizing Radiations. The effects on populations of exposure to low levels of ionizing radiation. Washington, D.C.: National Academy Press, 1980.
9. United Nations Scientific Committee on the Effects of Atomic Radiation Sources and Effects of Ionizing Radiation. Report to the General Assembly, 1977.
10. Brown WM, Doll R. Mortality from cancer and other causes after radiotherapy for ankylosing spondylitis. Br Med J. 1965; 2:1327–32.

11. Mettler FA, Hempelmann LH, Dutton AM, et al. Breast neoplasms in women treated with x-rays for acute postpartum mastitis. J Natl Cancer Inst. 1969; 43:803–11.

12. Cloutier RJ. Florence Kelley and the radium dial painters. Health Phys. 1980; 39:711–6.

13. Beebe GW, Kato H, Land CE. Studies of the mortality of A-bomb survivors: 6. mortality and radiation dose, 1950–1974. Radiat Res. 1978; 75:138–201.

14. Polhemus DW, Koch R. Leukemia and medical radiation. Pediatrics. 1959; 23:453–61.

15. Stewart A, Pennybacker W, Barber R. Adult leukaemias and diagnostic x-rays. Br Med J. 1962; 2:882–90.

16. Graham S, Levin ML, Lilienfeld AM, et al. Preconception, intrauterine, and postnatal irradiation as related to leukemia. Natl Cancer Inst Monogr. 1966; 19:347–71.

17. Gibson R, Graham S, Lilienfeld A, Schumann L, Dowd JE, Levin ML. Irradiation in the epidemiology of leukemia among adults. J Natl Cancer Inst. 1972; 48:301–11.

18. Bross ID, Ball M, Falen S. A dosage response curve for the one rad range: adult risks from diagnostic radiation. Am J Public Health. 1979; 69:130–6.

19. Boice JD, Land CE. Adult leukemia following diagnostic x-rays. Am J Pub Health. 1979; 69:137–45.

20. Ginevan ME. Nonlymphatic leukemias and adult exposure to diagnostic X-rays: the evidence reconsidered. Health Phys. 1980; 38:129–38.

21. Russell LB. Irradiation damage to the embryo, fetus and neonate. In: Fullerton GD, Kopp DT, Waggener RG, Webster EW, eds. Biological risks of medical irradiations. Medical Physics Monograph 5. New York: American Institute of Physics, 1980:33–54.

22. Dekaban AS. Abnormalities in children exposed to x-radiation during various stages of gestation: tentative timetable of radiation injury to the human fetus. J Nucl Med. 1968; 9:471–7.

23. Goldstein L, Murphy DP. Etiology of ill-health in children born after maternal pelvic irradiation; defective children born after postconception pelvic irradiation. Am J Roentgenol. 1929; 22:322–31.

24. Goldstein L, Murphy DP. Microcephalic idiocy following radium therapy for uterine cancer during pregnancy. Am J Obstet Gynecol. 1929; 18:189–95.

25. Miller RW. Delayed radiation effects in atomic-bomb survivors. Science. 1969; 166:569–74.

26. Miller RW, Mulvihill JJ. Small head size after atomic irradiation. Teratology. 1976; 14:355–7.

27. Yamazaki JN, Wright SW, Wright PM. Outcome of pregnancy in women exposed to the atomic bomb in Nagasaki. Am J Dis Child. 1954; 87:448–63.

28. Wood JW, Johnson KG, Omori Y. In utero exposure to the Hiroshima atomic bomb. An evaluation of head size and mental retardation: twenty years later. Pediatrics. 1967; 39:385–392.

29. Wood JW, Johnson KG, Omori Y, Kawamoto S, Keehn RJ. Mental retardation in children exposed in utero to the atomic bombs in Hiroshima and Nagasaki. Am J Public Health. 1967; 57:1381–9.

30. Brent R. Teratogenic and carcinogenic effects of in utero irradiation. In: Bolognese RJ, Schwarz RH, Schneider J, eds. Perinatal medicine. 2nd ed. Baltimore: Williams & Wilkins, 1982:85–107.

31. Stewart A. The carcinogenic effects of low level radiation. A re-appraisal of epidemiologists' methods and observations. Health Phys. 1973; 24:223–40.

32. Stewart A, Kneale GW. Radiation dose effects in relation to obstetric x-rays and childhood cancers. Lancet. 1970; 1:1185–8.

33. Stewart A, Webb J, Giles D, Hewitt D. Malignant disease in childhood and diagnostic irradiation in utero. Lancet. 1956; 2:447.

34. Stewart A, Webb J, Hewitt D. A survey of childhood malignancies. Br Med J. 1958; 1:1495–508.

35. Kato H. Mortality in children exposed to the A-bombs while in utero. Am J Epidemiol. 1971; 93:435–42.

36. Miller RW. Epidemiological conclusions from radiation toxicity studies. In: Fry RJM, Grahan D, Griem ML, Rust JH. Late effects of radiation. London: Taylor and Francis 1970.

37. Rugh R, Duhamel L, Skaredoff L. Relation of embryonic and fetal x-irradiation to life time average weights and tumor incidence in mice. Proc Soc Exp Biol Med. 1966; 121:714–8.

38. Brent RL, Bolden BT. The long term effects of low dosage embryonic irradiation. Radiat Res. 1961; 14:453–4. Abstract.

39. Brent RL, Bolden BT. Indirect effect of x-irradiation on embryonic development: utilization of high doses of maternal irradiation on the first day of gestation. Radiat Res. 1968; 36:563–70.

40. International Commission on Radiological Protection. Protection of the patient in X-ray diagnosis. ICRP Publication 16. New York: Pergamon Press, 1970.

41. Gray JE. The radiation hazard—let's put it in perspective. Mayo Clin Proc. 1979; 54:809–13.

42. Mole RH. Radiation effects on pre-natal development and their radiological significance. Br J Radiol. 1979; 52:89–101.

43. Executive Board, American College of Obstetricians and Gynecologists. Statement of Policy, May, 1977.

44. American College of Radiology. ACR policy on x-ray exams on fertile pregnant women. Radiol Times. December, 1977; p. 15.

45. Personal communication, William R. Hendee, PhD, Head, Department Radiology, University of Colorado Medical Center, Denver, Colorado.

46. Husak V, Weidermann M. Radiation absorbed dose estimates to the embryo from some nuclear medicine procedures. Eur J Nucl Med. 1980; 5:205–7.

47. Kereiakes JG, Thomas SR, Gelfand MJ, Maxon HR, Saenger EL. Dose evaluation in nuclear medicine. In: Fullerton GD, Kopp DT, Waggener RG, Webster EW, eds. Biological risks of medical irradiations. Medical Physics Monograph 5. New York: American Institute of Physics, 1980:125–53.

48. Winter W, Verdegaal W, Esseveld M, et al. Radio-nuclide fetal imaging. Eur J Nucl Med. 1979; 4:309–11.

49. Gaulden M. Comment. In: Fullerton GD, Kopp DT, Waggener RG, Webster EW, eds. Biological risks of medical irradiations. Medical Physics Monograph 5. New York: American Institute of Physics, 1980:282.

50. Honour AJ, Myant NB, Rowlands EN. Secretion of radioiodine in digestive juices and milk in man. Clin Sci. 1952; 11:449–62.

51. Miller H, Weetch RS. Excretion of radioactive iodine in human milk. Lancet. 1955; 2:1013.

52. Nurnberger CE, Lipscomb A. Transmission of radioiodine (I^{131}) to infants through human maternal milk. JAMA. 1952; 150:1398–1400.

53. Karialainen P, Penttila IM, Pystynen P. The amount and form of radioactivity in human milk after lung scanning, renography and placental localization by ^{131}I labelled tracers. Acta Obstet Gynecol Scand. 1971; 50:357–61.

54. Vagenakis AG, Abreau CM, Braverman LE. Duration of radioactivity in the milk of a nursing mother following ^{99m}Tc administration. J Nucl Med. 1971; 12:188.

55. Wyburn JR. Human breast milk excretion of radionuclides following administration of radiopharmaceuticals. J Nucl Med. 1973; 14:115–7.

56. International Commission on Radiological Protection (ICRP) Publication 9. London: Pergamon Press, 1966.

57. Kallinger W, Granninger W. The effect of a high gamma dose on a human foetus. Health Phys. 1979; 36:1–6.

58. Kalter H, Warkany J. Congenital malformations. Etiologic factors and their role in prevention I. N Engl J Med. 1983; 308:424–31.

The light of a candle is useful when it precedes you; it is useless when it trails behind.
—Talmud

9. CLINICAL CHEMISTRY
John E. Meyer

In recent years there has been a rapid and frequently bewildering expansion of laboratory capabilities in the United States and other countries. As the technical capability of measuring increasing numbers of blood constituents has developed, so too has the demand to apply this ability to both asymptomatic and symptomatic patients. In addition to the complete blood count (CBC) and urinalysis, the physician is now faced with the interpretation of the biochemical survey, which is often an additional component in the evaluation of a patient's health status.

Although values for normal range or reference intervals are usually provided with the patient results, the clinician must remember several important aspects of laboratory testing prior to interpreting any results. In most laboratories, the normal range is established by determining the level of the anylate in question in a series of individuals who are clinically felt to be free of disease. Blood donors are frequently used in this process. The mean of all of the measurements, plus or minus two standard deviations, then becomes the normal range. With this method, 95% of the healthy population should fall into this range, providing the population sampled was representative of the population as a whole. One would then expect 5% of the healthy people in this population to have values outside the range, and thus to be abnormal, even though they are clinically normal. As more tests are performed on the same patient, there is an increasing chance that the patient will have at least one abnormal result. For example, if 10 tests are performed, 40% of the healthy population would be expected to have at least one abnormal value. If 20 tests are performed, this figure rises to 64%.

In addition to being statistically imperfect, the establishment of normal ranges fails to take into account many preanalytic sources of variation, which are too numerous to fully evaluate in this chapter. Examples include variations due to exercise, stress, circadian rhythms, position of the subject when blood is drawn, relation to meals, prolonged tourniquet application, age, sex, and race.

Pregnancy, a physiologically altered but not abnormal state, is another important cause of variation in laboratory results from the stated normal ranges. A complete discussion of changes in blood constituents due to pregnancy is not possible in one brief chapter, but a general review of some of the more commonly ordered tests will be offered. This should save the busy and concerned physician from pursuing a lengthy evaluation of an isolated abnormal value, as well as alert him or her to the possibility that in some instances results in the normal range might actually be abnormal in the pregnant state.

The discussion will center around what might be considered a representative biochemical panel, the complete blood count and other hematologic measurements, and selected, specialized tests. The chapter is meant to serve as a resource for quick reference. A more detailed discussion of the physiology underlying the described changes can be found in the remaining chapters.

COMPLETE BLOOD COUNT AND OTHER HEMATOLOGIC MEASUREMENTS
Alterations in Blood Volume

Changes in blood volume throughout pregnancy partially explain changes in various blood constituents. It is clear that increases in plasma volume begin to be seen early in gestation and continue until 34 to 38 weeks, when a plateau is reached. Although plasma volume has traditionally been felt to decrease slightly in the last several weeks of pregnancy, there is evidence that this observed decrease may be due to procedural errors in measuring plasma volume. The maximum increase in plasma volume during pregnancy is variable from individual to individual, ranging from 25 to 80% of nonpregnant values (630–1,940 mL) [1]. The magnitude of increase may be related to the size of the fetus [1], the size of the mother [2], or parity. Twin pregnancies are associated with a larger increase in plasma volume.

Red cell volume also changes throughout pregnancy [10]. Taylor and Lind observed a decrease in red cell volume during the first trimester (av 100 mL), which was followed by a progressive increase thereafter [3]. An average rise of 180 mL of red cells was seen in 45 women. When folate and iron were given, this increment was 350 to 450 mL. The mechanism for the decrease early in pregnancy is poorly understood, but the subsequent increase is associated with increasing levels of erythropoietin. The stimulus for increased erythropoietin production is unknown.

Changes in Hemoglobin Concentration and Hematocrit

Hemoglobin concentration gradually decreases during pregnancy, and by late in gestation (36 weeks) values may drop to as low as 11 gm/dL [4,5]. If iron supplements are given, the decrease is less apparent, with mean values at 36 weeks being 12.66 gm/dL, as compared to average nonpregnant values of 13.5 gm/dL [3]. The hematocrit also decreases throughout pregnancy, reaching values of 35% at 36 weeks compared to a nonpregnant average of 39%. When iron therapy is given, the decrease is not so pronounced, reaching levels of 36% at 36 weeks. Hemoglobin levels of less than 11 gm/dL generally represent anemia during pregnancy and should be further investigated.

Changes in Red Cell Count

Red cell counts decrease from nonpregnant values of $4.6 \times 10^6/mm^3$ to $3.88 \times 10^6/mm^3$ at 36 weeks' gestation. This drop can begin as early as the first 12 weeks of pregnancy in women not receiving iron [3].

Changes in Red Cell Indices

Taylor and Lind have observed minimal increases in red cell volume (MCV) in pregnant women receiving iron supplements. In their series MCV averaged 89 μm^3 for pregnant women receiving supplemental iron compared to 86 μm^3 for pregnant women not receiving iron and 87 μm^3 in nonpregnant controls [4].

Neither the mean cell hemoglobin (MCH) nor the mean cell hemoglobin concentration (MCHC) changes significantly as a consequence of normal pregnancy [4].

Changes in White Blood Cell and Differential Counts

Leukocytosis has long been regarded as part of normal pregnancy, particularly late in gestation [7]. Kuvin and Brecher studied 88 normal pregnant women and found only 20% to have a white blood cell (WBC) of higher than 10,000 [6]. Whether or not the WBC is elevated, clinically normal pregnant women appear to have frequent abnormalities in the differential count. Myelocytes or metamyelocytes were found in 25% of this series of patients, which included both patients with a WBC above and patients with a WBC below 10,000. Total WBC rarely exceeds 12,000 during normal pregnancy.

Changes in Platelet Count

Some investigators have described increases in platelet counts during pregnancy; however, Pitkin and Witte [7] described progressively decreasing platelet counts throughout pregnancy in 23 women. The decrease (from initial mean of $322,000/mm^3$ in the first trimester to a mean of $278,000/mm^3$ in the third trimester) still left these patients within what is usually considered the normal range ($250,000–400,000/mm^3$). Platelet function does not change during normal gestation.

Serum Iron and Iron-Binding Capacity

Since serum iron levels vary considerably in nonpregnant, normal women (as much as 25–30% depending on time of day, menstrual cycle, etc.), the interpretation of iron levels in pregnancy is fraught with hazard [8]. Although iron levels have been documented to be higher in the first trimester in pregnant women than in nonpregnant controls, serum iron steadily decreases after the first trimester and reaches its lowest point in the third trimester [8,9]. At the same time, transferrin (iron-binding capacity) levels increase throughout pregnancy (60–90%), reaching the highest levels in the third trimester. The net effect of these changes is a decreased iron and percent saturation of transferrin, the pattern also seen in iron deficiency. Although specific levels of these anylates will vary depending on the method used in any given laboratory, in at least one study iron levels dropped from 90.9 μg per 100 dL to 56 μg per 100 dL during pregnancy [8]. For women treated with iron during pregnancy, decreases in serum iron and increases in transferrin are less pronounced.

Serum Ferritin

Several studies have documented a drop in serum ferritin during pregnancy. Ferritin is the storage form of iron, and serum levels are known to correlate with iron stores in the bone marrow. During pregnancy, ferritin levels increase by as much as 50% in the first trimester, after which they decrease, reaching a low point in the third trimester [9]. At their lowest levels, serum ferritin measurements may be in the range seen in iron deficiency (i.e., less than 20 ng/dL) even if the patient is not anemic. When supplemental iron is given, ferritin levels decrease throughout pregnancy but do not reach levels seen in iron deficiency. A ferritin level below 20 ng per mL should be considered evidence of iron deficiency whether or not the patient is anemic. It is clear from several studies that the finding of low ferritin levels in the presence of adequate hemoglobin levels (greater than 11 g/dL) is common during pregnancy [9].

Serum and Red Cell Folate
During early pregnancy, serum folate levels are comparable to those seen in nonpregnant controls. By 14 to 17 weeks, levels begin to decrease, and by term they have reached values averaging one-half of those found in nonpregnant women. Red cell folate concentrations are slightly lower than those seen in control subjects but the drop is not as marked as that observed in serum folate [11,12]. As a diagnostic tool to determine the presence of folate deficiency, red cell folate measurements are felt to be superior to serum folate measurements.

Vitamin B$_{12}$
B$_{12}$ levels generally decrease throughout pregnancy but do not reach deficient levels.

COAGULATION TESTS
Fibrinogen
Beginning at the end of the first trimester of pregnancy, fibrinogen levels gradually increase, reaching levels as high as 600 mg per deciliter. This change is due to increased synthesis [13].

Coagulation Factors
In the second and third trimesters factors VII and X are significantly increased to the 120 to 180% range. Factor VIII rises considerably as well, reaching levels of 200 to 300% by the third trimester. Slightly increased levels of factor IX are also seen. Antithrombin III levels remain normal or are slightly decreased during pregnancy [29].

Fibrin split products have been found to increase during pregnancy; however, there is no evidence of a generalized fibrinolysis [29].

In general, the routine coagulation screening tests, the activated partial thromboplastin time and prothrombin time, are not altered during normal pregnancy.

THE BIOCHEMICAL PANEL
The term biochemical panel means different combinations of tests to different physicians, depending on the capabilities of the hospital or reference lab being used. In this chapter the term will refer to a typical panel of tests offered at University of Colorado Health Sciences Center where it is referred to as the SMA-12. It includes the following tests: total protein, albumin, calcium, phosphorus, cholesterol, glucose, uric acid, creatinine, total bilirubin, alkaline phosphatase (ALP), lactic dehydrogenase (LDH), and SGOT (AST).

Total Protein and Albumin
Total protein concentrations fall during pregnancy, a phenomenon generally ascribed to hemodilution [15]. Several studies have documented an abrupt increase in protein prior to labor and a subsequent fall within 12 to 24 hours post partum. The latter is felt to be due to mobilization of extracellular fluid, which accumulates during pregnancy [14].

Albumin levels also decrease, although studies using radiolabeled albumin indicate that total body albumin and albumin synthesis are unchanged [16]. The concentration of albumin may drop as much as 25% [17,18].

Calcium
Total calcium levels fall during pregnancy, beginning shortly after conception and progressing until the third trimester [19,21]. This decrease is usually not marked, amounting to 5% of pregestation levels, and is probably related to decreased albumin. In contrast to total calcium, ionized calcium levels increase slightly (5%) as pregnancy progresses [20]. Some women show marked fluctuations in ionized calcium throughout pregnancy. Parathyroid hormone (PTH) becomes elevated by the third trimester of pregnancy, reaching levels up to 2.2 times those seen in the nonpregnant state [19]. This rise seems to parallel maximal calcification of the fetal skeleton. Persistent hypercalcemia in the presence of elevated PTH levels during pregnancy should suggest the possibility of hyperparathyroidism.

Phosphorus
Phosphorus decreases throughout early pregnancy by as much as 6% [19]. In the last trimester it may gradually rise to nonpregnant levels [22].

Cholesterol
Several studies have shown that serum total cholesterol decreases slightly early in pregnancy (first trimester), then increases throughout the second and third trimesters [23–25]. These changes have been shown to be unaffected by dietary manipulation. The baseline cholesterol value does not appear to affect this gradual increase since it is seen in women with low and high nonpregnant cholesterol levels.

Glucose

Maternal loss of glucose and gluconeogenic substrate to the fetus results in lowered fasting plasma glucose levels to 55 to 65 mg/dL, and a decrease in the mean plasma glucose to 80 to 87 mg/dL (whole blood values are approximately 15% lower than plasma values) [26]. Lowered fasting glucose levels persist throughout gestation, but fasting insulin levels may increase as much as 75% in response to the diabetogenic stress of pregnancy beginning around 24 weeks [27]. Criteria for altered glucose tolerance have been established by O'Sullivan and Mahan [28]. Their widely used standards defined an abnormal value following an oral 100-g glucose challenge as being more than two standard deviations above the mean from a large group of pregnant women with no features of potential diabetes. These criteria are listed in Chapter 11.

Reports vary regarding changes in concentrations of hemoglobin A_{1c} (HbA_{1c}) during normal pregnancy. Schwartz et al. could find no statistical difference in HbA_{1c} concentrations between nonpregnant normal women and pregnant normal women [30]. HbA_{1c} concentrations reflect mean blood glucose levels for the preceding 30 to 60 days and are proportionately elevated in gravidas with varying degrees of hyperglycemia. Most investigators agree that HbA_{1c} is not sensitive enough to serve as a screening test for gestational diabetes.

Uric Acid

There is an early decrease in the level of uric acid during pregnancy, but this constituent gradually increases as pregnancy progresses, approaching nonpregnant values by the time of delivery [31].

Creatinine

The serum creatinine decreases early in pregnancy up to the eighth week and thereafter remains stable. The magnitude of decrease varies but may be as much as 20% of the first-week value. Twenty-four-hour creatinine clearance increases dramatically during the first seven to ten weeks of pregnancy, with increases ranging from 20 to 80% above nonpregnant values [32,34]. Similar relative increases can be demonstrated in patients who have stable chronic renal disease, a normal single kidney, or even a transplanted kidney [33]. In addition to decreasing creatinine during pregnancy, urea (BUN) decreases early in pregnancy and remains at lower levels until term.

It is important for the clinician to be aware of these changes in renal function, since values considered normal for a nonpregnant woman may actually reflect renal impairment during pregnancy. It has been suggested that creatinine levels in excess of 0.8 mg per deciliter or BUN levels in excess of 13 mg per deciliter in the pregnant woman should alert the clinician to evaluate renal function further [35].

Bilirubin

Inconsistent variations in bilirubin level are seen in some women during pregnancy, but definite trends have not been documented. Serum bile acids (cholic and chenodeoxycholic acids) remain within normal levels throughout pregnancy [36,37].

Alkaline Phosphatase

The placenta is a well-known source of alkaline phosphatase, accounting for the increase in serum concentration of this enzyme during pregnancy. Placental alkaline phosphatase is responsible for 40 to 65% of the total serum levels in late pregnancy. The total alkaline phosphatase increase is seen most prominently in the third trimester and is generally higher than normal levels for most laboratories [38]. It should be noted that methods for measuring alkaline phosphatase (as well as many other enzymes) are not uniformly standardized; consequently, different methods may identify different fractions of alkaline phosphatase with varying degrees of efficiency. The clinician should be aware that differing results from different laboratories may or may not reflect a change in the clinical status of the patient [39].

Lactic Dehydrogenase

No consistent pattern of lactic dehydrogenase (LDH) change has been documented in pregnant women. Levels usually remain within the normal range, but some studies have discovered slightly elevated levels in late pregnancy in some women [31,38].

Aspartate Aminotransferase

Levels of aspartate aminotransferase (AST) (SGOT) remain in the normal range throughout pregnancy. The same is true of the other liver enzyme, glutamate pyruvate transaminase (SGPT), more recently referred to as alanine aminotransferase (ALT) [31].

OTHER CHEMICAL BLOOD CONSTITUENTS

Serum Electrolytes

Although serum sodium concentration decreases slightly during pregnancy, the quantity of change is so small that levels usually remain in the normal range given for nonpregnant women. Potassium also decreases slightly during pregnancy but remains in the normal range. Both sodium and potassium levels return to baseline values shortly after delivery [40].

The serum chloride levels do not change significantly during pregnancy. Bicarbonate concentrations decrease slightly [31,40].

Osmolality in the pregnant woman is lower by about 5 to 10 mOsm/kg than in the nonpregnant woman [40].

Other Commonly Measured Serum Enzymes

Creatine kinase (CK) decreases approximately 15% during early pregnancy when compared to nonpregnant values but returns to progestational levels during the second half of pregnancy [41]. This decrease is also seen in carriers of Duchenne muscular dystrophy. When screening for carriers of the disease, one should compare values to those seen in pregnant women at a comparable time in pregnancy.

Serum amylase is unchanged during pregnancy, but serum lipase decreases as much as 50%. Acid phosphatase is unaffected [31].

Thyroid Function Tests

As a result of estrogen-induced increase in thyroxine-binding globulin, total T_4 levels increase throughout pregnancy in a progressive manner. On the other hand, resin T_3 uptake decreases as the number of available binding sites increases. These offsetting changes cause the free thyroxine index (FTI) to remain constant in the euthyroid gravida [42,43]. Thyroid-stimulating hormone (TSH) levels do not change during normal pregnancy.

Serum Cortisol and ACTH

Although the circadian cortisol secretion patterns are preserved during pregnancy, serum cortisol concentrations are significantly higher when compared to those in nonpregnant women. In the third trimester, 8 A.M. mean values are as high as 40 mg/dL and 4 P.M. values as high as 20 to 25 mg/ml. Free serum cortisols follow a similar pattern [44].

Conversely, ACTH levels are decreased throughout pregnancy when compared to nonpregnant values although they are higher in late pregnancy than in earlier pregnancy. Several theories have been advanced, but the reason ACTH levels increase during pregnancy in the face of high serum cortisol levels is not clear [45].

REFERENCES

1. Hytten FE, Paintin DB. Increase in plasma volume during normal pregnancy. J Obstet Gynaecol Br Comm. 1963; 70:402–7.
2. Hutchins CJ. Plasma volume changes in pregnancy in Indian and European primigravidae. Br J Obstet Gynaecol. 1980; 87:586–9.
3. Taylor DJ, Lind T. Red cell mass during and after normal pregnancy. Br J Obstet Gynaecol. 1979; 86:364–70.
4. Taylor DJ, Lind T. Haematological changes during normal pregnancy: iron induced macrocytosis. Br J Obstet Gynaecol. 1976; 83:760–7.
5. Morgan EH. Plasma-iron and haemoglobin levels in pregnancy. Lancet. 1961; 1:9–12.
6. Kuvin SF, Brecher G. Differential neutrophil counts in pregnancy. N Engl J Med. 1962; 266:877–8.
7. Pitkin RM, Witte DL. Platelet and leukocyte counts in pregnancy. JAMA. 1979; 242:2696–8.
8. Zilva JF, Patston VJ. Variations in serum-iron in healthy women. Lancet. 1966; 1:459–62.
9. Puolakka J, Jänne O, Pakarinen A, Järvinen PA, Vihko R. Serum ferritin as a measure of iron stores during and after normal pregnancy with and without iron supplements. Acta Obstet Gynecol Scand [Suppl]. 1980; 95:43–51.
10. Chesley LC. Plasma and red cell volumes during pregnancy. Am J Obstet Gynecol. 1972; 112:440–50.
11. Landon MJ. Folate metabolism in pregnancy. Clin Obstet Gynaecol. 1975; 2:413–30.
12. Ek J, Magnus EM. Plasma and red blood cell folate during normal pregnancies. Acta Obstet Gynecol Scand. 1981; 60:247–51.
13. Bonnar J. Hemostatic function and coagulopathy during pregnancy. Obstet Gynecol Annu. 1978; 7:195–217.
14. Reboud P, Groulade J, Groslambert P, Colomb M. The influence of normal pregnancy and the postpartum state on plasma proteins and lipids. Am J Obstet Gynecol. 1963; 86:820–8.
15. Joseph JC, Baker C, Sprang ML, Bermes EW. Changes in plasma proteins during pregnancy. Ann Clin Lab Sci. 1978; 8:130–41.
16. Honger PE. Albumin metabolism in preeclampsia. Scand J Clin Lab Invest. 1968; 22:177–84.
17. Studd J. The plasma proteins in pregnancy. Clin Obstet Gynaecol. 1975; 2:285–300.
18. King JC. Protein metabolism in pregnancy. Clin Perinatol. 1975; 2:243–54.
19. Pitkin RM. Calcium metabolism in pregnancy: a review. Am J Obstet Gynecol. 1975; 121:724–37.
20. Fogh-Andersen N, Schultz-Larsen P. Free calcium ion concentration in pregnancy. Acta Obstet Gynecol Scand. 1981; 60:309–12.
21. Anast CS. Parathyroid hormone during pregnancy and effect on offspring. Prog Clin Biol Res. 1976; 10:235–48.
22. Watney PJ, Rudd BT. Calcium metabolism in pregnancy and in the newborn. J Obstet Gynaecol Br Comm. 1974; 81:210–9.

23. Green JG. Serum cholesterol changes in pregnancy. Am J Obstet Gynecol. 1966; 95:387–93.

24. De Alvarez RR, Gaiser DF, Simkins DM, Smith EK, Bratvold GE. Serial studies of serum lipids in normal human pregnancy. Am J Obstet Gynecol. 1959; 77:743–59.

25. Cramer K, Aurell M, Pehrson S. Serum lipids and lipoproteins during pregnancy. Clin Chim Acta. 1964; 10:470–2.

26. Gillmer MD, Beard RW, Brooke FM, et al. Carbohydrate metabolism in pregnancy. Part I. Diurnal plasma glucose profile in normal and diabetic women. Br Med J. 1975; 3:399–402.

27. Lind T, Billewicz WZ, Brown G. A serial study of changes occurring in the oral glucose tolerance test during pregnancy. J Obstet Gynaecol Br Comm. 1973; 80:1033–9.

28. O'Sullivan JB, Mahan CM. Criteria for the oral glucose tolerance test in pregnancy. Diabetes. 1964; 13:278–85.

29. Howie PW. Blood clotting and fibrinolysis in pregnancy. Postgrad Med J. 1979; 55:362–6.

30. Schwartz HC, King KC, Schwartz AL, Edmunds D, Schwartz D. Effects of pregnancy on hemoglobin A1c in normal, gestational diabetic, and diabetic women. Diabetes. 1976; 25:1118–22.

31. Lind T. Clinical chemistry of pregnancy. Adv Clin Chem. 1980; 21:1–24.

32. Davison JM, Noble MC. Serial changes in 24 hour creatinine clearance during normal menstrual cycles and the first trimester of pregnancy. Br J Obstet Gynaecol. 1981; 88:10–7.

33. Katz AI, Davison JM, Hayslett JP, Singson E, Lindheimer MD. Pregnancy in women with kidney disease. Kidney Int. 1980; 18:192–206.

34. Davison JM, Dunlop W, Ezimokhai M. 24-hour creatinine clearance during the third trimester of normal pregnancy. Br J Obstet Gynaecol. 1980; 87:106–9.

35. Lindheimer MD, Katz AI. Kidney function and disease in pregnancy. Philadelphia: Lee & Febiger, 1977:22.

36. Samuelson K, Thomassen PA. Radioimmunoassay of serum bile acids in normal pregnancy and in recurrent cholestasis of pregnancy. Acta Obstet Gynecol Scand. 1980; 59:417–20.

37. Heikkinen J, Maentausta O, Ylostalo P, Janne O. Changes in serum bile acid concentrations during normal pregnancy, in patients with intrahepatic cholestasis of pregnancy and in pregnant women with itching. Br J Obstet Gynaecol. 1981; 88:240–5.

38. Meade BW, Rosalki SB. Serum enzyme activity in normal pregnancy and the newborn. J Obstet Gynaecol Br Comm. 1963; 70:693–700.

39. Sadovsky E, Zuckerman H. An alkaline phosphatase specific to normal pregnancy. Obstet Gynecol. 1965; 26:211–4.

40. Macdonald HN, Good W. Changes in plasma sodium, potassium and chloride concentrations in pregnancy and the puerperium, with plasma and serum osmolality. J Obstet Gynaecol Br Comm. 1971; 78:798–803.

41. King B, Spikesman A, Emery AE. The effect of pregnancy on serum levels of creatine kinase. Clin Chim Acta. 1972; 36:267–9.

42. Souma JA, Green PJ, Loppage AT, Donner RS, Hogg AL. Changes in thyroid function in pregnancy and with oral contraceptive use. South Med J. 1981; 74:684–7.

43. Burrow GN. The thyroid in pregnancy. Med Clin North Am. 1975; 59:1089–98.

44. Nolten WE, Lindheimer MD, Rueckert PA, Oparil S, Ehrlich EN. Diurnal patterns and regulation of cortisol secretion in pregnancy. J Clin Endocrinol Metab. 1980; 51:466–72.

45. Carr BR, Parker CR, Madden JP, MacDonald PC, Porter JC. Maternal plasma adrenocorticotropin and cortisol relationships throughout human pregnancy. Am J Obstet Gynecol. 1981; 139:416–22.

... to venture forth on the uncharted sea of the endocrines ... even the most wary mariner may easily lose his way as he seeks to steer his bark amid the glandular temptations whose siren voices have proved the downfall of many who have gone before.
—William Boyd
Pathology for the Surgeon

10. ENDOCRINE DISORDERS
Mervyn L. Lifschitz

THYROID GLAND

Abnormalities of thyroid function are among the most common endocrine disorders encountered during pregnancy. When dealing with thyroid dysfunction during pregnancy, one should keep in mind several special considerations. First, signs and symptoms of disordered thyroid function can be mimicked by pregnancy itself. Second, pregnancy-induced increases in thyroid-binding proteins alter standard thyroid function tests. Third, placental transfer of most thyroid hormones is minimal. Finally, easy passage of antithyroid drugs to the fetus must be considered in any medical treatment.

Normal Thyroid Function During Pregnancy

It has long been known that thyroid function changes during normal pregnancy [1]. Four of the major thyroid alterations that occur during pregnancy are listed in Table 10-1, and discussed briefly.

Thyroid Gland Enlargement

Pregnancy is often accompanied by some degree of thyroid gland enlargement. Women living in regions of the world where dietary iodide intake is relatively low have been shown to have the greatest increase in thyroid gland size [2]. Burrow has provided histologic evidence of large follicles and abundant colloid, suggestive of active formation and secretion of thyroid hormones [3].

Alterations in Iodide Handling

The renal clearance of iodide is increased during normal pregnancy. Renal losses of iodide are compounded by an increased volume of distribution for iodide, and maternal losses to the fetus. Radioactive iodide uptake studies performed in women scheduled for abortion have demonstrated an increased avidity of the thyroid gland for iodide.

Renal iodide clearance rate and thyroid iodide uptake are increased in a compensatory fashion. T_4 turnover studies have confirmed that the net thyroxine turnover and hormonal requirements are unchanged by pregnancy [4].

Alterations in Thyroid-Binding Globulin and Thyroid Hormones

Plasma concentrations of thyroid-binding globulin (TBG), T_4, and T_3 increase during pregnancy but the magnitude and time course of these increases vary [5]. During the first trimester, estrogen-stimulated hepatic synthesis can approximately double plasma levels of TBG. After the first trimester, levels of TBG increase only slowly. On the other hand, total T_3 is not significantly altered until the third trimester when it is increased about 1.5 times. During active labor, serum T_3 increases to twice the level found in nongravid women, but rapidly returns to normal within the first postpartum week. In contrast, T_4 and TBG do not return to normal levels for 4 to 6 weeks postpartum. Reports have varied regarding pregnancy-induced changes in thyroid-stimulating hormone (TSH) levels and the response of TSH to the intravenous administration of thyrotropin-releasing hormone (TRH) [5–7].

Placental Thyrotropins

The placenta has been shown to produce at least three glycoproteins with thyroid-stimulating effects: (1) human chorionic gonadotropin (HCG), (2) human chorionic thyrotropin (HCT), and (3) human molar thyrotropin (HMT). HCG is a weak thyroid stimulator with approximately 1/4,000 the thyrotropic activity of TSH. HCT is similar in molecular size to TSH, but it has a short duration of action and is found in small amounts in normal placenta. HCT is unlikely to have a significant effect on the control of thyroid function. HMT can be produced in large amounts by hydatidiform

Table 10-1. Thyroid alterations
during normal pregnancy

1. Enlargement of the thyroid gland
2. Alterations in iodide handling
3. Increase in thyroid-binding proteins
4. Placental production of substances with a direct effect on thyroid function

moles and choriocarcinoma. It is now thought that HMT is a precursor for HCT.

Placental Passage of Thyroid Hormones

Placental transfer of T_4, T_3, and TSH is extremely limited at physiologic concentrations, although several studies have suggested that at high concentrations some transfer of T_4 and T_3 does occur. On the other hand, iodide freely crosses the placenta and has resulted in neonatal goiter when mothers have been given iodide-containing drugs. Other antithyroid drugs such as imidazole derivatives and propylthiouracil readily cross the placenta. Finally, thyroid-stimulating immunoglobulin crosses the placenta and, as will be discussed later, can affect fetal thyroid development.

Fetal Thyroid Development

The fetal hypothalamic-pituitary-thyroid system develops and functions autonomously. At no time during gestation do fetal and maternal levels of T_3, T_4, or TSH correspond. The thyroid gland develops between the second and seventh weeks, but colloid and follicle formation begins during the tenth to eleventh week. It is between the tenth and eleventh weeks that the fetal thyroid begins to concentrate iodide and to synthesize thyroid hormone. Therefore, it is at this same time that the fetal thyroid becomes vulnerable to exogenous iodide and antithyroid drugs [8].

TSH is not yet present in the fetal circulation at the end of the first trimester; nevertheless, fetal T_4 is produced in its absence. During weeks 18 to 24 there is an abrupt rise in fetal TSH and a corresponding increase in fetal T_4 production. Ultimately, fetal free T_4 exceeds maternal free T_4 at term. Fetal T_3 levels are undetectable in the first and second trimesters but increase during the third trimester. The major source of T_3 is the peripheral monodeiodination of T_4. This deiodination process also produces a substance called reverse triiodothyronine (rT_3). The exact importance of rT_3 remains unclear. Despite the relative biologic inactivity of rT_3, fetal deiodination favors its production over the more active T_3.

At birth, there is an abrupt increase in TSH as well as enhanced conversion of T_4 to T_3. Reverse

T_3 levels return to adult levels within 10 to 14 days, suggesting a maturation of the converting enzyme that allows the conversion of T_4 to T_3, rather than to rT_3.

Thyroid Function Tests during Pregnancy

Serum T_4 and Resin T_3 Uptake

The key to understanding the changes in thyroid function tests during normal pregnancy is an awareness that the T_4 level can be altered by changes not only in its production but also by the serum level of the proteins that transport it. Thus, serum T_4 level is increased during normal pregnancy as a result of increased hepatic production of TBG.

During pregnancy or any condition that alters serum levels of TBG, the resin T_3 uptake (RT_3U) becomes an important adjunct for interpreting thyroid function. RT_3U measures the competitive binding of labeled T_3 between TBG in the subject's serum and an artificial resin. The extent of binding to the artificial resin is inversely proportionate to the number of unoccupied thyroxine-binding sites in the patient's serum. Increased levels of TBG in pregnancy result in increased levels of T_4 and increased unoccupied binding sites for the added radioactive T_3. Thus, the proportion of the unbound radioactive T_3 that can be taken up by the artificial resin and measured is decreased. The reciprocal changes in T_4 level and RT_3U are best understood by use of the free thyroxine index.

Free Thyroxine Index

The free thyroxine index (FTI), derived from the values for T_4 concentration and RT_3U, is an indirect approximation of the free hormone concentration and compensates for the alterations of TBG associated with pregnancy. This calculated value remains unchanged during pregnancy and is a reliable routine test of thyroid function. It should be emphasized that the RT_3U is not an actual measure of thyroid hormone concentration. It is useful only in conjunction with serum T_4 concentration for the calculation of FTI. In order to calculate FTI, the normal values for T_4 and RT_3U for a particular laboratory must be known. A low FTI is consistent with hypothyroidism. An elevated index suggests hyperthyroidism.

T_3 by Radioimmunoassay

The total amount of T_3 can be measured by radioimmunoassay technique (T_3 by RIA). Normal values in nonpregnant patients have been reported between 70 and 200 ng/dL. This value may vary slightly at different laboratories depending on the method used. In pregnancy the normal values can increase up to 50%. Normal values have been reported up to 300 ng/dL [11]. The most important use of T_3 by RIA is for the diagnosis of an unusual condition called T_3 thyrotoxicosis. In this condition patients who are clinically hyperthyroid can demonstrate an elevated T_3 by RIA in the face of a normal FTI.

Thyroid-Stimulating Hormone
Measurement of thyroid-stimulating hormone (TSH) is the best single test for the recognition of hypothyroidism. In patients with normal thyroid function serum TSH levels will be less than 8 units/mL. Serum TSH will be increased in patients with primary malfunction of the thyroid gland. Thyroid dysfunction due to pituitary or hypothalamic disease will not demonstrate expected elevation of TSH. However, these are extremely rare causes for hypothyroidism during pregnancy. Serum TSH levels can be elevated even prior to any decrease in FTI as an early manifestation of thyroid failure. Serum TSH concentration is also useful for assessing the adequacy of thyroid hormone replacement therapy. TSH is not useful for recognition of hyperthyroidism.

Thyrotropin-Releasing Hormone
Basal thyroid-stimulating hormone (TSH) values do not always distinguish hypothyroid patients from normal individuals. Administration of synthetic thyrotropin-releasing hormone (TRH) elicits a brisker than normal release of TSH in nonpregnant hypothyroid patients. However, the response to TRH has been shown to vary during pregnancy [6,7].

Thyroid Antibodies
The determination of thyroid antibodies is useful in the diagnosis of Hashimoto's thyroiditis. Of the various kinds of thyroid antibodies, the antithyroglobulins and the antimicrosomal antibodies are the most commonly used. These autoantibodies are organ-specific immunoglobulins, and their presence correlates with histologic evidence of thyroiditis.

Tests for specific antibodies associated with Graves' disease are now available in research laboratories. Thyroid-stimulating immunoglobulin (TSI) is demonstrable in 80 to 90% of patients with the disease. Ultimately, TSI should become the specific immunologic marker for the diagnosis of Graves' disease.

Ultrasonography
The use of thyroid ultrasonography can be ex-

tremely helpful for differentiating a solid from a cystic thyroid nodule. This distinction has great clinical importance for deciding the proper approach to a thyroid nodule during pregnancy. The use of thyroid function tests during pregnancy is summarized in Table 10-2.

Hypothyroidism
Profound hypothyroidism is uncommonly encountered during pregnancy, because women with markedly impaired thyroid function often are infertile. The effect of mild thyroid dysfunction on fertility is less clear. Hypothyroidism can result from primary disorders of the thyroid gland or secondarily from pituitary or hypothalamic disorders. Common causes of hypothyroidism include Hashimoto's thyroiditis, destruction of the gland by radioactive iodine or surgery, antithyroid drugs, and iodine deficiency.

Consequences of maternal hypothyroidism include a higher than normal incidence of fetal wastage and malformation [9,10]. The reason for these problems is not clear since it is known that the fetal thyroid functions independently of the maternal system and the placental transfer of thyroid hormones is minimal.

The usual symptoms of hypothyroidism may be difficult to distinguish from symptoms associated with normal pregnancy. Typical symptoms include lethargy, weight gain, constipation, dry skin, and cold intolerance. Since none of these symptoms is invariably present or crucial for the diagnosis, the wary physician must exercise a high degree of suspicion. Certain groups of patients should be considered particularly vulnerable to thyroid dysfunction: (1) patients with goiter; (2) patients with thyroid nodules; (3) patients with Hashimoto's thyroiditis; (4) patients who have undergone previous thyroid surgery; (5) patients who have been previously treated with radioactive iodide; (6) patients who have received significant thyroid replacement in the past, even for dubious indications; and (7) patients who have been on suppressive thyroid therapy for any length of time regardless of the indication.

Confirmation of hypothyroidism is made by appropriate laboratory tests. Usually the RT_3U will be low, and the T_4 concentration will be lower than expected for pregnancy, albeit within the normal range for nonpregnant women. The FTI will usually be low. In cases of primary hypothyroidism the serum TSH level should be elevated. Elevation of serum TSH can antedate changes in T_4 concentration or RT_3U. An elevated TSH in the presence of a normal FTI indicates that the thyroid gland can

Table 10-2. Thyroid function tests during pregnancy

Test	Goal of test	Use during pregnancy
Total serum thyroxine (T_4)	T_4 level	Elevated during normal pregnancy due to increased TBG; further elevated in 90% of hyperthyroid patients
Resin T_3 uptake (RT_3U)	Clarifies whether alterations in T_4 are due to thyroid pathology or to alterations in TBG	Decreased during normal pregnancy
Free thyroxine index (FTI)	Compensates for pregnancy-induced reciprocal changes in T_4 and RT_3U	Values are unaltered in normal pregnancy, increased in hyperthyroidism, and decreased in hypothyroidism
Serum triiodothyronine (T_3 by RIA)	Measures actual T_3 level	Increased in unusual circumstance of T_3 thyrotoxicosis when FTI is normal
Thyroid-stimulating hormone (TSH)	Serum TSH level	May become elevated prior to low serum T_4 in hypothyroidism; useful for assessing adequacy of thyroid replacement therapy
Thyrotropin-releasing hormone test	TSH response to intravenous infusion of TRH	Brisker than normal response elicited in hypothyroidism; no response seen in hyperthyroidism; test has not been standardized for pregnancy
Serum antibodies	Antithyroglobulins, antimicrosomal antibodies	High titers suggest Hashimoto's thyroiditis
Radioactive iodide uptake (RAIU)	Extent of thyroid function	Contraindicated during pregnancy
Thyroid scan	Functional status of thyroid nodule	Contraindicated during pregnancy
Ultrasonography	Status of single nodules	90% reliable discrimination between cystic and solid nodules

produce normal levels of thyroid hormone only if stimulated by supranormal levels of TSH, and frank hypothyroidism may soon supervene.

Therapy for primary thyroid dysfunction during pregnancy is full thyroid hormone replacement. Most women will require 0.1 to 0.2 mg of L-thyroxine daily to remain euthyroid. When thyroid replacement is adequate, TSH levels will return to normal but may take up to eight weeks to do so. Excessive replacement will result in hypermetabolic symptoms, which can usually be elicited by a careful history. It has been my policy to continue thyroid hormone during pregnancy even if the indication for its use prior to conception was unclear. There is no current evidence to suggest that replacement doses of thyroid medication suppress fetal thyroid function. In fact, there is considerable evidence that intact T_3 and T_4 do not cross the placenta in any significant amounts [12].

Rare cases of pituitary-hypothalamic hypothyroidism can be confirmed by a low FTI and a low TSH. These patients should have further evaluation of the pituitary-hypothalamic axis.

Hyperthyroidism

In the past many women were mistakenly thought to be hyperthyroid during pregnancy on the basis of thyroid enlargement and an elevated basal metabolic rate. It is now known that basal metabolic rate increases during pregnancy as a result of the enhanced respiration of the fetal-maternal unit and increased cardiac output in the mother [13].

Graves' disease, characterized by a diffuse toxic goiter, is by far the most common cause of hyperthyroidism during pregnancy. The stimulus for goiter formation appears to be an IgG immunoglobulin called thyroid-stimulating immunoglobulin (TSI). TSI is known to cross the placenta and to affect the fetal thyroid. Other less common causes include toxic adenoma, multinodular goiters, subacute thyroiditis, hydatidiform mole, and factitious thyroid hormone ingestion.

Clinical recognition of hyperthyroidism during pregnancy may be difficult. Hypermetabolic symptoms such as heat intolerance, mild tachycardia, and nervousness can occur during normal gestation. Nevertheless, weight loss in the face of a good

Table 10-3. Drugs used for the management of hyperthyroidism

Drug	Action	Fetal effects
PTU	Inhibits thyroid hormone synthesis and peripheral conversion of T_4 to T_3	Freely crosses placenta and inhibits fetal thyroid hormone synthesis
Methimazole	Inhibits thyroid hormone synthesis but does not block conversion of T_4 to T_3	Freely crosses placenta and inhibits fetal thyroid hormone synthesis; associated with a congenital scalp defect (aplasia cutis)
Propranolol	Blocks peripheral action of thyroid hormone; no effect on synthesis	Crosses placenta and may cause fetal or neonatal bradycardia or hypoglycemia
Iodides	Inhibit organic iodine formation and block hormone release	Freely cross placenta and can cause fetal goiter

appetite, persistent tachycardia, hyperdefecation, and tremulousness should suggest thyrotoxicosis. The diagnosis is confirmed by elevated thyroid function tests. T_4 will increase beyond the expected level for a pregnant woman, and RT_3U will increase but often remains within the limits of normal for a nonpregnant patient. Rarely, a woman who is felt to be clinically hyperthyroid will have a normal FTI but an elevated T_3 by RIA. Levels of T_3 by RIA that are greater than 300 ng/dL are probably abnormal and consistent with the diagnosis of T_3 thyrotoxicosis.

Management of Hyperthyroidism

Management of hyperthyroidism during pregnancy is aimed at controlling maternal hyperthyroidism while minimizing any possible disruption of normal fetal thyroid development. Two important points require emphasis before specific treatment of hyperthyroidism is detailed: (1) Mild maternal hyperthyroidism appears to be well tolerated; and (2) antithyroid drugs freely cross the placenta and are active against the fetal thyroid. Since radioactive iodide therapy is contraindicated in pregnancy, therapeutic options include antithyroid drugs or surgery (Table 10-3).

PROPYLTHIOURACIL. Propylthiouracil (PTU) has long been the mainstay of medical therapy for hyperthyroidism. It inhibits thyroid hormone synthesis within the gland, as well as inhibiting peripheral conversion of T_4 to the more active metabolite T_3 [14]. Unquestionably, PTU can control maternal symptoms of thyrotoxicosis. However, PTU freely crosses the placenta and is active against the fetal thyroid. What remains unclear is the long-term effect of the drug on the offspring. Recently, Cheron et al. reported that modest doses of PTU (100–200 mg daily) given to women with Graves' disease significantly reduced serum thyroxine levels in their newborns [15]. The critical question is whether a mild, transient reduction of

T_4 is of any long-term consequence to the infant. Burrow et al. studied children who had been exposed in utero to PTU. Three of 15 children exposed to PTU had definite mental impairment [16]. The small size of the study precluded any definite conclusions. In a subsequent study intelligence tests administered to 24 children who had been exposed to PTU in utero and 32 nonexposed siblings showed no significant differences between the two groups [13].

Most researchers agree that PTU can be safely used during pregnancy. Nonetheless, it is appropriate to use the smallest dosage of the drug feasible in order to minimize the degree of potential fetal hypothyroidism. Although some hyperthyroid patients are successfully treated with a single daily dose of PTU, the drug has a short half-life and usually requires two to three doses. For patients with mild to moderate symptoms, initial doses of 50 to 100 mg of PTU every eight hours are usually sufficient. It should be kept in mind that pregnancy can ameliorate the symptoms of hyperthyroidism. Therefore, FTI should be measured at least monthly and the dosage of PTU reduced when the FTI falls to the normal range. Care should be exercised not to allow the FTI to fall into the hypothyroid range. A marked decrease in the FTI or failure of the FTI to rise after a reduction of the PTU dosage suggests that a further dosage reduction is indicated.

In the past some investigators have suggested giving thyroid supplement in combination with antithyroid drugs to prevent maternal hypothyroidism. Since we know that the placenta is freely permeable to PTU but relatively impermeable to T_3 and T_4, very little thyroid hormone will reach the fetus. Therefore, when thyroid hormone is added to the mother's regimen, it can only increase the need for PTU if she is to remain eumetabolic. Paradoxically, a combination of PTU and thyroid supplement increases maternal thyroid hormone levels but lowers fetal ones.

An important consideration in the management of Graves' disease during pregnancy is that TSI crosses the placenta and can cause neonatal hyperthyroidism. This can be a critical problem for the newborn [17,18]. Some authors have suggested giving a small dose of PTU to mothers with high TSI levels in an effort to prevent neonatal Graves' disease. Data to support this practice, especially in the euthyroid mother, are lacking [19].

Side effects of PTU include nausea, fever, skin rash, and pruritus. Little cross-reactivity occurs between PTU and methimazole. Therefore, if mild side effects occur, methimazole can be substituted for PTU. The most severe reaction to PTU is agranulocytosis. It occurs in approximately 0.1% of the patients treated with the agent, usually after one to two months of therapy [20]. Routine white blood cell counts are of limited value, since this complication can occur suddenly. Finally, several cases of neonatal goiter have been reported in newborns who were exposed to PTU in utero.

METHIMAZOLE. Like PTU, methimazole inhibits thyroid synthesis in both mother and fetus, but methimazole does not block the peripheral conversion of T_4 to T_3. This means that hyperthyroid symptoms are likely to be more rapidly controlled with PTU than with methimazole. Also, methimazole has been associated with a few cases of a congenital scalp defect called aplasia cutis [21]. However, such reports are few and should not stand as an absolute contraindication to use of the drug.

PROPRANOLOL. In nonpregnant patients propranolol has been shown to effectively block the peripheral action of thyroid hormone. It does not block the production of thyroid hormone synthesis or the peripheral conversion of T_4 to T_3. Nevertheless, there remains controversy over the safety of propranolol use during pregnancy. One double-blind study demonstrated that the offspring of women who had received propranolol were more depressed at birth than the offspring of those who had received placebos [22]. Other fetal and neonatal complications that have been attributed to propranolol include small placenta, intrauterine growth retardation, impaired responses to anoxic stress, postnatal bradycardia, and hypoglycemia [23]. Recently, the uses and complications of beta-blockers during pregnancy were reviewed by Rubin, who concluded that the drug can be safely used during pregnancy [24]. I have reserved its use in the treatment of hyperthyroidism from thyroid storm (discussed below), for patients who could not tolerate PTU or methimazole, or for patients about to undergo thyroidectomy. Experience with newer, more selective beta-blockers is lacking.

LITHIUM. The antithyroid effects of lithium became apparent when goiter or hypothyroidism developed in approximately 4% of patients treated with the drug for affective disorders [25]. The effect of lithium on the thyroid is similar to that of iodide, in that it decreases secretion of the preformed hormones. Like iodide, lithium crosses the placenta and can cause fetal goiter. Its use in pregnancy is not recommended.

SURGICAL MANAGEMENT. Surgical therapy of hyperthyroidism has become less popular in the past 35 years since effective medical therapy has been available. Nevertheless, in experienced hands, thyroidectomy is an effective and a safe procedure during pregnancy.

Surgery is usually reserved for patients with hypersensitivity to antithyroid drugs, for poorly compliant patients, and for the occasional patient in whom reasonable dosages of antithyroid drugs are ineffective. Also, patients with toxic uninodular or multinodular goiter may be resistant to medical therapy and require surgery.

Thyroid surgery has traditionally been performed during the second trimester. Preoperatively, thyrotoxicosis is controlled with propranolol, 20 to 60 mg given orally every six hours. Preoperative iodide therapy is avoided because of the tendency for iodide to cause fetal goiter. Surgery should be delayed until the patient's pulse is less than 90. The patient should be adequately sedated with diazepam, and induction of anesthesia should be performed as smoothly as possible in a quiet room. Anticholinergics should be omitted because they interfere with sweating and can lead to hyperthermia. Sodium thiopental is the agent of choice for induction and enflurane for maintenance since it does not sensitize the myocardium to catecholamines. Deep anesthesia is mandatory to prevent outpouring of catecholamines and consequent storm, which can develop up to 18 hours postoperatively. Other potential postoperative complications include carotid sinus reflex bradycardia, recurrent laryngeal nerve injury, and hypocalcemia. Finally, it must be remembered that patients with Graves' disease who are treated with thyroidectomy still may have high levels of thyroid-stimulating immunoglobulin; consequently, their offspring are vulnerable to neonatal Graves' disease.

Neonatal Hyperthyroidism

In 1964 McKenzie reported that high maternal levels of long-acting thyroid stimulator (LATS) were the rule in pregnancies whose outcome was a baby with neonatal hyperthyroidism [18]. Subsequently, other investigators have confirmed this observation. It has been shown that thyroid-stimulating immunoglobulin (which correlates well with LATS) readily crosses the placenta, resulting in virtually identical fetal and maternal levels [26]. Neonates exposed to high levels of TSI are vulnerable to thyrotoxicosis. Neonatal thyrotoxicosis occurs in 1% of babies born to mothers with Graves' disease and is more common in infants of mothers with ophthalmopathy and dermopathy.

TSI can persist in the mother who has been rendered euthyroid by surgery or antithyroid drugs. After approximately seven days the neonate will excrete the majority of any antithyroid drugs acquired transplacentally. It is at this time that the newborn might manifest thyrotoxicosis. Mortality for neonatal thyrotoxicosis has been reported to be as high as 16% [17]. Because the half-life of TSI in the infant is five to ten days, neonatal thyrotoxicosis usually remits within three months.

Prenatal treatment with PTU has been suggested for mothers with high levels of TSI in order to prevent neonatal thyrotoxicosis [19]. However, this approach has not been studied in any large series. If PTU is administered to the mother, the dosage should be titrated to maintain the fetal heart rate in the range of 120 to 160. Thyroid hormone supplementation may also be necessary for the euthyroid mother treated with PTU. Neonatal hyperthyroidism is treated with appropriate dosages of antithyroid drugs to the infant.

Thyroid Storm

Thyroid storm is a rare but life-threatening emergency characterized by hyperpyrexia, tachycardia, hypotension, agitation, and delirium. Storm can be precipitated by infection, surgery (thyroidal or nonthyroidal, including cesarean delivery), or even vaginal delivery.

Treatment is aimed at the immediate blocking of the peripheral effects of thyroid hormone as well as the reduction of thyroid hormone production. Propranolol is the drug of choice for reducing tachycardia and restlessness. It should be administered intravenously in a dose of 1 to 5 mg and titrated to reduce the maternal pulse to 100. Intravenous therapy should be followed by an oral maintenance dose of 20 to 80 mg every four hours. Control of thyroid storm can be achieved within a few hours by using propranolol. Since, as discussed previously, propranolol crosses the placenta, fetal heart rate requires careful surveillance.

Prompt reduction of thyroxine production can be achieved by giving aqueous iodide solution containing potassium iodide either intravenously or orally. The recommended dose is 0.1 to 0.5 mL every eight hours (36–180 mg of iodide) [27]. PTU should also be given immediately. The effect of PTU on thyroid hormone production is slower than that of potassium iodide. However, PTU has an additional effect on the peripheral conversion of T_4 to T_3. PTU can be given in doses up to 150 mg every six hours. Some theoretical evidence suggests that there is an inadequate response of adrenocorticotropic hormone (ACTH) during thyroid storm. Therefore, it has been recommended that hydrocortisone be administered immediately [27]. Adjunctive measures may also include cooling and sedation.

The Solitary Thyroid Nodule

Frequently, thyroid nodules are discovered during gestation. So common are simple nodules in women of childbearing age that it would be impossible to attempt to excise them all. Therefore, some sort of selection process is needed to recommend surgery.

A patient's history and physical exam may provide some suspicion of a malignant nodule. Features suggestive of malignancy include a history of prior irradiation to the head or neck, age less than 20 years, a family history of medullary thyroid carcinoma or other endocrine adenomatosis, a rock-hard nodule, or a nodule that did not decrease in size following suppressive therapy. However, several studies have pointed out that neither history nor physical exam can provide reliable differentiation of benign from malignant disease or even solitary nodules from multinodular goiters [28].

Since isotope scanning is contraindicated during pregnancy, other methods are necessary to predict malignancy. Ultrasonography in some centers can now provide as accurate anatomic information about a thyroid nodule as either palpation or radionuclide scanning [29]. Currently available equipment has shown intrathyroidal cystic lesions as small as 1 mm and solid lesions as small as 3 mm [30]. If a nodule is shown by ultrasound to be cystic, the chance of malignancy is considerably reduced. It must be remembered that ultrasound can provide only anatomic, not histologic, detail.

Needle biopsy, especially fine-needle aspiration, is safe and cost effective and has the best predictive value for differentiation of benign and malignant disease [31]. A recent review of the diagnostic approach to the thyroid nodule recommended that, if a medical center has experienced aspirators and cytologists, fine-needle aspiration should be the initial diagnostic step. Reliability of this technique has been reported to be approximately 97% [32].

Another approach to the thyroid nodule during pregnancy is thyroid suppressive therapy. This is based on the assumption that TSH initiates or promotes growth of thyroid nodules. The goal is to inhibit all TSH production by giving suppressive dosages of exogenous thyroid hormone and to observe the effect on the size of the nodule during a three- to six-month follow-up. This approach is often favored during the last trimester, with additional studies or surgery delayed until after delivery. It requires that the patient be followed monthly, to measure the size of the gland and to watch for the appearance of lymph nodes. If the lesion grows or does not diminish in size, it is considered to be autonomous and potentially malignant. A complete regression is strong evidence of a benign lesion. A partial regression is considered favorable, but most authors advise caution in such a case [31]. A lesion that is ultimately suspected to be malignant should be removed along with at least the entire lobe in which it occurs. Additional radioiodide ablative therapy should be delayed until post partum.

Autonomous Functioning Nodular Goiters

Hyperthyroidism can result from a single hyperfunctioning nodule or a multinodular goiter. The degree of hyperfunction is related to the mass of autonomously functioning follicles.

Treatment of the hyperfunctioning nodule during pregnancy is usually accomplished with antithyroid drugs (PTU or methimazole). Surgery or radioiodide therapy can be considered after childbirth. Spontaneous remission does not usually occur, and recurrence is common if medication is discontinued.

Hyperfunctioning Thyroid Cancer

Follicular carcinomas of the thyroid synthesize thyroid hormone very ineffectively and rarely cause hyperthyroidism. Hyperthyroidism is seen only with large tumors or with extensive metastasis. The approach in these rare circumstances should be surgical excision after the patient is rendered euthyroid with antithyroid drugs. Following delivery radioiodide ablation of any remaining neoplastic tissue is recommended. Thyroid suppressive therapy should be instituted following radioiodide therapy.

Subacute Thyroiditis

Subacute thyroiditis is an acute inflammation of the thyroid characterized by pain, swelling, and tenderness of the gland. It can also be accompanied by fever, malaise, and transient hyperthyroidism. Hyperthyroidism often lasts less than six weeks.

Treatment in the nonpregnant patient includes high-dose salicylates and antithyroid drugs. The use of high-dose salicylates during pregnancy is relatively contraindicated because of their prostaglandin-inhibiting effect. Corticosteroids are also very effective in diminishing acute inflammation of the gland and are preferable in pregnancy. Propranolol may be added if cardiovascular effects are prominent.

Transient Postpartum Thyrotoxicosis and Hyperthyroidism

Amino et al. have reported that 2.6% of postpartum Japanese women had transient thyrotoxicosis and that 2.8% of postpartum women had transient hypothyroidism. Associated with postpartum thyroid dysfunction was a high prevalence of antithyroid antibodies, suggesting that these abnormalities resulted from a postpartum exacerbation of subclinical autoimmune thyroid disease. All cases of postpartum thyrotoxicosis were self-limited, and thyrotoxic symptoms were transient. Three of the patients with postpartum thyrotoxicosis manifested symptoms compatible with so-called postpartum psychosis. In the majority of patients with postpartum hypothyroidism, thyroid function spontaneously returned to normal within four to six months [33]. The etiology of transient postpartum thyroid dysfunction is not clear. However, evidence implies a causal relationship involving abnormalities in both humoral and cellular immune systems. It has been suggested that suppression of humoral and cellular immunity during pregnancy, which allows survival of the antigenically foreign fetus, may rebound after delivery and lead to a variety of immunologic disorders, including thyroiditis [34].

Transient hyperthyroid symptoms may require control with propranolol. Antithyroid drugs such as PTU or methimazole are variably effective. Symptoms of thyroid inflammation can be treated with salicylates or corticosteroids. When symptoms of hypofunction are present, thyroid replacement may be used.

Hyperthyroidism Due to Trophoblastic Hormone

Molar pregnancies can be associated with excessive thyroid hormone production. Such pregnancies are accompanied by the production of a thyrotropin immunologically distinct from TSH. There is now strong evidence that human chorionic gonadotropin is the abnormal thyroid stimulator associated with hydatidiform moles. In fact, serum concentration of thyroid hormone appears to be proportional to the serum HCG level [35]. Thyrotoxicosis subsides rapidly once the offending tumor has been removed. Propranolol should be used to control cardiovascular manifestations of hyperthyroidism. Iodide is given preoperatively along with antithyroid drugs to block thyroid hormone production.

Choriocarcinomas produce thyrotropin similar to pituitary TSH and can be associated with thyrotoxicosis. Primary treatment is surgical removal of the tumor. However, it might also be necessary to control hyperthyroidism with propranolol or antithyroid drugs. Improvement of hyperthyroidism following removal of a choriocarcinoma is less rapid and more variable than that of a hydatidiform mole. Since patients can rapidly develop thyroid storm, it is reasonable to treat even those who have only biochemical evidence of hyperthyroidism.

Rarely, struma ovarii can cause thyrotoxicosis. In this event, the hyperthyroidism is accompanied by a low thyroidal uptake of radioiodide with a demonstrable increase in the uptake of radioiodide by the ovary. Struma is extremely unlikely to be associated with pregnancy.

PARATHYROID GLANDS
Normal Maternal Alterations of Calcium and Vitamin D Metabolism
A newborn skeleton contains 25 to 30 g of calcium, the greatest amount being acquired during the last trimester. Calcium deposition in the fetal skeleton occurs at a rate of 300 mg daily during this period. In order to meet fetal needs, calcium metabolism undergoes widespread changes in the gravida. Maternal gastrointestinal absorption of calcium increases as early as the twentieth week of pregnancy and becomes nearly twice normal by 25 to 30 weeks. This must be considered an anticipatory adjustment on behalf of the mother, as the increased absorption occurs prior to fetal skeletal mineralization. While calcium ions move freely across the placenta, serum PTH does not. This fetal-maternal transfer of calcium results in a new steady state in which fetal calcium requirements are met at the expense of maternal concentration. A study by Drake et al. reported that the biologically active calcium fraction, which represents 45% of total serum calcium, decreases at 21 to 25 weeks' gestation and remains low until term [36]. The new steady state suggests that pregnancy offers protection against hypercalcemia, but this protective effect is rapidly lost post partum.

Several investigators have described a "physiologic hyperparathyroidism" that occurs during normal gestation. It has been shown that parathyroid hormone concentration increases steadily throughout pregnancy because of either a decrease in serum ionized calcium or an increase in fetal demands for calcium or both [37,38]. It is as a result of the increased maternal parathyroid hormone that calcium can be reabsorbed from bone in the presence of 25-hydroxy vitamin D.

Fetal Calcium Metabolism
The relatively high serum calcium levels in the fetus, together with significant levels of inorganic phosphate, result in bone mineralization and accretion. Although fetal parathyroid tissue is recognizable in the fifth gestational week and functionally active by the thirteenth week, PTH secretion and fetal serum PTH levels are low or undetectable. This drop is possibly related to the fetal hypercalcemia that suppresses secretion of the hormone.

Serum calcitonin levels in the fetus are elevated because of fetal hypercalcemia. The rise enhances bone accretion and skeletal formation in the fetus but may be the cause of hypocalcemia observed in the first few days of life.

The high levels of 1,25-dihydroxy vitamin D in the fetus play an important role in calcium metabolism and bone mineralization during the neonatal period. The fact that hypocalcemia in the neonatal period can be prevented by the prophylactic use of vitamin D suggests that vitamin D plays a more important part than PTH in calcium homeostasis during the neonatal period.

Hyperparathyroidism
The occurrence of hyperparathyroidism during pregnancy is remarkably rare. Shangold et al. reviewed 159 pregnancies, of which 84 resulted in normal infants at term, 7 were interrupted by induced abortion, 13 terminated in spontaneous abortion, 11 resulted in intrauterine fetal death, 35 were followed by transient neonatal tetany, 1 child developed permanent hypoparathyroidism, and 4 resulted in neonatal death [39].

The fetus exposed to chronic maternal hypercalcemia becomes hypercalcemic, leading to suppression of fetal parathyroid glands. Parathyroid gland suppression often persists after birth and renders the neonate vulnerable to tetany when separated from the maternal source of calcium. In Shangold's review approximately 22% of the infants of mothers with hyperparathyroidism had transient tetany. Breast-milk supplies a higher concentration of calcium than either cow's milk or

*Table 10-4. Differential
diagnosis of hypercalcemia*

Hyperparathyroidism

Sarcoidosis

Hypervitaminosis D

Hypervitaminosis A

Malignancy

Milk-alkali syndrome

Renal tubular acidosis

Dysproteinemias

Prolonged bed rest

Paget's disease

evaporated milk and offers some potential protection against neonatal tetany [39].

Diagnosis

Although most patients are asymptomatic, women with a history of renal calculi, osteoporosis, peptic ulcer disease, bone pain, unexplained pancreatitis, protracted vomiting, or unexplained fetal wastage should be screened for hyperparathyroidism with a serum calcium determination.

The diagnosis rests primarily on the measurement of an elevated serum calcium in the face of inappropriately high levels of circulating PTH. Since total serum calcium is depressed because of physiologic hypoalbuminemia, any serum calcium level greater than 10 mg/dL should be considered elevated. The physiologic elevation of parathyroid hormone in normal pregnancies must be considered when establishing the diagnosis of hyperparathyroidism. However, significantly elevated levels of parathyroid hormone should not be found in patients with persistent hypercalcemia even during pregnancy. Approximately 85 to 90% of cases of primary hyperparathyroidism result from benign adenomas, and about 10% from parathyroid hyperplasia [40]. Additional causes of hypercalcemia are listed in Table 10-4.

Treatment

Patients with serum calcium levels greater than 12 mg/dL require emergency medical intervention. Immediate therapy includes intravenous infusions of isotonic saline, 4 to 5 liters per day, plus administration of a potent calciuretic agent such as furosemide. Several grams of calcium can be excreted daily with this regimen, resulting in rapid lowering of serum calcium. The beneficial effects result from the linkage of sodium and calcium transport in the kidney tubule. This form of therapy can be utilized only if renal function is normal. Strict records of intake and output must be kept to avoid fluid overload.

Recently, Montoro et al. employed oral phosphate therapy in two pregnant patients with hyperparathyroidism in whom surgery could not be performed [41]. Serum calcium was successfully decreased, and their infants remained normocalcemic throughout the neonatal period. Nevertheless, phosphate therapy increases the risk of widespread soft tissue calcifications and should not be used routinely.

Mithramycin, given as a single dose, may lower calcium to normal within several days. However, this drug has not been used during pregnancy and is potentially teratogenic.

Medical therapy for hyperparathyroidism is appropriate for short intervals only. Surgical exploration of the neck is the recommended treatment for a pregnant patient with rising serum calcium, worsening symptoms, or hyperparathyroid crisis unresponsive to medical therapy. Most authors agree that the high rate of maternal and neonatal complications for hyperparathyroidism makes surgery the treatment of choice even if the disease is mild. Most cases of hyperparathyroidism are associated with an adenoma that can be removed. If the glands are hyperplastic, it is recommended that three and a half glands be removed. Eighty percent of patients who undergo surgery have a normal outcome to their pregnancy in any trimester. Surgery should not be deferred because of pregnancy unless delivery is imminent. Surgical complications include the risk of anesthesia, transient postoperative hypocalcemia, premature labor, injury to either laryngeal nerve, and permanent hypoparathyroidism. Transient postoperative hypocalcemia can be managed with vitamin D and calcium. In rare instances in which hyperparathyroidism is associated with pancreatitis, surgery should be delayed until the pancreatitis subsides or the patient is stable. Initial therapy includes fluids and diuretics [42].

Hypoparathyroidism

Disorders of maternal hypocalcemia can be separated into those that are caused by decreased PTH secretion and those that are a result of inappropriate response of target organs to PTH (Table 10-5).

In the pregnant patient the concern is not only that abnormal concentrations of calcium will be injurious to the mother but that the fetus may suffer harm. There are several reports in the literature of infants born to hypoparathyroid mothers with changes consistent with hyperparathyroidism, including skeletal demineralization, subperiosteal

Table 10-5. Causes of hypocalcemia

Failure of PTH secretion
  Hypoparathyroidism
  Hypomagnesemia
Inadequate response of the target organ to PTH
  Vitamin D deficiency
  Abnormalities of vitamin D metabolism
  Pseudohypoparathyroidism

resorption of the cortices of the long bones, and osteitis fibrosa cystica [43,44].

In adults, hypoparathyroidism is usually a result of thyroid or parathyroid surgery. Hypocalcemia may produce many nonspecific symptoms such as lethargy, bone pain, or a generalized feeling of debilitation. When hypocalcemia is severe, tetany can result. However, it should be kept in mind that the most common cause of tetany during pregnancy is alkalosis secondary to hyperventilation. Latent tetany may be demonstrated by inflating a blood pressure cuff above systolic pressure for three minutes and noting the appearance of carpopedal spasm (Trousseau's sign). Hypoparathyroidism should be suspected in any woman with a low serum calcium and a normal or elevated inorganic phosphorus level. The diagnosis is confirmed by finding low levels of PTH concurrent with a low serum calcium.

Treatment

Frequently, the conventional treatment of hypoparathyroidism with massive doses of vitamin D is less than satisfactory. Variability of response to vitamin D makes it difficult to determine the correct therapeutic dosage. Furthermore, serum concentrations of calcium may fluctuate during pregnancy in an unpredictable manner. Several reports attest to the efficacy of the short-acting vitamin D preparation calcitriol (1,25-dihydroxycholecalciferol) [45]. A more rapid and predictable response occurs with calcitriol than with vitamin D. The usual dose of calcitriol in the nonpregnant hypoparathyroid woman is 1.5 ng per day. It is common for the pregnant woman with this problem to require twice that dosage. In addition, 1 to 2 g calcium carbonate should be administered orally in order to supply substrate for gastrointestinal absorption. Careful monitoring of serum calcium levels is necessary. The dosage of calcitriol should be adjusted to keep the serum calcium level in the low normal range.

Following delivery, the dosage of calcitriol used during pregnancy might cause maternal hypercalcemia since the fetal uptake of calcium ceases and the maternal level of estrogen falls. In mothers who breast-feed, no abrupt readjustment appears to be necessary because there is a continuing need for increased absorption of calcium from the gut. In mothers who choose not to breast-feed, it is important to reduce the dosage of calcitriol by half and to monitor serum calcium levels.

PITUITARY GLAND

Functional integrity of the pituitary gland is important for the achievement, maintenance, and successful outcome of pregnancy. This section focuses on (1) the effect of pregnancy on the normal pituitary gland, (2) management of the pregnant woman with a pituitary tumor, and (3) management of pituitary insufficiency during pregnancy.

Effect of Pregnancy on the Normal Pituitary Gland

It has long been known that during gestation the pituitary gland increases progressively in both size and weight. At term, the gland will normally have doubled in weight [46]. Most of the enlargement results from estrogen-induced hyperplasma of the acidophilic cells [47]. Estrogen is not only capable of enlarging the normal pituitary; it can also affect prolactin-secreting pituitary tumors and increase the probability that they will become symptomatic [48].

Hormonal function of the pituitary gland is also altered during pregnancy. Basal concentrations of human growth hormone do not change remarkably with advancing gestation. However, the maternal hypothalamic-hypophyseal growth hormone secretory mechanism does appear to be inhibited by human placental lactogen. As the human placental lactogen level rises, maternal growth hormone secretion in response to stress, hypoglycemia, or arginine infusion is blunted. Following parturition, with subsequent decreased human placental lactogen levels, hypophyseal regulation of growth hormone secretion eventually returns to normal [49]. Serum prolactin level rises throughout pregnancy and peaks at term. Thereafter, it either declines rapidly if the mother does not breast-feed or increases sharply with early breast-feeding episodes [50]. As months of breast-feeding ensue, these sharp rises in prolactin practically disappear.

Pituitary Tumors

In the past, pituitary tumors were thought to involve mainly the cells secreting polypeptide hormones such as growth hormone (in acromegaly), adrenocorticotropic hormone (in Cushing's disease), and prolactin (in amenorrhea-galactorrhea syndrome). Since it is now possible to identify specific tumor-secreted hormones, tumors have been shown to produce additional glycoprotein hormones such as follicle-stimulating hormone (FSH), luteinizing hormone (LH), and thyroid-stimulating hormone (TSH). The traditional classification of pituitary adenomas into acidophilic, basophilic, and chromophobe tumors is still used, despite its lack of specificity for hormone production. The chromophobe adenoma is the most common type, occurring in 85% of all pituitary tumors. Chromophobes are capable of secreting one or several hormones. However, 70% of chromophobes produce prolactin. Rarely, acidophilic tumors can produce excessive amounts of both growth hormone and prolactin. Other mixed hormone–producing tumors have also been reported [51].

For the purpose of considering pituitary tumors in pregnancy two groups can conveniently be defined. The first group of patients have macroadenomas (tumors greater than 10 mm in diameter) with or without associated endocrinopathy. These women become pregnant spontaneously or following ovulation induction and can experience visual impairment from compression of the optic chiasm as the tumor expands during gestation. The second group consists of patients with microadenomas (tumors measuring 10 mm or less in diameter), which can cause selective gonadotropin deficiency or hyperprolactinemia. Many of these tumors remain unsuspected for years, manifesting themselves only by amenorrhea. In recent years the use of drugs to induce ovulation has permitted pregnancy in these previously anovulatory patients.

Much of what is known about the clinical course and management of pituitary tumors and pregnancy comes from data collected by Gemzell and Wang [52]. They compiled the experience of several physicians active in this area. From these data they developed a protocol for the management of women with pituitary adenomas who wish to become pregnant.

Macroadenomas

The survey reported by Gemzell and Wang involved 46 women with previously untreated macroadenomas in whom 56 pregnancies occurred. In 91% of the pregnancies ovulation was induced. Sixty-four percent of these patients were asymptomatic throughout pregnancy. Headache alone occurred in 9%, headache and visual disturbances in 25%, and diabetes insipidus in 2%. Eighty-one percent of patients who had the combination of headache and visual disturbances received treatment. Those with headache alone

were not treated. Treatment consisted of yttrium-90 and corticosteroids, bromocriptine, or surgery during the pregnancy or puerperium. The authors concluded that the larger the tumor, the greater the risk of complications during pregnancy. From these observations they made the following recommendations:

1. Patients should be operated on or irradiated before attempting pregnancy.
2. Ovulation may be induced following surgery or radiation therapy.
3. Patients with persistently elevated posttreatment prolactin levels should be monitored monthly by visual field examination and repeat prolactin levels.
4. Thyroid or corticosteroid replacement may be necessary in some patients.
5. If a visual field defect appears during pregnancy, bromocriptine is the treatment of choice (discussed below). Termination of pregnancy may be necessary in some patients.
6. Radiographic study of the sella turcica should be performed post partum.

Microadenomas

Gemzell and Wang also reported on 91 pregnancies that occurred in 85 women with previously untreated pituitary microadenomas. Ninety-eight percent of these pregnancies required induction of ovulation. Symptoms occurred in only 5%: headache in 3%, headache and visual disturbance in 1%, and diabetes insipidus in 1%. On the basis of these data they recommended the following for women with prolactin-secreting microadenomas [52].

1. Ovulation may be induced with bromocriptine or HMG-HCG.
2. Patients should be monitored monthly during pregnancy by prolactin levels and visual field examination.
3. If a visual field defect appears during pregnancy, bromocriptine may be used. Pituitary surgery or radiotherapy is an alternative. In some patients, termination of pregnancy may be necessary.
4. Radiographic study of the sella turcica should be performed during the postpartum period.

Bromocriptine and Pregnancy

Bromocriptine is an ergot alkaloid and dopamine receptor stimulator capable of decreasing serum prolactin and causing disappearance of galactorrhea and return of menses in women with prolactin-secreting pituitary adenomas [53]. In several studies bromocriptine has also been demonstrated to reduce the size of pituitary adenomas [54–57].

The major controversies surrounding the use of bromocriptine involve its use in the treatment of anovulatory infertility and its use during pregnancy. Although prolactin can be lowered to within normal limits in most patients, values return to pretreatment levels almost immediately following discontinuation of the drug. Therefore, if pregnancy is desired, one cannot usually stop therapy and expect a good ovulation with a normal luteal phase to result. Since medication will probably continue after conception, if only until the patient is aware she is pregnant, it is important to know whether the course and outcome are likely to be affected. In a recent report on the outcome of 1,410 pregnancies in 1,335 women to whom bromocriptine had been given, the incidences of spontaneous abortions, extrauterine pregnancies, and minor and major malformations were comparable to those quoted for normal populations [58]. The data suggest that treatment with bromocriptine during pregnancy is not associated with an increased risk to the fetus.

Although the traditional alternatives for treatment of pituitary tumors have been radiotherapy or surgery (or both), further investigation and better understanding of the pathophysiology of these tumors might make it possible to select a few patients with small pituitary tumors who can be treated with bromocriptine without additional risk to the fetus.

Pituitary Insufficiency

Pituitary insufficiency usually arises from postpartum pituitary necrosis (Sheehan's syndrome), destruction of the gland by tumor, surgical hypophysectomy, or radiotherapy [59]. In all forms of hypopituitarism fertility is likely to be impaired. In Sheehan's syndrome, as in other types of hypopituitarism, hormonal deficiency may vary from loss of a single tropic hormone to classic panhypopituitarism. It is necessary to assay specific hormone levels and to study secretory reserve in order to evaluate the extent of pituitary damage.

Replacement therapy for pituitary insufficiency primarily involves thyroid and glucocorticoid hormones. Mineralocorticoids are usually unnecessary. Maintenance replacement of glucocorticoids can be provided by hydrocortisone, 25 mg every morning and 12.5 mg every evening, or prednisone, 5 mg every morning and 2.5 mg every evening. Delivery represents a major stress and requires supplemental amounts of glucocorticoid. Hydrocortisone, 250 mg, should be administered intravenously every six hours during labor or on the day of cesarean delivery. Adequate thyroid hormone replacement can usually be provided by L-thyroxine, 0.1 to 0.2 mg daily [60].

As previously discussed, patients with hypopituitarism resulting from a macroadenoma may demonstrate further tumor growth during pregnancy. Tumor enlargement may lead to visual impairment and require definitive treatment.

Diabetes Insipidus

Diabetes insipidus (DI) is a disorder of the neurohypophyseal system due to a deficiency of antidiuretic hormone (ADH). Its occurrence in pregnancy is rare, and the effect of pregnancy on the disease is variable. In a review of the literature by Hime and Richardson, 58% of the reported cases were shown to worsen during pregnancy [61]. Several explanations for the worsening of DI during pregnancy have been suggested [62,63]. Pregnancy appears to increase the requirement for ADH by increasing glomerular filtration rate. It can also be demonstrated that tubular sensitivity to ADH is diminished in some patients. Therefore, in patients with a partial lack of ADH, DI would predictably worsen as pituitary reserve would be inadequate to meet the increased ADH need during gestation.

The treatment of choice for DI is 1-deamino-8-D-arginine vasopressin (DDAVP), a synthetic analog of arginine vasopressin. Recently, Burrow et al. studied its use during pregnancy and the postpartum period. They concluded that DDAVP was appropriate for use during pregnancy. They also found that levels of DDAVP were low in breast milk, suggesting that mothers might also breastfeed [64].

A few cases of DI have been reported in which preeclampsia developed [61,65]. In these cases it was consistently observed that in the presence of preeclampsia the DI improved. The explanation for this observation is not yet apparent.

ADRENAL GLANDS
Pheochromocytoma

The association of pheochromocytoma and pregnancy has attracted special attention because of its inordinately high risk. Both maternal and fetal death rates have been reported to be as high as 50% [66]. The diagnosis of pheochromocytoma is rarely made during pregnancy. Presumably, many cases are overlooked or are mistakenly thought to be preeclampsia. In 1971 Shenker and Chowers reviewed a total of 112 pregnancies occurring in 89 patients with pheochromocytomas. In only 22 of these patients was the diagnosis made before delivery [66].

Clinical recognition of pheochromocytoma during pregnancy can be a formidable task. Palpitations, sweating, and headaches are common during normal pregnancy; and hypertension occurs more commonly in the absence of pheochromocytoma. If the tumors are to be identified during pregnancy, a high degree of suspicion is necessary. The diagnosis should be suspected in hypertensive gravidas with cardiac arrhythmias, postural hypotension, glucose intolerance, neurofibromatosis, seizures, or unexplained collapse, as well as in patients with the classic symptoms of pallor, sweating, headaches, and vasomotor phenomena. Recurrent intrauterine deaths, especially associated with hypertension, should also suggest the possibility of pheochromocytoma. A family history of multiple endocrine adenomas in the hypertensive woman should prompt a screening test for pheochromocytoma.

Laboratory diagnosis includes estimation of catecholamines and their metabolites in the urine or blood. Screening tests for vanillylmandelic acid (VMA) based on phenolic acid color reactions are notoriously unreliable. Urinary levels of VMA are elevated in 50 to 79% of patients with pheochromocytomas. However, urinary metanephrine and normetanephrine levels are elevated in 77 to 95% of patients, and supine plasma catecholamines are elevated in 92 to 100% of cases [67].

In the past, provocative pharmacologic tests were used to establish the diagnosis. These tests have been abandoned because of associated fetal and maternal deaths [68].

Once the presence of a tumor is suspected by biochemical tests, it is important to localize the tumor anatomically. Tests that require fetal radiation exposure such as intravenous pyelography, arteriography, and computed axial tomography are clearly necessary to localize this potentially lethal tumor. CT scan appears to be the most reliable technique for tumors exceeding 0.5 cm in size.

When the diagnosis of pheochromocytoma is confirmed, the tumor should be removed immediately regardless of the stage of pregnancy. The risk associated with labor and vaginal delivery is extremely great and should be avoided. Simultaneous cesarean delivery and removal of the tumor have been successfully carried out [66]. Preoperative stabilization and blood pressure control are mandatory and include the use of alpha-blocking agents followed by beta blockade. An appropriate regimen begins with the administration of phenoxybenzamine, 10 mg orally every 12 hours, increasing to 50 mg every 12 hours or until adequate blood pressure control is achieved. Next, propranolol is given in an oral dosage sufficient to control tachycardia and prevent catechol-induced arrhythmias. It has to be kept in mind that beta blockade should be delayed so as not to interfere with beta-mediated vasodilatation in the setting of alpha-adrenergic vasoconstriction. Hypertensive crisis resulting from pheochromocytoma has been successfully managed with nitroprusside together with adrenergic blocking agents [69]. Postoperatively, the anesthesiologist must be prepared to deal with possible hypotension.

Adrenal Insufficiency (Addison's Disease)

Patients with untreated Addison's disease most often are amenorrheic, and conception is rare. On the other hand, patients who have had the diagnosis of adrenal insufficiency established previously and are receiving corticosteroid replacement can conceive without difficulty. Classic symptoms and signs of adrenal insufficiency such as fatigue, weakness, anorexia, nausea, hypotension, and increased skin pigmentation can all occur during normal pregnancy. Addison's disease should be considered if any of these symptoms are unusually severe or persistent.

During the first trimester plasma cortisol levels are identical to those of nonpregnant women. From the second trimester onward levels increase steadily, reaching a peak at term [70]. By the end of gestation cortisol secretion rate is about double the normal value. A simultaneous rise in plasma corticosteroid-binding globulin renders most of the increased cortisol physiologically inactive. Plasma cortisol levels measured during pregnancy that are in the normal nonpregnant range should be considered low during late pregnancy.

Diagnosis can be established with an abbreviated ACTH stimulation screening test using synthetic ACTH. The initial sample for baseline plasma cortisol is drawn at 8 A.M., in order to receive the benefit of the normal maximal diurnal output of adrenal steroids, which is preserved during pregnancy. After the baseline sample is obtained, 0.25 mg of synthetic ACTH in 1 mL of saline is injected intravenously as a single dose. A second sample is obtained 60 minutes later. In normal women, plasma cortisol levels should increase at least twofold. This test does not distinguish individuals with primary adrenocortical insufficiency from those with secondary adrenal insufficiency (hypopituitarism).

In patients with adrenal insufficiency who are adequately treated and supervised, normal pregnancy and delivery should be readily achieved. Potential stresses on an inadequate adrenal reserve include electrolyte disturbances associated with first-trimester vomiting, infection, and delivery. In the absence of added stress, pregnancy itself does not necessitate any change in the maintenance dosage of steroids. In most cases adequate maintenance replacement of adrenocortical hormones is provided by hydrocortisone, 25 mg orally every morning and 12.5 mg every evening, or prednisone, 5 mg orally every morning and 2.5 mg every evening. It is essential that patients use a single reliable preparation of hydrocortisone, since differences have been noted in potency and absorption of some preparations. During periods of moderate stress or mild infections the dosage of corticosteroid should be at least doubled. Patients should be instructed in the use of intramuscular cortisone acetate if vomiting is present.

Delivery, either vaginal or cesarean delivery, is a major stress and requires increased amounts of hydrocortisone. At the onset of labor or early on the morning of a scheduled cesarean delivery the patient should be given hydrocortisone, 100 mg IM or IV. Throughout the next 24 to 48 hours 250 mg given IV in divided doses every six hours should be sufficient. Return to normal replacement dosage can take place gradually over the next seven to ten days.

Aldosterone deficiency is usually corrected by a daily maintenance dose of 9-fluorohydrocortisone, 0.05 to 0.2 mg. The response to mineralocorticoid therapy can be gauged by changes in blood pressure, body weight, presence of edema, and serum electrolytes. The dosage of 9-fluorohydrocortisone may need to be decreased if edema or hypertension develops. On the other hand, an increased dosage as well as increased salt intake may be helpful in hot weather when sweating is excessive.

One cannot overemphasize the need for emergency instructions and a kit containing medications for use by patients with chronic adrenal insufficiency during emergencies. Such a kit should be readily available, especially when patients are traveling. It should contain an identification card with usual treatment outlined and vials of injectable cortisone acetate. An injectable mineralocorticoid, deoxycorticosterone acetate, is also available.

Adrenal crisis is a rare but life-threatening occurrence. Women with untreated Addison's disease are most likely to develop crisis during the puerperium. Crisis is manifest by intractable nausea and vomiting, abdominal pain, somnolence, and hypotension. Treatment is primarily aimed at immediate administration of glucocorticoid and volume replacement with saline. In all patients, a precipitating cause for crisis should be sought. Intercurrent infection associated with failure to increase maintenance therapy is the most common setting.

Cushing's Syndrome

Amenorrhea and sterility are commonly associated with Cushing's syndrome; therefore its association with pregnancy is rare. Fewer than 30 cases of Cushing's syndrome complicating pregnancy have been reported [71].

Diagnosis of Cushing's syndrome can be difficult during pregnancy because many of the usual symptoms and signs such as weakness, weight gain, acne, striae, and edema can be normal findings during gestation. Furthermore, levels of plasma cortisol seen in normal pregnancy are sometimes as high as those seen in some patients with adrenocortical hyperfunction. When Cushing's syndrome is suspected clinically, laboratory evaluation is conducted in the same manner as it would be for a nonpregnant patient. The initial screening test should be an overnight dexamethasone suppression test. One milligram of dexamethasone is given orally at 11 P.M.; if the plasma cortisol at 8 the next morning is less than 5 mg/dL, the result is normal, and the endogenous overproduction of glucocorticoids is essentially excluded. If the plasma cortisol is greater than 5 mg/dL, a complete laboratory evaluation is warranted. When dexamethasone is given in a dosage of 2 mg every six hours for two to three days, most cases of adrenocortical hyperplasia will show a 50% reduction in plasma and urinary corticoids. Patients with the ectopic ACTH syndrome, large ACTH-secreting pituitary tumors, adrenocortical nodular hyperplasia, or adrenal tumors usually do not show suppression with the three-day dexamethasone test.

Cushing's syndrome appears to have an adverse effect on pregnancy. The incidence of abortion, prematurity, and stillbirth is high [72]. Adrenal insufficiency in the neonate has been reported [73]. Theoretically, fetal virilization is possible if maternal androgen levels are high [72].

The etiology of the syndrome must be determined before treatment can be planned. About 70% of cases of endogenous glucocorticoid excess are due to Cushing's disease (pituitary-dependent bilateral adrenal hyperplasia). Adrenal adenoma, adrenal carcinoma, and ectopic ACTH production (most often associated with bronchogenic carcinoma) each account for about 10% of the remaining cases. Once the diagnosis of an adrenal tumor has been established, surgical removal with appropriate steroid supplement should be performed. In pituitary-dependent disease bilateral adrenalectomy should be avoided during pregnancy [71]. Rather, treatment should be directed at the pituitary by transfrontal hypophysectomy. For milder cases external irradiation or a local implant may be sufficient. After removal of a unilateral adrenal adenoma the contralateral atrophic gland will eventually recover. However, no attempt to reduce the maintenance dosage of hydrocortisone should be made until after delivery.

Congenital Adrenal Hyperplasia

Congenital adrenal hyperplasia (CAH) actually represents a group of autosomal recessive disorders of metabolism affecting the adrenal cortex and resulting in defects in the biosynthesis of cortisol and aldosterone. Six varieties are recognized, the first of which (21-hydroxylase deficiency) is relatively common and the others are rare (the reader is referred to standard textbooks of endocrinology for more detailed discussion) [74]. These errors of metabolism result in a compensatory increase in ACTH secretion in order to maintain adequate cortisol levels. In addition, increased adrenal synthesis of androgens occurs, causing hirsutism or virilization. Treatment with steroids throughout childhood permits normal menstrual function and fertility. Inadequate treatment of CAH during pregnancy can rarely cause virilization or pseudohermaphroditism in female offspring [85].

Proper management with glucocorticoid therapy results in an uneventful pregnancy. As in patients with Addison's disease, supplemental steroids are needed during labor and delivery. Like other inborn errors of metabolism, congenital adrenal hyperplasia is inherited through autosomal recessive genes. A woman who has previously given birth to a child with congenital adrenal hyperplasia has approximately one chance in four of bearing an affected child in a subsequent pregnancy by the same father [71].

Primary Aldosteronism

Primary aldosteronism was first described by Conn in 1955 as hypertension caused by a solitary adrenal adenoma [75]. We are now aware that excessive production of aldosterone can also result from bilateral adrenal hyperplasia [76]. The association of primary aldosteronism and pregnancy has been reported in only a few cases [77–80]. Because so few cases have been reported, the effect of the disease on pregnancy and the fetus is not well characterized. On the other hand, several interesting observations have been made regarding the effect of pregnancy on the course of the disease.

Diagnosis of primary aldosteronism is complicated during pregnancy because plasma levels of aldosterone have been shown to rise progressively throughout normal gestation [81–82]. Normal pregnancy is characterized by elevated plasma renin levels, but it remains to be determined whether plasma renin activity during pregnancy can be suppressed by excessive aldosterone production in the same manner as in the nonpregnant state. Nevertheless, the diagnosis should be suspected in hypertensive gravidas with unexplained hypokalemia and concomitant increased urinary potassium excretion. Elevated aldosterone levels in the face of suppressed plasma renin activity further supports the diagnosis. An anomalous postural decline in plasma aldosterone concentration strongly suggests that a patient has a unilateral adrenal adenoma as opposed to bilateral adrenal hyperplasia [76].

In several reported cases of primary aldosteronism during pregnancy an amelioration of high blood pressure and hypokalemia has been demonstrated as gestation progresses [80]. Possible explanations for this observation include (1) pregnancy-induced increase in glomerular filtration rate and a resultant increased sodium excretion and (2) elevated levels of progesterone, known to have a natriuretic effect in patients with primary aldosteronism [83,84]. Following pregnancy blood pressure again rises and potassium concentration falls.

Medical treatment is directed toward control of blood pressure and maintenance of normal serum potassium concentration. This can be accomplished with spironolactone and appropriate potassium replacement. Because potassium loss may be ameliorated as gestation progresses, frequent determination of serum potassium level is necessary to prevent hyperkalemia. Where a unilateral adrenal adenoma can be localized, surgery should be considered. Within the first month postpartum blood pressure may rise and potassium concentration may fall precipitously.

REFERENCES

1. Feely J. The physiology of thyroid function in pregnancy. Postgrad Med J. 1979; 55:336–9.
2. Crooks J, Tulloch MI, Turnbull AC, Davidson D, Skulason T, Snaedal G. Comparative incidence of goitre in pregnancy in Iceland and Scotland. Lancet. 1967; 1:625–7.
3. Burrow GN. Hyperthyroidism during pregnancy. N Engl J Med. 1978; 298:150–3.

4. Dowling JT, Appleton WG, Nicoloff JT. Thyroxine turnover during human pregnancy. J Clin Endocrinol. 1967; 27:1749–50.

5. Malkasian GD, Mayberry WE. Serum total and free thyroxine and thyrotropin in normal and pregnant women, neonates, and women receiving progesterone. Am J Obstet Gynecol. 1970; 108:1234–8.

6. Burrow GN. Thyroid and parathyroid function in pregnancy. In: Fuchs F, Klopper A, eds. Endocrinology of pregnancy. 2nd ed. Hagerstown Md: Harper & Row, 1977:246–70.

7. Kannan V, Sinha MK, Devi PK, Rastogi GK. Plasma thyrotropin and its response to thyrotropin releasing hormone in normal pregnancy. Obstet Gynecol. 1973; 42:547–9.

8. Hobel CJ. Fetal thyroid. Clin Obstet Gynecol. 1980; 23:779–90.

9. Man EB, Holden RH, Jones WS. Thyroid function in human pregnancy. VII. Development and retardation of 4-year-old progeny of euthyroid and of hypothyroxinemic women. Am J Obstet Gynecol. 1971; 109:12–9.

10. Man EB, Shaver BA, Cooke RE. Studies of children born to women with thyroid disease. Am J Obstet Gynecol. 1958; 75:728–41.

11. Avruskin TW, Mitsuma T, Shenkman L, Sau K, Hollander CS. Measurements of free and total serum T_3 and T_4 in pregnant subjects and in neonates. Am J Med Sci. 1976; 271:309–15.

12. Innerfield F, Hollander CS. Thyroidal complications of pregnancy. Med Clin North Am. 1977; 61:67–87.

13. Burrow GN. Hyperthyroidism during pregnancy. N Engl J Med. 1978; 298:150–3.

14. Solomon DH. Antithyroid drugs. In: Werner SC, Ingbar SH, eds. The thyroid: a fundamental and clinical text. 4th ed. Hagerstown, Md: Harper & Row, 1978:814–21.

15. Cheron RG, Kaplan MM, Larsen PR, Selenkow HA, Crigler JF. Neonatal thyroid function after propylthiouracil therapy for maternal Graves' disease. N Engl J Med. 1981; 304:525–8.

16. Burrow GN, Bartsocas C, Klatskin EH, Grunt JA. Children exposed in utero to propylthiouracil. Subsequent intellectual and physical development. Am J Dis Child. 1968; 116:161–5.

17. Hollingsworth DR, Mabry CC. Congenital Graves' disease. In: Fisher DA, Burrow GN, eds. Perinatal thyroid physiology and disease. New York: Raven Press, 1975:163–83.

18. McKenzie JM. Neonatal Graves' disease. J Clin Endocrinol. 1964; 24:660–8.

19. Solomon DH. Pregnancy and PTU. N Engl J Med. 1981; 304:538–9. editorial.

20. Burrow GN. Medical complications during pregnancy. Philadelphia: Saunders, 1975.

21. Milham S, Elledge W. Maternal methimazole and congenital defects in children. Teratology. 1972; 5:125. letter.

22. Tunstall ME. The effect of propranolol on the onset of breathing at birth. Br J Anaesth. 1969; 41:792.

23. Gladstone GR, Hordof A, Gersony WM. Propranolol administration during pregnancy: effects on the fetus. J Pediatr. 1975; 86:962–4.

24. Rubin PC. Current concepts: beta-blockers in pregnancy. N Engl J Med. 1981; 305:1323–6.

25. Schou M, Amdisen A, Jensen SE, Olson T. Occurrence of goitre during lithium treatment. Br Med J. 1968; 3:710–3.

26. Munro DS, Dirmikis SM, Humphries H, Smith T, Broadhead GD. The role of thyroid stimulating immunoglobulins of Graves' disease in neonatal thyrotoxicosis. Br J Obstet Gynaecol. 1978; 85:837–43.

27. Lowy C. Endocrine emergencies in pregnancy. Clin Endocrinol Metab. 1980; 9:569–81.

28. Ashcraft MW, Van Herle AJ. Management of thyroid nodules. I. History and physical examination, blood tests, X-ray tests, and ultrasonography. Head Neck Surg. 1981; 3:216–30.

29. Tannahill AJ, Hooper MJ, England M, Ferris JB, Wilson GM. Measurement of thyroid size by ultrasound, palpation and scintiscan. Clin Endocrinol. 1978; 8:483–6.

30. Scheible W, Leopold GR, Woo VL, Gosink BB. High-resolution real-time ultrasonography of thyroid nodules. Radiology. 1979; 133:413–7.

31. Ashcraft MW, Van Herle AJ. Management of thyroid nodules. II. Scanning techniques, thyroid suppressive therapy, and fine needle aspiration. Head Neck Surg. 1981; 3:297–322.

32. Van Herle AJ, Rich P, Ljung BE, Ashcraft MW, Solomon DH, Keeler EB. The thyroid nodule. Ann Intern Med. 1982; 96:221–32.

33. Amino N, Mori H, Iwatani Y, et al. High prevalence of transient post-partum thyrotoxicosis and hypothyroidism. N Engl J Med. 1982; 306:849–52.

34. Shahady EJ, Meckler GM. Postpartum thyroiditis. J Fam Pract. 1980; 11:1049–52.

35. Higgins HP, Hershman JM. The hyperthyroidism due to trophoblastic hormone. Clin Endocrinol Metab. 1978; 7:167–75.

36. Drake TS, Kaplan RA, Lewis TA. The physiologic hyperparathyroidism of pregnancy. Is it primary or secondary? Obstet Gynecol. 1979; 53:746–9.

37. Cushard WG, Creditor MA, Canterburn J, Seiss E. Physiologic hyperparathyroidism during pregnancy. J Clin Endocrinol Metab. 1972; 34:767–71.

38. Pitkin RM, Reynolds WA, Williams GA, Hargis GK. Calcium metabolism in normal pregnancy: a longitudinal study. Am J Obstet Gynecol. 1979; 133:781–90.

39. Shangold MM, Dor N, Welt SI, Fleischman AR, Crenshaw MC. Hyperparathyroidism and pregnancy: a review. Obstet Gynecol Surv. 1982; 37:217–28.

40. Wells S. The parathyroid glands. In: Sabiston D, ed. Davis-Christopher textbook of surgery. Philadelphia: Saunders, 1972:656–67.

41. Montoro MN, Collea JV, Mestman JH. The management of hyperparathyroidism in pregnancy with oral phosphate therapy. Obstet Gynecol. 1980; 55:431–4.

42. Thomason JL, Sampson MB, Farb HF, Spellacy WN. Pregnancy complicated by concurrent primary hyperparathyroidism and pancreatitis. Obstet Gynecol. 1981; 57:34S–36S.

43. Bronsky D, Kiamko RT, Moncada R, Rosenthal IM. Intrauterine hyperparathyroidism secondary to maternal hypothyroidism. Pediatrics. 1968; 42:606–13.

44. Landing BH. Congenital hyperparathyroidism secondary to maternal hypoparathyroidism. J Pediatr. 1970; 77:842–7.

45. Russell RG, Smith R, Walton RJ, et al. 1,25-dihydroxycholecalciferol and 1 alpha-hydroxycholecalciferol in hypoparathyroidism. Lancet. 1974; 2:14–7.

46. Marshall JR. Pregnancy in patients with prolactin-producing pituitary tumors. Clin Obstet Gynecol. 1980; 23:453–63.

47. Saxena BB. Human prolactin. In: Fuchs F, Klopper A, eds. Endocrinology of pregnancy. Hagerstown, Md: Harper & Row, 1977:222.

48. Magyar DM, Marshall JR. Pituitary tumors and pregnancy. Am J Obstet Gynecol. 1978; 132:739–51.

49. Mintz DH, Stock R, Finster J, Taylor AL. The effects of normal and diabetic pregnancies on growth hormone responses to hypoglycemia. Metabolism. 1968; 17:54–61.

50. Jacobs LS, Daughaday WH. Physiologic regulation of prolactin secretion in man. In: Josimovich JB, Reynolds M, Cobo E, eds. Lactogenic hormones, fetal nutrition and lactation. New York: Wiley, 1974:351–77.

51. Zimmerman EA, Defedini R, Frantz AG. Prolactin and growth hormone in patients with pituitary adenomas: a correlative study of hormone in tumor and plasma by immunoperoxidase technique and radioimmunoassay. J Clin Endocrinol Metab. 1974; 38:577–85.

52. Gemzell C, Wang CF. Outcome of pregnancy in women with pituitary adenoma. Fertil Steril. 1979; 31:363–72.

53. Parkes D. Drug therapy: bromocriptine. N Engl J Med. 1979; 301:873–8.

54. McGregor AM, Scanlon MF, Hall K, et al. Reduction in size of a pituitary tumor by bromocriptine therapy. N Engl J Med. 1979; 300:291–3.

55. Landolt AM, Wuthrich R, Fellmann H. Regression of pituitary prolactinoma after treatment with bromocriptine. Lancet. 1979; 1:1082–3. letter.

56. Thorner MO, Martin WH, Rogol AD, et al. Rapid regression of pituitary prolactinomas during bromocriptine treatment. J Clin Endocrinol Metab. 1980; 51:438–45.

57. Spark RF, Baker R, Bienfang, DC, Bergland R. Bromocriptine reduces pituitary tumor size and hypersecretion. Requiem for pituitary surgery? JAMA. 1982; 247:311–6.

58. Turkalj I, Braun P, Krup P. Surveillance of bromocriptine in pregnancy. JAMA. 1982; 247:1589–91.

59. Sheehan HL, Murdoch R. Post-partum necrosis of the anterior pituitary. Effect of subsequent pregnancy. Lancet. 1983; 2:123.

60. Grimes HG, Brooks MH. Pregnancy in Sheehan's syndrome. Report of a case and review. Obstet Gynecol Surv. 1980; 35:481–8.

61. Hime MC, Richardson JA. Diabetes insipidus and pregnancy. Case report, incidence and review of literature. Obstet Gynecol Surv. 1978; 33:375–9.

62. Scheer RL, Raisz LG, Lloyd CW. Changes in diabetes insipidus during pregnancy and lactation. J Clin Endocrinol Metab. 1959; 19:805–11.

63. Warren JC, Jernstrom RS. Diabetes insipidus and pregnancy. Am J Obstet Gynecol. 1961; 81:1036–41.

64. Burrow GN, Wassenaar W, Robertson GL, Sehl H. DDAVP treatment of diabetes insipidus during pregnancy and the post-partum period. Acta Endocrinol (Copenh). 1981; 97:23–5.

65. Campbell JW. Diabetes insipidus and complicated pregnancy. JAMA. 1980; 243:1744–5.

66. Schenker JG, Chowers I. Pheochromocytoma and pregnancy. Review of 89 cases. Obstet Gynecol Surv. 1971; 26:739–47.

67. Bravo EL, Tarazi RC, Gifford RW, Stewart BH. Circulating and urinary catecholamines in pheochromocytoma. Diagnostic and pathophysiologic implications. N Engl J Med. 1979; 301:682–6.

68. Roland CB. Pheochromocytoma in pregnancy: report of a fatal reaction to phentolamine (Regitine) methanesulfonate. JAMA. 1959; 171:1806–9.

69. Lipson A, Hsu TH, Sherwin B, Geelhoed GW. Nitroprusside therapy for a patient with a pheochromocytoma. JAMA. 1978; 239:427–8.

70. Bayliss RIS, Browne JCM, Round BP, Steinbeck AW. Plasma 17-hydroxycorticosteroids in pregnancy. Lancet. 1955; 1:62–4.

71. Montgomery DA, Harley JM. Endocrine disorders. Clin Obstet Gynaecol. 1977; 4:339–70.

72. Grimes EM, Fayez JA, Miller GL. Cushing's syndrome and pregnancy. Obstet Gynecol. 1973; 42:550–9.

73. Kreines K, DeVaux WD. Neonatal adrenal insufficiency associated with maternal Cushing's syndrome. Pediatrics. 1971; 47:516–9.

74. Bondy PK, Rosenberg LE, eds. Metabolic control and disease. Philadelphia: Saunders, 1980.

75. Conn JW. Presidential address: painting background; primary aldosteronism: a new clinical syndrome. J Lab Clin Med. 1955; 45:3–17.

76. Weinberger MH, Grim CE, Hollifield JW, Kem DC, et al. Primary aldosteronism: diagnosis, localization, and treatment. Ann Intern Med. 1979; 90:386–95.

77. Biglieri EG, Slaton PE. Pregnancy and primary aldosteronism. J Clin Endocrinol Metab. 1967; 27:1628–32.

78. Crane MG, Andes JP, Harris JJ, Slate WG. Primary aldosteronism in pregnancy. Obstet Gynecol. 1964; 23:200–8.

79. Gordon RD, Fishman LM, Liddle GW. Plasma renin

activity and aldosterone secretion in a pregnant woman with primary aldosteronism. J Clin Endocrinol Metab. 1967; 27:385–8.

80. Aoi W, Doi Y, Tasaki S, Mitsuoka T, Suzuki S, Hashiba K. Primary aldosteronism aggravated during peripartum period. Jpn Heart. J1978; 19:946–53.

81. Jones JM, Lloyd-Jones R, Riondel A, Tait JF, Tait SAS, Bulbrook RD, Greenwood FC. Aldosterone secretion and metabolism in normal men and women in pregnancy. Acta Endocrinol (Copenh). 1959; 30:321.

82. Watanabe M, Meeker MI, Gray MJ, Sims EAH, Solomon S. Secretion rate of aldosterone in normal pregnancy. J Clin Invest. 1963; 42:1619–31.

83. Landau RL, Lugibihl K. Inhibition of the sodium retaining influence of aldosterone by progesterone. J Clin Endocrinol Metab. 1958; 18:1237–45.

84. Laidlaw JC, Ruse JL, Gornall AG. The influence of estrogen and progesterone on aldosterone excretion. J Clin Endocrinol Metab. 1962; 22:161–71.

85. Kai H, Nose O, Iida Y, Ono J, Harada T, Yabuuchi H. Female pseudohermaphroditism caused by maternal congenital adrenal hyperplasia. J Pediatr. 1979; 95:418–9.

*If a pregnant woman acquires diabetes, my
advice would be to allow the pregnancy to
continue ... if a diabetic becomes pregnant,
it is more serious.*
—Dr. Elliott Joslin
Treatment of Diabetes Mellitus

11. DIABETES MELLITUS

Richard S. Abrams, Walter A. Huttner, and Paul Wexler

In 1928 Dr. Priscilla White wrote, "Before insulin, coma was the end result of the pregnant diabetic" [1]. Dr. White and her mentor, Dr. Elliott Joslin, pioneered the development of successful treatment programs for the pregnant diabetic. Today we confront the occurrence of diabetes during pregnancy with a distinctly more optimistic view. Current understanding of maternal metabolism and its effect on fetal growth and development has allowed physicians to make a major impact on this most difficult medical complication of pregnancy. Meticulous care and rigid metabolic control of the diabetic woman during pregnancy have dramatically reduced maternal and fetal mortality [2,25].

Specific management protocols vary at different institutions. Regardless of minor differences, we feel that the most important principles of medical management are preconceptional control of diabetes, prompt recognition of gestational diabetes, rigid glycemic control, and close surveillance of mother and fetus throughout pregnancy. Management is best performed by a team of health care professionals including an obstetrician, a nurse, a nutritionist, a neonatologist, and a physician with special expertise in medical complications during pregnancy.

METABOLIC ALTERATIONS DURING NORMAL PREGNANCY

During nondiabetic pregnancy, maternal metabolism adapts to provide fuel for the growing fetoplacental unit as well as the mother. At term, the human fetus has a daily glucose requirement of approximately 30 g [3]. This requirement is four times greater per kilogram of body weight than that of a normal adult [4]. In order to meet this need, the fetus continually siphons glucose from the maternal compartment [5]. While the fetus may be in a constant state of feeding, the mother will be feeding at some times and fasting at others. Therefore, if fetal glucose levels are to be maintained within narrow limits, the maternal pancreas must meticulously regulate maternal glucose levels.

Glucose reaches the fetus by a process called facilitated diffusion; that is, it crosses the placenta at a rate faster than would be predicted on physiochemical grounds alone. Maternal mechanisms to preserve glucose levels within narrow limits include increased protein catabolism, activation of hepatic gluconeogenesis, and accelerated renal gluconeogenesis [6,7].

Amino acids are actively transported to the fetal circulation against a concentration gradient. This process of active transport results in a fetal concentration of amino acids approximately one to four times higher than in the maternal plasma [9]. Particularly important to the maintenance of maternal blood glucose level is the gluconeogenic amino acid, alanine. As a result of the active transport of amino acids, alanine concentrations are decreased in the mother [10].

Thus, maternal loss of glucose and gluconeogenic substrate to the fetus occurs concomitantly and conspires to cause maternal hypoglycemia in early pregnancy.

At approximately 24 weeks' gestation the so-called diabetogenic effect of pregnancy begins. At this time the mother switches from primarily a glucose-based energy economy to a lipid-based energy economy derived either from circulating fats or from stored adipose tissue in order to spare glucose for fetal growth [6]. Also at this time, the contrainsulin hormones, human placental lactogen, prolactin, and cortisol are produced in amounts proportional to the growing placenta [11–15,19–21].

These metabolic and hormonal alterations create a "stress" which the insulin-dependent diabetic or the woman with borderline pancreatic reserve is unable to meet. The insulin-dependent diabetic will require additional exogenous insulin. The woman with inadequate pancreatic reserve or abnormal insulin utilization will become overtly diabetic. Maternal glucose assimilation becomes more sluggish in the presence of the diabetogenic stress. When this condition ensues, the maternal plasma compartment becomes a conduit of excessive substrate for the developing fetus. Moreover, in the diabetic pregnancy, it appears that not only glucose but other circulating nutrients have the potential for increased placental transport to the fetus. Any or all of these nutrients could contribute to altered cellular development.

FETAL EFFECTS OF ALTERED METABOLISM

In 1952 Pedersen proposed an explanation for the observed high morbidity and mortality of infants of diabetic mothers (Fig. 11-1). According to his hypothesis, maternal hyperglycemia caused fetal hyperglycemia and fetal hyperinsulinemia. Fetal hyperinsulinemia resulted in increased fetal body fat (macrosomia) and also possibly inhibited the pulmonary maturation process required for surfactant production [31].

Freinkel and Metzger have expanded Pedersen's classic hypothesis to explain how metabolic disturbances might result in abnormal organogenesis and cellular development (Fig. 11-2). They concluded that

pregnancy represents a type of tissue culture in which the conceptus develops *de novo* and the composition of the tissue culture medium is determined by the maternal fuels which gain access to the conceptus. As in all tissue culture exercises, the developing cells may be greatly influenced by the nature of the incubation medium. For many developing fetal cells, this carries few long range implications since they will be undergoing continuous renewal throughout the lifetime of the offspring. Other cells, however, are more "terminal" structures. They have limited replicative capacity and some of the total endowment and function of these cells in the offspring may be influenced by intrauterine and perinatal events. These include brain cells, fat cells, muscle cells and perhaps the beta cell of the pancreatic islets [8] (Fig. 11-3).

Thus, Freinkel and Metzger's expanded hypothesis goes beyond the original hyperglycemia-hyperinsulinemia model to include additional substrates available to the fetus and their effect on all stages of cellular development.

PERINATAL MORBIDITY AND MORTALITY

The fetus of a diabetic woman, for reasons that remain uncertain, can die suddenly and unexpectedly in the last trimester of pregnancy. Stillbirths can occur 10 to 20 times more frequently than in the nondiabetic population [22]. Third-trimester perinatal mortality has most often been attributed to (1) prematurity as a result of preterm delivery, functional immaturity, or both; (2) traumatic vaginal delivery; and (3) unexpected intrauterine death [23]. The deaths appear to be most common in patients with poor control, in association with fetal macrosomia, in pregnancies complicated by preeclampsia, and in women who have had a previous stillbirth.

It is now clear that previously reported high perinatal mortality associated with diabetic pregnancies can be dramatically reduced. Improved obstetric care, combined with rigid control of maternal glucose levels, has lowered perinatal mortality in one study to approximately 6.5% during the years 1976 to 1979, as compared to 18% during the years 1950 to 1970 [24]. This decrease in perinatal mortality has also been demonstrated by the extensive experience of Molsted-Pedersen's group in Copenhagen. Their study of 1,995 infants of diabetic mothers extending from 1946 to 1978 permits two conclusions. First, they showed that perinatal death rates have fallen from 22% to 4.4% during this 32-year period. Second, the distribution of patients by the White classification has not changed. Therefore, one cannot attribute the decreased mortality to less severe maternal disease [25]. A review of the major published research on diabetic pregnancies during the last 60 years reveals that the key to this improvement is normalization of maternal blood sugars [25,26,40].

Despite the marked improvement in fetal survival, the incidence of congenital anomalies in infants of diabetic mothers remains three times greater than the incidence in the general population. Anomalies incompatible with life have continued to occur six times as frequently [27]. No less than 40% of the perinatal mortality encoun-

Fig. 11-1. The classic hyperglycemia-hyperinsulinemia hypothesis of Pedersen. (Adapted from Freinkel and Metzger [8].)

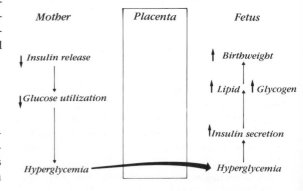

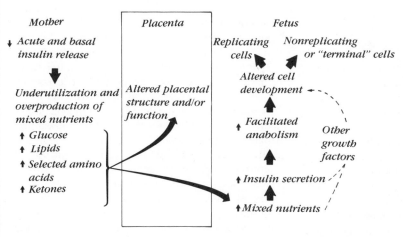

Fig. 11-2. The Pedersen hypothesis as expanded by
Freinkel and Metzger. (Adapted from Freinkel and
Metzger [8].)

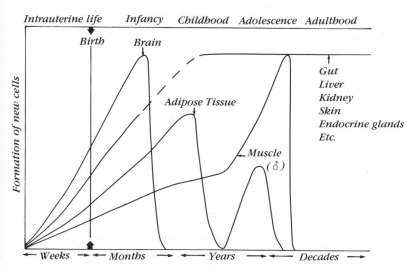

Fig. 11-3. Cycles of cell development. (From Freinkel
and Metzger [8].)

tered at present results from fetal congenital malformations [28]. Recent studies have suggested
that metabolic perturbations are responsible for
the high incidence of congenital malformations as
well as the growth problems that occur in late
pregnancy. Studies using measurements of hemoglobin A_{1c} (HbA$_{1c}$) in early pregnancy imply that
when organogenesis occurs in the setting of
hyperglycemia the incidence of congenital
anomalies is significantly increased [29,30].

GENERAL MANAGEMENT PRINCIPLES
Preconception Control
In their study of 115 insulin-dependent diabetics,
Miller et al. obtained retrospective evidence that
women delivering infants with major congenital
anomalies had significantly higher levels of HbA$_{1c}$
during the first trimester than did diabetics who
delivered infants free of anomalies [29]. On the
basis of these data we have asked diabetic women
who are planning pregnancy to begin rigid blood
sugar control, assessed by home glucose monitoring, while they continue contraception. Only
when HbA$_{1c}$ levels are less than 8.5% do we advise
them to discontinue contraceptive measures. Patients are asked to measure and record daily basal
body temperatures. Women who have not had any
menstrual bleeding 16 days after a rise in basal
body temperature are instructed to report for a
serum pregnancy test. They are also instructed to
report for pregnancy testing in the event their
menstrual periods do not occur on schedule. Be-

Table 11-1. The White classification

Gestational diabetes	Diabetes discovered for the first time during pregnancy
Class A	Diet controlled; any duration or onset
Class B	Onset—age 20 or older; duration—less than 10 years
Class C	Onset—age 10–19; duration—10–19 years
Class D	Onset—before age 10; duration—over 20 years
Class R	Background retinopathy; proliferative retinopathy or vitreous hemorrhage
Class F	Diabetic nephropathy
Class RF	Retinopathy and nephropathy
Class G	Multiple reproductive failures (habitual abortions and/or stillbirths)
Class H	Arteriosclerotic heart disease, clinically evident
Class T	Prior renal transplantation

Table 11-2. Prognostic bad signs during pregnancy

Clinical pyelonephritis
Diabetic ketoacidosis
Pregnancy-induced hypertension
Lack of antenatal care

Table 11-3. O'Sullivan criteria for detection of diabetes during pregnancy (100 g oral GTT)

Interval	Whole blood* (mg/dL)	Plasma* (mg/dL)
Fasting	90	105
1 hr	165	190
2 hr	145	165
3 hr	125	140

*Values represent two standard deviations above the mean.

cause of the variability in menstrual periods, a careful review with each patient at the time of initial evaluation is helpful in determining at what time she should consider a menstrual period late.

Classification

For many years the White classification has been accepted worldwide as the standard categorization of diabetes during pregnancy. This classification is based on the duration of diabetes, the age of onset, and the presence of vascular disease (Table 11-1).

Some confusion has occurred when an attempt has been made to fit women with gestational dia-

betes into these classes. The White classification was originally intended to be used for women with glucose intolerance recognized prior to pregnancy. Thus, class A was never intended to be synonymous with gestational diabetes. In a recent clarification, Dr. White proposed that "gestational diabetes be separately considered whether insulin treated or not." She defined gestational diabetes as diabetes discovered for the first time during pregnancy. Class A diabetics have had glucose intolerance established prior to pregnancy but they do not require insulin to achieve glycemic control. It was recognized that some women's diabetes will be discovered during pregnancy for the first time despite probable prior glucose intolerance. Nevertheless, in the absence of data obtained when not pregnant, the diagnosis of gestational diabetes may be presumed, though not firmly established [37].

An additional classification scheme for diabetes during pregnancy was proposed by Pedersen. In Pedersen's series a high mortality was encountered if any of the "prognostic bad signs during pregnancy" (Table 11-2) were present in each of White's classifications except F.

Gestational Diabetes

The incidence of gestational diabetes has been reported to be 1 to 2% of pregnant women [35]. Despite improvement in the outcome of diabetic pregnancies in general, gestational diabetes continues to present significant perinatal risks. Evidence is accumulating that this risk can be reduced by a systematic approach to identification and management of this disease [32].

The generally accepted criteria for abnormal glucose tolerance during pregnancy were established by O'Sullivan and Mahan in 1964 and revised in 1973 [35] (Table 11-3). These criteria were based on the results of administering a 100-g oral glucose load to 751 unselected pregnant women. Normal limits were defined as two standard deviations above the mean for each of four values determined. The O'Sullivan criteria have been validated by follow-up of gestational diabetics, which revealed a 16-year cumulative incidence of diabetes, by life table, of 60% [33]. Unfortunately, the 3-hour glucose tolerance test is expensive, time-consuming, and not easily tolerated by many women. In order to select a group of pregnant women with the greatest likelihood of glucose intolerance several screening methods have been suggested. It is clear that any effective screening test for gestational diabetes must be extremely sensitive.

Traditionally, women thought to be at high risk

Table 11-4. Risk factors for gestational diabetes

History of gestational diabetes

History of large babies

Family history of diabetes

Symptoms of diabetes

Recurrent moniliasis

Recurrent urinary tract infections or pyelonephritis

Glycosuria

Excessive weight gain during pregnancy

Hypertension during pregnancy

Obstetric history of stillbirths, prematurity, or
polyhydramnios (past or present)

for gestational diabetes were identified by clinical criteria (Table 11-4). In fact, if clinical history alone is used to determine the need for a 3-hour glucose tolerance test, 38% of gestational diabetics will not be identified [35].

In 1973, O'Sullivan proposed the use of a 1-hour screening test following a 50-g glucose load. A whole blood glucose value greater than 130 mg/dL or 143 mg/dL by plasma glucose was considered abnormal and obligated a complete 100-g glucose load, 3-hour glucose tolerance test. The sensitivity and specificity of this screening method were 79% and 87% respectively, in the general population, and 88% and 82%, respectively, among pregnant women 25 years of age or older [35]. In an attempt to identify an even more efficient screening threshold Carpenter and Coustan administered a 50-g glucose load to 381 gravidas 25 years of age or older [34]. They identified three diagnostic zones: (1) a zone where the 1-hour plasma glucose

Fig. 11-4. An algorithm for detection of abnormal glucose tolerance during pregnancy.

1 hr 50 g glucose screen
performed at 22–26 wk

plasma glucose $\geq$ 135 mg/dL*

↓

3 hr OGTT (O'Sullivan Criteria)

┌──────────────┴──────────────┐

Abnormal   *Normal*

↓   ↓

Diet   Repeat 3 hr OGTT
or   at 32 wk
begin insulin if:
FBS > 105 mg/dL and/or
2 hr postprandial > 120 mg/dL

*1 hr screening test should be repeated at 32 wk for selected high risk patients with a normal screen at 24 wk.

value was below 135 mg/dL, with less than 1% probability of diabetes; (2) a zone where the plasma glucose was above 182 mg/dL, with more than 95% probability of diabetes; and (3) a central zone of uncertainty where the plasma glucose was between 135 mg/dL and 182 mg/dL. Thus, these data suggest that the threshold for further testing be lowered from that suggested by O'Sullivan (143 mg/dL by plasma glucose determination or 130 mg/dL by whole-blood glucose determination) to 135 mg/dL of plasma glucose.

Another proposed screening method for gestational diabetes is the determination of glycosylated hemoglobin. It has been reasoned that, since the level of glycosylated hemoglobin reflects the mean blood glucose level over the previous 4 to 8 weeks, it may be a sensitive screening device. Shah et al. tested this hypothesis in a prospective study of 90 subjects [36]. The sensitivity and specificity of HbA_1 determination alone were 27% and 86.5%, respectively. These data suggest that glycohemoglobin determination is not sensitive enough to be used as a screening method.

An outline for detection of abnormal glucose tolerance during pregnancy is presented in Figure 11-4. The 50-g glucose load is easily tolerated and can be administered anytime of day without any specific dietary preparation [35]. In general, we recommend that this test be performed at 22 to 26 weeks gestation, when most patients demonstrate insulin resistance. The test can be performed earlier if clinical criteria strongly suggest diabetes. Likewise, a 1-hour screen should be repeated at 32 weeks for selected high risk patients even if a prior screen was normal.

Women determined to be gestational diabetics should be counseled regarding diet and taught home glucose monitoring. We usually begin insulin therapy when fasting blood sugar values consistently exceed 105 mg/dL or postprandial values are greater than 120 mg/dL determined by home monitoring.

Achievement of Glycemic Control

It has been emphasized in this chapter as well as many reviews that the most significant contribution to the successful outcome of a diabetic patient is rigid, near-normal glycemic control [13,25, 30,40,48]. This goal is applicable to both insulin-dependent and non-insulin-dependent diabetics. For the insulin-dependent diabetic rigid control combines careful balancing of diet, energy expenditure in daily activity, and an insulin regimen designed to achieve efficient energy utilization while avoiding extremes of either hyperglycemia or hypoglycemia. For the non-insulin-dependent diabetic it is critical to recognize when she can no longer be satisfactorily managed with diet alone, thus becoming insulin dependent for the remainder of her pregnancy.

Home Glucose Monitoring

Home glucose monitoring is the present cornerstone of rigid glycemic controls for all patients with glucose intolerance. Adjustments in insulin dosage can be made even on a daily basis utilizing this technique. We instruct patients to measure and record blood sugars at least twice each day. The timing of the measurements can be random or specifically designed to check certain times of the day when control for that individual has been most difficult. On occasion we have instructed patients to awaken from sleep in the early morning and check blood sugar. This technique has allowed us to recognize asymptomatic nocturnal hypoglycemia.

Most home glucose monitors approximate plasma glucose rather than whole blood glucose since only the plasma of the capillary whole blood applied to the strip permeates the reagent pad to react with the glucose oxidase. Some variations have been reported with the reflectance meters of various manufacturers [47].

Our experience has been that of uniform acceptance of this approach by our pregnant diabetics. In addition to the requisite information obtained, we have found the use of home glucose monitoring to be a major motivational factor that encourages active participation of our patients in their own rigid control. In almost every instance this careful glycemic control has become the new standard for which our patients strive even after pregnancy.

Glycosylated Hemoglobin

In 1968 an abnormal hemoglobin was found in the red cells of diabetics. It was later shown that this was a modification of hemoglobin A in the presence of persistent hyperglycemia [43]. Hemoglobin A_{1c} (HbA_{1c}) is a normal minor hemoglobin that is distinguished from HbA by the addition of a glucose moiety to the amino-terminal valine of the beta chain. Glycosylation of the HbA occurs during circulation of the red cell. The level of HbA_{1c} is dependent on the average concentration of glucose to which the red cell has been exposed during its life cycle. Measurement of HbA_{1c} provides an integrated, retrospective index of glucose control during the previous 30 to 60 days [54].

We have utilized the measurement of HbA_{1c} during pregnancy for two major reasons. First, monthly samples have provided us with a mean glucose assessment in addition to home monitoring. Elevated values, inconsistent with a patient's home glucose determinations, alert us to inaccurate technique, inadequate or poorly timed sampling, or possibly false reporting. On the other hand, the technique of HbA_{1c} measurement does not permit the clinician the security of relying on a normal or slightly low HbA_{1c} as the sole indication of good control [55]. Second, we have used the measurements of HbA_{1c} to assess preconceptional glycemic control in order to achieve optimum circumstances for planned conception. Because of the degree of overlap between HbA_{1c} levels from a population of diabetic patients and levels in the normal range, HbA_{1c} has not been recommended as a screening device for gestational diabetes [36]. Some diabetic patients will be missed if the HbA_{1c} level is the only tool used for detection [55]. Screening techniques are usually permitted a small degree of false positivity; however, even a small degree of unrecognized diabetes in pregnancy is unacceptable.

Diet

All too frequently dietary instructions for pregnant women, whether diabetic or not, have been empiric and at times irrational. For instance, there is no rationale for stringent limitations on weight gain during pregnancy. The Committee on Maternal Nutrition—Food and Nutrition Board has suggested an optimal weight gain for pregnancy: for the normal patient an initial weight gain of 0.9 to 1.8 kg in the first trimester and then a steady weight gain of 0.23 to 0.46 kg per week to a total of 10.0 to 13.7 kg during the course of gestation [38,39].

Many gestational diabetics are overweight prior to pregnancy. Principal goals for these patients are to meet the nutritional needs of both mother and fetus and to avoid hyperglycemia. Although caloric restriction might prevent hyperglycemia, without adequate carbohydrate intake fat metabolism will occur, resulting in maternal ketonemia. Mintz et al. have stated that "pregnancy is not the time to initiate a weight reduction program." Their overweight patients were prescribed a diet adequate to support the usual pattern of weight gain, but excessive (greater than 3 kg per month) weight gain was "firmly discouraged" [40].

Mothers with inadequate weight gain are at risk for pregnancy-induced hypertension, antepartum hemorrhage, and low-birth-weight infants [41]. These patients require careful and repeated dietary consultations. Occasionally hospital confinement is needed to ensure adequate nutrition.

For the insulin-dependent diabetic, whether obese or not, a dietary regimen must be predicated on a careful diet history. A clear understanding of a woman's dietary preferences, activity, and mealtimes can avoid dietary instructions that are likely not to be followed. In many cases insulin therapy can be designed to achieve rigid glycemic control while a patient's "usual" diet is followed.

In general we recommend that a diet contain approximately 30 to 35 kcal/kg ideal body weight. In order to avoid ketonemia, at least 45% of the total calories should be carbohydrate [42]. Carbohydrate intake can be divided into convenient portions (i.e., 25% at each meal). Smaller amounts of carbohydrate should be eaten as midmorning and evening snacks. The evening snack is particularly important in order to avoid nocturnal hypoglycemia. Additional nutritional requirements include a total daily protein intake of approximately 30 g and a total fat intake of 40 to 60 g. Special gestational requirements for mineral and vitamin supplements have been discussed in Chapter 4 and in several recent reviews [44–46]. Recently there has also been growing enthusiasm for the addition of dietary fiber to flatten the postprandial glycemic response, apparently by reducing the rate of gastric emptying and slowing intestinal absorption of carbohydrate.

If a patient has symptoms of hypoglycemia, she is instructed to eat a snack containing both carbohydrate and protein (e.g., 4–6 oz milk and two crackers with cheese or peanut butter). If hypoglycemic symptoms have not abated in 10 to 15 minutes, an additional 4 oz of milk should be drunk. We find that these specific instructions prevent the temptation to ingest large amounts of carbohydrates (e.g., candy or orange juice laced with sugar), which can cause blood sugar to overcompensate. The protein content of supplemental snacks tends to maintain normoglycemia longer than would pure carbohydrate.

As important as the content of meals is timing of meals. All meals and snacks should be monotonously constant. If timing consistency is maintained, insulin adjustments can be made simple to compensate for blood sugar changes.

A characteristic feature of non-insulin dependent diabetes, including many gestational diabetics, is that endogenous insulin secretion is delayed. Nevertheless, most gestational diabetics mount a sufficient insulin response to restore postprandial blood glucose levels to their basal levels within 4 or 5 hours. Meals should be adequately spaced to permit restoration of basal (preprandial) glucose levels before additional food is consumed. Except for a bedtime snack to prevent morning ketosis, we ask gestational diabetics to avoid between meal snacks and to space meals by approximately 5 hours.

Activity

When there are no specific medical or obstetric contraindications, we encourage our patients to continue prepregnancy daily activities. We attempt to design a diet and insulin regimen that permits continued employment or daily exercise until late in gestation.

At least two potential complications of exercise in diabetes should be kept in mind. First, exercise in the insulin-dependent diabetic can cause significant episodes of hypoglycemia. The tendency to exercise-induced hypoglycemia can be ameliorated by (1) ingestion of supplemental carbohydrate prior to exercise, (2) using a nonexercised area of the body for insulin injection, and (3) lowering the dosage of insulin. Unfortunately, the amount of extra carbohydrate needed or the amount by which the insulin dosage requires reduction can be determined only empirically. Second, exercise-induced elevations of counterregulatory hormones (glucagon, catecholamines, and growth hormone) are exaggerated in diabetes if insulin treatment is less than optimal. In the setting of inadequate insulin therapy, exercise can worsen rather than improve glycemic control. Exercise should be considered an adjunct to rather than a substitute for proper management of diabetes with insulin. We underscore the need for consistency in the amount and timing of daily exercise to avoid frequent dietary and insulin adjustments.

Insulin Therapy

Most insulin-dependent diabetics will require multiple doses of insulin each day. The physician must individualize therapy and anticipate the changing insulin requirements at various stages of gestation. During early pregnancy, fasting hypoglycemia and decreased insulin requirements can be expected. As pregnancy progresses, insulin requirements will increase to overcome contra-insulin factors. The more severe diabetics have greater excursions in blood sugars above and below daily mean values, frequently associated with nocturnal hypoglycemia and possibly ketosis [50].

The goal of any insulin program must be to achieve efficient energy utilization while avoiding extremes of either hyperglycemia or hypoglycemia. In the nondiabetic individual there is a constant or basal level of insulin secretion supplemented by additional or bolus secretion in response to meals. The ideal insulin regimen

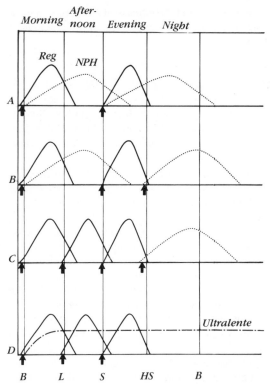

Fig. 11-5. Four multiple-component insulin regimens discussed in text. Symbols used in regimens A–D are: B, breakfast; L, lunch; S, supper; HS, bedtime snack; Reg, regular or short-acting insulin; and NPH, intermediate-acting insulin. Arrows indicate the time of insulin injection. (Adapted from Skyler, et al. [48]. Reproduced with permission from Skyler, et al. the American Diabetes Association, Inc.)

should be designed to mimic this pattern. Clearly, single-dose insulin therapy cannot provide a continuous basal insulinemia throughout the day and night. We feel that the vast majority of insulin-dependent diabetics will require multiple-component insulin regimens in order to achieve rigid glycemic control.

Skyler et al. have suggested four multiple-component insulin regimens useful for achieving rigid glycemic control [48]. These regimens are schematically depicted in Figure 11-5. Regimen A involves a twice-daily injection of a mixture of short-acting and intermediate-acting insulin. As a guideline, we have found that two-thirds of the total daily dose (one part short-acting mixed with two parts intermediate-acting) given in the morning and one-third of the total (equal parts short- and intermediate-acting) given before the evening meal provides good control for many patients. However, this regimen can produce nocturnal hypoglycemic episodes if the intermediate-acting

insulin given before the evening meal has its peak action during the middle of the night. Regimen B attempts to obviate the problem of nocturnal hypoglycemia by delaying the evening injection of intermediate-acting insulin until bedtime. This schedule results in peak insulin action coinciding with awakening and breakfast. Regimen C is composed of multiple injections of short-acting insulin preceding each meal and intermediate-acting insulin given at bedtime. This regimen can achieve good glycemic control but requires four daily injections. Regimen D is a multiple-dose program providing preprandial short-acting insulin and basal insulin as long-acting, relatively peakless ultralente insulin. Although the figure depicts all the ultralente being mixed with the morning short-acting insulin, Skyler suggests providing half of the total ultralente dose with the pre-supper short-acting insulin, in order to reduce the total volume of injection and to provide smoother action. Algorithms for adjustment of these various regimens have been described by Skyler et al. [48].

Oral hypoglycemic agents should not be used to manage diabetes during pregnancy. Sulfonylureas have been reported to cause intractable hypoglycemia in infants of diabetic mothers [49].

On the premise that the ultimate glycemic control is to mimic normal pancreatic insulin release, some diabetics are now using portable, battery-driven insulin infusion pumps. These pumps provide a basal rate of insulin infusion with pulse-dose increments before meals. Tamborlane et al. have shown that these devices can considerably improve glycemic control [52]. The same investigators have also demonstrated the efficacy and feasibility of the insulin infusion pump during pregnancy [53]. In their group of seven patients (White classes D–RF), they were able to reduce mean blood sugars from 135 to 104 mg/dL during pump treatment. All infants were born at term and had no macrosomia or neonatal problems. Insulin infusion devices are rapidly being improved with respect to miniaturization, safety, and ease of use. The reader is referred to specific product instructions for actual use.

Recently, a study done by Reeves et al. demonstrated that comparably rigid glycemic control could be achieved with continuous subcutaneous insulin infusion or with intensification of conventional therapy using one of the regimens described above [51]. Their data suggest that the method of insulin delivery (infusion pump versus multiple injections) contributes less to rigid control than such factors as home glucose monitoring, carefully controlled diet and exercise, and continual availability of the physician in order to make adjustments of insulin dosage promptly. It should be emphasized that the safety of utilizing continuous insulin infusion during pregnancy has yet to be established.

SPECIAL PROBLEMS IN DIABETIC PREGNANCIES
Diabetic Ketoacidosis

Fortunately, severe ketoacidosis is encountered with decreasing frequency during pregnancy. Ketoacidosis at any time during pregnancy has been associated with fetal death. Drury et al. noted 11 intrauterine deaths in 13 women who experienced ketoacidosis [57]. During the first trimester diabetic ketoacidosis could probably cause major fetal malformations. As previously discussed, the latter half of gestation can be associated with marked deterioration in glucose control and ketosis. Patients most likely to develop ketoacidosis are those who are unsophisticated or unconcerned about diabetic management. Ketoacidosis and subsequent fetal death have also been reported during sympathomimetic therapy for premature labor in an insulin dependent diabetic [58].

There are many acceptable protocols for insulin administration to correct ketoacidosis. One approach has been to give a priming dose of regular insulin, 0.2 units/kg intravenously, followed by an infusion of 0.1 to 0.15 units/kg/hour. We give all insulin intravenously, but protocols using subcutaneous and intramuscular routes can be equally effective. Initial insulin is administered in normal saline. We give glucose only when the blood sugar falls below 150 mg/dL. Glucose is important at this point, since the effect of the insulin continues as the infusion is discontinued.

Although total body stores of potassium are usually low, serum levels can be initially high. We add potassium at approximately 40 mEq/L once it is established that the glucose level is falling. A falling glucose is a safe indicator that the potassium level is also falling; therefore it is not necessary to wait for laboratory confirmation of a falling potassium before giving intravenous potassium. An exception is made when a patient is admitted with acidemia and a low serum potassium, in which case potassium should be administered immediately.

Patients with ketoacidosis usually present with anorexia, nausea, and vomiting, coupled with polyuria, tachypnea, and, in severe cases, altered consciousness. Treatment must be individualized, with immediate attention to correction of metabolic disturbances and determination of the underlying cause.

Diabetic Retinopathy

Extensive experience with pregnant diabetic women at the Joslin Clinic reveals that perinatal loss remains high in diabetics with known vascular disease [62]. One form of vascular disease, diabetic retinopathy, has been a major concern because of the fear that pregnancy may cause further retinal damage. The prognosis for vision in the presence of diabetic retinopathy relates both to duration of disease and to the status of visual acuity at the time retinopathy was first discovered. Background retinopathy is present in up to 25% of pregnant diabetics. It worsens and remits periodically regardless of pregnancy. A prospective study of 279 diabetic patients by Horvat et al. has shown that pregnancy does not cause progression of vascular lesions of the retina [59]. They suggest that the presence of diabetic retinitis is not an indication for elective early termination of pregnancy.

Patients should have a careful ophthalmologic exam early in pregnancy or, ideally, prior to conception. Patients with background retinopathy should be followed expectantly, whereas those with proliferative changes should receive laser photocoagulation treatment as early in pregnancy as possible. Consideration of pregnancy termination should be restricted only to patients with severe neovascular changes or to women showing a marked progression of retinopathy despite first-trimester photocoagulation therapy. Finally, although pregnancy does not appear to accelerate retinopathy, a young diabetic woman with extensive retinopathy contemplating pregnancy should be aware that she may have to contend with the progression of her disease and its threat of blindness during the same period of life she devotes to child rearing.

Diabetic Nephropathy

A study by Kitzmiller et al. concluded that "pregnancy is not associated with permanent worsening of renal function in the majority of diabetic patients with nephropathy" [60]. Nevertheless, diabetic nephropathy is a relentlessly progressive disease. End-stage uremia occurs within two to four years of the onset of clinical signs in nearly all patients. The diagnosis of diabetic nephropathy during pregnancy is made on the basis of persistent proteinuria of greater than 400 mg per 24 hours occurring in the first half of pregnancy in the absence of a urinary tract infection [60]. The current prevalence of diabetic nephropathy during pregnancy at the Joslin Clinic is reported to be 9.6% [60]. At the same clinic, perinatal survival for class F pregnancies attaining 24 weeks' gestation was 88.9% for the years 1975 to 1978, compared

Table 11-5. Management of diabetic renal disease

Clinical syndrome	Laboratory data	Management
Stage 1. Early diabetic nephropathy Essentially asymptomatic Rare hypertension	Occasional proteinuria	Sodium restriction if hypertensive
Stage 2. Early renal failure (Cr clearance > 30 mL/min) Occasional edema Hypertension Difficult control of diabetes	Proteinuria BUN $\simeq 40$ mg/dL Cr $\simeq 2$–4 mg/dL PO_4 elevation	Sodium restriction Phosphate binders Antihypertensive drugs
Stage 3. Advanced renal failure (Cr clearance < 30 mL/min) Hypertension Fluid overload Anemia Weakness Diabetes very difficult to control	BUN > 50 mg/dL Cr $\simeq 4$–5 mg/dL PO_4 elevation Calcium low Anemia Hyperkalemia	Sodium restriction Potassium restriction Protein restriction PO_4 binders Maintain calcium levels Control hypertension Creation of AV fistula Tissue typing

Decision for hemodialysis or renal transplant made when creatinine clearance < 10 mL/min, BUN > 100 mg/dL, or serum creatinine > 10 mg/dL, or earlier.

Cr = creatinine; BUN = blood urea nitrogen; AV = arteriovenous.
From J. L. Kitzmiller et al. Diabetic vascular disease complicating pregnancy. *Clin Obstet Gynecol.* 1981; 24:109.

to 71% for the years 1963 to 1975 and 59% for the years 1938 to 1958 [60]. These improved perinatal survival figures presumably related to more careful glycemic and blood pressure control, willingness of patients to accept prolonged bed rest, and improved obstetric management.

Kitzmiller's data suggest that creatinine clearance is not worsened by the course of pregnancy in the majority of women with diabetic nephropathy. However, women with nearly normal creatinine clearances in early pregnancy did not show the expected increase in creatinine clearance seen in normal gestation [60]. Hypertension continues to be thought of as possibly the most important exacerbating factor in diabetic nephropathy. In the Joslin Clinic study, hypertension was related to increased proteinuria, decreased creatinine clearance, and decreased fetal growth [60].

Treatment of renal disease in diabetics may be considered in two stages. In the early stage of the disease salt and water restriction and appropriate diuretic therapy may help control edema and congestion associated with the nephrotic syndrome. Bed rest and additional antihypertensive medication should be used when indicated. During pregnancy it is impossible to diagnose preeclampsia without renal biopsy, since accelerating hypertension and proteinuria are common features of both disorders. In the later stage, when severe renal insufficiency ensues, appropriate dietary restrictions and ultimately dialysis or transplantation may be required. Table 11-5 summarizes the approach to management of diabetic renal disease at the Joslin Clinic.

Questions regarding pregnancy in renal transplant recipients are arising with increased frequency. Rudolph et al. conducted a questionnaire survey and review of the literature on this subject [61]. With therapeutic abortions excluded, 71% of 308 pregnancies in renal transplant recipients resulted in full-term infants. Kidney rejection episodes occurred in 9% of these pregnancies. No predicted pattern or triggering mechanism could be identified that might have indicated which patients were likely to develop a rejection episode. Hypertension and proteinuria were also found to increase in frequency during gestation. Major fetal complications were prematurity and growth retardation. The authors concluded that it was their "general policy to discourage pregnancy in these patients. However, if the patient very much desires pregnancy, it may be permitted providing that good renal function has been present and stable on low dose maintenance immunosuppression for one year, or preferably two, and that the patient's renal disease is not inheritable" [61].

GENERAL PRINCIPLES OF OBSTETRIC MANAGEMENT

Fetal Assessment and Timing of Delivery

Detailed description of obstetric management is beyond the purpose of this chapter. Nevertheless, it is necessary for the nonobstetrician to have some awareness of the problems of fetal assessment, fetal maturity, and timing of delivery. The application of fetal assessment techniques to the insulin-dependent diabetic can provide the clinician information about the intrauterine environment. Either vascular compromise or an abnormal metabolic maternal state can place the fetus in jeopardy. Careful determination of gestation age and size, and evaluation of the intrauterine environment are essential if the welfare of both mother and infant is to be maintained.

Ultrasonography should be done early in gestation to assess gestational sac size and crown–rump measurements, which can be compared to standardized charts. Follow-up ultrasonography at 16 to 22 weeks and at 25 to 30 weeks will allow detection of some fetal anomalies and establish measurements of fetal growth and placental aging, which can be compared with expected changes for gestational age. Thereafter, the examinations should be performed at least monthly.

Another important aspect of fetal assessment in diabetic pregnancies is the prenatal detection of neural tube defects. Data from the Joslin Clinic revealed a tenfold increase in the frequency of neural tube defects in the offspring of diabetic women. On the basis of these data it has been strongly suggested that "the normal standard of care for diabetic pregnancy should include serum alphafetoprotein screening between 16 and 18 weeks' gestation" [16].

Daily fetal movement charts should be kept beginning at 30 weeks' gestation. Weekly unconjugated plasma estriol levels should also be determined, beginning at 30 weeks, to establish a baseline for later comparison. At 34 weeks' gestation, an estriol level should be measured daily (earlier if glycemic control has been poor or if gestation has been complicated by polyhydramnios, preeclampsia, or vascular disease). Biweekly nonstress tests (NST) or weekly contraction stress tests (CST) are performed beginning at 34 weeks in connection with estriol measurements. Likewise, these tests may be initiated earlier for women with complications that may place the fetus at increased risk. If a normal estriol pattern has been established and a 35 to 50% decrease is recorded and confirmed, the NST or CST is used to make a decision regarding the performance of aminocentesis for fetal lung maturation testing. In the absence of accurate plasma estriol determination, several centers are employing daily NSTs. If the NST is nonreactive, a CST is done. Whether biophysical testing alone will yield similar outcome data to combined biophysical and biochemical monitoring is unknown.

If it is likely that the infant is mature and there is concern for fetal well-being, amniocentesis should be performed to analyze for lecithin/sphingomyelin ratios (L/S) and phosphatidyl glycerol/phosphatidyl inositol ratios (PG/PI). If the tests confirm the probability of lung maturity, the patient should be delivered. In the absence of fetal lung maturity, amniocentesis may be performed weekly. If all the tests performed fail to confirm fetal well-being, most clinicians would choose to deliver the patient without laboratory evidence of fetal lung maturity. Significant decreases in fetal movement patterns mandate the performance of another biophysical test (NST or CST).

If all measurements suggest fetal well-being, the patient should be delivered as close to 39 weeks' gestation as possible. Amniocentesis should be performed at 37 to 38 weeks and delivery effected when the infant's lungs can be expected to be mature. Although it has been said that the L/S ratio should be greater than 2, the incidence of respiratory distress syndrome (RDS) (30%) in infants of diabetic mothers was not statistically different from that in infants of nondiabetics, with ratios greater than 2 when the mean gestational age for both groups was 38 weeks [17]. The presence of phosphatidyl glycerol in more than trace amounts is additional assurance that RDS due to hyaline membrane disease will not ensue.

Neonatal complications other than those due to pulmonary immaturity can affect outcome. Intensive fetal surveillance is required in the first few days of life. Because of the impact of corticosteroids on the maternal diabetes as well as their unproved efficacy in accelerating fetal lung maturation, corticosteroids are not usually used in diabetic patients if delivery needs to be effected before lung maturity is assured.

Insulin Therapy During Labor and Delivery

In the past it was common practice to simply withhold insulin the morning of delivery. This practice was based on the knowledge that removal of the placenta and thus the source of human placental lactogen (HPL) rendered the mother vulnerable to hypoglycemia in the immediate postpartum period. As pointed out by Mintz et al., this approach has at least two major problems [40]. First, even with induction of labor the exact timing of delivery cannot always be accurately predicted. Induction may frequently require longer than a single day. Second, withholding of insulin for a prolonged time obviously predisposes the mother to varying degrees of hyperglycemia. The metabolic control achieved throughout gestation is lost. Fetuses exposed to maternal hyperglycemia will become hyperinsulinemic and, consequently, hypoglycemic when ultimately separated from the maternal source of glucose. The long periods without insulin may also result in maternal and fetal ketonemia and acidemia.

At most institutions glycemic control during labor is achieved with a combined infusion of glucose and insulin. Previously, our regimen utilized an infusion of 1.0–2.0 units of regular insulin per hour given simultaneously with 5–10 g of dextrose per hour. However, the caloric consumption during labor can be as much as 1.8 kcal/min during the second stage of labor [56]. To meet the energy needs of labor, 15–25 g of dextrose per hour may be required. Using a solution of 10% dextrose, 10–20 g of glucose can be infused hourly in combination with an appropriate dosage of regular insulin (usually 2.0–4.0 units/hr). Despite a theoretically inadequate caloric supply, this regimen can achieve glycemic control without detectable ketonuria. Larger amounts of hourly glucose would require the use of 20% hypertonic dextrose solution. Many authors prefer to administer dextrose and insulin separately using an infusion pump. This method permits adjustments in the infusion rate of insulin or dextrose or both without mixing new solutions. On the other hand, mixing insulin and dextrose in the same bottle gives an added measure of safety, because if the infusion rate inadvertently changes, the ratio of insulin to dextrose remains constant. A blood sugar should be determined 1 to 2 hours after the infusion is begun and appropriate changes in insulin delivery made. We attempt to maintain blood sugars between 80–120 mg/dL.

If a trial of labor induction is discontinued in the evening, we discontinue the infusion, allow the patient to eat dinner, and give a subcutaneous dose of insulin. The next morning the infusion is resumed. At the time of delivery the insulin-containing solution is discontinued while a dextrose infusion is maintained. Following delivery it is often unnecessary to give subcutaneous insulin for 24 to 72 hours. When the patient's blood sugar remains greater than 200 mg/dL we generally resume her prepregnancy dosage of insulin. We have also used this regimen successfully for diabetic pregnancies scheduled for cesarean delivery.

GENETIC COUNSELING FOR DIABETICS

Current research efforts are giving clues to the genetics of the many disease entities that constitute diabetes mellitus [63,64]. Studies utilizing the human leukocyte antigen (HLA) system have provided significant new information on the genetic heterogeneity of diabetes. Although HLA typing remains a research tool, specific types—HLA-DR3, DR4, B8, and B15—have been linked with diabetes, and it may soon be possible to identify individuals at risk within a family. Nevertheless, the practicing physician's approach to questions asked by the family must rely on empirical risk figures.

The counseling physician must stress to the family that diabetes is a heterogeneous disease. It is clearly important to distinguish between insulin-dependent diabetes mellitus (IDDM) and non-insulin-dependent diabetes mellitus (NIDDM). In a given family the risk relates only to the specific disease seen in that family. If a child has IDDM, the risk of his or her sibling's contracting the same disease is approximately 5 to 10%. If a parent has IDDM, the risk to the offspring is 1 to 5%. As with most empirical risk figures, the risk increases slightly when more than one person in the family is affected. The exact risk to the child of two IDDM parents is not known.

The risk to the child of two parents with NIDDM is only approximately 10%. Thus, most geneticists take exception with the 1965 World Health Organization's recommendation that two diabetics should not have children together.

The determination of a new subgroup of NIDDM, maturity onset diabetes of the young (MODY), has provided some of the best evidence for etiologic heterogeneity in diabetes. This subgroup has clearly been shown to conform to autosomal dominant transmission.

In addition to the genetic susceptibility for diabetes, the autoimmune pathogenesis of at least some forms of IDDM has been emphasized by the high frequency of other autoimmune endocrine diseases in some patients. Other endocrine diseases associated with IDDM include Grave's disease, Hashimoto's thyroiditis, Addison's disease, and pernicious anemia [65,66].

What is inherited in diabetics may be the susceptibility or increased vulnerability to certain pancreatotoxic viral infections or to pancreatic damage resulting from immune overreaction. The end result is severe beta cell destruction.

Future research holds forth the promise that genetic identification of individuals at risk for diabetes may make it possible to prevent the disease through specific immunization or to treat the disease at the very onset with agents such as anti-lymphocyte globulin. As Dr. White wrote in 1952, "Only when the entire genetic and vascular problem of diabetes is solved will our total experience be equal to the best in non-diabetic pediatric and obstetrical experience" [18].

REFERENCES

1. White P. Diabetes in pregnancy. In: Joslin EP, ed. The treatment of diabetes mellitus. 4th ed. Philadelphia: Lea & Febiger, 1928:861–72.
2. Gabbe SG. Application of scientific rationale to the management of the pregnant diabetic. In: Merkatz IR, Adam PAG, eds. The diabetic pregnancy: a perinatal perspective. New York: Grune & Stratton, 1979.
3. Crenshaw C. Fetal glucose metabolism. Clin Obstet Gynecol. 1970; 13:579–85.
4. Pagliara AS, Karl IE, Haymond M, Kipnis DM. Hypoglycemia in infancy and childhood. J Pediatr. 1973; 82:365–79.
5. Haworth JC. Carbohydrate metabolism in the fetus and the newborn. Pediatr Clin North Am. 1965; 12:573–84.
6. Freinkel N, Metzger BE, Nitzan M, et al. "Accelerated starvation" and mechanisms for the conservation of maternal nitrogen during pregnancy. Isr J Med Sci. 1972; 8:426–39.
7. Gillmer MDG, Beard RW, Brook FM, Oakley NW. Carbohydrate metabolism in pregnancy. Part I. Diurnal plasma glucose profile in normal and diabetic women. Br Med J. 1975; 3:399–402.
8. Freinkel N, Metzger BE. Pregnancy as a tissue culture experience: the critical implications of maternal metabolism for fetal development. In: Ciba Foundation Symposium 63 (New Series). Pregnancy, metabolism, diabetes and the fetus. Amsterdam: Excerpta Medica, 1979:3–28.
9. Young M, Prenton MA. Maternal and fetal plasma amino acid concentrations during gestation and in growth retarded fetal growth. J Obstet Gynaecol Br Comm. 1969; 76:33–4.
10. Felig P, Kim YJ, Lynch V, Hendler R. Amino acid metabolism during starvation in human pregnancy. J Clin Invest. 1972; 51:1195–1202.
11. Oakey RE. Progressive increase in estrogen production in human pregnancy: an appraisal of the factors responsible. Vitam Horm. 1970; 28:1–36.
12. Kalkhoff RK, Kim YJ. The influence of hormonal changes of pregnancy on maternal metabolism. In: Ciba Foundation Symposium 63 (New Series). Pregnancy, metabolism, diabetes and the fetus. Amsterdam: Excerpta Medica, 1979:29–56.
13. Gabbe SG, Quilligan EJ. Fetal carbohydrate metabolism: its clinical importance. Am J Obstet Gynecol. 1977; 127:92–103.
14. Josimovich JB, Kosor B, Bocella L, Mintz DH, Hutchinson DL. Placental lactogen in maternal serum as an index of fetal health. Obstet Gynecol. 1970; 36:244–50.
15. Kyle GC. Diabetes and pregnancy. Ann Intern Med. 1963; 59(Suppl 3):1–82.
16. Milunsky A, Alpert E, Kitzmiller JL, Younger MD, Neff RK. Prenatal diagnosis of neural tube defects. Am J Obstet Gynecol. 1982; 142:1030–2.
17. Gabbe SG, Lowensohn RI, Mestman HJ, Freeman RK, Gobbelsmann U. Lecithin/sphingomyelin ratio in pregnancies complicated by diabetes mellitus. Am J Obstet Gynecol. 1977; 128:757–60.
18. White P. Pregnancy complicating diabetes. In: Joslin EP, Root HF, White P, Marble A, eds. The treatment of diabetes mellitus. 4th ed. Philadelphia: Lea & Febiger, 1952:676.
19. Kalkhoff RK, Kissebah AH, Kim HJ. Carbohydrate and lipid metabolism during normal pregnancy: relationship to gestational hormone action. In: Merkatz IR, Adam PAJ, eds. The diabetic pregnancy: a perinatal perspective. New York: Grune & Stratton, 1979.
20. Freinkel N, Metzger BE. Some considerations of fuel economy in the fed state during late human pregnancy. In: Camerini-Davalos RA, Cole HS, eds. Early diabetes in early life. New York: Academic Press, 1976:289–302.
21. Daniel RR, Metzger BE, Freinkel N, Faloona GR, Unger RH, Nitzan M. Carbohydrate metabolism in pregnancy. XI. Response of plasma glucagon to overnight fast and oral glucose during normal pregnancy and in gestational diabetes. Diabetes. 1974; 23:771–6.
22. Hagbard L. Pregnancy and diabetes mellitus; a clinical study. Acta Obstet Gynecol Scan [Suppl 1]. 1956; 35:1–180.
23. Gabbe SG, Quilligan EJ. General obstetric management of the diabetic pregnancy. Clin Obstet Gynecol. 1981; 24:91–105.
24. Gabbe SG. Medical complications of pregnancy. Management of diabetes in pregnancy: six decades of experience. In: Pitkin RM, Zlatnik FJ, eds. Yearbook of obstetrics and gynecology. Chicago: Year Book, 1980:37–49.
25. Molsted-Pedersen L. Pregnancy and diabetes: a survey. Acta Endocrinol (Copenh). 1980; 94(Suppl 238):13–19.
26. Roversi GD, Gargiulo M, Nicolini U, et al. A new approach to the treatment of diabetic pregnant women. Am J Obstet Gynecol. 1979; 135:567–76.
27. Pedersen J. The pregnant diabetic and her newborn: problems and management. 2nd ed. Baltimore: Williams & Wilkins, 1977:191–7.
28. Pedersen J. Goals and end-points in management of diabetic pregnancy. In: Camerini-Davalos RA, Cole HS, eds. Early diabetes in early life. New York: Academic Press, 1976:381–90.

29. Miller E, Hare JW, Cloherty JP, et al. Elevated maternal hemoglobin A_{1c} in early pregnancy and major congenital anomalies in infants of diabetic mothers. N Engl J Med. 1981; 304:1331–4.

30. Fuhrmann K, Reiher H, Semmler K, Fischer F, Fischer M, Glöckner E. Prevention of congenital malformations in infants of insulin-dependent diabetic mothers. Diabetes Care. 1983; 6:219–23.

31. Pedersen J. Diabetes and pregnancy; blood sugar of newborn infants during fasting and glucose administration. Copenhagen: Danish Science Press, 1952.

32. Mestman JH. Outcome of diabetes screening in pregnancy and perinatal morbidity in infants of mothers with mild impairment in glucose tolerance. Diabetes Care. 1980; 3:447–52.

33. O'Sullivan JB. Long term follow up of gestational diabetics. In: Camerini-Davalos RA, Cole HS, eds. Early diabetes in early life. New York: Academic Press, 1976;503–19.

34. Carpenter MW, Constan DR. Criteria for screening tests for gestational diabetes. Am J Obstet Gynecol. 1982; 144:768–73.

35. O'Sullivan JB, Mahan CM, Charles D, et al. Screening criteria for high-risk gestational diabetic patients. Am J Obstet Gynecol. 1973; 116:895–900.

36. Shah BD, Cohen AQ, May C, Gabbe SG. Comparison of glycohemoglobin determination and the one-hour oral glucose screen in the identification of gestational diabetes. Am J Obstet Gynecol. 1982; 144:774–7.

37. Hare JW, White, P. Gestational diabetes and the White classification. Diabetes Care. 1980; 3:394.

38. Committee on Maternal Nutrition—Food and Nutrition Board. Maternal nutrition and the course of pregnancy. National Academy of Sciences–National Research Council, Washington, D.C., 1970.

39. National Research Council. Committee on Dietary Allowances. Recommended dietary allowances. 8th ed. Washington, D.C.: National Academy of Sciences, 1974.

40. Mintz DH, Skyler JS, Chez RA. Diabetes mellitus and pregnancy. Diabetes Care. 1978; 1:49–63.

41. Hibbard LT. Perinatal mortality in private obstetric practice. Obstet Gynecol. 1974; 43:73–80.

42. A guide for professionals: the effective application of "exchange lists for meal planning." New York and Chicago: American Diabetes Association and American Dietetic Association, 1970.

43. Trivelli LA, Ranney MH, Lai HT. Hemoglobin components in patients with diabetes mellitus. N Engl J Med. 1971; 289:353–7.

44. Pitkin RM. Vitamins and minerals in pregnancy. Clin Perinatol. 1975; 2:221–32.

45. Pitkin RM. Calcium metabolism in pregnancy. A review. Am J Obstet Gynecol. 1975; 121:724–37.

46. Kitay DZ, Harbort RA. Iron and folic acid deficiency in pregnancy. Clin Perinatol. 1975; 2:255–73.

47. Nelson JD, Woelk MA, Sheps S. Self glucose monitoring: A comparison of the Glucometer, Glucoscan, and Hypocount B. Diabetes Care. 1983; 6:262–7.

48. Skyler JS, Skyler DL, Seigler DE, O'Sullivan MJ. Algorithms for adjustment of insulin dosage by patients who monitor blood glucose. Diabetes Care. 1981; 4:311–8.

49. Adam PAJ, Schwartz R. Diagnosis and treatment: should oral hypoglycemic agents be used in pediatric and pregnant patients? Pediatrics. 1968; 42:819–23.

50. Rigg L, Cousins L, Hollingsworth D, Brink G, Yen SS. Effects of exogenous insulin on excursions and diurnal rhythm of plasma glucose in pregnant diabetic patients with and without residual beta cell function. Am J Obstet Gynecol. 1980; 136:537–44.

51. Reeves ML, Seigler DE, Ryan EA, Skyler JR. Glycemic control in insulin-dependent diabetes mellitus. Am J Med. 1981; 72:673–80.

52. Tamborlane WV, Sherwin RS, Genel M, Felig P. Reduction to normal of plasma glucose in juvenile diabetes by subcutaneous administration of insulin with a portable infusion pump. N Engl J Med. 1979; 300:573–8.

53. Rudolf MC, Coustan DR, Sherwin RS, et al. Efficacy of the insulin pump in the home treatment of pregnant diabetics. Diabetes. 1981; 30:891–5.

54. Dunn PJ, Cole RA, Soeldner JS, et al. Temporal relationship of glycosylated hemoglobin concentrations to glucose control in diabetics. Diabetologia. 1979; 17:213–20.

55. O'Shaughnessy R. Role of the glycohemoglobins (hemoglobin A_1) in the evaluation and management of the diabetic pregnancy. Clin Obstet Gynecol. 1981; 24:65–71.

56. Benerjee B, Khen KS, Saha N, Ratnam SS. Energy cost and blood sugar level during different stages of labor and duration of labor in Asiatic women. J Obstet Gynecol Br Cmwl. 1971; 78:927–9.

57. Drury MI, Greene AT, Stronge JM. Pregnancy complicated by clinical diabetes mellitus. Obstet Gynecol. 1977; 49:519–22.

58. Schilthnis MS, Aaronduse JG. Fetal death associated with severe ritodrine induced ketoacidosis. Lancet. 1980; 2:1145–6.

59. Horvat M, Maclean H, Goldberg L, Crock GW. Diabetic retinopathy in pregnancy: a 12-year prospective survey. Br J Ophthalmol. 1980; 64:398–403.

60. Kitzmiller JL, Brown ER, Phillippe M, et al. Diabetic nephropathy and perinatal outcome. Am J Obstet Gynecol. 1981; 141:741–51.

61. Rudolph JE, Schweizer RT, Bartus SA. Pregnancy in renal transplant patients: a review. Transplantation. 1979; 27:26–9.

62. Hare JW, White P. Pregnancy in diabetes complicated by vascular disease. Diabetes. 1977; 26:953–5.

63. Kobberling J, Tattersall R. The genetics of diabetes mellitus. London: Academic Press, 1982.

64. Rotter JI, Anderson CE, Rimoin DL. Genetics of diabetes mellitus. In: Ellenberg M, Rifkin H, eds. Diabetes mellitus: theory and practice (3rd ed.). New York: Medical Examination Publishing, 1982:481–503.

65. Riley WJ, Maclaren NK, Lezotte DC, Spillar KP, Rosenbloom AL. Thyroid autoimmunity in insulin dependent diabetes mellitus: the case for routine screening. J Pediatr. 1981; 98:350–4.

66. Samloff IM, Varis K, Shamaki T, Siurala M, Rotter JI. Relationships among serum pepsinogen. I. Serum pepsinogen. II. Gastric micosal histology. Gastroenterology. 1982; 83:204–9.

It is no exaggeration to say that the composi-
tion of the blood is determined not by what
the mouth takes in but by what the kidneys
keep.
—Homer Smith

12. RENAL DISEASE
Robert G. Benedetti and Tomas Berl

The interrelation of pregnancy and renal disease has long concerned physician and patient alike. Of the nonreproductive organs, the kidney is the most directly affected by the major alterations in body fluids associated with gestation. Pregnancy is accompanied by anatomic and functional changes in the kidney and lower urinary tract, so that many biochemical and clinical measurements that would be considered normal in the nonpregnant woman are abnormal in the gravida. An understanding of the basis for these changes is essential in order to properly diagnose and manage renal disease during pregnancy.

ANATOMIC CHANGES

Renal length is increased by approximately 1 cm during pregnancy [1]. This increase in size is thought to be due to increased renal vascular volume [2]. Microscopic examination of renal biopsies reveals enlarged glomeruli [3], but they are otherwise similar to those of nonpregnant women [4]. The most striking morphologic change is calyceal, pelvic, and ureteral dilatation, which occurs in the first trimester and is maintained until term [5–8]. The hydronephrosis and hydroureter are more prominent on the right side. Controversy abounds over the relative importance of mechanical and humoral factors in producing this change; both probably contribute.

These anatomic changes have direct clinical consequence as stasis of urine probably contributes to the propensity to develop pyelonephritis following asymptomatic bacteriuria in pregnant women. Furthermore, ureteral obstruction caused by a gravid uterus has even been reported to result in acute renal failure [9].

The increase in renal size and dilatation of the collecting system may persist up to 12 weeks following delivery. Therefore, clinical interpretation of excretory urography, ultrasonography, or angiography must be done with an awareness of these alterations (Fig. 12-1).

FUNCTIONAL CHANGES
Renal Hemodynamics

Homer Smith recognized the unique effects of pregnancy on renal function when he noted, "A pregnant woman is a very interesting phenomenon; I do not know any other way to increase the filtration rate by 50% or better for prolonged periods." In fact, both renal blood flow and glomerular filtration rate are dramatically increased throughout most of gestation [10]. This effect was recognized more than 30 years ago when inulin and paraaminohippurate clearances were measured to assess glomerular filtration rate (GFR) and effective renal plasma flow (ERPF) during gestation [11, 12]. Though methodologic and technical difficulties have impaired collection and interpretation of data by these techniques [12], for clinical purposes the measurement of endogenous creatinine clearance performed with a 24-hour urine collection at high urine flow rates provides a reasonable index of filtration rate [10].

The increase in glomerular filtration rate, as measured by creatinine clearance, occurs as early as four weeks after the last menstrual period [10]. Though some studies indicated that the initial increase in glomerular filtration and renal plasma flow declined to the normal range by the third trimester [11], current opinion holds that when lateral recumbency is maintained throughout the period of study no significant decrease in renal plasma flow can be found in the third trimester [13]. A summary of four studies that serially measured glomerular filtration rate and renal plasma flow during pregnancy and post partum is shown in Figure 12-2. Such a summary reveals that during most of pregnancy plasma flow increases more than glomerular filtration rate, leading to a decrease, rather than the increase in filtration fraction frequently alluded to.

The mechanism involved in these hemodynamic alterations remains speculative. Though cardiac output [14] and total blood volume [15] are increased in pregnancy, the greatest rise in renal

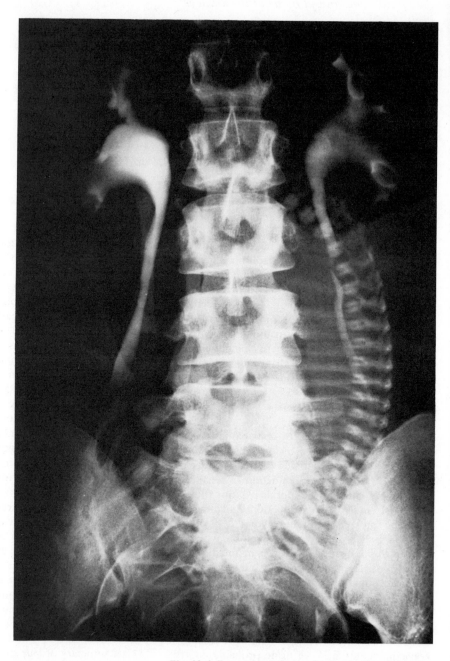

Fig. 12-1. Excretory urogram demonstrating dilatation of the mid right ureter and mild hydronephrosis.

blood flow is seen prior to the maximal volume expansion [16]. A decrease in plasma albumin concentration is seen early in pregnancy and may contribute to the increase in glomerular filtration rate by diminishing glomerular oncotic pressure [17]. Experiments studying the glomerular dynamics in pregnancy have emphasized the important role of the increased plasma flow as a mediator of the increase in glomerular filtration rate [18,19]. This increase in plasma flow is a consequence of both an increase in plasma volume and renal vasodilata-

tion. It is of interest that many of the early renal hemodynamic changes seen in the pregnant rat are also seen in the pseudopregnant rat (mated with sterile male), suggesting that the mechanism is maternal and not fetoplacental in origin [19]. In this regard, a number of humoral factors may contribute to the increase in glomerular filtration rate. Thus, pregnancy is associated with an increased secretion of several hormones, including prolac-

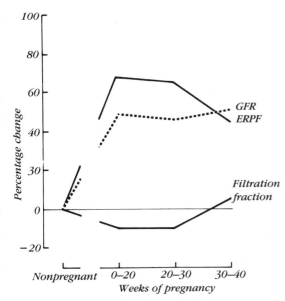

Fig. 12-2. Relative changes in renal hemodynamics during normal human pregnancy. (From Davison and Dunlop [10].)

tin, cortisol, and progesterone, which can alter renal hemodynamics, but the contribution of these hormones to the observed hemodynamic alterations remains unknown [20,21].

Clinical assessments of renal function in pregnancy must be made with awareness of the elevation of glomerular filtration rate. Creatinine and urea production does not increase, and as a consequence plasma concentrations and urea decrease in pregnancy. Therefore, a value for serum creatinine or urea that would be normal in a nonpregnant patient may be abnormally high in pregnancy; values of serum creatinine above 0.8 mg/dL or blood urea nitrogen above 13 mg/dL warrant further investigation.

Acid-Base Balance

Plasma bicarbonate values decrease by approximately 4 mEq/L during pregnancy in response to mild hyperventilation and resultant respiratory alkalosis (mean arterial pH 7.44). Filtered bicarbonate reclamation and urinary acidification have been shown to be normal in the third trimester of pregnancy [22].

Water and Sodium Metabolism: Volume Homeostasis

Of the 12 to 14 kg of body weight gained by the average woman during pregnancy, approximately 6 to 8 kg is accounted for by an increase in total body water. Furthermore, an average woman retains nearly 950 mEq of sodium in the course of a

normal pregnancy [23,24]. Though alterations of salt and water are of impressive magnitude during normal gestation, regulation of volume remains poorly understood.

Increase in total body water in excess of the increase in total body sodium [25] accounts for the decrease in serum sodium concentration and a 5- to 10-mOsm/kg decrease in osmolality seen in pregnancy [26,27]. From observations in pregnant rats that parallel those in human gestation, it has recently been shown that in pregnancy there is a "resetting" of the osmoreceptors controlling antidiuretic hormone release so that concentrating and diluting mechanisms remain intact but at a lower set point for serum osmolality. Figure 12-3 reflects the displacement of the arginine vasopressin–plasma osmolality to the left in pregnant rats. The sensitivity (slope) is unchanged. It is likely that the increase in extracellular fluid volume is the mediator of this resetting. While the alteration in antidiuretic hormone secretion in large measure accounts for the hypotonicity of pregnancy, an additional contribution of increased water intake is probably also operant [28].

The factors that maintain sodium homeostasis in pregnant women are intricate but can be best conceptualized as an interplay between forces that increase sodium excretion and forces that increase sodium retention. Sodium excretion is enhanced by the increase in glomerular filtration responsible for an estimated 5,000 to 10,000 mEq per day of additional sodium delivered to the reabsorptive portion of the nephron. Progesterone, markedly elevated in pregnancy, acts to inhibit the sodium-retaining influence of aldosterone on the distal tubule [29], and other hormones (antidiuretic hormone, prostaglandins, natriuretic factor) may affect sodium excretion in ways yet to be determined [30,31]. Finally, alteration of capillary Starling forces by lowered serum albumin concentration and decreased renal vascular resistance augments sodium excretion [32].

Despite the forces that enhance sodium excretion, net sodium reabsorption occurs throughout pregnancy at a rate of approximately 2 to 3 mEq per day. Aldosterone increases sodium reabsorption at the distal tubule and in third-trimester gravidas is present in serum concentrations 10 to 20 times those of nonpregnant women [24,33]. Despite these high levels of circulating aldosterone, secretion of the hormone is regulated by normal mechanisms during pregnancy. Pregnant women remain sensitive to the sodium-retaining effect of exogenous mineralocorticoids [24], and dietary salt loading or diuretic-induced volume depletion leads to appropriate changes in the aldo-

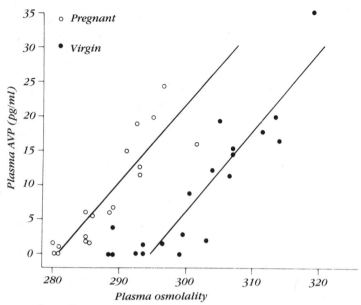

Fig. 12-3. Arginine vasopressin–plasma osmolality relationship in pregnant and virgin rats. Note displacement of intercept to a lower plasma osmolality with no change in slope. (From Durr et al. [28].)

sterone secretion rate in pregnancy [33,34]. Supine and upright positions also have a marked effect on sodium excretion [35].

Sodium homeostasis in pregnancy, therefore, is a complicated interplay of hormonal and physical factors that act as if they are responding to a decreased effective blood volume and serve to return the gravida to a new, higher "euvolemic" state. As with the reset osmostat described above, the pregnant women can be viewed as having a "reset barostat" whose set point for total body sodium increases throughout pregnancy. Thus, although interstitial and plasma volumes are markedly increased, these alterations are perceived as normal by maternal volume receptors. The understanding of this sodium homeostasis is linked with the shifting opinion as to whether diuretics or sodium restriction should be used in pregnancy. A number of investigators have strongly advised against such practice [36]. Although sodium-conserving mechanisms are stimulated by diuretics and low sodium intake, these may still lead to undesirable volume depletion. Since diuretics do not reduce the incidence of preeclampsia, such agents present risks without known benefits and their use during pregnancy should be discouraged.

Glucose

Glucosuria is more common in pregnancy than in the nongravid state. Usually, it reflects alterations of renal handling of filtered glucose rather than derangements in carbohydrate metabolism. Nonpregnant women excrete less than 100 mg of glucose per day, but during gestation this level is surpassed in as many as 70% of gravidas [37]. Ex-

cretion increases soon after conception and peaks between 8 and 11 weeks of gestation but is extremely variable from day to day [10,38]. The pathogenesis of this glucosuria remains enigmatic. The increase in glomerular filtration rate seen in pregnancy will lead to an increased filtered load of glucose which has classically been thought to exceed the tubular reabsorptive ability for glucose [39]. However, when examined carefully with improved techniques, all women demonstrate decrements in fractional tubular reabsorption of glucose in pregnancy as compared to the nonpregnant state [40]. There is no evidence that gestational glucosuria in the absence of altered carbohydrate metabolism portends the development of diabetes mellitus, nor is it associated with the perinatal complications that accompany diabetes mellitus. Conversely, patients with overt hyperglycemia will have increased glucosuria in pregnancy and the attendant complications of an osmotic diuresis.

Uric Acid

In normal pregnancy the serum uric acid concentration falls by at least 25%, especially in the first and second trimesters [41]. It returns to near-normal levels in the third trimester [42] (Fig. 12-4). The hypouricemia of early pregnancy is probably due to increased clearance of urate as glomerular filtration rate is increased and reabsorption de-

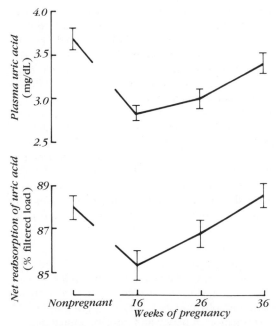

Fig. 12-4. *Plasma uric acid levels and net reabsorption of uric acid during normal pregnancy. (From Dunlop and Davison [42].)*

creased in the setting of volume expansion. Owing to factors that are not fully understood, reabsorption of urate again increases in the latter stages of gestation. Interpretation of serum uric acid concentration is important in diagnosis of preeclampsia. Values above those expected for the appropriate time in pregnancy may be one of the earliest signs of preeclampsia and relate to both the severity of the process and fetal prognosis [43,44].

CLINICAL EVALUATION OF RENAL DISEASE
Symptoms
Symptoms associated with renal disease in pregnancy may be obscured by normal physiologic alterations. The increase in glomerular filtration rate mentioned above may lead to frequency, polyuria, and nocturia. Symptoms of anemia, nausea and vomiting, malaise, alteration in the diurnal sleep cycle, and pruritus occur in pregnancy for reasons unrelated to renal dysfunction. Therefore, when renal disease produces symptoms in pregnancy, the manifestations are predominantly those of the primary disease (e.g., septic shock, hemorrhage with hypovolemia, hypertension, and intravascular coagulation) [45,46].

Signs
Similarly, the signs of renal disease in pregnancy are typically those of the underlying disease.

Asymptomatic edema occurs at some time during pregnancy in most gravidas; however, marked edema or a sudden change in the amount of edema may reflect a decrease in renal function or hypoalbuminemia from the development of proteinuria in the nephrotic range. Any acute deterioration of renal function, particularly one associated with tissue necrosis or systemic ischemia, will lead to decreased potassium excretion and hyperkalemia. Signs of hyperkalemia such as muscle weakness, decreased deep tendon reflexes, and cardiac arrhythmias may ensue [46]. Hypertension is commonly associated with renal disease in pregnancy; it is discussed in Chapter 13.

Laboratory Evaluation
Because of the lack of specificity of signs and symptoms, the discovery of renal disease in pregnancy is frequently made through identification of an abnormal laboratory test.

Measures of Glomerular Filtration Rate
Serum creatinine and blood urea nitrogen concentrations are useful measures of renal function in a steady state. However, the normal values for pregnancy are lower than for the nongravid state, and small, but significant, decrements of renal function may not be readily apparent. Creatinine clearance is the most clinically useful measurement of glomerular filtration rate. As the excretion of creatinine is maintained at a steady state during pregnancy (approximately 20 mg of creatinine/kg/day), this test retains its clinical importance during pregnancy [47]. If the pregnant patient increases her water intake in order to produce urine volumes adequate to minimize the error associated with the increase in ureteral dead space, endogenous creatinine clearance performed with a 24-hour urine collection provides a reasonable index of filtration rate [12,48,49].

Urinalysis
Urinalysis is an important noninvasive method to assess the presence and activity of parenchymal renal disorders. It is equally useful in pregnancy despite the fact that quantitative standardization remains to be agreed upon [46]. For example, both increased [49] and similar [50] rates of leukocyte excretion compared to nongravidas have been reported in pregnant women. However, the presence of more than five white blood cells per high-powered field should prompt a urine culture. Few attempts have been made to standardize red blood cell excretion and cylindruria in normal pregnancy [51]. However, in hypertensive gravidas substantial hematuria, pyuria, or the presence of

cellular casts should suggest a diagnosis other than preeclampsia as urine sediment is usually normal in this disorder [4,52,53].

The evaluation of proteinuria is probably the most important aspect of the urinalysis. Normal nongravidas excrete less than 100 mg of protein in the urine daily. During pregnancy the amount may increase threefold. Since the sensitivity of the reagent for albumin on a urine dipstick measures "trace" at a concentration of 20 mg of protein per 100 mL of urine, this increased amount of albuminuria may go undetected in most routine screening procedures [54]. However, orthostatic proteinuria, a condition affecting approximately 2% of young adults [55], may be initially detected in pregnancy and is exacerbated during the third trimester by the accentuated lordotic posture [56]. This finding may evoke consideration of preeclampsia, but the absence of hypertension and marked edema in close follow-up should exclude that diagnosis. Furthermore, the urine may be tested for albumin on a first voided morning specimen obtained while the patient is still recumbent. A decreased concentration of albumin in the specimen, compared to one obtained when the patient is ambulatory, indicates that the proteinuria is orthostatic in nature. While proteinuria does not invariably accompany preeclampsia, this disorder is the most common cause of proteinuria in pregnancy. Although protein excretion in preeclampsia is usually mild or moderate, it is also the most common cause of the nephrotic syndrome (i.e., heavy proteinuria) during gestation [51]. The proteinuria in preeclampsia is characterized by its extreme quantitative and qualitative variability [57, 58]. Finally, it must be noted that the presence of proteinuria in the early stages of gestation more probably reflects underlying parenchymal renal disease.

Radiologic Tests

Excretory Urography

For the typical five-film excretory urogram an average of 500 milliroentgens is delivered to the female gonads [59]. To reduce the risk of radiation damage to the developing fetus, urography in pregnancy should be done to evaluate a problem that cannot be investigated by ultrasonography or nuclear scanning. In the situation in which urography is needed (e.g., unexplained hematuria and persistent flank pain) radiation exposure can be reduced by taking a single 30-minute film confined to the renal areas with appropriate shielding [60].

Renal Nuclear Scan

Renal scanning performed in pregnancy using ^{131}I-Hippuran exposes the fetal kidneys and gonads to less than 2 milliroentgens and less than 0.5 milliroentgen, respectively [61]. After intravenous injection the isotope is both filtered at the glomerulus and secreted by the tubules, providing an estimation of renal blood flow and tubular function. In pregnancy, this test has been clinically utilized most frequently to estimate the physiologic significance of hydronephrosis. However, because of the "reservoir effect" of the dilated collecting system in pregnancy [62], and the decreased secretion seen when the renogram is performed in the supine position [63], evaluation of hydronephrosis by renal nuclear scanning should be performed cautiously [64]. Technetium can also be used as a scanning isotope and does not expose the fetal thyroid to [131]I.

Ultrasonography

Similar patterns of dilatation of the upper urinary tract in pregnancy have been demonstrated by ultrasonography and conventional pyelography [8]. Investigation of pelvic and intraabdominal masses in pregnancy with ultrasound is able to identify purely cystic masses, which need no intervention unless their size or location may cause mechanical problems with delivery [65]. Placement of percutaneous nephrostomy tubes is possible under ultrasound guidance without exposing the fetus to radiation [66]. Perhaps the greatest clinical use may come in the evaluation of acute flank pain in pregnancy, when one can frequently differentiate acute hydronephrosis caused by a renal stone from nonrenal causes such as abruptio placentae, torsion of an ovarian cyst, or appendiceal abscess [8,66]. Finally, ultrasonography may also be useful in the assessment of fetal renal function [67].

Renal Biopsy

Percutaneous renal biopsy has been utilized in clinical assessment of renal disease for more than 30 years [68]. The contributions made by this technique in pregnancy are exemplified in the diagnosis of preeclampsia. Renal biopsies performed on 62 primagravidas at the University of Chicago clinically felt to have preeclampsia revealed that 16 (26%) had chronic renal disease and only 44 (71%) actually had the renal lesion of pure preeclampsia (i.e., glomerular endotheliosis) [4]. Lindheimer et al. propose that open renal biopsies be performed (1) when acute or chronic renal dysfunction occurs prior to the 34th gestational week if the precise diagnosis is important in the management of the patient [69] (the nephrotic syndrome of undetermined origin may be the only example of such a situation since identification of a steroid-responsive lesion will alter therapy) or (2) to provide information useful in counseling women desirous of future pregnancies, since more than 20% of women presenting with preeclampsia have another renal disease that may complicate future pregnancies. It must be noted, however, that since the latter patients frequently have persistent renal dysfunction or hypertension post partum, a histologic diagnosis can be made at that time. The indications for an antepartum biopsy, therefore, are very few, and the procedure is only rarely performed.

Contraindications to renal biopsy are similar in pregnant and nonpregnant patients. An uncooperative patient, the presence of a single kidney, or a bleeding diathesis is an absolute contraindication. In addition, contraindications in pregnancy include uncontrolled hypertension and a gestation beyond the thirty-fourth week, since the biopsy results will be unlikely to alter therapy. It has been noted that kidney biopsy performed during cesarean delivery is associated with a significant bleeding risk and should not be undertaken [69].

The risks of renal biopsy in pregnancy were initially thought to be increased [70], but subsequent series have been unable to corroborate this assumption, providing the contraindications previously mentioned are strictly observed [69,71]. Complications include gross hematuria (1.2–5.2%) and nephrectomy for uncontrolled bleeding (0.1%). The reported mortality from renal biopsy is 0.05 to 0.1%.

ACUTE RENAL FAILURE IN PREGNANCY
The incidence of obstetric acute renal failure is estimated at between 1 per 1,400 and 1 per 1,500 pregnancies [72,73]. Despite this relatively low incidence, in two series of patients with acute renal failure studied in the 1960s obstetric patients represented 8 to 24% of the total population [74,75]. It appears, however, that the incidence of obstetric acute renal failure has decreased dramatically in countries where medical care is readily available [76]. Thus, a review by Chapman and Legrain noted that, while obstetric acute renal failure accounted for 40% of all cases of acute renal failure in 1960, by 1979 it accounted for only 4.5% in the same patient population [76]. It is in fact remarkable that at one time these authors observed no cases of acute renal failure in 12,000 consecutive pregnancies. This decrease almost certainly reflects the virtual elimination of septic abortion and its attendant renal complications. Unfortunately, the decline in incidence is not shared by all societies; in less-developed countries incidence continues to be high [77].

The recognition of renal injury in pregnancy requires awareness of the normal alterations in renal function and anatomy that attend the gravid state. As previously mentioned, an apparently normal serum creatinine or blood urea nitrogen in the pregnant woman may in fact be inappropriately high.

The distribution of acute renal failure in pregnancy appears to be bimodal [78], as depicted in Figure 12-5. The early peak occurred at 16 weeks and in most studies in the 1950s and 1960s accounted for about 60% of obstetric acute renal failure. The late peak occurred at 38 weeks, in the remaining 40%. Significant temporal overlap was found between the two groups. A third high-incidence peak in the first one to four weeks post partum has been described by Robson et al. [82]. While postpartum renal failure has been a subject of great interest, it comprises a minuscule fraction of renal failure in pregnancy. It must also be pointed out that approximately 95% of cases of obstetric acute renal failure result from the pregnant state per se, and only about 5% occur coincidentally with the pregnancy (e.g., from drug ingestion, acute glomerulonephritis) [78].

Acute Renal Failure in Early Pregnancy
In the first trimester a complication of abortion is the underlying cause of acute renal failure in at least 95% of cases [77–79]. These abortions are almost invariably "septic" and not spontaneous. A variety of mechanisms have been postulated for the acute renal failure seen in these patients.

Septic Shock
Sepsis, with its hypotensive effect, is the most common cause of acute renal failure in association with

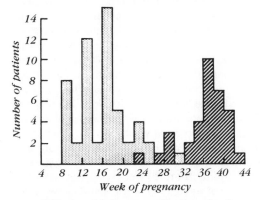

Fig. 12-5. Bimodal distribution of acute renal failure during pregnancy. (From Smith et al. [78].)

Renal failure complicating abortion

Renal failure in late pregnancy

nontherapeutic abortions [83]. In fact, septic abortions represent the major source of septicemia during pregnancy, as pyelonephritis, chorioamnionitis, and puerperal infections rarely culminate in sepsis. Gram-negative organisms, usually *Escherichia coli,* are cultured from the uterus of approximately half of these patients, but positive blood cultures are obtained in only 20% [79]. Another common infection leading to acute renal failure in early pregnancy is clostridial infection. While the incidence of septicemia with clostridia is not known, other complications such as myonecrosis with myoglobinuria or intravascular hemolysis with hemoglobinuria may cause decrease in renal function.

Disorders of coagulation occur frequently in patients with septic abortion [84]. In fact, one series reported thrombocytopenia and increased fibrin degradation products in almost half of the patients with septic abortion and acute renal failure [79].

Nephrotoxins

A number of substances used in the setting of nontherapeutic abortions can cause acute renal failure. Soaps and phenols are the most common abortifacients, but a wide variety of substances such as potassium permanganate, heavy metals, and ergot alkaloids have also been employed [83]. In addition to direct nephrotoxic effects, abortifacients, usually administered as hypotonic solutions, may induce hemolysis. Furthermore, nephrotoxic antibiotics such as aminoglycosides have frequently been utilized in this setting.

Volume Contraction

A major cause of volume contraction in early pregnancy is hyperemesis gravidarum. Fifty percent of women experience nausea and vomiting during pregnancy, which typically peaks at 4 weeks and regresses by 12 weeks. While the cause is unclear, there is a close temporal relationship to peak gonadotropin levels. In a small minority, a syndrome of truly intractable nausea and vomiting occurs; the etiology of this so-called hyperemesis gravidarum is not fully understood [85]. Significant volume depletion and electrolyte abnormalities may ensue. A number of cases of otherwise unexplained renal failure have developed in this setting but have not always responded to volume repletion. It is noteworthy that in a large series of patients with hyperemesis gravidarum the onset of renal failure was not restricted to early pregnancy but ranged from 14 to 23 weeks of pregnancy [86]. Pathologic examination in these patients revealed, in addition to nonspecific tubular necrosis and fatty infiltration, some vacuolization, which is

probably a consequence of potassium depletion.

The mortality of acute renal failure associated with septic abortion is 20 to 25% [77–79,83]. Cortical necrosis occurs in only 2%, a figure comparable to that with nonobstetric acute renal failure; hence return of function is anticipated in most survivors. The mortality in patients with acute renal failure in the setting of volume contraction is even lower, and the azotemia is usually readily reversible.

In summary, acute renal failure in early pregnancy occurs largely as a consequence of septic abortion, has a good prognosis for survival, and has a low incidence of residual renal dysfunction. Although adequate data are not yet available, it seems probable that liberalized abortion policies are making this a vanishing entity.

Acute Renal Failure in Late Pregnancy

The settings in which acute renal failure supervenes in late pregnancy are severe preeclampsia or eclampsia and uterine bleeding, usually caused by abruptio placentae [77–80]. It is not always possible to differentiate these two etiologies. Hypertension can be a major risk factor for abruption, being present in approximately 50% of cases; conversely, hemorrhage may conceal the presence of undiagnosed antecedent hypertension.

There is reason to believe that with improved medical management the incidence of acute renal failure associated with eclampsia may be decreasing. In one series of 154 consecutive cases of eclampsia only a single episode of acute renal failure occurred [87]. Similarly, a 1% incidence of renal failure in 365 cases of eclampsia was reported in another series [88]. In two series of patients it has been noted that a large percentage of hypertensive patients who developed acute renal failure were multiparous and that their average age was 27 to 30 years [75,80]. Perhaps, therefore, many of these patients were not truly "preeclamptic" but had underlying hypertensive disease. The mechanism whereby severe preeclampsia leads to acute renal failure is unclear. The possibility that swelling of the endothelial cells leads to ischemia has been suggested, but there is no evidence that the endothelial swelling is more severe in patients with eclampsia who developed renal failure [89]. Alternatively, tubular obstruction with hemolytic anemia and diffuse intravascular coagulation has also been implicated [90].

Hemorrhage, particularly in the setting of abruptio placentae, is another common predisposing factor for the development of acute renal failure. In fact, in one series 5 to 10% of patients with severe abruptio placentae experienced acute renal failure [91]; in many of them bilateral cortical necrosis developed. It must be emphasized that the degree of antepartum hemorrhage is not always externally obvious. Furthermore, pregnancy appears to enhance the propensity for renal failure to develop in response to hemorrhage. This may well be due to alterations in the coagulation system that accompany the pregnant state [92].

Bilateral Cortical Necrosis

Mortality in obstetric acute renal failure is relatively low (approximately 20%). However, permanent impairment of renal function in patients who survive is not, primarily because of the high incidence (10–30%) of cortical necrosis in obstetric acute renal failure [77,81]. In fact, obstetric complication is the most common cause of acute cortical necrosis and in one large series accounted for 70% of the total group [81].

On pathologic examination, this entity is characterized by destruction of the renal cortex with relative sparing of the medulla as well as a thin rim of subcapsular tissue. The lesion may be either diffuse or patchy.

The pathogenesis of acute cortical necrosis is not entirely known. However, a pathologically similar lesion may be produced by the so-called generalized Shwartzman reaction (sequential injections of endotoxin 24 hours apart). In the pregnant state, a generalized Shwartzman reaction may be induced by a single dose of endotoxin. Most cases of cortical necrosis have been associated with increases in clotting factors V, VIII, X, decreased plasminogen activity, decreased antithrombin III levels, and decreased platelet count [92,93]. It is not surprising, therefore, that while acute cortical necrosis has been associated with shock, sepsis, and toxins at least 50 to 60% of cases have occurred in late pregnancy [94]. Kleinknecht et al. compared 18 cases of obstetric cortical necrosis with 20 cases of obstetric acute tubular necrosis and found no difference in the amount of blood loss or initial hypotension [81]. Surprisingly, while the fibrinogen level was lower in the cortical necrosis group, there were no differences in platelet count, thrombin, or fibrin degradation products. Bilateral renal cortical necrosis occurred earlier in pregnancy (28 versus 34 weeks) and was in fact associated with a lower incidence of eclampsia (16 versus 60%). Thus, the specific risk factors for a given case of acute cortical necrosis in pregnancy remain unclear. Factors such as underlying nephrosclerosis or prolonged renal vasoconstriction could also be playing a role in the pathogenesis of this disorder [94]. Abruptio placentae is the most common setting in which bilateral cortical necrosis occurs, but it has also been reported with overwhelming septic abortions, preeclampsia, amniotic fluid embolization, and retained fetal products.

Cortical necrosis is suggested clinically by the presence of anuria or by the presence of prolonged oliguria. Occasionally the diagnosis can be made by the appearance of a rim of cortical calcification on a roentgenogram of the abdomen 18 to 60 days after the initial event. Otherwise the diagnosis is established by biopsy or renal arteriography, in which the cortical nephrogram may be absent (diffuse cortical necrosis) or "patchy" (patchy cortical necrosis) [81]. Approximately half of the cases have the so-called patchy variety, and in this group of patients there was delayed return of function and continuation of dialysis for up to one year after the original insult. A case with progressively increased function over a three-year period has also been described [95]. The long-term prognosis may be less optimistic as five of the ten patients with patchy cortical necrosis eventually resumed hemodialysis.

Acute Renal Failure Associated with Acute Fatty Liver of Pregnancy

Approximately 60 cases of idiopathic fatty liver of pregnancy have been reported [96,97]. The etiology of this disorder is not known. Nutritional deficits, viral infection, and acquired enzymatic defects have all been implicated. Twelve cases have been reported in association with parenteral tetracycline therapy [98], and a similar number with preeclampsia [99]. While 90% of cases occur in the third trimester, isolated cases are seen in the second trimester or in the postpartum period. One-third of all cases of acute renal failure in the third trimester present with jaundice [80]. Therefore, the diagnosis of fatty liver should be made only on the basis of pathologic data. Most cases demonstrate severe hyperbilirubinemia (3–26 mg/dL), with variably increased alkaline phosphatase and moderately increased serum glutamic oxaloacetic transaminase. This is a multisystem disorder with central nervous system dysfunction, hemorrhagic pancreatitis, ischemic colitis, and renal impairment. Ninety percent of cases are associated with azotemia, although renal failure is rarely the cause of death. Renal biopsy has variously shown no abnormalities, tubular necrosis, or fatty infiltration. In the only patient from whom such data are available, the urinary sodium was 3 mEq/L and the urinary osmolality 550 mOsm/kg [100]. Thus, it is unclear whether this entity is a functional derangement and should be included in the so-called hepatorenal syndrome or a true anatomic injury. The prognosis is poor, with an 85% mortality; early delivery does not favorably alter the outcome. In the few (three) patients in whom recovery and subsequent pregnancy have taken place, no recurrence has been noted.

Acute Pyelonephritis

Acute pyelonephritis occurs in 1 to 2% of all pregnancies. Untreated asymptomatic bacteriuria leads to pyelonephritis in 33% of cases in the third trimester. There are numerous case reports of acute renal failure in this setting [86]. While it is impossible to exclude volume depletion or gram-negative sepsis as the etiology, there are data to suggest a depression of renal function by acute pyelonephritis per se in the setting of pregnancy. When 130 patients with third-trimester pyelonephritis were examined, in 25% the glomerular filtration rate was less than 80 mL per minute, in 10% it was less than 60 mL per minute, and in one case it was 20 mL per minute. All patients were treated for volume depletion, and all were restudied in the postpartum period and found to have a normal glomerular filtration rate, excluding underlying renal disease [101].

Obstructive Uropathy

Dilatation of the ureters, pelvis, and calyces is a physiologic response to pregnancy; however, in an occasional patient with multiple gestations or polyhydramnios, a massively enlarged gravid uterus may mechanically obstruct the ureters and impair renal function. This phenomenon has been documented by sequential ultrasonographic examinations [9,102].

Management of Acute Renal Failure in Pregnancy

The management of acute renal failure in pregnancy is in general the same as in nonpregnant patients: meticulous attention to fluid and electrolyte status, maintenance of adequate nutrition, and careful observation for the complications of sepsis and gastrointestinal bleeding. Problems specific to pregnancy include the following: (1) Concealed placental hemorrhage can occur; hence blood loss is often underestimated in the correction of volume deficits. (2) Cortical necrosis with anuria is frequent; thus the possibilities for fluid overload and hyperkalemia are magnified.

When acute renal failure is coincidental to pregnancy, it is now clear that gestation need not always be terminated. There are three documented cases of pregnant females treated with acute hemodialysis for drug intoxication and four cases with coincidental acute renal failure. Six of these

seven cases have had normal full-term deliveries. There have been no fetal malformations or maternal mortality. Optimal dialysis for the patient with renal failure remains inadequately defined. This is even more uncertain in the pregnant state, but thus far complications have not been frequent [103].

Postpartum Renal Failure

Approximately 50 cases of an entity designated postpartum renal failure have now been reported in the literature under a variety of terms including *malignant nephrosclerosis in women postpartum, idiopathic postpartum renal failure,* and *postpartum hemolytic-uremic syndrome* [82].

This illness can occur from the time of delivery to seven months later; 80% of cases have occurred within the first month after delivery. In about 50% the patients are primigravidas, and 75% follow an uncomplicated delivery [104]. Antecedent events have included preeclampsia, use of ergot alkaloids or oxytocin at the time of delivery, administration of oral contraceptives post partum, and a preceding upper respiratory infection. Since each of these has been present in only a small minority of cases, a causal relationship remains to be established. Presenting complaints are variable and range from headache, nausea, vomiting to acute oliguria and a bleeding diathesis. Initially, only about 40% have hypertension, but frequently malignant hypertension ensues during the course of the illness. Renal failure is rapidly progressive, with end-stage renal disease developing in weeks. Extrarenal manifestations in the form of central nervous system and myocardial dysfunction are the rule. Laboratory examination reveals azotemia, microangiopathic hemolytic anemia, thrombocytopenia, reticulocytosis, and hyperbilirubinemia. Fibrin degradation products are increased, but no consistent abnormalities of the prothrombin time, partial thromboplastin time, thrombin time, or fibrinogen occur. The Coombs test is negative, total and individual complement components are normal, and cryoglobulins are not detectable [105].

Renal biopsy performed during the first month of the disease reveals abnormalities identical to those in the hemolytic uremic syndrome of childhood. Light microscopy shows intimal proliferation, subintimal fibrin deposition, and intravascular thrombosis of the interlobular and afferent arterioles. Fibrinoid necrosis may occasionally be seen. The glomerular endothelial cells are also swollen, and subendothelial fibrin deposition gives rise to a double contour appearance of the basement membrane. Proliferative changes occur rarely, and intracapillary thrombi are seen in 50%

Table 12-1. Results of therapy in postpartum renal failure

Modality	Number of cases	Deaths	End stage renal disease	Partial remission	Complete remission
None	19	14	2	1	2
Heparin	24	9	4	9	2
Dipyridamole	7	2	1	4	0
Antimetabolites	3	2	0	1	0
Corticosteroids	7	4	1	2	0
Streptokinase	1	1	0	0	0
Antithrombin III	1	0	0	0	1
Nephrectomy	4	0	4	—	—
Transplant	4	2	0	1	1

Source: Kelleher and Berl [109].

of cases. Electron microscopy demonstrates a subendothelial lucent space containing granular material with a periodicity consistent with an atypical or incompletely polymerized form of fibrin. Immunofluorescent studies have been performed in 12 cases; all have been positive for fibrin, 50% have shown deposition on the third component of complement, and immunoglobulin deposition has been unusual. Biopsy performed late in the course may reveal only sclerotic changes. A recent review of 20 cases of adult hemolytic uremic syndrome, including five patients with postpartum renal failure, found that abnormalities of the small vessels, namely, intimal thickening of the interlobular and afferent arterioles, rather than glomerular abnormalities or clinical features, could be used to predict subsequent recovery of renal function [106]. It should be noted that bleeding complicated renal biopsy frequently. Four patients had major retroperitoneal hemorrhages, and nephrectomy was required in two.

The etiology of postpartum renal failure remains obscure. The abnormalities of coagulation associated with pregnancy and the enhanced susceptibility to the generalized Shwartzman reaction have already been noted, but it is unclear that these represent the primary process. The precipitating factor may be some as yet unrecognized infection, immunologic event, or drug reaction; further study is obviously needed.

In the 50 cases of postpartum renal failure reported in the literature, there have been 30 deaths and 20 survivors. Of the survivors, six patients are apparently disease free, eight have significant hypertension or renal insufficiency but do not require dialysis, six had end-stage renal disease requiring chronic hemodialysis, and one has had a successful transplantation [107]. Recovery of renal function, if it is to occur, is usually seen in the first 30 days, but return of glomerular filtration rate has been seen as late as 13 months after the initial event. In a patient who had a complete remission, the syndrome recurred and remitted in a subsequent pregnancy [108].

Treatment protocols have been completely uncontrolled, and many patients have received multiple modalities [109]. The results of these treatments are summarized in Table 12-1. Plasmapheresis has been suggested but apparently not yet attempted. Survival has been higher in patients treated with heparin. However, all patients receiving dipyridamole, corticosteroids, and antimetabolites have also received heparin. Thus, no firm conclusions can be drawn from these data.

CHRONIC RENAL DISEASE AND PREGNANCY

The relationships between chronic renal disease and the outcome of pregnancy lack universal acceptance in spite of active interest and investigation for more than 20 years. The major problems that confound interpretation of reported series are lack of histologic renal diagnosis from which to make population comparisons, the preponderance of retrospective reports, and the fact that many studies originate from tertiary referral centers where selected patients with more severe renal disease are seen [110]. Despite these difficulties, some consensus emerges from the debate, serving to aid clinical management of pregnancy in women with underlying renal disease.

A history of antecedent renal disease in childhood that has apparently healed with no functional renal impairment (e.g., poststreptococcal glomerulonephritis or pyelonephritis) has no effect on fertility or maternal outcome of pregnancy [111]. Conversely, women with underlying renal disease who manifest moderately severe pregestational decrease in glomerular filtration rate (serum creatinine greater than 3 mg/dL and blood urea nitrogen greater than 30 mg/dL) have markedly reduced abilities to conceive and maintain a viable pregnancy [112]. In one report, only 2 of 13 women who had creatinine clearances less than 20 mL per minute had regular menstrual periods [113].

The major determinants for the outcome of pregnancy in gravidas with chronic renal disease are (1) the presence of hypertension, (2) the severity of pregestational renal insufficiency, and (3) the type of primary renal disease. The dissociation of these three factors as independent variables is extremely difficult. Nonetheless, each will be discussed individually.

Effect of Hypertension

The critical importance of hypertension in the outcome of pregnancy was best dramatized by Mackay's report in 1963 [112]. In 19 of 39 patients (50%) with "abnormal renal function tests" whose blood pressure was less than 175/110 a deterioration of renal function during pregnancy was evidenced by an increase in blood urea nitrogen of 10 mg/dL or greater. The fetal loss in this group was 40%. In 25 patients with "abnormal renal function tests" and blood pressure exceeding 175/110, deterioration of renal function occurred in 61% of patients and fetal loss was 60%. The development of preeclampsia in these patients was not reported. Though the association of hypertension with a poor outcome in pregnancy has been confirmed in subsequent studies, the magnitude of untoward effects (i.e., 60% incidence of fetal loss and 60% incidence of deterioration of renal function) may reflect the classification of a "normal" blood pressure as a diastolic of less than 110 mm Hg. This overestimation of maternal morbidity has led to the unjustified conclusion that the presence of hypertension is probably an absolute contraindica-

tion to pregnancy in a woman with underlying renal disease [114].

In 1968 Felding reported that of patients with a blood urea nitrogen greater than 40 mg/dL and a blood pressure greater than 140/90 mm Hg 41% developed superimposed preeclampsia during pregnancy. This figure compared to a 6% development of preeclampsia in gravidas with a similar level of renal insufficiency whose blood pressure was less than 140/90 [115]. Likewise, perinatal mortality was much higher in the hypertensive group (31%) when compared to the normotensive group (6%).

Ferris reviewed eight series comprising the experience of 385 gravidas with chronic glomerulonephritis during the years 1956 to 1969 [116]. The development of preeclampsia in normotensive and hypertensive gravidas was found to be 17% and 57%, respectively, and fetal loss increased more than six times (7% in normotensive versus 45% in hypertensive gravidas). A recent series addressing this issue was reported by Katz et al. in 1980 [117]. In that series of 121 pregnancies in 89 women, all of whom had a renal biopsy as a prerequisite for inclusion, antenatal hypertension was noted in 15 (17%). Sixty percent of these 15 women were clinically diagnosed as having preeclampsia, though only half of them had the characteristic glomerular changes of preeclampsia on postpartum renal biopsy. This finding compares to a 13% incidence of preeclampsia in previously normotensive gravidas. Likewise, as in earlier studies perinatal mortality was much higher in women who were hypertensive before delivery (47% versus 6% for normotensive women).

Table 12-2 reveals that hypertension in gravidas with preexisting renal disease is associated with an incidence of perinatal mortality and clinical preeclampsia of 42% and 54%, respectively, as compared to 6% and 11% in normotensive gravidas with underlying renal disease. The presence of hypertension is clearly the major determinant of

Table 12-2. Effect of hypertension on the outcome of pregnancy in women with chronic renal disease

| Reference | Normotensive patients | | Hypertensive patients | |
	Perinatal mortality	Preeclampsia*	Perinatal mortality	Preeclampsia*
Felding [115] (1968)	6% (2/33)	6% (2/33)	31% (9/29)	41% (12/29)
Ferris [116] (1975)	7% (12/176)	17% (20/176)	45% (55/123)	57% (70/123)
Katz et al. [117] (1980)	6% (6/106)	13% (13/106)	47% (7/15)	60% (9/15)
Combined	6% (20/315)	11% (35/315)	42% (71/167)	54% (19/167)

*Defined by worsening hypertension in third trimester.

Table 12-3. Degree of pregestational renal insufficiency and obstetric prognosis

Reference	Creatinine < 1.5 mg/dL Creatinine clearance > 80 mL/min		Creatinine > 1.5 mg/dL Creatinine clearance < 80 mL/min	
	Perinatal mortality	Associated hypertension*	Perinatal mortality	Associated hypertension*
Studd and Blainey [118] (1969)	0/8	5/8	2/6	4/6
Bear [119] (1976)	1/36	9/36	0/7	7/8
Hayslett and Lynn [120] (1980)	8/60	14/60	3/5	3/5
Katz et al. [117] (1980)	2/70	16/70	1/4	3/4
Combined	5%	24%	27%	78%

*Either onset of hypertension during pregnancy or exacerbation of preexisting hypertension.

pregnancy outcome for women with chronic renal disease.

Severity of Renal Insufficiency Prior to Pregnancy

The severity of renal insufficiency also impacts significantly on the outcome of pregnancy in women with underlying renal disease. Table 12-3 summarizes the combined data from four studies in which the level of serum creatinine or the creatinine clearance in the nonpregnant state was known [117–120]. The table reveals that pregnancies in women with a serum creatinine concentration of greater than 1.5 mg/dL or a creatinine clearance of less than 80 mL per minute are associated with a marked increase in both perinatal mortality and the onset or worsening of hypertension. Thus, while perinatal mortality in patients with renal disease who have relatively normal glomerular filtration rates is 5%, it increases to 27% for those with diminished filtration. Likewise, hypertension ensues or is worsened in 24% of patients with creatinine less than 1.5 mg/dL while complicating the pregnancies of 78% of the patients with pregestational serum creatinine greater than 1.5 mg/dL. It must be noted that some of the increased maternal and fetal risk associated with decreased renal function may be attributed to the accompanying hypertension. However, analysis of the available data suggests that hypertension is not solely responsible for the increased risk and that glomerular filtration rate probably represents an independent variable.

Effect of Specific Renal Disorders

Primary Glomerular Disease

Diffuse and focal glomerulonephritis is associated with greater fetal wastage and, along with arteriolar nephrosclerosis, accounts for the major incidence of significant hypertension [117]. A marked deterioration of renal function and an alarmingly high incidence of maternal death in women with membranoproliferative glomerulonephritis have been reported [121]. However, some investigators have found no association between membranoproliferative glomerulonephritis and obstetric prognosis [117,118]. Similarly, lipoid nephrosis and membranous nephropathy are lesions unassociated with increased risk during pregnancy [117–119, 122]. Isolated nephrotic-range proteinuria, unaccompanied by renal functional impairment or hypertension, has no effect on the outcome of pregnancy [118,122,123].

Lupus Nephropathy

Though systemic lupus erythematosus occurs frequently in women of childbearing age, the relationship of pregnancy and lupus nephropathy remains uncertain. Three large retrospective series [120,124,125] concluded that (1) active clinical disease, either renal or nonrenal, within six months of conception is associated with four times higher incidence of fetal wastage than that of pregnancies conceived in a period of clinical remission for more than six months (30% versus 8%); (2) onset of systemic lupus erythematosus during pregnancy has a similarly poor fetal prognosis; (3) treatment of clinically active systemic lupus erythematosus with steroids or cytotoxic agents is associated with no adverse fetal effects; (4) the course of lupus nephropathy is unaffected by pregnancy; and (5) intrapartum and postpartum intensification of steroid therapy reduces postpartum exacerbations to clinically active renal and nonrenal systemic lupus erythematosus.

Diabetic Nephropathy

Despite the fact that diabetes is one of the most common medical disorders encountered during pregnancy, surprisingly few series are available reporting pregnancy outcome in diabetic mothers with overt renal disease [126–129]. One large series found that, as in other patients with chronic renal diseases, diabetic gravidas with nonproliferative renal disease demonstrate an increase in glomerular filtration rate throughout pregnancy [130].

Nephropathy manifested solely as proteinuria does not accelerate in pregnancy despite an increase in the level of proteinuria to greater than 3 grams per 24 hours in 69% and the onset of hypertension in 57% [129]. However, pregnancy may aggravate the nephropathy in patients with moderate or severe pregestational impairment of renal function or in patients who are hypertensive prior to conception [128]. The success of pregnancy appears to correlate with the severity of diabetes as described by the White classification. Classes A and B and gestational diabetes had 100%, 87%, and 94% fetal survival, respectively, compared to 60% successful pregnancy in class F gravidas [130].

Chronic Interstitial Nephritis
It is now recognized that most patients previously classified as having chronic pyelonephritis have renal disease unrelated to infection. Reflux nephropathy and analgesic abuse are thought to be major causes of acquired chronic nonglomerular renal disease. The outcome of pregnancy in the patients is related to the presence of hypertension and the degree of renal insufficiency [117].

Polycystic Kidney Disease
Clinical manifestations of polycystic kidney disease appear at an average of 40 years. Therefore, most women with polycystic kidneys remain undetected during pregnancy. In 81 patients with polycystic kidneys from four series, 126 pregnancies were followed and 116 live babies were delivered—a fetal survival rate of 92% [131–134]. It appears that despite occasional reports of hypertensive crises and pyelonephritis, normotensive patients with this disease have no increase in complications during pregnancy. It is also of interest that, despite the frequent association of polycystic kidney disease and intracranial aneurysms, there were no reports of cerebral hemorrhage in the four series mentioned above.

Urolithiasis
Renal stones may be the most common cause of nonobstetric abdominal pain [135]. The prevalence varies between 0.03 and 0.35% [136,137]. A careful review by Coe et al. of 78 women with urolithiasis who had a total of 148 pregnancies revealed that stone disease has no adverse effect on pregnancy except for an increased frequency of urinary tract infections [138]. Although none of the patients in the series were subjected to instrumentation, one recent report suggests that endoscopic basket extraction can be performed safely if a stone needs to be removed [139].

Effect of Pregnancy on the Course of Chronic Renal Disease
The effect of pregnancy on the natural history of the underlying renal disease is still controversial. Most reports cite no adverse relationship between pregnancy and postpartum renal function [116,118,119,122]. A recent study found that renal function decreased in 16% of gravidas with a variety of renal diseases, and that more than 50% of the women in whom the decrease occurred had diffuse glomerulonephritis [117]. Furthermore, all but 15% of these patients had a complete recovery of prepregnancy renal function. In contrast, Fairley et al., in a rigorous study including renal biopsy before, during, and after pregnancy in patients with diffuse glomerulonephritis and membranous nephropathy found a sudden and irreversible deterioration in renal function in 7 of 22 patients [121]. The reasons for these divergent findings remain unknown. However, the consensus holds that any deterioration of renal function during pregnancy is a coincidental exacerbation of the primary disease [110].

In summary: Successful pregnancy is possible in women with underlying renal disease, but hypertension, pregestational renal insufficiency, active renal disease, and a proliferative histologic picture adversely affect the likelihood of a successful outcome. The presence of two or more of these risks should deter any attempt at pregnancy.

PREGNANCY AND HEMODIALYSIS
Hemodialysis has been used in women with chronic renal failure from a variety of causes who either become pregnant while on maintenance hemodialysis or require maintenance hemodialysis because of end-stage renal disease developed during pregnancy [140–154]. These cases are summarized in Table 12-4. In addition, hemodialysis has been employed in pregnant patients with acute renal failure or drug overdoses [155–159]. The following conclusions can be drawn from the available data: (1) Almost all infants were born prematurely (i.e., less than 37 weeks), (2) hypotension and vaginal bleeding have been noted during hemodialysis, and (3) premature contractions occurred frequently during or immediately after dialysis. It is obvious that experience with

Table 12-4. Patients with chronic renal failure dialyzed during pregnancy

Reference	Length of pregnancy at which dialysis starts (wk)	Complication	Fetal outcome
Orme et al. [142]	30	None	Alive
Herwig et al. [143]	26	Unavailable	Alive
Pepperell et al. [144]	24	Premature contractions	Dead
Confortini et al. [145]	Onset	Unavailable	Premature
Beaudry et al. [146]	Onset	Premature contractions	Dead
Unzelman et al. [147]	Onset	Premature contractions	Premature
Ackrill et al. [148]	Onset	Vaginal bleeding	Premature
Sheriff et al. [150]	Onset	None	Premature
Johnson et al. [151]	29	Premature contractions	Premature
Robinson et al. [152]	Onset	Premature contractions	Premature
Naik et al. [153]	20	None	Premature
Nissenson [154]	36	Premature contractions	Alive

Source: Adapted from Nissenson [154].

hemodialysis in pregnancy is limited and not likely to be subjected to controlled research. The largest reported experience in pregnancy with maintenance hemodialysis comes from Europe [160]. According to these data, 1 in 200 women on chronic dialysis becomes pregnant. Of 75 reported pregnancies, 7 ended in live births, 32 had therapeutic abortions, and 36 ended in spontaneous abortion.

The following modifications in the dialysis procedure may be of value for the pregnant patient [154]. Hypotension on dialysis should be treated with albumin rather than saline since the patient is frequently hypoalbuminemic and salt overloaded. Ultrafiltration and dialysis should not be performed simultaneously because peripheral vascular resistance is already diminished in pregnancy and could be exacerbated when ultrafiltration and dialysis are combined. What constitutes adequate dialysis in the pregnant patient is unclear though some authors urge intensive dialysis to "normalize" the blood urea nitrogen [142,148].

PREGNANCY FOLLOWING RENAL TRANSPLANTATION

In contrast to patients on hemodialysis, pregnancy being possible in approximately 1 out of 200 women, fertility may be restored to 1 out of 50 women after a successful renal transplant [161]. Menstruation reappears within six months after transplantation [162–164].

Table 12-5 summarizes the outcome of pregnancy following renal transplantation in 151 women from three large series. Two series report the results from a single center [162,164], and one is a compilation of data from more than 20 centers [163]. Successful pregnancy occurred in 86% of the total. Maternal deterioration of renal function was reported in 7 to 40% of patients. This deterioration typically occurred in the third trimester and was reversible. Preeclampsia developed in 30% of women with a functioning renal transplant, or approximately four times the incidence in a nontransplant pregnant population. Furthermore, patients who have received a renal transplant are subject to an increased risk of urinary and pulmonary infection [165]. Those treated with immunosuppressive drugs are at even greater risk.

Fetal hazards include a 45% incidence of prematurity, and one-third of neonates will have complications including respiratory distress syndrome, congenital anomalies, adrenocortical insufficiency, septicemia, hyperviscosity, and seizures.

In summary, both mother and child are at high risk in pregnancy following renal transplantation. Women receiving this form of therapy for end stage renal disease should be informed of the risks. The high incidence of therapeutic abortion in this population suggests that many pregnancies are accidental and may result from inadequate patient education about restored fertility [161].

Table 12-5. Outcome of pregnancy following renal transplantation

Reference	Live births	Preeclampsia
Penn et al. [162]	43/49 (7 TAB)	15/56
Rifle and Traeger [163]	77/87 (22 TAB)	11/38
Sciarra et al. [164]	10/15 (2 TAB)	7/17
Combined	130/151 (86%)	33/111 (30%)

TAB = therapeutic abortion.

REFERENCES

1. Bailey RR, Rolleston GL. Kidney length and ureteric dilatation in the puerperium. J Obstet Gynaecol Br Comm. 1971; 78:55–61.
2. Davison JM, Lindheimer MD. Changes in renal haemodynamics and kidney weight during pregnancy in the unanaesthetized rat. J Physiol (Lond). 1980; 301:129–36.
3. Sheehan HL, Lynch JB. Pathology of toxaemia of pregnancy. Edinburgh: Churchill Livingstone, 1973:47–52.
4. Pollak VE, Nettles JB. The kidney in toxemia of pregnancy, a clinical and pathologic study based on renal biopsies. Medicine (Baltimore). 1960; 39:469–526.
5. Fainstat T. Ureteral dilatation in pregnancy: a review. Obstet Gynecol Surv. 1963; 18:845–60.
6. Roberts JA. Hydronephrosis of pregnancy. Urology. 1976; 8:1–4.
7. Dure-Smith P. Pregnancy dilatation of the urinary tract. The iliac sign and its significance. Radiology. 1970; 96:545–50.
8. Fried AM. Hydronephrosis of pregnancy: ultrasonographic study and classification of asymptomatic women. Am J Obstet Gynecol. 1979; 13:1066–70.
9. Homas DC, Harrington JT. Acute renal failure caused by ureteral obstruction by a gravid uterus. JAMA. 1981; 246:1230–1.
10. Davison JM, Dunlop W. Renal hemodynamics and tubular function in normal human pregnancy. Kidney Int. 1980; 18:152–61.
11. Bucht H. Studies on renal function in man with special reference to glomerular filtration and renal plasma flow in pregnancy. Scand J Clin Lab Invest [Suppl 3]. 1951; 3:1–64.
12. Sims EA, Krantz KE. Serial studies of renal function during pregnancy and the puerperium in normal women. J Clin Invest. 1958; 37:1764–74.
13. Pippig L. Clinical aspects of renal disease during pregnancy. Med Hyg. 1969; 27:181–91.
14. Bader RA, Bader ME, Rose DG, Braunwald E. Hemodynamics at rest and during exercise in normal pregnancy as studied by cardiac catheterization. J Clin Invest. 1955; 34:1524–36.
15. Berlin NI, Goetsch C, Hyde GM, Parsons RJ. The blood volume in pregnancy as determined by P32 labeled red blood cells. Surg Gynecol Obstet. 1953; 97:173–6.
16. Walters WW, Lim YL. Blood volume and haemodynamics in pregnancy. Clin Obstet Gynaecol. 1975; 1:301–20.
17. Lindheimer MD, Katz AI. Renal function in pregnancy. In: Wynn R., ed. Obstet Gynecol Annu. 1972; 1:139–176.
18. Baylis C. The mechanism of the increase in glomerular filtration rate in the twelve-day pregnant rat. J Physiol (Lond). 1980; 305:405–14.
19. Baylis C. Glomerular ultrafiltration in the pseudopregnant rat. Am J Physiol. 1982; 242:F300–F305.
20. Katz AI, Lindheimer MD. Actions of hormones on the kidney. Annu Rev Physiol. 1977; 39:97–133.

21. Berl T, Better OS. Renal effects of prolactin, estrogen and progesterone. In: Brenner BM, Stein JH, eds. Contemporary issues in nephrology. Vol 4, Hormonal function and the kidney. New York: Churchill Livingstone, 1980:192–214.
22. Lim VS, Katz AI, Lindheimer MD. Acid-base regulation in pregnancy. Am J Physiol. 1976; 231:1764–9.
23. Hytten FE, Leitch I. The physiology of human pregnancy. 2nd ed. Oxford: Blackwell Scientific, 1971.
24. Nolten WE, Ehrlich EN. Sodium and mineralocorticoids in normal pregnancy. Kidney Int. 1980; 18:162–72.
25. Gray MJ, Munro AB, Sims EA, et al. Regulation of sodium and total body water metabolism in pregnancy. Am J Obstet Gynecol. 1964; 89:760–5.
26. Davison JM, Vallotton MB, Lindheimer MD. Alterations in plasma osmolality (Posm) during human pregnancy. Clin Res. 1980; 28:442A. abstract.
27. Macdonald HN, Good W. The effect of parity on plasma sodium, potassium chloride and osmolality levels during pregnancy. J Obstet Gynaecol Br Comm. 1972; 79:441–9.
28. Durr JV, Stamoutsos B, Lindheimer MD. Osmoregulation during pregnancy in the rat. J Clin Invest. 1981; 68:337–46.
29. Landau RL, Lugibihl K. Inhibition of the sodium-retaining influence of aldosterone by progesterone. J Clin Endocrinol Metab. 1958; 18:1237–45.
30. Torres C, Schewitz LJ, Pollak VE. The effect of small amounts of antidiuretic hormone on sodium and urate excretion in pregnancy. Am J Obstet Gynecol. 1966; 94:546–58.
31. Bay WH, Ferris TF. Studies of the circulation during pregnancy. Clin Res. 1975; 23:468A. abstract.
32. Schrier RW, DeWardener HE. Tubular reabsorption of sodium ion: influence of factors other than aldosterone and glomerular filtration rate. N Engl J Med. 1971; 185:1231–43.
33. Nolten WE, Lindheimer MD, Oparil S, Ehrlich EN. Desoxycorticosterone in normal pregnancy: sequential studies of the secretory patterns of desoxycorticosterone, aldosterone, and cortisol. Am J Obstet Gynecol. 1978; 132:414–20.
34. Bay WH, Ferris T. Factors controlling renin and aldosterone during pregnancy. Hypertension. 1979; 1:410–15.
35. Lindheimer MD, Ehrlich EN. Postural effects on renal function and volume homeostasis during pregnancy. J Reprod Med. 1979; 12:135–41.
36. Lindheimer MD, Katz AI. Sodium and diuretics in pregnancy. N Engl J Med. 1973; 288:891–4.
37. Fine J. Glycosuria of pregnancy. Br Med J. 1967; 1:205–10.
38. Davison JM. Proceedings: changes in renal function and other aspects of homeostasis in early pregnancy. J Obstet Gynaecol Br Comm. 1974; 81:1003–9.
39. Welsh GW, Sims EA. The mechanism of renal glucosuria in pregnancy. Diabetes. 1960; 9:363–9.
40. Davison JM, Hytten FE. The effect of pregnancy on the renal handling of glucose. Br J Obstet Gynaecol. 1975; 82:374–81.

41. Semple PF, Carswell W, Bayle JA. Serial studies on the renal clearance of urate and inulin during pregnancy and after the puerperium in normal women. Clin Sci Mol Med. 1974; 47:559–65.

42. Dunlop W, Davison JM. The effect of normal pregnancy upon the renal handling of uric acid. Br J Obstet Gynaecol. 1977; 84:13–21.

43. Lancet M, Fisher IL. The value of blood uric acid levels in toxaemia of pregnancy. J Obstet Gynaecol Br Comm. 1956; 63:116–9.

44. Redman CW, Beilin LJ, Bonnar J, Wilkinson RH. Plasma urate measurements in predicting fetal death in hypertensive pregnancy. Lancet. 1976; 1:1370–3.

45. Berl T, Schrier RW. Renal function in pregnancy. In: Schrier RW, ed. Renal and electrolyte disorders. 2nd ed. Boston: Little, Brown, 1980:471–99.

46. Lindheimer MD, Katz AI. Kidney disease in pregnancy. Part I. In: Lindheimer MD, Katz AI, eds. Kidney function and disease in pregnancy. Philadelphia: Lea & Febiger, 1977:106–45.

47. Clark LC, Thompson H, Beck, EI. The excretion of creatine and creatinine during pregnancy. Am J Obstet Gynecol. 1951; 62:576–83.

48. Davison JM, Hytten FE. Glomerular filtration during and after pregnancy. J Obstet Gynaecol Br Comm. 1974; 81:588–95.

49. Kincaid-Smith P, Bullen M. Bacteriuria in pregnancy. Lancet. 1965; 1:395–9.

50. Little PJ. The incidence of urinary infection in 5000 pregnant women. Lancet. 1966; 2:925–8.

51. Lindheimer MD, Katz AI. The renal response to pregnancy. In: Brenner BM, Rector FC Jr, eds. The kidney. 2nd ed. Philadelphia: Saunders, 1981: 1762–1815.

52. Katz AI. Clinical tests of renal function. In: Lindheimer MD, Katz AI, eds. Kidney function and disease in pregnancy. Philadelphia: Lea & Febiger, 1977:77–105.

53. Gallery ED, Gyory AZ. Urinary concentration, white blood cell excretion, acid excretion, and acid-base status in normal pregnancy: alterations in pregnancy-associated hypertension. Am J Obstet Gynecol. 1979; 135:27–36.

54. Kark RM, Lawrence JR, Pollak VE, Pirani CL, Muehrcke RC, Silva H. A primer of urinalysis. 2nd ed. New York: Harper & Row, 1963:29.

55. Glassock RJ. Postural (orthostatic) proteinuria: no cause for concern. N Engl J Med. 1981; 305:639–41. editorial.

56. Boodt PJ, Van Kessel H, Stolte LAM, Janssens J. Postural proteinuria in pregnancy. Eur J Obstet Gynaecol Reprod Biol. 1973; 3:19–23.

57. Robson JS. Proteinuria and the renal lesion in preeclampsia and abruptio placentae. In: Lindheimer MD, Katz AI, Zuspan FP, eds. Hypertension in pregnancy. New York: Wiley, 1976:61–73.

58. Lorincz AB, McCartney CP, Pottinger RE, Li KH. Protein excretion patterns in pregnancy. Am J Obstet Gynecol. 1961; 81:252–9.

59. Witten DM, Myers GH, Utz DC. Emmett's clinical urography. Philadelphia: Saunders, 1977:45–6.

60. Shanks SC, Kerley P. A textbook of x-ray diagnosis. 4th ed. Vol 5. Philadelphia: Saunders, 1970:440–1.

61. Laakso L. Isotope renography on parturients. Acta Obstet Gynecol Scand [Suppl]. 1967; 46:1–104.

62. Bergstrom H. Renographic evaluation of renal excretion in hydronephrosis of pregnancy. Acta Obstet Gynecol Scand. 1975; 54:203–8.

63. Baird DT, Gasson PW, Doig A. The renogram in pregnancy. Am J Obstet Gynecol. 1966; 95:597–603.

64. Nieminen U, Pollanen L, Kiviniitty K. Isotope renography during pregnancy. Ann Chir Gynaecol Fenn. 1970; 59:67–70.

65. Peat KW, Fried AM. Hydronephrosis masquerading as ovarian pathology. Obstet Gynecol. 1981; 57:533–6.

66. Baron RL, Lee JK, McClenna BL, Melson GL. Percutaneous nephrostomy using real-time sonographic guidance. AJR. 1981; 136:1018–9.

67. Campbell S, Wladimiroff JW, Dewhurst CJ. The antenatal measurement of fetal urine production. J Obstet Gynaecol Br Comm. 1973; 80:680–6.

68. Iversen P, Brun C. Aspiration biopsy of the kidney. Am J Med. 1951; 11:324–30.

69. Lindheimer MD, Spargo BH, Katz AI. Renal biopsy in pregnancy induced hypertension. J Reprod Med. 1975; 15:189–94.

70. Schewitz LJ, Friedman IA, Pollak VE. Bleeding after renal biopsy in pregnancy. Obstet Gynecol. 1965; 26:295–304.

71. Dennis EJ, McIver FA, Smythe CM. Renal biopsy in pregnancy. Clin Obstet Gynecol. 1968; 11:473–86.

72. Knapp RC, Hellman LM. Acute renal failure in pregnancy. Am J Obstet Gynecol. 1959; 78:570–7.

73. Kerr DN, Elliott W. Renal disease in pregnancy. Practitioner. 1963; 190:459–67.

74. Hall JW, Johnson WJ, Maher FT, et al. Immediate and long-term prognosis in acute renal failure. Ann Intern Med. 1970; 73:515–21.

75. Kennedy AC, Burton JA, Luke RG, et al. Factors affecting the prognosis in acute renal failure. Q J Med. 1973; 42:73–86.

76. Chapman A, Legrain M. Acute tubular necrosis and interstitial nephritis. In: Hamburger J, Crosnier J, Grunfeld KP, eds. Nephrology. New York: Wiley, 1979:383–410.

77. Chugh KS, Singhal PC, Sharma BK, et al. Acute renal failure of obstetric origin. Obstet Gynecol. 1976; 48:642–6.

78. Smith K, Browne JC, Shackman R, et al. Renal failure of obstetric origin. Br Med Bull. 1968; 24:49–58.

79. Harkins JL, Wilson DR, Muggah HF. Acute renal failure in obstetrics. Am J Obstet Gynecol. 1974; 118:331–6.

80. Grunfeld JP, Ganeval D, Bournerias F. Acute renal failure in pregnancy. Kidney Int. 1980; 18:179–91.

81. Kleinknecht D, Grunfeld JP, Cia Gomez P, et al. Diagnostic procedures and long-term prognosis in bilateral renal cortical necrosis. Kidney Int. 1973; 4:390–400.

82. Robson JS, Martin AM, Ruckley V, et al. Irreversible postpartum renal failure. A new syndrome. Q J Med. 1968; 37:423–35.

83. Czernobilsky B. Pathology of septic abortion. In: Schwarz RH. Septic abortion. Philadelphia: Lippincott, 1968:23–54.

84. Clarkson AR, Sage RE, Lawrence JR. Consumption coagulopathy and acute renal failure due to gram-negative septicemia after abortion. Complete recovery with heparin therapy. Ann Intern Med. 1969; 70:1191–9.

85. Willson JR, Carrington ER. Obstetrics and gynecology. St. Louis: Mosby, 1979:297–9.

86. Ober WE, Reid DE, Romney SL, Merrill JP. Renal lesions and acute renal failure in pregnancy. Am J Med. 1956; 21:781–810.

87. Pritchard JA, Pritchard SA. Standardized treatment of 154 consecutive cases of eclampsia. Am J Obstet Gynecol. 1975; 123:543–52.

88. Lopez-Llera M, Linares GR. Factors that influence maternal mortality in eclampsia. In: Lindheimer MD, Katz AI, Zuspan FP, eds. Hypertension in pregnancy. New York: Wiley, 1976:41–9.

89. Sheehan HL, Lynch JB. Pathology of toxaemia of pregnancy. Edinburgh: Churchill Livingstone, 1973.

90. Brain NC, Kuah KB, Dixon HG. Heparin treatment of haemolysis and thrombocytopenia in pre-eclampsia. J Obstet Gynaecol Br Comm. 1967; 74:702–11.

91. Pritchard JA, MacDonald PC. Williams obstetrics. 15th ed. New York: Appleton-Century-Crofts, 1976:406–416.

92. Kleiner GJ, Greston WM. Current concepts of defibrination in the pregnant woman. J Reprod Med. 1976; 17:309–17.

93. Bonnar J. Blood coagulation and fibrinolytic systems during pregnancy. Clin Obstet Gynecol. 1975; 2:321–44.

94. Matlin RA, Gary NE. Acute cortical necrosis. Am J Med. 1974; 56:110–8.

95. Effersoe P, Raaschou F, Thomsen AC. Bilateral renal cortical necrosis. A patient followed up over 8 years. Am J Med. 1962; 33:455–8.

96. Nash DT, Dale JT. Acute yellow atrophy of the liver in pregnancy. NY State J Med. 1971; 71:458–65.

97. Holzbach RT. Jaundice in pregnancy—1976. Am J Med. 1976; 61:367–76.

98. Kunelis CT, Peters JL, Edmondson HA. Fatty liver of pregnancy and its relationship to tetracycline therapy. Am J Med. 1965; 38:359–77.

99. Nardone AA, Stroup PE, Gill RJ. Acute fatty metamorphosis of the liver in pregnancy. Am J Obstet Gynecol. 1960; 80:158–62.

100. Mackenna J, Pupkin M, Crenshaw C, McLeod M, Parker RT. Acute fatty metamorphosis of the liver. Am J Obstet Gynecol. 1977; 127:401–4.

101. Whalley PJ, Cunningham FG, Martin FG. Transient renal dysfunction associated with acute pyelonephritis of pregnancy. Obstet Gynecol. 1975; 46:174–7.

102. O'Shaughnessy R, Weprin SA, Zuspan FP. Obstructive renal failure by an overdistended pregnant uterus. Obstet Gynecol. 1980; 55:247–9.

103. Schreiner GE. Dialysis and pregnancy. JAMA. 1976; 235:1725. editorial.

104. Churg J, Koffler D, Paronetto F, Rorat E, Barnett RN. Hemolytic uremic syndrome as a cause of postpartum renal failure. Am J Obstet Gynecol. 1970; 108:253–61.

105. Finklestein FO, Kashgarian M, Hayslett JP. Clinical spectrum of postpartum renal failure. Am J Med. 1974; 57:649–54.

106. Morel-Maroger L, Kanfer A, Solez K, Sraer JD, Richet G. Prognostic importance of vascular lesions in acute renal failure with microangiopathic hemolytic anemia (hemolytic-uremic syndrome): clinico-pathologic study in 20 adults. Kidney Int. 1979; 15:548–58.

107. Segonds A, Louradow N, Suc JM, Orfila C. Postpartum hemolytic uremic syndrome: a study of three cases with a review of the literature. Clin Nephrol. 1979; 12:229–42.

108. Race MH, Fortune RA, Christiano A. Recurrent postpartum hemolytic uremic syndrome. Lancet. 1980; 1:449.

109. Kelleher SP, Berl T. Acute renal failure in pregnancy. Semin Nephrol. 1981; 1:61–8.

110. Lindheimer MD, Katz AI. Kidney disease and pregnancy. Part II. In: Lindheimer MD, Katz AI, eds. Kidney function and disease in pregnancy. Philadelphia: Lea & Febiger, 1977:146–87.

111. Leppert P, Tisher CC, Cheng SC, Harlan WR. Antecedent renal disease and the outcome of pregnancy. Ann Intern Med. 1979; 90:747–51.

112. MacKay EV. Pregnancy and renal disease. Aust NZ J Obstet Gynaecol. 1963; 3:21–34.

113. Goodwin NJ, Valenti C, Hall JE, Friedman EA. Effects of uremia and chronic hemodialysis on the reproductive cycle. Am J Obstet Gynecol. 1968; 100:528–35.

114. Hull AR. Pregnancy and renal disease. Dallas: Southwestern Medical School, Department of Medicine Grand Rounds, 1977:23.

115. Felding C. The obstetric prognosis in chronic renal disease. Acta Obstet Gynecol Scand. 1968; 47:168–72.

116. Ferris TF. Renal disease. In: Burrow GN, Ferris TF, eds. Medical complications during pregnancy. Philadelphia: Saunders, 1975:1–52.

117. Katz AI, Davison JM, Hayslett JP, Singson E, Lindheimer MD. Pregnancy in women with kidney disease. Kidney Int. 1980; 18:192–206.

118. Studd JW, Blainey JD. Pregnancy and the nephrotic syndrome. Br Med J. 1969; 1:276–80.

119. Bear RA. Pregnancy in patients with renal disease. Obstet Gynecol. 1976; 48:13–8.

120. Hayslett JP, Lynn RI. Effect of pregnancy in patients with lupus nephropathy. Kidney Int. 1980; 18:107–20.

121. Fairley KF, Whitworth JA, Kincaid-Smith P. Glomerulonephritis and pregnancy. In: Kincaid-Smith

P, Mathew TH, Becker EL, eds. Glomerulonephritis. New York: Wiley, 1973:997–1011.

122. Strauch BS, Hayslett JP. Kidney disease and pregnancy. Br Med J. 1974; 4:578–82.

123. Kaplan AL, Smith JP, Tillman AJ. Healed acute and chronic nephritis in pregnancy. Am J Obstet Gynecol. 1962; 83:1519–25.

124. Barnett BV, Danovitch GM, Lieb SM. In: Fine LG, moderator. Systemic lupus erythematosus in pregnancy. Ann Intern Med. 1981; 94:667–77.

125. Jungers P, Douglas M, Pelissier C, Kuttenn F, Tron F, Lesavre P, Bach J. Lupus nephropathy and pregnancy. Report of 104 cases in 36 patients. Arch Int Med. 1982;142:771–6.

126. Oppe TC, Hsia D, Gellis SS. Pregnancy in the diabetic mother with nephritis. Lancet. 1957; 1:353-6.

127. Sims EA. Serial studies of renal function in pregnancy complicated by diabetes mellitus. Diabetes. 1961; 10:190–7.

128. White P. Pregnancy and diabetes, medical aspects. Med Clin North Am. 1965; 49:1015–24.

129. Kitzmiller J, Brown E, Phillippe M, Acker D, Kaldany A, Singh S, Hare J. Diabetic nephropathy and perinatal outcome. Am J Obstet Gynecol. 1981; 141:741–51.

130. Sims EA. The kidney in pregnancy complicated by diabetes mellitus. Clin Obstet Gynecol. 1962; 5:462–81.

131. Higgins CC. Bilateral polycystic kidney disease; review of ninety-four cases. Arch Surg. 1952; 65:318–29.

132. Landesman R, Scherr L. Congenital polycystic kidney disease in pregnancy. Obstet Gynecol. 1956; 8:673–80.

133. Millar WG. Pregnancy and polycystic disease of the kidneys. J Obstet Gynecol Br Emp. 1953; 60:868–71.

134. Morris N. Pregnancy complicated by congenital polycystic disease of the kidneys. J Obstet Gynaecol Br Emp. 1952; 59:822–8.

135. Folger GK. Pain and pregnancy. Obstet Gynecol. 1955; 5:513–8.

136. Harris RE, Dunnihoo DIR. The incidence and significance of urinary calculi in pregnancy. Am J Obstet Gynecol. 1967; 99:237–41.

137. Roopnarinesingh S. Renal calculi in pregnancy. West Indian Med J. 1972; 21:35–9.

138. Coe FLC, Parks JH, Lindheimer MD. Nephrolithiasis during pregnancy. N Engl J Med. 1978; 298:324–6.

139. Swanson SK. Personal communication and Trans Am Urol Assoc. 1981.

140. De Los Rios JE, Perez JJP, Perez SC, Avendono LH. Successful pregnancy and advanced renal failure. Lancet. 1978; 1:861.

141. Joglar F, Burgos R. End-stage renal disease and pregnancy. Dial Transplant. 1981; 10:833–6.

142. Orme BM, Ueland K, Simpson DP, Scribner BH. The effect of hemodialysis on fetal survival and renal function in pregnancy. Trans Am Soc Artif Intern Organs. 1968; 14:402–4.

143. Herwig KR, Merrill JP, Jackson RL, Oken DE. Chronic renal disease and pregnancy. Case report of azotemia, hemodialysis, and delivery of a viable infant. Am J Obstet Gynecol. 1965; 92:1117–21.

144. Pepperell RJ, Adam WR, Dawborn JK. Haemodialysis in the management of chronic renal failure during pregnancy. Aust NZ J Obstet Gynaecol. 1970; 10:180–6.

145. Confortini P, Galanti G, Ancona G, Giongo A, Bruschi E, Lorenzini E. Full term pregnancy and successful delivery in a patient on chronic hemodialysis. Proc Eur Dial Transplant Assoc. 1971; 8:74–80.

146. Beaudry C, Carriere S, Barcelo R. Hémodialyse chronique: résultats observés au cours de six années d'expérience (plus de 8,000 traitements par le rein artificiel de Kolff). Union Med Can. 1971; 100:100–12.

147. Unzelman RF, Alderfer GR, Chojnacki RE. Pregnancy and chronic hemodialysis. Trans Am Soc Artif Intern Organs. 1973; 19:14–9.

148. Ackrill P, Goodwin FJ, March FP, Stratton D, Wagman H. Successful pregnancy in patient on regular dialysis. Br Med J. 1975; 1:172–4.

149. Marwood RP, Ogg CS, Coltart TM, Klopper AI. Plasma oestrogens in a pregnancy associated with chronic haemodialysis. Br J Obstet Gynaecol. 1977; 84:613–7.

150. Sheriff MH, Hardman M, Lamont CA, Shepherd R, Warren DJ. Successful pregnancy in a 44-year-old haemodialysis patient. Br J Obstet Gynaecol. 1978; 85:386–8.

151. Johnson TR Jr, Lorenz RP, Menon KM, Nolan GH. Successsful outcome of a pregnancy requiring dialysis. Effects on serum progesterone and estrogens. J Reprod Med. 1979; 22:217–8.

152. Robinson CD, Unzelman RF, Chojnacki RE. Survival of an infant of a mother dependent on hemodialysis. J Pediatr. 1973; 82:537–8.

153. Naik RB, Clark AD, Warren DJ. Acute proliferative glomerulonephritis with crescents and renal failure in pregnancy successfully managed by intermittent hemodialysis. Case report. Br J Obstet Gynaecol. 1979; 86:819–22.

154. Nissenson AR. The use of hemodialysis to treat end-stage renal failure during pregnancy. In: Fine LG, moderator. Systemic lupus erythematosus in pregnancy. Ann Intern med. 1981; 94:667–77.

155. Theil GB, Richter RW, Powell MR, Doolan PD. Acute dilantin poisoning. Neurology (Minneap). 1961; 11:138–42.

156. Kurtz GG, Michael UF, Morosi HJ, Vaamonde CA. Hemodialysis during pregnancy. Report of a case of glutethimide poisoning complicated by acute renal failure. Arch Intern Med. 1966; 118:30–2.

157. Goldsmith JH, Menzies DN, DeBoer CH, Caplan W, McCandless A. Delivery of healthy infant after five weeks' dialysis treatment for fulminating toxaemia of pregnancy. Lancet. 1971; 2:738–41.

158. Vaziri ND, Kumar KP, Mirahmadi K, Rosen SM. Hemodialysis in treatment of acute chloral hydrate poisoning. South Med J. 1977; 70:377–8.

159. Nemoto R, Sugiyama Y, Kuwahara M, Kata T, Tsuchida S. Successful delivery of a patient on hemodialysis for acute renal failure: a case report and review of the literature. J Urol. 1977; 118:673–4.

160. Jacobs C, Brunner FP, Chantler C, et al. Combined report on regular dialysis and transplantation in Europe VIII, 1976. Proc Eur Dial Transplant Assoc. 1977; 14:3–69.

161. Editorial. Pregnancy after renal replacement. Br Med J. 1976; 1:733–4.

162. Penn I, Makowski EL, Harris P. Parenthood following renal transplantation. Kidney Int. 1980; 18:221–33.

163. Rifle G, Traeger J. Pregnancy after renal transplantation. An international survey. Transplant Proc. 1975; 7 (Suppl 1):723–8.

164. Sciarra JJ, Toledo-Pereyra LH, Bendel RP, Simmons RL. Pregnancy following renal transplantation. Am J Obstet Gynecol. 1975; 123:411–25.

165. Rudolph JE, Schweizer RT, Bartus SA. Pregnancy in renal transplant patients. Transplantation. 1979; 27:26–9.

13. HYPERTENSION AND PREECLAMPSIA

Lawrence E. Feinberg

Hypertension has emerged as the most common serious antenatal complication of pregnancy. Although this incidence of hypertension complicating pregnancy is subject to racial and socioeconomic factors, it remains important in any practice setting. Hypertension is a major cause of morbidity and mortality in both mother and fetus. The maternal mortality attributed to hypertension in the United States is approximately 3 to 5 per 100,000 live births. Maternal hypertension is associated with 12.5% of all perinatal deaths, principally because of fetal growth retardation and the need for preterm delivery.

The overall risk that a primigravida will have pregnancy-induced hypertension is 7 to 8%, being highest for teenagers or older nulliparas, and two to three times higher for those entering pregnancy with chronic hypertension. Hypertension is common in the general population (e.g., 7% incidence in white women, ages 20–29), and essential hypertension accounts for about one-third of cases of hypertension in pregnancy [1]. Blood pressure elevation during pregnancy is closely related to perinatal mortality. The Collaborative Perinatal Project examined the course of more than 50,000 women and found a sharp rise in perinatal mortality when the blood pressure (BP) rose to about 125/75 mm Hg at week 36, a BP level considered normal in the nonobstetric setting [2]. Fortunately, good prenatal supervision, early detection of the signs and symptoms of pregnancy-induced hypertension, and appropriate treatment can prevent many fetal losses and result in a satisfactory outcome for mother and baby.

PHYSIOLOGIC CHANGES OF BLOOD PRESSURE DURING PREGNANCY

An increase in cardiac output provides the uteroplacental circulation with the extra blood flow that is required to support fetal development. In spite of a 25 to 50% rise in resting cardiac output, mean arterial blood pressure declines until midpregnancy, then rises toward prepregnancy levels as term approaches (Fig. 13-1). Diastolic BP is lowered by an average of 5 to 10 mm Hg by the sixteenth week of gestation, so that a representative average BP among gravidas during late second trimester is 115/66 mm Hg [3]. At the beginning of the third trimester, BP slowly rises toward prepregnancy levels, and, despite considerable variation, there are increases of at least 3 to 5 mm Hg for systolic BP and 6 to 10 mm Hg for the diastolic blood pressure (DBP) from the beginning to the end of the third trimester. Any sustained rise in blood pressure exceeding 30 mm Hg systolic or 15 mm Hg diastolic is considered abnormal.

The normal fall in blood pressure during early and midpregnancy must be related to a decrease in peripheral vascular resistance since cardiac output normally increases and blood volume expands, progressively, until 30 to 34 weeks' gestation. There are two mechanisms for the decrease in resistance: One is vasodilatation in the maternal vascular tree; the other is the increasing fraction of cardiac output that passes through the uteroplacental circulation. Vasodilatation is evident by the tenth week of gestation and results from a decreased responsiveness of vascular smooth muscle to angiotensin II and other pressor substances [4].

Concurrent with systemic vasodilatation, many factors, including progesterone-induced relaxation of capacitance veins and estrogen-induced synthesis of angiotensinogen, combine to activate the renin-angiotensin-aldosterone system [5]. Marked increases in plasma renin activity and plasma aldosterone promote a gradual cumulative retention of 700 to 900 mEq of sodium during the course of pregnancy. Plasma volume reaches an average level of 140% of nonpregnant levels in the third trimester [6]. Similar expansion of maternal plasma volume and augmentation of cardiac output are observed in gravidas with uncomplicated mild essential hypertension.

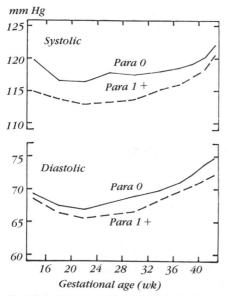

Fig. 13-1. Mean systolic and diastolic blood pressures by gestational age and parity (white gravidas, ages 25–34, who delivered single, live term births). Note average BP at midpregnancy = 115/66 mm Hg; BP consistently rises during last trimester. (From Christianson [3].)

The magnitude of the increase in maternal blood volume and the development of edema correlate with fetal and placental growth and the eventual birth weight of the infant. Maternal edema may be physiologic, and edema involving the hands and face occurs in one-third of women by the thirty-eighth week of pregnancy. In addition to physiologic sodium retention, compression of the inferior vena cava by the gravid uterus promotes lower-extremity edema. Occasionally, normal women in late pregnancy experience marked hypotension in the supine recumbent position because of this effect of the gravid uterus, which interferes with venous return to the heart. The hemodynamic, renal, and other physiologic changes associated with pregnancy are summarized in Table 13-1.

CLASSIFICATION AND DIAGNOSIS OF HYPERTENSION IN PREGNANCY

The classification of hypertensive disorders in pregnancy, first proposed by Chesley and modified by Gant and Worley [7,8], remains an excellent framework for discussion of the subject. The classification is as follows:

A. Pregnancy-induced hypertension
   1. Preeclampsia, mild or severe
   2. Eclampsia
B. Chronic hypertension preceding pregnancy (any etiology)
C. Chronic hypertension with superimposed pregnancy-induced hypertension
D. Late, transient, or unclassifiable hypertension

The development of high blood pressure during pregnancy, in a previously normotensive woman, categorizes pregnancy-induced hypertension. When hypertension with proteinuria arises de novo, the condition is called preeclampsia; when preexisting hypertension is intensified by pregnancy and is accompanied by proteinuria, the condition is referred to as superimposed preeclampsia. If the pregnancy-induced hypertensive disorder causes convulsions, the condition is called eclampsia [9].

Table 13-1. Changes in normal pregnancy and preeclampsia

Function or value	Normal pregnancy	Preeclampsia (relative to normal pregnancy)
Hemodynamics		
Plasma volume	Expanded	Decreased
Total body sodium	Increased	Increased
Cardiac output	Increased	Unchanged
Peripheral resistance	Reduced	Increased
Vascular reactivity	Reduced	Increased
Uterine blood flow		Decreased
Renal function		
Blood flow	Increased	Decreased
Glomerular filtration	Increased	Decreased
Hormonal changes		
Plasma renin activity	Increased	Decreased
Plasma aldosterone	Increased	Decreased
Plasma PGI_2 (prostacyclin)	Increased	Decreased

Source: Adapted from Kaplan [16].

Pregnancy-Induced Hypertension

Preeclampsia

Preeclampsia is diagnosed on the basis of hypertension with proteinuria and edema, which develop after the 24th week of gestation. Approximately 75% of cases are documented after the thirty-seventh week of pregnancy. The first clinical signs may arise during labor or during the first 48 to 72 hours post partum. Preeclampsia is primarily a disease of the primigravida. When it is observed in the multipara, one of the following clinical conditions is usually present: chronic hypertension, diabetes mellitus, renal disease, multiple gestations, hydramnios, fetal hydrops, hydatidiform mole. Among multiparas diagnosed as having preeclampsia in the absence of these conditions, the true underlying disorder often is latent essential hypertension or subclinical renal disease. Even in primigravidas, up to 25% of women given the diagnosis of preeclampsia have renal lesions suggestive of chronic glomerulonephritis or essential hypertension [10,11].

The blood pressure criterion for mild preeclampsia is one or both of the following: systolic pressure of 140 mm Hg or greater, or an increment of 30 mm Hg above baseline levels; a diastolic pressure of 90 mm Hg or greater, or an increase of 15 mm Hg over baseline levels. These elevations must be present on two or more occasions at least six hours apart, when measured on a patient in the left lateral decubitus position.

Proteinuria almost always develops later than hypertension. In early preeclampsia, proteinuria may be minimal or entirely lacking. Significant proteinuria is defined as the presence of > 500 mg in a 24-hour urine collection (or > 300 mg/liter) or a random protein dipstick measurement of 2 + or greater. Although trace or 1 + amounts are common (13.3% of nearly 140,000 urine samples in the United States Collaborative Perinatal Study), the combination of significant proteinuria and hypertension during pregnancy reflects a serious pathophysiologic disturbance and is associated with an increase in perinatal mortality. In one analysis of more than 3,000 pregnancies, the presence of proteinuria and DBP ≥ 85 mm Hg was associated with one and a half times the perinatal mortality observed in gravidas who had higher blood pressure (i.e., DBP ≥ 95 mm Hg) but *no* proteinuria [12].

Edema is observed in more than 85% of cases of preeclampsia. Since even generalized edema is such a common finding in women who remain normotensive (30%), it is of minimal value in the differential diagnosis of the hypertensive disorders of pregnancy or in the prediction of outcome.

Table 13-2. Clinical and laboratory features of severe preeclampsia

BP ≥ 160 mm Hg systolic or ≥ 110 mm Hg diastolic or an increase of ≥ 60 mm Hg systolic or ≥ 30 mm Hg diastolic over baseline levels

Proteinuria of ≥ 5 g/24 hr or 3–4 + by dipstick

Oliguria (< 400 mL/24 hr)

Cerebral or visual disturbances, i.e., lethargy, headache, scotomata, blurred vision

Extreme hyperreflexia or clonus

Epigastric or right upper quadrant pain

Abnormal liver function tests

Hemoconcentration

Pulmonary edema

Thrombocytopenia

Microangiopathic hemolysis; disseminated intravascular coagulation (DIC)

Characteristically, preeclampsia progresses in the following manner: Edema, primarily of the hands and face, first appears clinically, and excessive weight gain is noted. Next, a significant increase in blood pressure occurs, which is followed by the onset of proteinuria. Some patients progress to severe illness and ultimately to eclampsia. In others, the condition may ameliorate with bed rest or other treatment or by termination of the pregnancy. Clinical and laboratory features of severe preeclampsia are listed in Table 13-2.

Eclampsia

Eclampsia refers to the occurrence of one or more generalized seizures in a woman with preeclampsia. Signs and symptoms of severe preeclampsia often precede a convulsion. However, in a large series of eclamptic patients, one-fourth of the patients were classified as having *mild* preeclampsia prior to the onset of seizures while in 22% of eclamptic women, SBP had never been recorded above 140 mm Hg [13]. Since a patient with seemingly "mild" preeclampsia and trace proteinuria may suddenly have a convulsion, the terms *mild* and *severe* preeclampsia may be misleading. Blood pressure alone is not a reliable indicator of severity. In about 50% of cases, a seizure first appears before labor. The other 50% are equally divided between seizures occurring during labor and those first appearing in the postpartum period [8]. Because nearly all cases of postpartum eclampsia appear within 24 hours, any seizure occurring more than 48 hours post partum is likely to be caused by a separate metabolic or structural process affecting the brain [8]. There are, however, reports of otherwise unexplained seizures having their onset up to seven days post partum [14].

The diagnosis of eclampsia is usually not difficult, but other causes of seizures such as idiopathic epilepsy, intracerebral hemorrhage, cerebral embolism or thrombosis (arterial or venous), CNS infection, brain tumor, water intoxication, idiosyncratic reaction to local anesthetics, hypoglycemia, and lupus cerebritis should not be overlooked. In the chronically hypertensive gravida with extreme hypertension and retinal hemorrhages and exudates, the development of seizures probably reflects hypertensive encephalopathy. Malignant hypertensive disease simulating eclampsia is also a well-recognized manifestation of pheochromocytoma in pregnancy.

Chronic Hypertension
The diagnosis of chronic hypertension in the pregnant woman is suggested by the following features:

1. A well-authenticated history of hypertension, BP $\geq$ 140/90 prior to the current pregnancy [8]
2. Hypertension, BP $\geq$ 140/90 before the twentieth week of gestation (DBP $\geq$ 80 mm Hg between weeks 10 and 20 is also suggestive of hypertension preceding pregnancy) [8]
3. Severe hypertension (SBP $\geq$ 200 mm Hg), particularly with signs of left ventricular hypertrophy or hypertensive retinopathy
4. Multiparity or the presence of hypertension without proteinuria in a previous pregnancy
5. Presence of renal insufficiency, diabetes mellitus, systemic lupus erythematosus

Commonly the pregnant patient does not present to a physician until the middle of the second trimester, when the blood pressure is, physiologically, lower. Even patients with chronic hypertension may demonstrate normal blood pressures. A subsequent elevation in the late second or third trimester may be attributed to pregnancy-induced hypertension and the underlying chronic hypertension might not be recognized.

While the vast majority of hypertension is primary or essential and many cases are obesity related, the secondary causes of hypertension should be considered: renovascular disease, coarctation of the aorta, primary aldosteronism, Cushing's syndrome, pheochromocytoma, chronic glomerulonephritis, connective tissue disease with renal involvement, and diabetic nephropathy.

Chronic Hypertension with Superimposed Preeclampsia
Women with chronic hypertension are predisposed to preeclampsia and may experience increasing blood pressures, proteinuria, and edema earlier in pregnancy than observed in previously normotensive women.

The diagnosis of superimposed preeclampsia should depend on the acute elevation of either the systolic blood pressure of $\geq$ 30 mm Hg or the diastolic blood pressure of $\geq$ 15 mm Hg and the development of proteinuria in a patient with documented hypertension.

Using a DBP rise of at least 15 mm Hg and proteinuria $\geq$ 3 + as criteria, Chesley estimates that a minimum of 5.7% of chronically hypertensive gravidas will manifest preeclampsia [7]. Higher estimates (15–25%) reflect less strict criteria for this diagnosis, such as minimal proteinuria. The studies of McCartney and others indicate that only 14 to 25% of multiparas with chronic hypertension and a clinical diagnosis of superimposed preeclampsia have the characteristic renal lesions of preeclampsia on postpartum renal biopsy [10,11].

Late, Transient, or Unclassifiable Hypertension
Some cases of gestational hypertension include transient BP elevations, unaccompanied by proteinuria, which occur in late pregnancy, during labor, or within the first 24 hours post partum. The BP returns to normal within ten days after delivery, although in selected cases recurrence in successive pregnancies has been reported. The underlying mechanism is uncertain, but latent essential hypertension or mild pregnancy-induced hypertension may be responsible.

Overall, the relative prevalence of the hypertensive disorders of pregnancy is as follows: preeclampsia/eclampsia 70%; chronic hypertension 15 to 25%; chronic hypertension with superimposed preeclampsia 6 to 7%; and chronic glomerulonephritis and other causes 3 to 4% [15].

PATHOPHYSIOLOGY OF PREECLAMPSIA
No single mechanism for preeclampsia is yet established, but its increasing incidence as term approaches, the rapid resolution after delivery, and most of the disease's manifestations are explained best by the concept of inadequate uteroplacental function [7,8,16,17]. Placental degeneration may arise from an imbalance between placental mass and uterine blood flow, possibly aggravated by conditions with a large placental mass (molar pregnancy, twins, diabetes, primigravidas destined to develop preeclampsia) or associated with vascular disease (hypertension, diabetes). Presum-

ably, a factor(s) released from the compromised uteroplacental unit acts to increase vascular reactivity and initiate the events of vasospasm and organ injury. Clinically relevant pathophysiology is summarized below.

Vasoconstriction and Hypertension

In contrast to normotensive gravidas who have diminished peripheral vascular resistance, most women destined to develop pregnancy-induced hypertension become abnormally sensitive to pressor substances such as angiotensin II after the twenty-second week of gestation, a full 10 to 18 weeks before high blood pressure develops (Fig. 13-2) [4]. This increase in vascular responsiveness is likewise noted (usually by week 30) in chronically hypertensive women who subsequently manifest superimposed preeclampsia at weeks 36 to 40 [18].

Vasodilatation and enhancement of uteroplacental flow during normal pregnancy may be regulated by the action of prostaglandins (PG). Increasing evidence suggests that derangements of prostaglandin synthesis, catabolism or action at the arteriolar level, may contribute to the vasospastic tendency of preeclampsia [19]. Vasodilatory prostaglandins, PGE_1 and particularly PGI_2 (prostacyclin), appear to mediate the increments of uterine blood flow in pregnant experimental animals and humans. In the pregnant sheep, PGI_2 is an especially potent vasodilator of the uterine vasculature and produces dose-related increases in uterine blood flow in late-term ewes. In humans, Everett et al. observed that vascular responsiveness to angiotensin II was greater when prostaglandins were inhibited by the administration of indomethacin or aspirin during pregnancy [20]. Maternal blood obtained late in pregnancy contains elevated levels of prostacyclin metabolites, but in preeclamptic pregnancies, decreased prostacyclin activity has been consistently found in maternal and fetal blood and in amniotic fluid [21–24].

Vascular constriction increases the resistance to blood flow and promotes arterial hypertension. Vasospasm damages vessels themselves by impairing the circulation of the vasa vasorum; the resulting endothelial injury probably leads to subendothelial fibrin and platelet deposition, which, together with vasospasm, promotes tissue hypoxia, hemorrhage, necrosis, and compromised perfusion to vital organs, particularly kidney, brain, and placenta.

Sodium Retention and Volume Abnormalities

Patients in whom preeclampsia develops have a normal expansion of blood volume until 25 to 28 weeks. By the middle of the third trimester, prior to becoming hypertensive, two-thirds of these gravidas have plasma volumes lower than expected for that stage of pregnancy [25]. This plasma volume contraction is closely correlated with the severity of hypertension and the degree of intrauterine growth retardation. The vasoconstriction of pregnancy-induced hypertension is associated with an increased vascular permeability and a shift of fluid from the intravascular to the

Fig. 13-2. Comparison of mean angiotensin II doses (ng/kg/min) required to evoke a pressor response in 120 primigravidas who remained normotensive and 72 primigravidas who ultimately had pregnancy-induced hypertension. The nonpregnant mean is shown as a broken line. The difference between the two groups became significant after week 23 (p < 0.01). (From Gant et al. [4]. Reproduced from The Journal of Clinical Investigation, 1973; 52:2682–9, *by copyright permission of* The American Society for Clinical Investigation.*)*

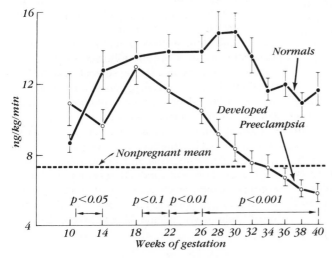

extravascular space. The result is an average decrease of plasma volume of approximately 10% (300–400 mL) in mild preeclampsia. In severe disease, total blood volume may be only 60 to 70% of normal, making the woman with severe preeclampsia or eclampsia unduly sensitive to blood loss at delivery. The intravascular compartment is contracted but not underfilled because the capacity of the vascular bed is diminished. As a result, these patients are also sensitive to vigorous fluid administration.

Renal Abnormalities

Vasospasm of afferent and efferent arterioles and glomerular lesions of endothelial swelling, mesangial cytoplasmic proliferation, and fibrin deposition result in enlargement of the capillary tuft and narrowing of the vessel lumen leading to ischemia [26]. Decreased renal blood flow and glomerular filtration rate and increased glomerular capillary membrane permeability explain the renal insufficiency and proteinuria.

Coagulation Abnormalities

The severe vasospasm accompanying preeclampsia is thought to injure vascular endothelium, causing exposure of subendothelial collagen and subsequent platelet adherence and fibrin strand deposition within small vessels. In this manner thrombocytopenia and, less commonly, microangiopathic hemolysis may develop. Although intravascular fibrin deposition probably occurs, the plasma fibrinogen level and the titer of fibrin degradation products are normal in almost all cases of pregnancy-induced hypertension; clinical evidence of disseminated intravascular coagulation (DIC) is a rare complication of severe preeclampsia or eclampsia (0–3%) [27].

The arterial hypertension, vasospasm, and secondary tissue hypoxia associated with preeclampsia may cause hemorrhage, necrosis, and ischemic injury in the placenta or other maternal organs. Potential consequences to mother and fetus are reviewed in the following sections (Table 13-3).

EFFECTS OF PREGNANCY-INDUCED HYPERTENSION ON THE MOTHER

Hypertensive disease is one of the four major causes of maternal death in the United States. Nearly all of this mortality is associated with eclampsia and with preeclampsia superimposed on chronic hypertensive vascular disease. The incidence of eclampsia is probably one in every 1,000 to 1,500 deliveries; the maternal death rate associated with eclampsia in the United States still approaches 5%.

Table 13-3. Maternal consequences of severe preeclampsia

A. CNS complications
  1. Eclampsia
      Seizures
      Encephalopathy and coma
      Psychosis, self-limited
  2. Cerebral hemorrhage
B. Cardiopulmonary complications
  1. Pulmonary edema
      Usually noncardiogenic
      Left ventricular failure possible
      Potential for superimposed bacterial or
          aspiration pneumonia
  2. Pleural, pericardial effusions; ascites
  3. Cardiovascular collapse (shock)
      Rare complication within first 24 hours post
          partum
      Possible contributing role of diuretic therapy
          and unappreciated degree of hemorrhage,
          fluid loss
C. Renal disease (major manifestations)
  1. Acute renal failure
  2. Nephrotic syndrome
D. Abruptio placentae
E. Hematologic complications
  1. Thrombocytopenia
  2. Microangiopathic hemolysis
  3. DIC
F. Liver disease
  1. Mild functional abnormalities
  2. Subcapsular hemorrhage with pain (rare hepatic
      rupture)
G. Retinal detachment

In 50 to 60% of women who die of eclampsia, petechiae or multiple focal hemorrhages can be found in the cerebral cortex, white matter, and midbrain. Larger hemorrhages, which may rupture into the subarachnoid space, are found in the white matter, basal ganglia, and pons [7]. Fortunately, patients who recover from eclampsia rarely have residual neurologic impairment. Repeated eclamptic seizures may be followed by encephalopathy or frank coma lasting several days. In 5%, a self-limited psychosis may persist for one to two weeks. Bacterial or aspiration pneumonitis may complicate the course of the disease.

Cardiac failure arises as a consequence of markedly increased peripheral resistance (increased afterload). Focal necrosis and hemorrhage within the myocardium and conduction system, as well as coronary arterial spasm, may further contribute to left ventricular dysfunction [7,28]. A tendency toward pulmonary edema is aggravated by the pathologic expansion of the extracellular fluid volume and the increase of capillary permeability associated with preeclampsia. Massive sodium retention, cardiac dysfunction, renal insufficiency, and possible nephrotic syndrome may lead to anasarca, with pleural and pericardial effusions and ascites.

Preeclampsia-induced glomerular disease is the most common cause of nephrotic syndrome in pregnancy. Although glomerular filtration rate (GFR) decreases approximately 25% in mild preeclampsia, this value may remain above pregravid levels and the decrement in renal function may not be appreciated. A significant decrease in the GFR is accompanied by rising creatinine, oliguria, and often rapidly worsening hypertension and edema (i.e., acute renal failure). Rarely, prolonged vasospasm and ischemia produce extensive thrombosis of intralobular arteries and infarction resulting in bilateral renal cortical necrosis.

Abruptio placentae occurs in 10 to 12% of women with early-onset preeclampsia, presumably because of occlusive disease of placental vessels and thrombosis and necrosis of the decidua. Abruption may cause life-threatening uterine hemorrhage and may release thromboplastic substances into the maternal circulation resulting in spontaneous hemorrhage or DIC. In the absence of abruptio placentae (or fetal death in utero) overt DIC is rare in preeclampsia or eclampsia [29,30].

Severe preeclampsia may involve the liver, wherein hemorrhagic and necrotic lesions contribute to mild disturbance of liver function, subcapsular hemorrhage, and, rarely, rupture of the hepatic capsule with hemorrhage into the peritoneal cavity.

Visual symptoms associated with severe preeclampsia (i.e., blurring or scotomata) are secondary to retinal ischemia and edema and are associated with ophthalmoscopic findings of irregular arteriolar spasm and a diffuse retinal sheen. Retinal detachment may result in patients with severe preeclampsia or eclampsia. Visual impairment is usually reversible, and normal vision returns within three weeks.

EFFECTS OF PREGNANCY-INDUCED HYPERTENSION ON THE FETUS

Hypertension complicating pregnancy is a major cause of preterm birth and perinatal death. When mild essential hypertension in the absence of proteinuria complicates pregnancy, fetal outcome is virtually normal. However, when preeclampsia is superimposed on chronic hypertension or when severe preeclampsia or eclampsia occurs, intra-uterine growth is often retarded and the perinatal mortality increases to 10 to 30%.

The grave threat that pregnancy-induced hypertension poses to fetal well-being is accounted for by a decrease in maternal uterine blood flow and placental reserve. Uteroplacental blood flow may be reduced by 40 to 60% in preeclamptic women as compared to normotensive gravidas [8,31]. Prospective studies by Gant et al. of adolescent primigravidas and multigravidas with chronic hypertension showed that uteroplacental perfusion began to decrease three to four weeks before the development or acceleration of hypertension [32]. These data suggest that preeclampsia is a chronic disease in pregnancy, a concept further supported by the findings of enhanced vascular responsiveness to angiotensin II, increased platelet turnover, subnormal plasma volume, subnormal estriol excretion, and intrauterine growth retardation, which can all occur in preeclamptic pregnancies *prior to the recognition of hypertension or proteinuria.*

Morphologic studies have shown occlusive lesions in decidual spiral arterioles in preeclampsia (mean diameter of 200 μm versus 500 μm in normal pregnancy) [33]. The placental vessels show changes of acute arteriosclerosis with atheroma-like lesions in the decidual and myometrial segments. Similar changes are noted in chronically hypertensive women, but, when preeclampsia supervenes, placental vascular disease is exaggerated so that complete destruction of spiral arteries and thrombosis of the decidua may occur. Not surprisingly, preeclamptic pregnancies that result in fetal demise are associated with a 42% incidence of large placental infarcts and consistent retardation of fetal growth. Uteroplacental perfusion is further impaired by the increase in myometrial tone and contractility associated with preeclampsia. Even moderate contraction patterns may be sufficient to evoke fetal distress.

Fetal growth averages approximately 4% less per week in infants born to preeclamptic mothers, the average infant weight being approximately 250 g lighter than those born to healthy mothers. Accordingly, the time of onset of preeclampsia is crucial to the outcome of the newborn. Fetal growth retardation is common, and perinatal mortality exceeds 10% if the disease manifests itself before the thirty-seventh gestational week. Spontaneous or induced preterm delivery invites the neonatal problems of respiratory distress, apnea, hypoglycemia, hypocalcemia, jaundice, sepsis, cerebral hemorrhage, and circulatory instability. When the onset of preeclampsia begins after 37 weeks of gestation, there is no apparent growth retardation and perinatal mortality is less than 1%.

CLINICAL EVALUATION AND MANAGEMENT

The management of pregnancy complicated by preeclampsia or chronic hypertension is based largely on clinical assessment. The nature and severity of the hypertensive process and the maturity and well-being of the fetus are the key issues. The rationale and practical aspects of evaluation and management can be divided into four clinical settings: chronic hypertension, preeclampsia (or severe hypertension) remote from term, preeclampsia near term, and eclampsia. This method of organizing the material is modeled after the excellent monograph by Gant and Worley [8].

Chronic Hypertension

Principles
Eighty-five percent of women entering pregnancy with hypertension will do well. Patients with mild hypertension tolerate pregnancy well unless preeclampsia supervenes. Women with moderate to severe hypertension, particularly when complicated by hypertensive heart disease or nephrosclerosis (creatinine clearance < 50 mL/minute) have a poor prognosis. Abortion may be considered in these patients.

High blood pressure in pregnancy has the same maternal risks as in the nonpregnant subject (i.e., stroke, cardiac failure, and renal failure) [34]. In the absence of severe hypertension, antihypertensive drug therapy is unlikely to alter the outlook for a young hypertensive woman during the relatively brief 40-week gestational period and provides only modest benefit for those with diastolic blood pressure less than 100 mm Hg. Although moderate hypertension in pregnancy may predispose to aortic dissection, bleeding from cerebral aneurysms, or myocardial infarction, the extreme rarity of these complications in pregnancy does not, alone, justify the treatment of all these patients. The major risk for the mother and fetus is superimposed preeclampsia [35].

Arias and Zamora demonstrated that treatment of moderate hypertension (DBP ≥ 95 mm Hg) minimized exacerbations of hypertension late in gestation (13 of 29 untreated gravidas had pregnancy-aggravated hypertension as against 4 of 29 treated) [36]. The effect of superimposed preeclampsia could not be derived from this study; all mothers did well. All but one of the 17 patients in whom pregnancy-aggravated hypertension developed acquired this complication after the thirty-seventh week of gestation. This study concurs with findings by Redman et al. suggesting that hypotensive therapy in gravidas with mild chronic hypertension is effective in reducing the incidence of severe hypertension late in gestation [37]. In a more recent study, Sibai et al. analyzed 211 pregnancies complicated by mild chronic hypertension. The majority (83%) were not taking antihypertensive drugs at the time of the first prenatal visit, and the remainder had their antihypertensive medications discontinued. The incidence of superimposed preeclampsia (10%) and of exacerbation of hypertension (13%) was similar to that reported in other series [36,37]. Furthermore, the perinatal mortality for the untreated chronic hypertensives who did not become preeclamptic was similar to that of the general obstetric population [39].

The effect of lowering maternal blood pressure on fetal health remains controversial, in part, because of inadequate clinical studies and inadequate understanding of the human placental circulation. The weight of evidence, based on animal and human studies, suggests that uteroplacental perfusion in normal pregnancy varies as a function of the maternal perfusion pressure. Transient reductions of placental blood flow, if marked, could jeopardize the fetus, particularly if uterine flow is already subnormal in hypertensive pregnant women. Gant and others have demonstrated decreases of 20 to 50% in uteroplacental blood flow when diuretics, vasodilators, or other antihypertensive drugs are instituted during pregnancy [8]. In this regard, the study of Welt et al. suggested that antihypertensive therapy could reduce the incidence of preeclampsia among women with chronic hypertension, but such therapy was associated with a higher incidence of small-for-gestational-age infants [38].

Other studies suggest that long-term hypotensive treatment does not retard fetal growth in spite of blood pressure reduction. Arias and Zamora examined fetal outcome in women receiving antihypertensive drugs compared with women who remained untreated for moderate hypertension in pregnancy. No difference was found in birth weights, Apgar scores, or numbers of small-for-gestational-age infants [36]. British clinicians showed that treatment of women with long-standing hypertension with methyldopa was associated with an improved survival rate for the fetus [37].

Currently, the value of treating DBP ≥ 100 mm Hg in chronically hypertensive pregnant women remains uncertain; more studies are necessary. There is no evidence that diuretics alone can prevent the superimposition of preeclampsia in these patients [2]. Therefore, diuretic agents should not

Table 13-4. Evaluation of pregnant hypertensive patients

Chronic hypertension	Preeclampsia or severe hypertension (remote from term)	Preeclampsia/eclampsia (mature fetus)
Thorough initial H & P, empha-sizing retinal, cardiovascular, and neurologic exams	Thorough initial H & P looking for signs and symptoms of severe preeclampsia (Table 13-2)	MILD PREECLAMPSIA Thorough initial H & P looking for signs and symptoms of severe preeclampsia (Table 13-2)
Standardized method of BP determination	Initial lab evaluation CBC Urinalysis Serum creatinine, uric acid 24-hr urine protein, creatinine clearance, meta-nephrine	Assess fetal maturity Fetal monitoring for signs of distress
Initial lab evaluation CBC Urinalysis Urine culture Electrolytes 1-hr 50 g glucose screen Serum creatinine	Consider molar pregnancy if onset prior to wk 24	Initial lab evaluation CBC, platelet count, urinalysis, serum creatinine, uric acid Serial maternal monitoring BP, weight, sensorium, fundoscopy, chest exam, reflexes, edema
Additional testing in those with severe hypertension, end-organ changes, or abnormal initial tests 24-hr urine for protein, creatinine clearance, and metanephrine Electrocardiogram	Assess fetal maturity via dates, uterine size, sonogram Serial fetal monitoring (refer to Chap. 5)	Intake and output Urine protein CBC, platelet count, uric acid SEVERE PREECLAMPSIA/ECLAMPSIA
Baseline sonogram of fetus by week 20	Serial maternal monitoring Daily review of symptoms BP Weight Fundoscopy Chest exam Reflexes Pelvic exam Urine protein 3 times/week CBC once weekly 24-hr urine protein and creati-nine clearance 1–2 times/wk	Intensive nursing care Initial lab evaluation Platelet count, blood smear, DIC screen, liver function tests, CBC, urinalysis, chest roentgenogram, electrocardiogram
Serial maternal monitoring Symptoms BP Weight Edema Urine protein		Monitor $MgSO_4$ therapy: respi-rations, reflexes, urine output, seizures. Consider checking serum Mg^{++} levels Consider Swan-Ganz catheter to monitor pulmonary capillary wedge pressure
Hospitalize if signs of preeclampsia occur		Workup seizures associated with focal signs, fever, stiff neck (i.e., electrolytes, glucose, CT scan, LP)

be started at any time during pregnancy for the purpose of blood pressure control.

Evaluation

Chronically hypertensive women should have careful assessment of end-organ changes, with history focused on past cardiovascular events and the course of prior pregnancies. Examination is oriented to the retinal vessels (retinopathy) and the cardiovascular and nervous systems. The arterial blood pressure should be measured using the same arm and appropriately sized cuff, with the pa-tient in a sitting position. If not established earlier, the possibility of secondary causes of hypertension should be evaluated. A minimum, cost-effective evaluation of hypertensive patients is summarized in Table 13-4.

The presence of severe hypertension, end-organ changes on exam, or abnormalities of basic laboratory tests should warrant determination of 24-hour urine protein excretion and creatinine clearance, baseline electrocardiogram, and other individualized studies. Urine collection for meta-nephrines to diagnose pheochromocytoma has been recommended for severe hypertensives (see Chap. 10).

Ultrasonography should be performed during the first half of all pregnancies complicated by essential hypertension for baseline fetal measurements, which can be used to determine possible fetal growth retardation later in pregnancy (see Chap. 5).

During the last half of pregnancy, meticulous monitoring of weight, edema, urine protein, blood pressure, and fetal well-being should be carried out. In the chronically hypertensive patient, blood pressure typically rises toward baseline during the last trimester. Distinguishing this common and innocent trend from the rising blood pressure associated with superimposed preeclampsia may be difficult. Serial uric acid determinations, supine pressor response ("roll over") testing, or the blood pressure response to angiotensin II infusion do not have high enough predictive values or practical utility to advocate their routine use in pregnant patients with hypertension. When signs of definite superimposed preeclampsia are recognized, hospitalization is indicated.

Management

Women of childbearing age being treated for essential hypertension should be counseled prior to conception. If no reliable contraception is being employed or if pregnancy is planned in the near future, the antihypertensive drug regimen should be reviewed. It would seem wise to substitute antihypertensives with established safety records (e.g., methyldopa) for agents such as reserpine, clonidine, prazosin, or the newly marketed beta-adrenergic blockers. Women with mild or borderline hypertension who have been controlled by nonpharmacologic methods or have not been treated should be carefully observed. In general, women whose hypertension is effectively controlled by drugs prior to conception should continue on antihypertensive medication (Table 13-5).

Once pregnancy is diagnosed, a regular program of rest should be prescribed. During one- or two-hour-long periods of rest each day the woman should lie on her left side to minimize possible compromise of the uteroplacental circulation (in later pregnancy, uteroplacental blood flow is diminished by 20 to 30% in supine position versus left lateral recumbent). Dietary management is similar to that of all pregnant women; 1,500 to 2,500 calories per day depending on height and weight; protein intake at 1.3 to 2.0 g/kg/day and moderate intake of sodium (women should be ad-

Table 13-5. Management of women with chronic hypertension during pregnancy

Optimal nutrition is necessary, with customary sodium intake.

Prescribe rest—left lateral decubitus position.

Discourage cigarette smoking and heavy alcohol intake.

Continue ongoing antihypertensive drug regimen, including diuretic.

Propranolol or metoprolol can be continued (see text p. 170).

Methyldopa or hydralazine should be substituted for other second-step drugs.

Maintain average DBP less than 95 mm Hg during pregnancy; if treatment has begun, goal should be DBP ≤ 90 mm Hg.

vised to salt their food according to taste). Severe sodium restriction of less than 2 g per day should never be imposed as the expansion of maternal plasma volume is important for a successful gestation. The hypertensive gravida should abstain from cigarette smoking or heavy alcohol ingestion as such practice may contribute to fetal growth retardation. In addition, nonsteroidal antiinflammatory drugs should be avoided, if possible, in the interest of maintaining normal prostaglandin homeostasis.

If a patient is taking a thiazide diuretic at the time she becomes pregnant, it is recommended that she continue to take the drug. Multidrug regimens may be continued with the consideration noted above for antihypertensive drugs having had limited trials in pregnancy. Propranolol (or other beta-blocker) may be continued if it has effectively controlled BP prior to pregnancy, particularly if the woman has severe hypertension, end-organ complications, renal disease, or other compelling indications for beta blockade (i.e., arrhythmias, idiopathic hypertrophic subaortic stenosis or incapacitating migraine).

When a woman treated with a diuretic alone manifests an average DBP ≥ 95 mm Hg during pregnancy, additional drug therapy should be considered. The author recommends beginning methyldopa at 250 mg orally twice daily, increasing the dose (and frequency of administration to t.i.d.) on a weekly basis, if necessary. Blood pressure response and side effects from the drug determine the dosage. Maximum dosage is 2 g per day. Oral hydralazine is a safe and effective alternative (Table 13-6). If blood pressure control is still inadequate, methyldopa and hydralazine should be combined.

Average diastolic pressures exceeding 100 mm Hg, in spite of excellent drug compliance, are uncommon during the first half of pregnancy and warrant hospitalization. If blood pressures do not improve after hospitalization, the possibility of a secondary etiology for the hypertension should be reconsidered. Substitution of propranolol (or metoprolol) for methyldopa or, rarely, the addition of an oral diuretic might be justified. Substitution or addition of other sympathetic depressant drugs such as clonidine, prazosin, or reserpine is not likely to be effective for women with resistant hypertension and has had limited trials (prazosin, clonidine) or caused troublesome problems (reserpine) during pregnancy. Patients with refractory hypertension should be counseled about the high risk of continuing pregnancy.

Preeclampsia (or Severe Hypertension) Remote from Term

Principles

When signs of preeclampsia appear before the thirty-seventh gestational week, fetal survival becomes a major concern. Early-onset preeclampsia often requires premature delivery and is associated with a high incidence of fetal growth retardation and perinatal death. Evidence of fetal distress or severe growth retardation, recurrence or worsening of hypertension or proteinuria, declining creatinine clearance, or other signs and symptoms of severe preeclampsia may necessitate delivery. The acute onset of preeclampsia will not be accompanied by the same degree of intrauterine growth retardation as chronic hypertension. It should be noted that, in the presence of either of these conditions, there may be an earlier appearance of fetal pulmonary stabilizing phospholipids to "mature" values at 32 to 33 weeks rather than at 35 weeks' gestation (see Chap. 5).

Evaluation

Development of hypertension and proteinuria before the 24th week of pregnancy may be seen with molar pregnancy or fetal hydrops.

When hypertension complicates pregnancy before the thirty-fourth week, hospitalization and rest may allow delivery to be deferred until the fetus is mature.

During the hospitalization, superimposed or worsening preeclampsia must be detected early and the fetal status monitored. The gestational age, by dates, is reassessed and a sonogram is obtained.

Subsequent sonograms should be performed every two to three weeks. If gestational dates are uncertain in a patient with persistent hypertension, in spite of hospitalization and rest, amniocentesis should be performed to measure phospholipids. The health of the fetoplacental unit may be further assessed with nonstress tests (NSTs) or contraction stress tests (CSTs), as discussed in Chapter 5. If both infant and mother remain stable and fetal lung maturation is *not* present, delivery may be postponed. During this critical period of fetal observation, maternal assessment should focus on signs and symptoms of advancing preeclampsia, with serial exams and laboratory testing performed according to the guidelines in Table 13-4.

Management

Hospitalization is advocated for women with mild preeclampsia or resistant essential hypertension who are remote from term. Often, a spontaneous diuresis, decrease in weight, and improvement in blood pressure are noted in the first 24 hours of hospitalization. Gilstrap, Cunningham, and Whalley noted that up to 85% of nulliparous women who became hypertensive in the latter half of pregnancy demonstrated a lowering of blood pressure to less than 140/90 mm Hg within five days of hospitalization. In their experience, 9% of preeclamptic women showed only modest BP reductions after admission, but in the absence of other signs and symptoms of severe preeclampsia and with evidence of favorable fetal growth, pregnancy could continue. In 6% the disease either remained severe or worsened, and delivery was necessary [40].

Antihypertensive therapy of women remote from term was described previously. When pregnancy-induced hypertension is being treated with oral medications, the nocturnal worsening of hypertension should be anticipated by a drug schedule that provides the largest doses at night [35].

The high perinatal mortality arising from preeclampsia remote from term has stimulated several experimental forms of treatment. In three reported cases prostacyclin was administered by intravenous infusion and appeared to ameliorate maternal hypertension [19,24]. However, in two cases intrauterine death occurred without warning after 4 to 12 days of infusion. In the third instance cesarean delivery had to be performed after three days of therapy because of fetal distress.

A preliminary experience with plasma exchange therapy in severe preeclampsia cited improvement in renal function and BP control of sufficient

Table 13-6. Selected aspects of antihypertensive drugs used in pregnancy

Drug	Mechanism of action	Dosage	General indications

Diuretics
  Thiazides and
    related diuretics
	Plasma volume contraction;
	  decrease in total peripheral
	  resistance
		50–100 mg
		(equivalent of
		hydrochlorothiazide)
			Continuation of prepregnancy
			  antihypertensive regimen

Potassium-sparing
  diuretics
  Amiloride
  Spironolactone
  Triamterene			

Furosemide	Potent loop diuretic
	Acute sodium, water diuresis—
	  plasma volume contraction
		20–40 mg as initial
		  intravenous dose
		20–80 mg b.i.d. or
		  greater orally
			Parenteral diuretic for severe
			  pulmonary edema
			Rarely as ongoing oral diuretic
			  in severe renal insufficiency

Beta-adrenergic
  blocking agents
  Propranolol
  Metoprolol
  Nadolol
  Timolol
  Atenolol
  Pindolol
	Mechanism of sustained hypo-
	  tensive effect uncertain
	Initial reduction of cardiac
	  output and peripheral vascular
	  resistance
		Propranolol,
		  20–240 mg b.i.d.
		Metoprolol,
		  25–300 mg b.i.d.
		
		Limited use of beta-blockers other
		than propranolol and metoprolol
			Continuation of prepregnancy
			  antihypertensive regimen; BP
			  control during pregnancy

Clonidine	↓ CNS sympathetic outflow ↓ total peripheral resistance Occasional ↓ c.o. and heart rate		

Methyldopa	Same as clonidine	250 mg–1000 mg p.o.
		  b.i.d.–t.i.d.
			Drug of choice for longer-term
			  BP control
			Onset of action too slow for urgent
			  parenteral use

Prazosin			
Reserpine			

Diazoxide	Direct relaxation of
	  arteriolar smooth
	  muscle
		Initial 30–60 mg IV bolus;
		  wait 10–15 min between
		  successive boluses
			Emergency treatment of life-
			  threatening hypertension

Effects on fetus or neonate	Excretion into breast milk	Common maternal side/adverse effects	Comments
Rare association with neonatal thrombocytopenia, hypovolemia, electrolyte depletion Association with fetal growth retardation when started in late pregnancy	Yes Pharmacologically insignificant amounts No adverse effects reported in human infants Manufacturers recommend avoiding use during nursing	Hypokalemia, hyperuricemia, ↓ glucose tolerance, hypovolemia, thrombocytopenia, photosensitivity, pancreatitis, gastric intolerance	Do not start during pregnancy
Limited use in pregnancy			Do not start during pregnancy; discontinue if part of a prepregnancy regimen
Teratogenic and embryotoxic potential in rabbits Rare hyponatremia in newborn	Yes Effects unknown	Hypokalemia Metabolic alkalosis Hypovolemia Glucose intolerance Ototoxicity in patients with impaired renal function	Not to be used for BP control or to reverse oliguria 2′ preeclampsia For severe pulmonary edema: Swan-Ganz catheterization may be indicated
Retrospective studies and anecdotes suggest: intrauterine growth retardation, neonatal bradycardia and hypoglycemia Prospective studies suggest: safe for fetus, few neonatal problems	Trace—slight amounts of propranolol No known harmful effects	Contraindications: asthma, CHF, insulin-dependent diabetes mellitus (relative) CNS: listlessness, fatigue, depression, insomnia Diarrhea Cold extremities	Use propranolol or metoprolol; substitute for other beta-blockers Methyldopa or hydralazine still favored as drugs to be started during pregnancy See text for further discussion (pp. 179)
Limited use in pregnancy No untoward effects known to date	No information	Taper off drug over 5–7 days to prevent withdrawal syndrome and/or rebound ↑ BP	Would substitute methyldopa, etc., when pregnancy planned or first diagnosed
Overall, no adverse effects May decrease fetal wastage, possibly via effect on myometrial tone	Yes No apparent adverse effects	Drowsiness, fatigue, dry mouth, + Coombs test (10% after 6 months) Potential difficulty cross-matching blood Rare hemolytic anemia Rare hepatitis (↑ AST 10%) Rebound hypertension after sudden withdrawal (rare)	See text, pp. 179
Extremely limited use in pregnancy			Avoid Substitute when conception is planned or when pregnancy first diagnosed
Possibly impaired implantation in rabbits; abortions and teratogenicity in rats at high doses Neonatal syndrome of lethargy, bradycardia, hypothermia, nasal congestion; can cause respiratory difficulties			Avoid Substitute when conception is planned or when pregnancy first diagnosed
Excessive abrupt fall in blood pressure could jeopardize fetus; one report of severe persistent postnatal hyperglycemia in a premature infant exposed in utero; four infants reported with alopecia	Unknown	Abrupt hypotensive response → organ ischemia Reflex tachycardia Sodium retention Hyperglycemia	Nitroprusside favored for Rx of hypertensive crises; diazoxide is, however, more convenient and more rapidly initiated

Table 13-6 (Continued)

Drug	Mechanism of action	Dosage	General indications
Hydralazine	Direct relaxation of arteriolar smooth muscle	Initial 5 mg IV; effect begins within 15 min; if no effect, repeat—10 mg IV bolus; once BP lowered, maintenance infusion at 5 mg/hr to maintain DBP 90—100 mm Hg; effect of initial bolus may last 3–4 hr Oral: 10–25 mg b.i.d.–t.i.d. to maximum 200 mg/day	Drug of choice as parenteral treatment of severe hypertension prior to delivery Alternative to methyldopa as oral antihypertensive for long-term use in pregnancy
Minoxidil			
Nitroprusside	Arteriolar and venous smooth muscle relaxation (resistance and capacitance vessels)	Continuous IV infusion, started at 0.1 µg/kg/min to 10 µg/kg/min or higher Nearly immediate onset of action	Emergency treatment of life-threatening hypertension and complications such as cerebral hemorrhage, pulmonary edema
Captopril			

degree and duration to allow delivery of two healthy infants [41]. The use of plasma volume expansion has been advocated by Gallery et al., who used rapid single infusion of 500 mL of a plasma protein solution in 14 women with pregnancy-induced hypertension who had failed to respond to 48 hours of bed rest in the hospital [42]. Twelve of these patients (86%) showed a significant rise of plasma volume and a fall in blood pressure, which persisted for at least 48 hours. Nonetheless, when hypertension complicating pregnancy becomes severe or when fetal jeopardy complicates the picture, delivery is indicated, almost regardless of the stage of gestation.

Preeclampsia (Mature Fetus)
Principles
Preeclampsia is not preventable at the present time. The major threat posed by preeclampsia near term is to the mother, as the incidence of eclampsia is 3 to 7%. Careful management of preeclampsia after 37 weeks' gestation results in perinatal mortality as low as 0.6%. This is accounted for by a supernormal uteroplacental blood flow, which occurs during much of pregnancy in women destined to have pregnancy-induced hypertension [32]. In these cases, uteroplacental perfusion usually decreases to normal and then to subnormal levels two to four weeks before hypertension ap-

pears. Since most hypertension develops later in gestation, the period of subnormal perfusion is probably too short to reverse the earlier growth-enhancing effects of high blood flow.

Evaluation
If the fetus is judged to be mature, the patient is admitted and delivery effected. If signs or symptoms of severe preeclampsia are present (Table 13-2), the mother should be stabilized prior to proceeding with delivery.

During delivery and the immediate postpartum period, blood loss is often increased. Any degree of hemorrhage is less well tolerated because of the volume-contracted state. Accordingly, an abrupt fall in blood pressure or hematocrit soon after delivery most often indicates serious hypovolemia rather than immediate relief of the vasospasm or hemoconcentration associated with preeclampsia. In the event that epidural or spinal anesthesia is employed, the resultant sympathetic blockade may lead to peripheral pooling of blood and an additional tendency to lowered blood pressure.

Management [8,9]
Upon admission, the rate of intravenous fluid administration is adjusted according to urine output. A central line capable of measuring central venous pressure is advised for patients with severe dis-

Effects on fetus or neonate	Excretion into breast milk	Common maternal side/adverse effects	Comments
High doses are teratogenic in mice, possibly rabbits No definite adverse effects in humans	No information Probably safe to nurse	Reflex tachycardia, headache, nausea, vomiting, flushing, rash Chronic: SLE-like syndrome, usually > 200 mg/day	See text, pp. 179–180
Limited use in pregnancy			Avoid
Potential fetal cyanide toxicity with prolonged antepartum infusion Infusion should be limited to 30–60 min prior to delivery	Unknown	Possible headache, nausea, vomiting, palpitations, restlessness, sweating secondary to rapid ↓ BP Thiocyanate toxicity: lethargy, muscle spasms, disorientation, psychosis; blood cyanide may accumulate in patients with hepatic disease Check thiocyanate level if infusion continues beyond 72 hr	Most rational pharmacologic approach to cardiogenic pulmonary edema; Swan-Ganz catheter indicated; ICU monitoring
Limited use in pregnancy Adverse effect on viability of fetal lamb; single report of congenital malformation in human case			Avoid

ease. Jugular venous pressure should be maintained at 8 to 10 cm H_2O.

Prevention of convulsions is achieved with parenteral magnesium sulfate. Magnesium sulfate is effective, yet not overly sedative to the mother, and can be administered so as not to depress the already compromised fetus. Magnesium sulfate may be given slowly intravenously (2–4 g of a 10 or 20% solution initially), followed by 0.5 to 2.0 g per hour by continuous IV infusion. The infusion rate is adjusted according to neurologic irritability, titrating to normoreflexia. If signs of magnesium toxicity (i.e., respiratory depression—less than 14 respirations per minute) or the disappearance of peripheral reflexes (e.g., patellar, biceps) is noted or if the urinary volume decreases (<25–30 mL/hour), the infusion rate should be reduced or temporarily discontinued. Patients with well-preserved renal function may require infusions of 1.5 to 3.0 g/hr in order to provide appropriate magnesium concentrations and prevent seizures [43].

Serum magnesium levels should be used to guide therapy. The therapeutic range, described by Pritchard, is 4.8 to 8.4 mEq/L. An initial 4-g intravenous dose (10–20% solution) given over four minutes raises the plasma concentration to approximately 7 to 9 mEq/L. Maintenance infusion stabilizes the plasma magnesium level at 4 to 7 mEq/L. The first warning of impending toxicity in the mother is loss of peripheral reflexes at plasma concentrations between 7 and 10 mEq/L. If the loss of peripheral reflexes is ignored and the plasma concentration increases much beyond 10 mEq/L, impairment of the muscles of respiration can cause dangerous hypoxia. Calcium gluconate, 10 mL of a 10% solution injected intravenously over three minutes, is an effective antidote for hypermagnesemia-induced respiratory depression. Serum magnesium concentrations of approximately 30 mEq/L may cause cardiac arrest.

Although the intravenous route is preferred for administration of magnesium sulfate, it requires the constant attendance of a nurse or physician. In the absence of constant observation, 5 g of magnesium sulfate (10 mL of a 50% solution) may be given deeply in the upper outer quadrant of each buttock. A long needle is used. A small volume of local anesthetic may be drawn into each syringe to reduce the discomfort to the patient. Subsequently, 10 mL of a 50% solution (5 g) may be administered at three- to four-hour intervals if peripheral reflexes are present and the patient is not manifesting respiratory depression or oliguria. If six or more hours have elapsed between doses, the full 10-g dose may be used if required.

Intramuscular administration of magnesium sulfate reduces the time required for monitoring by personnel. However, because of the dynamic, often precipitous changes that can occur, consideration should be given to transport of these seriously ill patients unless adequate surveillance can be provided. If close monitoring of the pregnant woman and the infant is carried out, the risk of toxicity from intramuscular administration of magnesium sulfate is low. Sciatic nerve damage can occur, and pain at the injection sites is common [8].

The initial intramuscular loading dose (10 g) will usually result in plasma levels of 3.5 to 6.0 mEq/L. When 5-g doses are used at four-hour intervals, plasma levels can be maintained in the low therapeutic level. Once begun, magnesium sulfate will usually need to be maintained for at least 24 hours [8].

Contrary to the view of many clinicians, the use of magnesium sulfate to prevent convulsions does not promote significant BP reduction. Instead, hydralazine is used to treat severe maternal hypertension. Hydralazine should be given if blood pressure is above 160 mm Hg systolic or greater than 110 mm Hg diastolic. An initial intravenous dose of 5 mg may reduce DBP to the range of 90 to 100 mm Hg. If the desired BP level is not reached within 15 minutes of injection, a repeat dose of 10 mg is given and blood pressure is monitored at five-minute intervals. Usually, a cumulative dose of 5 to 50 mg will stabilize the blood pressure. Thereafter, a constant infusion of 5 mg per hour (40 mg hydralazine diluted to 50 mL infused via constant infusion pump at 6 mL/hour) is titrated to maintain DBP in the 90 to 100 mm Hg range. Side effects may accompany continuous intravenous infusion. Because these can include headache, vomiting, shakiness, and even hyperreflexia, they can mimic impending eclampsia. Alternatively, repeated bolus injections of hydralazine for DBP above 110 mm Hg is an acceptable method of treatment.

Severe hypertension may persist for several days after delivery. Hydralazine, 10 mg given intramuscularly every four to six hours, is usually adequate for BP control. Other complications, such as pulmonary edema or acute renal failure, may appear during this time. Their management is reviewed in the next section.

Eclampsia
Principles
Convulsions superimposed on preeclampsia threaten the life of the mother and the fetus. Even with excellent care, the maternal mortality in eclampsia may range between 0 and 5%; perinatal loss in antenatal eclampsia ranges between 12 and 25%. The occurrence of seizures signifies cerebral

vasospasm and suggests generalized vasospastic disease severe enough to provoke renal failure, cardiac decompensation, thrombocytopenia, DIC, or placental insufficiency. The hostile intrauterine environment of the fetus is further aggravated by hypoxemia and acidosis associated with maternal seizure activity. The recognition of eclampsia should initiate a stepwise plan of management: treatment of convulsions, control of blood pressure, stabilization of the mother, and delivery [8,9].

Evaluation
If eclampsia develops in spite of magnesium sulfate prophylaxis, all aspects of the drug's preparation and administration must be rechecked. A serum magnesium level is obtained in order to better estimate the patient's maintenance infusion requirement. Further evaluation proceeds as in preeclampsia (Table 13-4), except that extra attention must be devoted to other systemic complications of preeclampsia and to other causes and sequelae of the patient's seizure. The general trend of laboratory findings in preeclampsia/eclampsia is summarized in Table 13-7.

Physical examination and the chest roentgenogram serve to detect pulmonary edema. Cardiac failure may be the underlying cause of pulmonary edema, but in the majority of cases it is due to excessive intravenous fluid administration in a patient with oliguria and underlying anasarca. Since clinical examination cannot reliably distinguish cardiogenic from noncardiogenic pulmonary edema, insertion of a Swan-Ganz catheter is advised to document and monitor pulmonary capillary wedge (PCW) pressure in cases of severe pulmonary edema [44,45]. Noncardiac causes of pulmonary edema that can occur in the obstetric setting include aspiration pneumonitis, sepsis, transfusion reactions, severe allergic reactions, DIC, amniotic fluid embolism, as well as severe preeclampsia.

A differential diagnosis of major motor seizures must be considered before it is concluded that eclampsia alone is responsible. Diagnostic possibilities have been discussed on page 164. Relevant tests, such as serum electrolytes, glucose, computed tomography of the brain, and lumbar puncture, should be performed if focal neurologic findings, fever, nuchal rigidity, or other signs suggest a process other than eclampsia.

Management
General supportive measures include use of a padded tongue blade, modest physical restraint, positioning to prevent aspiration, suctioning, and

Table 13-7. Trend of laboratory findings in pregnancy-induced hypertension

Condition	Uric acid	Creatinine	Proteinuria	Liver enzymes	Platelet count
Normal	↓	0.4–0.6	0–trace	Normal	Normal
Mild preeclampsia	↓	0.4–0.6	1–2 +	Normal	Normal
Severe preeclampsia	↑	0.6–0.8	2–4 +	Normal	↓(15%)*
Eclampsia	↑↑	Above 0.8	3–4 +	Elevated	↓(15%)*

*Platelet count < 100,000.

oxygen administration. Immediate intravenous injection of 4 g of magnesium sulfate over a three- to four-minute period is followed by a constant intravenous infusion administered according to the protocol described previously.

Proper use of magnesium sulfate will usually arrest convulsions, but up to 20% of women may have additional seizures, usually within 20 minutes after the initial loading dose is given. If a seizure occurs after this interval, an additional 2 to 4 g of magnesium sulfate, depending on body size, should be given slowly, intravenously. If seizures persist, the slow intravenous injection of up to 10 to 20 mg of diazepam or 250 mg of sodium amobarbital should control the convulsive tendency. These agents have more CNS depressant effect on both mother and fetus and they further jeopardize the soon-to-be-delivered infant. Therefore, except for the rare case, magnesium sulfate remains the drug of choice.

Hypertension in the eclamptic woman is managed in the same way as in the preeclamptic patient. After severe hypertension and seizures are controlled, it is necessary to allow time before delivery for both the mother and the fetus to recover from the hypoxemia and acidosis associated with a grand mal seizure. Recovery may be expected within four to eight hours following the last seizure and will be signaled by the increased responsiveness and orientation of the mother. During this time, the patient is observed in a quiet, darkened, emotionally supportive environment. Frequent observations should be made of vital signs and urine output via Foley catheter. Periodic evaluations should include sensorium, hepatic tenderness, focal neurologic signs, and signs of aspiration pneumonitis or pulmonary edema. Fetal heart tones should be monitored closely.

The treatment of severe pulmonary edema depends on its etiology. If left ventricular failure is responsible, afterload reduction with sodium nitroprusside more effectively reverses the underlying pathophysiology as compared to furosemide diuresis and digitalization. Vasodilator therapy reduces the impedance to ventricular emptying; cardiac output and contractility increase, and pulmonary congestion is relieved [46]. If a pulmonary artery catheter is in place and hydralazine has been discontinued, nitroprusside infusion can safely be initiated at 0.1 micrograms/kg/minute with rapid upward adjustments in dosage guided by the patient's symptomatic response, cardiopulmonary findings, measurements of blood pressure (via arterial line), PCW pressure, urine output, and oxygenation as measured by arterial blood gas determinations. In response to nitroprusside, rapid and marked improvement in cardiogenic pulmonary edema has been observed, corresponding to a 10 to 20% drop in mean systemic BP [46].

The blood pressure should not be allowed to drop precipitously in the antepartum patient. In addition, the duration of nitroprusside infusion should be limited to 30 minutes prior to delivery for fear of promoting cyanide toxicity in the fetus (see Selected Antihypertensive Drugs). During the early postpartum period, continued pulmonary artery balloon catheter monitoring may guide the expected decrease in fluid requirements and help identify individuals with impending circulatory overload caused by the mobilization of fluid from the extravascular space. These patients are best managed by diuretic therapy. Expectant treatment with diuretics is appropriate for the large number of severely preeclamptic patients who do not require Swan-Ganz monitoring.

Intravenous furosemide, 20 to 40 mg, administered 24 to 36 hours post partum, can ameliorate the markedly increased circulating blood volume and potential for pulmonary edema in these patients. These patients transiently improve in response to intravenous furosemide, but oxygen, rest, and careful observation may be adequate for all but the most severely affected women.

When urinary output falls to less than 25 mL/hour, serum magnesium sulfate levels should be rechecked and the rate of infusion decreased to prevent toxicity. Oliguria in the peripartum period suggests severe vasospasm and glomerular disease; hence, optimal fluid balance is critical. Volume loading or diuretic therapy is not recommended.

Fluid replacement should be guided by careful measurement of urinary output. Most instances of severe oliguria occur in labor or during the first 24 hours post partum. Conservative management is often sufficient to guide these ill women through this self-limited phase of their disease.

SELECTED ANTIHYPERTENSIVE DRUGS

The drugs used for ambulatory blood pressure control during pregnancy and the drugs reserved for urgent control of severe hypertension are outlined in this section. Table 13-6 describes relevant clinical pharmacology. The reader is referred to more comprehensive reviews of antihypertensive drugs and is reminded of the limited experience with some of these drugs [49–52].

Diuretics
Thiazide Diuretics
These agents are the single most common blood pressure–lowering drugs taken by hypertensive women prior to pregnancy. The hypotensive effect of thiazides involves reduction of extracellular and plasma volumes concurrent with a slight reduction in cardiac output. When administered later in pregnancy, thiazide therapy may aggravate the already contracted plasma volume of patients with incipient or established preeclampsia and compromise the fetus by decreasing uterine blood flow. Gant et al. have shown a 40 to 50% decrease in placental perfusion on the seventh day of thiazide therapy in nine of ten women treated in late pregnancy [51]. Diuretics initiated between weeks 20 and 30 of pregnancy are associated with decreased maternal weight gain, decreased birth weight, and increased perinatal mortality. It is, therefore, not advisable to begin diuretics during pregnancy, although patients on thiazides months or years before conception may safely continue their use. There are no convincing data to suggest that the normal expansion of blood volume or uteroplacental blood flow will be compromised.

Furosemide
This potent diuretic may be part of a prepregnancy antihypertensive regimen in women with severe renal insufficiency or with past intolerance to thiazide diuretics (e.g., gastric intolerance, photosensitivity). Otherwise, furosemide is not routinely used for blood pressure control during pregnancy. Its use is limited to treatment of severe pulmonary edema secondary to cardiac failure or selected noncardiac causes (i.e., nephrotic syndrome, iatrogenic fluid overload, or prevention of pulmonary edema during the early postpartum period).

Sympathetic Depressant Drugs
Methyldopa
Methyldopa has proved effective when used during pregnancy. It prevents severe exacerbations of chronic hypertension in late pregnancy. In the prospective controlled trial of Redman et al. on 117 gravidas treated with methyldopa through most of their pregnancies, there were fewer pregnancy losses [37]. Methyldopa was found to have no adverse effect on growth in utero, as the birth weight and maturity of the viable infants were comparable to those in the control group. Patients who began methyldopa between weeks 16 and 20 did give birth to infants with slightly smaller head circumferences. For this reason, advise that methyldopa therapy not be started between the sixteenth and twentieth weeks of gestation. However, extensive follow-up examinations of these children at the age of 7½ years have shown no difference in mean intelligence quotients or in other areas of mental or motor development [52]. Methyldopa is the only drug for which satisfactory long-term follow-up of "treated" children is available.

Beta-Adrenergic Antagonists
Propranolol, metoprolol, nadolol, timolol, atenolol, and pindolol are all effective antihypertensive drugs taken by chronic hypertensive women prior to pregnancy. Hemodynamic response to beta-blockers has not been well studied in pregnancy, but in nonpregnant individuals these agents depress cardiac output and transiently increase peripheral vascular resistance (pindolol excepted).

Three reports describing 50 pregnancies of propranolol-treated women with moderately severe hypertension and poor obstetric histories documented an improved incidence of live births (88%) and a low incidence of neonatal problems [53]. Oxprenolol, a nonselective blocker with intrinsic sympathomimetic activity, has been shown to be as effective and safe as methyldopa for treatment of gravidas with moderately severe hypertension [54]. In another large controlled trial, perinatal mortality was significantly lowered in metoprolol-treated hypertensive pregnancies when compared to those given hydralazine treatment [53].

Propranolol therapy has been associated with intrauterine growth retardation. An overall trend of slightly lower birth weight as well as four small-for-gestational-age babies have resulted from 41 prospectively followed propranolol-treated pregnancies [55]. Beta-blockers have been associated with transient neonatal bradycardia and hypoglycemia, and respiratory depression in the neonate has been observed when propranolol was administered, intravenously, at the time of induction of anesthesia, for cesarean delivery [56]. Overall, beta-blocker treatment of hypertension in pregnancy is relatively safe, and at least two beta-blockers, oxprenolol and metoprolol, have appeared to improve the fetal outcome in comparison to traditional antihypertensive therapy.

Although the hypotensive effect of all beta-blockers is similar, the advantage of the intrinsic sympathomimetic activity of oxprenolol and pindolol remains to be determined. At present, the new beta-antagonists are not recommended for use during pregnancy. Women taking any of these beta-blockers at the outset of pregnancy are advised to switch to propranolol (or metoprolol, if cardioselectivity is needed). Patients entering pregnancy with chronic hypertension controlled with propranolol may continue this drug throughout pregnancy.

Vasodilators
Hydralazine
Hydralazine is the recommended agent for urgent control of severe pregnancy-induced hypertension. This drug decreases vascular resistance secondary to direct relaxation of arteriolar smooth muscle. The decreased blood pressure that accompanies peripheral vasodilatation activates a baroreceptor-mediated increase in sympathetic discharge, resulting in an increase in heart rate and cardiac output.

The literature contains conflicting reports on the effect of hydralazine on the uteroplacental circulation. Ladner et al. observed decreased uterine blood flow in response to hydralazine administration in normotensive sheep. Gant and colleagues observed that hydralazine given to eight chronic hypertensive women near term was followed by a mean 23.5% decrease in uteroplacental perfusion [57,58]. However, this decrement in uterine flow was accompanied by a 47% decrease in diastolic blood pressure, which represents drastic overtreatment for the gravida near term. Several investigators have reported significant increases in the uterine blood flow when hydralazine was given to hypertensive sheep [59]. The vast experience with acutely administered hydralazine in preeclampsia has not suggested any tendency to provoke fetal distress [60].

The protocol for use of parenteral hydralazine was reviewed earlier (page 176). When hydralazine is used without a sympathetic depressant agent, the reflex increase in sympathetic activity may add to the already hyperdynamic circulation of the pregnant hypertensive patient and result in bothersome tachycardia and palpitations. However, most pregnant women tolerate the drug well. Its chronic use is not advised in hypertensive patients with systemic lupus erythematosus because of the known propensity of the drug to aggravate or induce a lupus-like syndrome, particularly at dosages of > 200 mg/day.

Sodium Nitroprusside
Sodium nitroprusside [46] is the most potent and predictably effective agent for treatment of hypertensive emergencies (preeclampsia-induced cardiac failure, cerebral hemorrhage, myocardial infarction, aortic dissection, etc.). It dilates both resistance and capacitance vessels with resulting change in cardiac output and heart rate, depending on the preexisting state of cardiac performance. In heart failure, nitroprusside diminishes ventricular afterload and preload, promoting increased cardiac output and lessening of pulmonary congestion.

Nitroprusside infusion is begun at 0.1 μg/kg/min. Its onset of action is very rapid and its administration must be monitored in an intensive care unit. The desired initial 10 to 15% reduction in DBP is usually achieved with an infusion rate of less than 10 μg/kg/min. Patients receiving this drug are ordinarily asymptomatic unless they are made excessively hypotensive. Prolonged administration can cause thiocyanate toxicity in the mother (see Table 13-6). Because the placenta is readily permeable to nitroprusside and the drug combines with sulfhydryl groups in tissues to liberate cyanide, fetal cyanide toxicity can occur. One study in fetal lambs showed marked accumulation of fetal cyanide, which was dose related to maternal nitroprusside levels and was associated with fetal death in utero [61]. For this reason, nitroprusside infusion should be limited to 30 minutes prior to delivery; postpartum infusion may be required for 24 to 48 hours.

Diazoxide
Diazoxide is a potent, rapidly acting, direct arteriolar vasodilator employed as an alternative to nitroprusside treatment for extreme hypertension. Diazoxide-induced reductions in arterial pressure promote reflex increases in heart rate and cardiac output. When administered to normotensive pregnant sheep, the drug provokes moderate hypotension, but little change in uterine blood flow. For clinical use, the standard dose of 300 mg, by rapid intravenous injection, is excessive and may cause

serious hypotension. The tendency to hypotension is accentuated by the plasma volume depletion and often concurrent use of sympathetic blocking drugs. Intermittent administration of 30 to 60 mg is preferable and effective. After diazoxide injection, the maximum response is usually observed within two to five minutes [62].

Side effects include reflex tachycardia, hyperglycemia in the mother and the fetus and sodium retention. Because diazoxide may abolish or inhibit spontaneous uterine contractions, oxytocin must often be employed to stimulate labor.

SHORT- AND LONG-TERM PROGNOSIS

High blood pressure aggravated or induced by pregnancy usually stabilizes by the third postpartum day. Many gravidas with preeclampsia become normotensive within 48 hours of delivery, although an elevated blood pressure may be observed for up to six weeks. Should hypertension persist beyond 12 weeks, chronic hypertension should be formally diagnosed and evaluated.

Most preeclamptic primigravidas become normotensive shortly after delivery. According to the studies of Chesley and others, the outlook for future pregnancies is favorable [7,63]. The occurrence of preeclampsia or eclampsia in a first pregnancy is associated with a recurrence risk of less than 5% in the next pregnancy. On the other hand, the previously normotensive multipara who manifests hypertension or preeclampsia may have latent essential hypertension or renal disease and has a 20% chance of having the next pregnancy complicated by hypertension. Future pregnancies in these multiparous patients are associated with an increased incidence of abruptio placentae, preterm birth, and perinatal death.

Women with chronic hypertension experience approximately a 20% risk of superimposed preeclampsia. Careful review of their course in a previous pregnancy may allow finer prognostication about the risk of a subsequent pregnancy. If, in the previous gestation, preeclampsia supervened early, was severe, and required premature delivery, it is more likely that future pregnancies will evolve similarly. If, however, a prior case of superimposed preeclampsia was mild and had its onset near term, the prospect for future gestations is more favorable. As discussed earlier, women with severe, resistant hypertension, particularly those with heart disease, renal insufficiency, diabetes mellitus, or a history of superimposed preeclampsia, face an excessive risk of maternal and fetal complications during subsequent pregnancies.

Table 13-8 estimates the risk for hypertension or preeclampsia in a pregnancy from blood pressure findings in a previous pregnancy. The risk in any specific case cannot be determined from these data, but they may help the family to arrive at a decision regarding future pregnancies, family planning, or sterilization.

Preeclampsia and eclampsia seldom, if ever, cause chronic hypertension in women who otherwise never would have had it. If pregnancy-induced hypertension develops during a first pregnancy, future childbearing should not be restricted. A woman who has experienced pregnancy-induced hypertension as a multigravida must be educated about the increased risk to her and to the fetus. Future pregnancy should be discouraged in women with essential hypertension who suffered severe superimposed preeclampsia.

The use of oral contraceptive steroids should be avoided by women with essential hypertension and by multiparas who have experienced preg-

Table 13-8. Risk of hypertension or preeclampsia based on blood pressure response during previous pregnancy

Status	Approximate future risk of hypertension induced or aggravated by pregnancy
Never previously pregnant; now primigravida	7–9% for first pregnancy
Normotensive during first pregnancy	1%
Preeclampsia, first pregnancy	5% in second pregnancy
Preeclampsia as multipara[a]	10–20% chance of next pregnancy complicated by hypertension
Chronic hypertension	20% chance of superimposed preeclampsia
Other factors present in a first eclamptic pregnancy[b] Hypertension persisting 10 days post partum Obesity Onset of preeclampsia before week 36 Average SBP > 160 mm Hg during eclampsia	Presence of any two of these factors associated with approximately 50% chance that future pregnancy will be complicated by hypertension

[a]Includes hypertension as multipara, without proteinuria.
[b]Presumed to apply to women manifesting severe preeclampsia in first pregnancy.

nancy-induced hypertension. Their use by the young primiparous woman with a history of pregnancy-induced hypertension is acceptable, as the incidence of high blood pressure brought on by these agents is not significantly greater than that observed in control women [64]. Low-dose medication is recommended. Regular follow-up is mandatory, initially at three-month intervals and thereafter every six months.

REFERENCES

1. Stamler J, Stamler R, Riedlinger WF, et al. Hypertension screening of one million Americans. JAMA. 1976; 235:2299–306.
2. Naeye RL. Maternal blood pressure and fetal growth. Am J Obstet Gynecol. 1981; 141:780–7.
3. Christianson RE. Studies on blood pressure during pregnancy I. Influence of parity and age. Am J Obstet Gynecol. 1976; 125:509–13.
4. Gant NF, Daley GL, Chand S, Whalley PJ, MacDonald PC. A study of angiotensin II pressor response throughout primigravid pregnancy. J Clin Invest. 1973; 52:2682–9.
5. Wilson M, Morganti AA, Zervoudakis I, et al. Blood pressure, the renin-aldosterone system and sex steroids throughout normal pregnancy. Am J Med. 1980; 68:97–104.
6. Pritchard JA. Changes in blood volume during pregnancy and delivery. Anesthesiology. 1965; 26:393–9.
7. Chesley LC. Hypertensive disorders in pregnancy. New York: Appleton-Century-Crofts, 1978.
8. Gant NF, Worley RJ. Hypertension in pregnancy: concepts and management. New York: Appleton-Century-Crofts, 1980.
9. Pritchard JA. Management of preeclampsia and eclampsia. Kidney Int. 1980; 18:259–66.
10. Fisher KA, Luger A, Spargo BH, Lindheimer MD. Hypertension in pregnancy: clinical-pathological correlations and remote prognosis. Medicine (Baltimore). 1981; 60:267–76.
11. McCartney CP. Pathological anatomy of acute hypertension of pregnancy. Circulation. 1964; 30 (Suppl 2):37–42.
12. Naeye RL, Friedman EA. Causes of perinatal death associated with gestational hypertension and proteinuria. Am J Obstet Gynecol. 1979; 133:8–10.
13. Chesley LC. Orientation. In: Chesley LC. Hypertensive disorders in pregnancy. New York: Appleton-Century-Crofts, 1978:1–15.
14. Sibai BM, Schneider JM, Morrison JC, Lipshitz J, Anderson GD, Shier RW, Ditts PV. The late postpartum eclampsia controversy. Obstet Gynecol. 1980; 55:74–8.
15. de Alvarez RR, Welt SI. Hypertension complicated by pregnancy. In: Iffy L, Kaminetzky HA, eds. Principles and practice of obstetrics and perinatology. New York: Wiley, 1981:1241–64.
16. Kaplan NM. Clinical hypertension. 2nd ed. Baltimore: Williams & Wilkins, 1978:325–51.
17. Davidson JN, Lindheimer MD. Hypertension in pregnancy. In: Sciarra JJ, Depp R, Eschenbach DA, eds. Gynecology and obstetrics. Vol. 3. New York: Harper & Row, 1981:1–20.
18. Gant NF, Jimenez JM, Whalley PJ, Chand S, MacDonald PC. A prospective study of angiotensin II pressor responsiveness in pregnancies complicated by chronic essential hypertension. Am J Obstet Gynecol. 1977; 127:369–75.
19. Speroff L. Prostaglandins and reproduction. Fertil Steril. (in press).
20. Everett RB, Worley RJ, MacDonald PC, Gant NF. Effect of prostaglandin synthetase inhibitors on pressor response to angiotensin II in human pregnancy. J Clin Endocrinol Metab. 1978; 46:1007–10.
21. Goodman RP, Killam AP, Brash AR, Branch RA. Prostacyclin production during pregnancy: comparison of production during normal pregnancy and pregnancy complicated by hypertension. Am J Obstet Gynecol. 1982; 142:817–22.
22. Lewis PJ, Boylan P, Friedman LA, Hensby CN, Downing I. Prostacyclin in pregnancy. Br Med J. 1980; 280:1581–2.
23. Stuart MJ, Clark DA, Sunderji SG, Allen JB, Yambo I, Elrad H, Slott JA. Decreased prostacyclin production: a characteristic of chronic placental insufficiency syndromes. Lancet. 1981; 1:1126–8.
24. Lewis PJ, Shepherd GL, Ritter J, et al. Prostacyclin and preeclampsia. Lancet. 1981; 1:559.
25. Assali NS, Vaughn DL. Blood volume in preeclampsia: fantasy and reality. Am J Obstet Gynecol. 1977; 129:355–9.
26. Sheehan HL. Renal morphology in preeclampsia. Kidney Int. 1980; 18:241–52.
27. Pritchard JA, Cunningham FG, Mason RA. Coagulation changes in eclampsia: their frequency and pathogenesis. Am J Obstet Gynecol. 1976; 124:855–64.
28. Bauer TW, Moore GW, Hutchins GM. Morphologic evidence for coronary artery spasm in eclampsia. Circulation. 1982; 65:255–9.
29. Gedekoh RH, Hayashi TT, MacDonald HM. Eclampsia at Magee-Women's Hospital, 1970 to 1980. Am J Obstet Gynecol. 1981; 140:860–6.
30. Sibai BM, McCubbin JH, Anderson GD, Lipshitz J, Silts PV. Eclampsia. I. Observations from 67 recent cases. Obstet Gynecol. 1981; 58:609–13.
31. Lunell NO, Nylund LE, Lewander R, Sarby R. Uteroplacental blood flow in pre-eclampsia: measurements with indium-113m and a computer-linked gamma camera. Clin Exp Hypertens. 1982; B1:105–17.
32. Gant NF, Hutchinson HT, Siiteri PK, MacDonald PC. Study of the metabolic clearance rate of dehydroisoandrosterone sulfate in pregnancy. Am J Obstet Gynecol. 1971; 111:555–63.
33. Robertson WB, Brosens I, Dixon G. Maternal uterine vascular lesions in the hypertensive complications of pregnancy. In: Lindheimer MD, Katz AI, Zuspan FP, eds. Hypertension in pregnancy. New York: Wiley, 1976:115–27.

34. Sullivan JM. Blood pressure elevation in pregnancy. Prog Cardiovasc Dis. 1974; 16:375–93.

35. Redman CW. Treatment of hypertension in pregnancy. Kidney Int. 1980; 18:267–78.

36. Arias F, Zamora J. Antihypertensive treatment and pregnancy outcome in patients with mild chronic hypertension. Obstet Gynecol. 1979; 53:489–94.

37. Redman CW, Beilin LJ, Bonnar J. Treatment of hypertension in pregnancy with methyldopa: blood pressure control and side effects. Br J Obstet Gynaecol. 1977; 84:419–26.

38. Welt SI, Dorminy JH, Jelovsek FR, Crenshaw MC, Gall SA. The effects of prophylactic management· and therapeutics on hypertensive disease in pregnancy: preliminary studies. Obstet Gynecol. 1981; 57:557–65.

39. Sibai BM, Abdella TN, Anderson GD. Pregnancy outcome in 211 patients with mild chronic hypertension. Obstet Gynecol. 1983; 61:571–6.

40. Gilstrap LC, Cunningham FG, Whalley PJ. Management of pregnancy-induced hypertension in the nulliparous patient remote from term. Semin Perinatol. 1978; 2:73–81.

41. d'Apice AJ, Reit LL, Pepperell RJ, Fairley KF, Kincaid-Smith P. Treatment of severe pre-eclampsia by plasma exchange. Aust NZ J Obstet Gynaecol. 1980; 20:231–5.

42. Gallery ED, Delprado W, Györy AZ. Antihypertensive effect of plasma volume expansion in pregnancy-associated hypertension. Aust NZ J Med 1981; 11:20–4.

43. Sibai BM, Lipshitz J, Anderson GD, Dilts PV. Reassessment of intravenous $MgSO_4$ therapy in preeclampsia-eclampsia. Obstet Gynecol. 1981; 57:199–202.

44. Rafferty TD, Berkowitz RL. Hemodynamics in patients with severe toxemia during labor and delivery. Am J Obstet Gynecol. 1980; 138:263–70.

45. Benedetti TJ, Cotton DB, Read JC, Miller FC. Hemodynamic observations in severe pre-eclampsia with a flow-directed pulmonary artery catheter. Am J Obstet Gynecol. 1980; 136:465–70.

46. Cohn JN, Burke LP. Nitroprusside. Ann Intern Med. 1979; 91:752–7.

47. Kaplan NM. Clinical hypertension. 2nd ed. Baltimore: Williams & Wilkins, 1978.

48. McMahon FG. Management of essential hypertension. Mount Kisco, N.Y.: Futura, 1978.

49. Berkowitz RL. Anti-hypertensive drugs in the pregnant patient. Obstet Gynecol Surv. 1980; 35:191–204.

50. Redman CW. The use of antihypertensive drugs in hypertension in pregnancy. Clin Obstet Gynaecol.

1977; 4:685–705.

51. Gant NF, Madden JD, Siiteri RP, MacDonald PC. The metabolic clearance rate of dehydroisoandrosterone sulfate. III. The effect of thiazide diuretics in normal and future pre-eclamptic pregnancies. Am J Obstet Gynecol. 1975; 123:159–63.

52. Cockburn J, Moar VA, Ounsted M, Redman CW. Final report of study on hypertension during pregnancy: the effects of specific treatment on the growth and development of the children. Lancet. 1982; 1:647–9.

53. Rubin PC. Current concepts: beta-blockers in pregnancy. N Engl J Med. 1981; 305:1323–6.

54. Gallery EDM, Saunders DM, Hunyor SN, Györy AZ. Randomised comparison of methyldopa and oxprenolol for treatment of hypertension in pregnancy. Br Med J. 1979; 1:1591–4.

55. Redmond GP. Propranolol and fetal growth retardation. Semin Perinatol. 1982; 6:142–7.

56. Tunstall ME. The effect of propranolol on the onset of breathing at birth. Br J Anaesth. 1969; 41:792.

57. Ladner C, Brinkman CR, Weston P, Assali NS. Dynamics of uterine circulation in pregnant and nonpregnant sheep. Am J Physiol. 1970; 218:257–63.

58. Gant NF, Madden JD, Siiteri PK, MacDonald PC. The metabolic clearance rate of dehydroisoandrosterone sulfate. IV. Acute effects of induced hypertension, hypotension, and natriuresis in normal and hypertensive pregnancies. Am J Obstet Gynecol. 1976; 124:143–8.

59. Brinkman CR, Assali NS. Uteroplacental hemodynamic response to antihypertensive drugs in hypertensive pregnant sheep. In: Lindheimer MD, Katz AI, Zuspan FP, eds. Hypertension in pregnancy. New York: Wiley, 1976:363–75.

60. Pritchard JA, Pritchard SA. Standardized treatment of 154 consecutive cases of eclampsia. Am J Obstet Gynecol. 1975; 123:543–52.

61. Lewis PE, Cefalo RC, Naulty JS, Rodkey FL. Placental transfer and fetal toxicity of sodium nitroprusside. Gynecol Invest. 1977; 8:46. abstract.

62. Ram CV, Kaplan NM. Individual titration of diazoxide dosage in the treatment of severe hypertension. Am J Cardiol. 1979; 43:627–30.

63. Chesley LC, Annitto JE, Cosgrove RA. The remote prognosis of eclamptic women. Am J Obstet Gynecol. 1976; 124:446–59.

64. Pritchard JA, Pritchard SA. Blood pressure response to estrogen-progesterone oral contraceptive after pregnancy-induced hypertension. Am J Obstet Gynecol. 1977; 129:733–9.

Her o'erflowing heart, which pants
with all it granted,
with all it grants.
—Byron
Don Juan

14. CARDIOVASCULAR DISORDERS
Phillip S. Wolf

Virtually every facet of the heart and circulatory system may be affected by pregnancy. An understanding of the effects of pregnancy on the heart, and of maternal heart disease on gestation should begin with an appraisal of the normal circulatory adjustments in pregnancy.

NORMAL CARDIOVASCULAR ADJUSTMENTS IN PREGNANCY
Cardiac Output

Cardiac output rises in all pregnant women. The magnitude of the rise is known only approximately since the methods to measure output during pregnancy are imprecise. The earliest detectable rise in cardiac output begins during the first trimester and is well under way by midgestation (Table 14-1). The peak rise, about 30 to 50% over nonpregnant levels, occurs by the twentieth to twenty-fourth week of pregnancy [1,75].

Whether or not cardiac output falls in late pregnancy is a subject of controversy [1,2]. When a decline in output is measured, the mechanism is thought to result from venacaval compression by the gravid uterus when the patient lies supine [3–5]. The resulting entrapment of blood in the lower limbs reduces circulating blood volume and cardiac output. Some women with venacaval compression experience actual hypotension in this setting, known as the supine hypotensive syndrome. Moreover, caval compression is almost universal in late pregnancy, and the few women who experience symptomatic hypotension are apparently those who fail to develop adequate venous collaterals around the obstructed cava [6–8,76].

Most of the increase in cardiac output during pregnancy can be attributed to an increase in stroke volume. Echocardiography confirms that heart size and stroke volume increase progressively throughout gestation [9]. Cardiac output is further augmented by a rise in heart rate that averages 10 to 15%, an increase that begins early in gestation and continues until term [10].

The basis for the increased cardiac output associated with pregnancy is uncertain. An early

theory held that the placenta acts as an arteriovenous fistula and produces a hyperdynamic circulation. This concept has been discounted by the detection of circulatory changes earlier than placental development [1]. Changes in cardiac output are likewise not related to the hypervolemia of pregnancy as the time course of increased blood volume and cardiac output are not parallel. The increased cardiac output may have a hormonal basis. Estrogens given to pregnant ewes produce an increase in cardiac output, heart rate, and blood flow to the breasts, uterus, and skin and a fall in peripheral vascular resistance. These changes closely resemble those of human pregnancy [11]. The estrogen effect may represent a direct action on myocardial contractile proteins [12].

Early in pregnancy, the arterial pressure, especially the diastolic level, declines and tends to return to nonpregnant levels near term. Peripheral arterial resistance and mean arterial blood pressure are lowest when cardiac output is maximal at 20 to 24 weeks' gestation [10].

In the pulmonary circulation there is no change in either systolic or diastolic pressure as pregnancy progresses. The normal pressures and elevated cardiac output indicate that pulmonary vascular resistance has fallen. The right ventricle, like the left, produces an increased stroke volume but ejects this load at a normal systolic pressure. The increased work performed by both ventricles thus represents pure volume overload [2,13].

A portion of the increased cardiac output is distributed to the renal circulation (which rises 30% over nonpregnant levels), the breasts, the uterus, and the skin, especially the skin of the hands [11]. The increase in uterine flow provides a rich supply of well-oxygenated blood to the fetus at its early stages of development, before the placental circulation has been fully established.

Blood Volume

Maternal blood volume increases in all patients [14]. First noted to rise at six weeks' gestation, blood volume increases progressively to reach a peak level at 24 weeks, then rises more slowly

Table 14-1. Circulatory changes during pregnancy

Cardiovascular adjustment	Earliest rise	Maximal rise	Changes during labor	Changes following labor
Blood volume	6 weeks	↑40% at 24 wk	↓600 mL with vaginal delivery ↓1,100 mL with cesarean delivery	↓16% 3 days post partum
Cardiac output	1st trimester	↑30–50% at 20–24 wk	↑15–20% with uterine contractions	↑10–20% 1st and 2nd wk post partum
Blood flow to uterus, breasts, skin, renal circulation	1st trimester	↑30%	Not known	Not known

until it reaches a plateau in the last trimester. Most of the increase in circulating volume is due to an increase in plasma volume [3,14,77]. Red cell mass increases an average of 20% throughout pregnancy, but its rise in early pregnancy is proportionately less than the rise in plasma volume; hydremia results. In late gestation as red cell mass continues to increase and the plasma volume stabilizes, the blood hemoglobin level will rise [1].

The average increase in blood volume over nonpregnant levels is 40%, but there is considerable variability in normal women [14]. The increase does not correlate well with maternal size but in primigravidas does correlate with the birth weight of the infant. Women with twins show a significantly greater increase in plasma volume than women with a single fetus, and in women bearing triplets the expansion is even greater. On the other hand, mothers with a small increase in plasma volume tend to deliver babies of low birth weight [15].

Labor and Delivery

Labor produces transient but dramatic changes in cardiac output. Each uterine contraction ejects blood from the uterine veins, and cardiac output rises about 15 to 20% in supine patients. The sudden rise in output is associated with an increase in arterial pressure and a reflex bradycardia. When the patient lies supine, the venous return (and, hence, cardiac output) exceeds that which occurs when the patient lies in a lateral position. It has also been shown that uterine contraction causes significant compression of the aorta and distal iliac arteries, resulting in a redistribution of the maternal cardiac output to the extremities and head [16]. Anesthesia also influences cardiac output, but a discussion of the effects of anesthesia is beyond the scope of this section [17].

Prior to delivery, most of the increase in blood volume is thought to be distributed to the uterine

veins and the lower extremities. Following delivery, blood volume abruptly declines. Blood loss is estimated to be approximately 600 mL for patients undergoing vaginal delivery and approximately twice that for patients having cesarean delivery [14]. A remarkable tolerance for blood loss at delivery has been shown, making it appear that hypervolemia acts as a safeguard against excessive blood loss during delivery. Within three days after delivery, approximately a 16% decline in blood volume can be demonstrated whether the woman had either a vaginal or a cesarean delivery [14].

Effects of Exercise

Light to moderate exercise during normal pregnancy produces an appropriate rise in cardiac output [18–20]. In a healthy woman, the fetus appears to be in no jeopardy from the extra demands imposed by this level of exercise. Such may not be the case if cardiac output is insufficient to meet the demands, as is possible in women with heart disease.

Although information on the benefits and hazards of exercise in pregnancy is incomplete, the physician's advice to the pregnant woman with regard to exercise should probably be based on common sense. If the woman has excellent health and has followed a regular exercise routine, it appears reasonable to allow her to continue her activities. Some curtailment of exercise may be advisable for women with more than one fetus because of the larger hemodynamic demands placed on the circulation. On the other hand, women with impaired cardiac function may require severe exercise restriction during gestation.

CLINICAL EVALUATION
Normal Findings

Healthy pregnant women often display signs and symptoms that mimic heart disease. The circulatory adjustments already described may account for these findings. Shortness of breath (at rest as well as with exertion), easy fatigue, and reduced effort tolerance are relatively common symptoms in healthy pregnant women. The supine hypotensive syndrome can cause lightheadedness and even syncope. Edema of the legs is very common in most gravidas. Basilar rales that clear with deep breathing may be observed especially after bed rest. In the neck, the venous pressure is more easily visible although the actual level of pressure is normal. Taken together, these signs may erroneously suggest heart disease [2].

Auscultation

The first heart sound is normally prominent during pregnancy and is split because of early mitral valve closure. The second heart sound in late pregnancy tends to exhibit wider than usual splitting and normal intensity of aortic and pulmonic components. A physiologic third heart sound is very commonly heard in pregnant women, as it is in young people generally. The increased rate of blood flow across the tricuspid and mitral valves tends to augment the intensity of a third sound during gestation. Fourth heart sounds, by contrast, are rare [21,22].

Systolic Murmurs

Systolic murmurs are found in more than 90% of pregnant women. Typical of innocent murmurs, they occur in early or mid systole and usually do not exceed grade 3 in intensity on a scale of 1 to 6. The murmurs tend to be heard along the left sternal border but may be widely propagated and difficult to localize. Often they have a buzzing or vibratory quality. Peak incidence is reached during midpregnancy [21–23].

Diastolic Murmurs

Diastolic murmurs almost always indicate underlying heart disease. Two exceptions occur in normal pregnancy, and in neither case do these murmurs originate from the heart [21,24]. A venous hum, heard in nearly all cases in which it is specifically sought, is best listened for over the lateral supraclavicular fossa with the patient seated. The murmur, which is continuous through systole and diastole, may extend beneath the clavicle and cause confusion with a patent ductus arteriosus. Gentle finger pressure over the jugular vein on that side will obliterate the murmur.

A mammary souffle is heard in some women in the latter months of pregnancy and especially during lactation [21]. It is usually maximal in the second or third intercostal space and shows very little radiation. It may be heard on the right or left side

or both. It may be purely systolic or systolic with some diastolic component and usually is of fairly high pitch. The intensity varies from time to time, and the murmur is most obvious when the patient is lying flat; it often disappears if the patient sits up or if pressure over the site of the murmur is applied with the stethoscope or a finger. The uterine souffle is a continuous murmur heard over the lower abdomen in the last trimester. It is produced in the uterine arteries and is of no clinical significance.

Electrocardiography

The electrocardiogram does not show characteristic changes during pregnancy. In contrast to earlier observations, the mean QRS axis tends to remain within the normal range as the diaphragm elevates with advancing pregnancy [25]. Premature beats, atrial or ventricular, are relatively common. Reentrant supraventricular tachycardia occurs most commonly in normal young women, and pregnancy lowers the threshold for recurrences in susceptible patients [26].

Chest Roentgenography

There are no characteristic changes on the chest roentgenogram associated with normal pregnancy. The same criteria for interpretation of films should be applied to chest roentgenograms during pregnancy as in nonpregnant women [27]. Obviously, care should be exercised to properly shield the uterus and to limit the field of exposure.

Echocardiography

This highly useful and safe technique for diagnosis has found increasing application for cardiac disorders in pregnancy [28]. Normal pregnancy is characterized by a progressive increase in the internal dimensions of the heart. Velocity of circumferential shortening and ejection fraction increase as pregnancy progresses [4]. Echocardiography confirms that cardiac output increases in late pregnancy when the patient is evaluated in the lateral recumbent position. In the supine position, cardiac output falls almost to nonpregnant levels [4,9].

Increasingly, echocardiography has gained acceptance as a substitute for cardiac catheterization. In contrast to angiography, echocardiography produces no known adverse effects on the fetus. A recent report indicates that echocardiography may be used in lieu of fluoroscopy in the performance of right heart catheterization [29].

SPECIFIC CARDIAC DISORDERS

It is generally agreed that heart disease is the major nonobstetric cause of maternal death and that the largest number of patients dying will have had pulmonary congestion from preexisting rheumatic heart disease [30]. The scope of heart disease in pregnancy, however, is changing. Rheumatic valvular disease, which once accounted for 90% of cardiac disease in pregnancy, now represents no more than 60 to 75% of the total [30–32]. Moreover, the severe forms of rheumatic heart disease are at present seen less often. Congenital heart disease, on the other hand, has increased in importance as corrective surgery has permitted young women to reach childbearing age.

In the pregnant woman with heart disease, the lives of two individuals are at stake. The fetus depends on a normal uterine blood flow and a normal oxygen delivery. Thus, maternal heart disease (which may reduce uterine blood flow) and maternal cyanosis (which reduces the available oxygen to the fetus) pose a significant threat to the viability, growth, and development of the fetus. As a result, the vast majority of infants born to mothers with heart failure or cyanosis are preterm or small for gestational age. There is also a high rate of spontaneous abortion, the incidence of which tends to parallel the degree of cyanosis.

Optimally, the time to consider the effects of heart disease is prior to pregnancy, a time when the patient and her physician should mutually decide whether pregnancy should be attempted. If the cardiac patient becomes pregnant, the problem must be carefully individualized as to whether the pregnancy should continue and what method of care is applicable [33].

Therapy for the mother with heart disease centers around prevention and management of congestive heart failure, arrhythmias, thromboembolism, and infective endocarditis. Any treatment for the pregnant woman must also reckon with the effects of treatment on the fetus. As a general rule, the fetus is more vulnerable to the effects of therapy, whether medical or surgical, than the mother. For example, successful treatment of congestive heart failure in the mother may alleviate maternal symptoms and improve placental blood flow, but too drastic a diuresis will deplete plasma volume and place the fetus in jeopardy [53]. Anticoagulant therapy is mandatory in the pregnant woman with a mechanical prosthetic heart valve, but the fetal morbidity and mortality are inordinately high [70]. Most cardiac operations can be performed during gestation with a low maternal mortality, but the rate of fetal wastage is excessive [67]. Therapy, then, requires considering each case individually and mandates a close working relationship between patient, obstetrician, and cardiologist.

Valvular Heart Disease

Mitral Stenosis

Mitral stenosis is by far the most common rheumatic valvular lesion encountered in pregnant women. Because of the expected increase in heart rate, blood volume, and transmitral flow, the severity of mitral stenosis tends to be accentuated during gestation. Severe mitral stenosis is especially likely to run a complicated course during pregnancy. The most common problems include the following: acute pulmonary edema, hemoptysis (rupture of endobronchial varicosities), infective endocarditis, atrial fibrillation, and arterial and pulmonary embolization. Most patients with mild to moderate mitral stenosis can be successfully managed throughout pregnancy by restricting activity and sodium intake, and in severe cases placing the mother at strict bed rest until term [33–35].

The diagnosis of mitral stenosis can usually be made by careful physical examination. Characteristically, a "rumbling" low-frequency diastolic murmur can best be appreciated at the area of the apical impulse, especially after turning the patient to her left side. The murmur should be sought in any young patient with unexplained atrial fibrillation, arterial emboli, or pulmonary congestion. When the diagnosis is in question, echocardiography offers a reliable indicator of the presence, although not necessarily the severity, of the lesion.

Mitral Regurgitation

Rheumatic mitral regurgitation imposes a volume overload on the left ventricle. Changes associated with pregnancy pose no great threat except in very severe cases. In such instances, the additional volume overload of pregnancy can produce overt congestive heart failure. Pregnancy may alter the auscultatory findings of rheumatic mitral regurgitation [36,37]. The murmur frequently becomes less intense or even inaudible, presumably as the diminished peripheral vascular resistance of pregnancy reduces the flow through the incompetent valve. The murmur may be ignored or the clinical severity underestimated.

Aortic Valve Disease

For practical purposes, rheumatic aortic valve disease does not occur in the absence of mitral valve disease. The mitral valve disease may previously not have been clinically apparent but become manifest because of the additional hemodynamic burdens of pregnancy. The findings of isolated pure aortic stenosis and regurgitation are discussed later.

Mitral Valve Prolapse

Mitral valve prolapse is now considered the most common cause of mitral regurgitation and is frequently encountered in young women [38]. A recent study found that mitral valve prolapse was well tolerated in pregnant women [37]. The incidence of antepartum and postpartum complications, and fetal distress resulting from mitral valve prolapse are not greater than in pregnant patients with no known cardiac disorders. Pregnancy does alter the usual findings of the midsystolic click and systolic murmur characteristic of mitral prolapse. Both the click and the murmur may soften or disappear during pregnancy only to reappear following delivery [39]. Patients with mitral valve prolapse are at risk for infective endocarditis; most authorities agree that antibiotic prophylaxis is indicated at delivery for the patient with mitral valve prolapse [139].

Congenital Heart Disease

The incidence of congenital heart disease has remained relatively constant (0.3–0.8 per 100 live births) [2,40]. Because of a declining incidence of rheumatic heart disease, congenital heart disease has become relatively more prevalent during pregnancy. In addition, successful heart surgery in childhood or young adulthood has allowed many patients with congenital lesions to reach childbearing age. In this chapter, only the more common congenital lesions are discussed.

Atrial Septal Defect (ASD)

ASD is one of the more frequent congenital heart defects. This interatrial shunt produces a high pulmonary blood flow relative to systemic. Unless pulmonary hypertension is present (and it seldom is in young pregnant women), atrial septal defect is well tolerated during pregnancy [2].

Ventricular Septal Defect (VSD)

VSD, a very common congenital lesion in childhood, is rarely seen in adults. This lesion can produce early pulmonary hypertension (in which case there is a high mortality in childhood), or undergo spontaneous closure, or produce right ventricular outflow obstruction. In a given case the pathologic consequences of VSD depend on which of these complications has occurred. In the absence of pulmonary hypertension or large left-to-right shunts, the lesion is usually well tolerated in pregnancy [2].

Patent Ductus Arteriosus (PDA)

Patent ductus arteriosus is either well tolerated or associated with left ventricular failure in pregnancy, depending on the magnitude of the left-to-right shunt. A large ductus coupled with the normal volume expansion of pregnancy may overburden the left ventricle and produce overt cardiac failure. Through early recognition and relatively simple operation of ductus ligation, most patients with patent ductus arteriosus have had the lesion corrected in childhood [2].

Pulmonary Valvular Stenosis (PVS)

PVS creates obstruction to right ventricular outflow and, in some cases, right ventricular failure. Pregnancy accentuates the severity of this lesion by increasing transvalvular flow. Except when the defect is severe, it is usually well tolerated during pregnancy [2].

Tetralogy of Fallot

In tetralogy of Fallot, a ventricular septal defect is associated with stenosis at or below the pulmonic valve. Right-to-left shunting occurs in all but the mildest cases and causes cyanosis. The fetus tolerates an unsaturated arterial blood supply poorly. Retarded fetal growth and a high rate of spontaneous abortions result. Patients with tetralogy and other congenital lesions producing venous to arterial admixture are especially vulnerable at the time of labor and delivery. Risks such as sudden reduction in systemic vascular resistance may cause intense cyanosis, syncope, and sometimes death [53].

Eisenmenger's Syndrome

The Eisenmenger syndrome is defined as a right-to-left or bidirectional shunt at the atrial, ventricular, or aortopulmonary level coupled with a very high pulmonary vascular resistance. Some women survive this defect and become pregnant, but the risks of pregnancy with this disorder are formidable. Maternal mortality averages 35% [41–43]. A number of the physiologic alterations associated with pregnancy threaten both the mother with Eisenmenger's syndrome and her fetus. A drop in systemic vascular resistance can suddenly increase the right-to-left shunt and produce marked arterial oxygen desaturation. Straining during labor sharply reduces cardiac output and causes syncope and sometimes death [44]. The high mortality associated with Eisenmenger's syndrome mandates early interruption of pregnancy, or preferably avoidance of pregnancy (Table 14-2).

Congenital Aortic Stenosis

Congenital aortic stenosis accounts for about 5% of all cases of congenital heart disease in children

*Table 14-2. Cardiac conditions
in which pregnancy should be avoided*

Pulmonary hypertension
Eisenmenger's syndrome
Marfan's syndrome with overt cardiovascular disease
Cardiomyopathy with persistent cardiac enlargement

and young adults. Syncope, chest pain, and dyspnea progressing to left ventricular failure occur in severe cases. The development of these symptoms, when associated with hemodynamically significant aortic stenosis, portends a poor prognosis; about half of the patients are dead after four years of medical follow-up [45]. The diagnosis depends on finding a rough systolic murmur at the right base and left sternal border and an ejection click heard at the cardiac apex. ECG signs of left ventricular enlargement are present in severe cases and echocardiography confirms concentric left ventricular enlargement and a heavy band of echoes within the aortic root. Cardiac catheterization is necessary, however, to establish the severity of aortic stenosis and is justified when symptoms of left ventricular failure or syncope develop during pregnancy. In mild to moderate aortic stenosis, medical therapy is preferable. Open heart surgery with valvular replacement is reserved for cases in which maternal health is in jeopardy [46].

Aortic Regurgitation
Aortic regurgitation hemodynamically resembles mitral regurgitation. The effect is one of volume overload, generally well tolerated by the left ventricle. Pregnancy, by reducing total systemic resistance, usually reduces the intensity of the murmur of aortic regurgitation or may eliminate it completely [36]. Rarely, in a patient with advanced aortic regurgitation, pregnancy may further expand an already dilated left ventricle. Should heart failure develop, standard treatment is appropriate. When aortic insufficiency occurs as a result of infective endocarditis, acute left ventricular failure may result and require emergency valve replacement [47].

Primary Pulmonary Hypertension
This entity is an acquired syndrome of unknown etiology. It shares with the Eisenmenger syndrome the pathophysiology of a high pulmonary vascular resistance and an association with high maternal mortality (greater than 50%). The hazards at the time of delivery or in the early puerperium are especially severe. Every attempt should be made to avoid pregnancy or to terminate pregnancy under the best possible operative conditions

(Table 14-2) [2]. In those women who reach term, it is highly desirable to place a thermodilution Swan-Ganz catheter into the pulmonary artery so that pressures and cardiac output can be closely monitored. A cardiologist should be available throughout labor and delivery. Monitoring of the maternal and fetal heart rate is essential, and every attempt should be made to maintain adequate venous return [48]. Pharmacologic measures as well as oxygen may be useful to lower pulmonary vascular resistance. Anticoagulant therapy has been used post partum to reduce the risks of pulmonary vascular thrombosis, but the value of this form of therapy has been questioned [42].

Diseases of the Aorta and Great Vessels
Coarctation of the Aorta
Coarctation of the aorta is most often recognized (and surgically corrected) in childhood, but an occasional woman may have the lesion recognized for the first time during pregnancy. The major complications of coarctation include cardiac failure, infective endocarditis, aortic dissection or rupture, and intracranial hemorrhage. The latter is usually due to rupture of an aneurysm of the circle of Willis. A very high correlation with an abnormal, bicuspid aortic valve has been noted. In women with uncorrected coarctation, the maternal mortality averages 3.5%. Surgical correction during pregnancy has been successful [49,50].

Aortic Dissection
Aortic dissection is uncommon in nonhypertensive young women, but when it does occur it is associated with pregnancy at least one-half of the time. Advances in vascular surgery have made correction of aortic dissection feasible, but surgery is still likely to be palliative and not curative. Operation is most effective for dissection involving the ascending aorta. On the other hand, if dissection occurs distal to the left subclavian artery, medical management with beta-blockers and vasodilating drugs is usually tried first; surgery is reserved for patients with distal dissections in whom complications develop [59].

Marfan's syndrome, one of the causes of aortic dissection and rupture in young women, is also associated with myxomatous degeneration of the aortic and mitral valves. Valvular regurgitation and infective endocarditis may result. The dreaded complications of aortic dissection and rupture are probably exacerbated by pregnancy because of structural alterations in the aorta and the widened pulse pressure that increases stress on the aorta [51–53]. Pregnancy is ordinarily contraindicated for women with Marfan's syndrome (Table 14-2).

A recent report indicates a more favorable prognosis for women with Marfan's syndrome who lack major cardiovascular involvement [138]. Pregnancy was well tolerated if an aortic root diameter of less than 4 cm (determined echocardiographically) or major valvular regurgitation was absent. It should be kept in mind that Marfan's syndrome is an autosomal dominant disease, and 50% of offspring will inherit it.

Coronary Artery Dissection
Dissection of the coronary arteries is another uncommon entity, which has a strong predilection for the peripartum period. This lesion leads almost invariably to sudden death from acute myocardial infarction [54,55].

Coronary Artery Disease
Myocardial infarction has been reported during pregnancy. Although atherosclerosis is uncommon in women of childbearing age, the risk is enhanced by hyperlipidemia, smoking, and prior use of oral contraceptive agents. Women who suffer myocardial infarction tend to have had preeclampsia and present with severe chest pain or meet sudden death [56,57]. Coronary artery spasm may play a role in some cases, and isolated coronary arteritis has been reported as a rare cause of acute myocardial infarction [58].

Cardiomyopathy
Idiopathic Hypertrophic Subaortic Stenosis (IHSS)
IHSS is a genetic disorder that produces variable and changing levels of obstruction to left ventricular outflow. Increasing left ventricular diastolic volume, which occurs with normal pregnancy, tends to improve the condition; the normal diminution in systemic vascular resistance and in venous return due to caval compression in late pregnancy tends to accentuate the obstruction [60,61].

Labor offers its special hazards for these patients. Care should be taken to avoid hypotension from rapid blood loss, violent expulsive efforts, fatigue, and cardiac stimulation from inotropic agents. The lateral decubitus position for delivery is preferable. Oxytocin may be used to facilitate delivery and may actually reduce outflow obstruction. Antibiotic coverage for infective endocarditis (which occurs on the mitral valve) is indicated prior to delivery [60,61].

Peripartum Cardiomyopathy
The term *peripartum cardiomyopathy* refers to a form of congestive cardiomyopathy that develops in the last half of gestation or the early postpartum period. The etiology is unknown, but the risk of peripartum heart disease is increased for multiparas older than 30 years. It is also more common in women with twin gestations and in women with preeclampsia. Autopsy studies reveal cardiac dilatation and hypertrophy, degeneration and fibrosis of muscle fibers, and mural thrombi. The presenting signs are those of a low cardiac output with cool, dusky limbs, elevated jugular venous pressure, cardiomegaly, a third heart sound, and often murmurs of mitral or tricuspid regurgitation. Management is the same as that for any form of congestive heart failure. Early induction of labor and epidural anesthesia may be advantageous. The need for cesarean delivery is determined by the usual obstetric indications [64–66].

The prognosis is variable, but poorest when cardiomegaly is persistent. Women who have persistent cardiac enlargement for longer than six months post partum (about half the patients) have a very poor prognosis, and subsequent pregnancies are associated with recurrent cardiac failure and should be avoided. On the other hand, patients whose heart size returns to normal may carry future pregnancies with a relatively favorable outlook [65].

Infective Endocarditis
Infective endocarditis is a potential hazard for any woman with valvular heart disease. Nevertheless, the incidence of endocarditis appears to be low during pregnancy and the puerperium. Although approximately one gravida in 80 has some form of heart disease, the estimated frequency of infective endocarditis is approximately 1 out of 8,000 cases [62]. Current recommendations hold that antibiotics need not be given for patients with uncomplicated vaginal delivery, but in view of the simplicity of prophylaxis and the dire consequences of endocarditis, it seems prudent to use prophylaxis in susceptible patients. An antibiotic regimen for prophylaxis against endocarditis is presented in Table 14-3 [63].

Table 14-3. Antibiotic prophylaxis for patients with heart disease*

Ampicillin 1.0 g IM or IV	Given 30–60 min before delivery; then repeated
Gentamicin 1.5 mg/kg IM or IV	every 8 hr for 2 additional doses
For patients allergic to penicillin	
Vancomycin 0.5–1.0 g IV	Given 30–60 min before delivery; then repeated
Streptomycin 1.0 g IM	once 12 hr later

*For patients with most congenital heart lesions, acquired valvular disease, IHSS, or mitral valve prolapse.

Cardiac Surgery

Strides in cardiac surgery have been enormous. The physician will probably encounter cardiac surgery after the fact—that is, in the setting of a young woman who has had corrective surgery for rheumatic or congenital heart disease prior to pregnancy. As a rule, corrective cardiac surgery prior to pregnancy enhances the likelihood of a successful pregnancy [67,68]. Mitral valve repair in particular reduces the risk of complications of mitral stenosis during pregnancy. When tetralogy of Fallot has been corrected, there is evidence that the mother may complete several subsequent pregnancies without complications [69]. However, not all cardiac operations are curative, and the risks to mother and fetus must be individualized.

Recent experience with women who begin pregnancy with prosthetic cardiac valves indicated no antepartum mortality in a series of 106 cases. Six maternal deaths occurred following delivery, five of which were due to cerebral emboli in mothers who had not received anticoagulant therapy. However, only half the pregnancies resulted in live normal infants [70]. The data from this and similar investigations indicate a clear need for anticoagulant therapy during and after pregnancy for patients with prosthetic heart valves [78].

Ideally, the question of cardiac surgery should be considered prior to pregnancy. However, when surgery is required during pregnancy, the optimal time is before the hemodynamic burden becomes greatest (e.g., before the twenty-fifth week of gestation) [34,53,71]. The patient most likely to require cardiac surgery during pregnancy is the one with mitral stenosis who has unremitting pulmonary congestion or hemoptysis despite optimal medical management. The initial management of such a patient is appropriately conservative: hospitalization, strict bed rest, sodium restriction, diuretics, and control of any rhythm disturbances. Cardiac catheterization should be reserved for those cases in which surgery appears imminent or there is major uncertainty about the extent and severity of the cardiac lesion.

Experience at several leading centers indicates that open heart surgery including prosthetic valve replacement can be accomplished with exceedingly low maternal mortality [67]. Fetal death rate is another matter. Overall fetal mortality has been reported to be as high as 33%. Fetal heart rate monitoring during cardiopulmonary bypass is essential. Slowing of the fetal heart rate and loss of beat-to-beat variation indicate fetal distress [72,

73]. Using high perfusion rates during cardiopulmonary bypass appears to restore normal fetal heart rate. Reports of successful valve repair and delivery of a normal infant at term are seen with increasing frequency. In the rare event of maternal death near term, consideration must be given to immediate postmortem cesarean delivery. There have been several reported cases of fetal salvage in such situations [74].

Cardiac Arrhythmias

Young women commonly have atrial and ventricular premature beats as well as supraventricular tachycardia. Pregnancy lowers the threshold for reentrant supraventricular tachycardia [26]. Fortunately, most rhythms are well tolerated, and, when not subjectively disabling or associated with underlying heart disease, no specific therapy is indicated. On the other hand, with heart disease such as mitral stenosis, atrial septal defect, or cardiomyopathy, supraventricular tachycardia (and sometimes atrial fibrillation or flutter) may be hazardous. A special situation arises in the pregnant woman with Wolff-Parkinson-White syndrome, who may develop extremely rapid ventricular rates. Even in the absence of heart disease, rates in excess of 200 beats per minute may place the mother and fetus in jeopardy [79].

Pharmacologic therapy after the first trimester is essentially the same as for the nonpregnant patient (see below) [80–84]. Cardioversion has led to no apparent adverse consequences [85–87].

Complete heart block is rarely encountered in pregnancy. Mothers usually fare well with this rhythm and bear live, healthy babies [88]. Permanent cardiac pacing is seldom needed; indications for pacing are the same as for nonpregnant patients.

Fetal tachycardia is being detected with increasing frequency as a result of continuous electronic monitoring of the fetal heart rate. Most cases have been recognized when the mother perceives decreased fetal movement, the physician detects very rapid fetal rates (in the range of 200–280/min), or the sonogram reveals fetal hydrops or congestive heart failure [97].

Several attempts at pharmacologic conversion of fetal tachycardia have been successful. Digitalis has been used successfully; when given to the mother in usual adult dosages it produces slowing of the fetal heart rate to 120 to 140 beats per minute and gradual clearing of fetal hydrops [98]. Propranolol, another drug that crosses the placenta with facility, is an alternative agent [99].

DRUG THERAPY

As a matter of principle, it is best to avoid all cardioactive medications during the first trimester. Thereafter, many antiarrhythmic medications, including digitalis glycosides and quinidine, can be given without adversely affecting the fetus (Table 14-4).

Digitalis

Digitalis is the drug of first choice for supraventricular tachycardia, atrial fibrillation, or atrial flutter unless these rhythms are secondary to the Wolff-Parkinson-White syndrome. Rapid transmission of atrial impulses down the accessory pathway in this disorder may be facilitated by digitalis and produce extremely rapid heart rates with circulatory collapse.

Digitalis preparations freely cross the placenta. Serum levels in pregnant women are reduced to about one-half compared with the level obtained one month post partum, while the serum level of the newborn approximates that of the mother [94]. Digitalis does not appear to be teratogenic and is well tolerated by the fetus in ordinary doses.

Quinidine Sulfate

Quinidine is an antiarrhythmic drug that has been used extensively in pregnant women. Maternal and fetal blood levels of quinidine are approximately equal and remain stable throughout gestation. In general, quinidine appears to be safe for use during pregnancy. However, there have been isolated reports of associated neonatal thrombocytopenia and damage to the eighth nerve of the fetus. Quinidine is also known to have mild oxytocic properties. The drug is found in breast milk at a concentration similar to that in serum. Women who require quinidine therapy post partum should be advised against breast-feeding because of the potential accumulation of quinidine in the immature liver [81].

Verapamil

Verapamil is one member of the group of drugs known as calcium antagonists. Given intravenously it can be useful for the treatment of supraventricular tachycardia. To date verapamil has not been used to any significant extent during pregnancy. There are animal studies to suggest that each of the calcium antagonists has some tocolytic properties.

Propranolol

Propranolol crosses the placenta freely. Although it causes no obvious teratogenic effect, the drug has been implicated in a number of cases of transient fetal bradycardia, hypoglycemia, and respiratory depression. In addition, there is evidence from animal studies that propranolol reduces umbilical blood flow and increases uterine tone. The data in humans are conflicting, but the reduced uterine blood supply and increased tone could result in infants of small birth weight. Fetal growth retardation has been found in some, although not all, studies [89–93]. If it is necessary to use propranolol, it is essential that a neonatologist be in attendance immediately following delivery.

Disopyramide

Disopyramide is an oral antiarrhythmic agent with electrophysiologic actions similar to those of quinidine and procainamide. Relatively little information is available regarding its use in pregnancy. One report described a case in which the drug appeared to be responsible for initiating uterine contractions [95]. In view of the greater experience with quinidine during pregnancy, disopyramide should be reserved for arrhythmias unresponsive to quinidine. If the drug is used, careful monitoring should be instituted to avoid adverse maternal and fetal effects.

Procainamide

Little is known about the use of procainamide during pregnancy. It should be reserved for arrhythmias unresponsive to quinidine.

Diuretics

Diuretics have been extensively used in pregnancy for management of edema. Abundant evidence indicates that these agents should be used with extreme caution. Diuretics in early pregnancy deplete plasma volume, an effect that potentially reduces uterine blood flow and placental perfusion [53]. Further, diuretics do not prevent development of preeclampsia, nor are they of proven benefit in established preeclampsia [100]. In fact, the administration of diuretics to patients with preeclampsia has been shown to aggravate hypovolemia and to cause significant deterioration in the disease [53].

For the present, diuretics are recommended only for a very few specific clinical indications such as congestive heart failure and pulmonary edema and in certain forms of renal disease [100].

THROMBOEMBOLISM

Thromboembolism is properly regarded as one of the most feared complications of pregnancy and

Table 14-4. Antiarrhythmic drugs

Drug	Route of administration	Clinical application	Therapeutic concentration	Placental transfer[a]	Excretion into breast milk[b]	Use in pregnancy	Comments
Digoxin	Oral, parenteral	Paroxysmal supraventricular tachyarrhythmias; rate control in chronic atrial fibrillation and flutter	1–2 μg/mL	1.0	~1.0	Safe	Adjust dosage when quinidine or verapamil are given concomitantly
Quinidine	Oral	Prophylaxis in atrial and ventricular tachyarrhythmias	2–5 μg/mL	1.0	~1.0	Relatively safe	Excessive doses may lead to premature labor
Procainamide	Oral, parenteral	Termination and prophylaxis in atrial and ventricular tachyarrhythmias	4–8 μg/mL (+NAPA[c] 8–20 μg/mL)	0.25	?	Relatively safe	High incidence of maternal antinuclear antibodies and lupus-like syndrome with chronic use
Disopyramide	Oral, parenteral	Atrial and ventricular tachyarrhythmias	3–7 μg/mL	0.4	~1.0	Probably safe[d]	One report documents uterine contractions
Beta-adrenergic blocking agents	Oral, parenteral	Termination and prophylaxis in atrial and ventricular tachyarrhythmias; rate control in chronic atrial fibrillation	Variable	~1.0	~4.0–5.0	Relatively safe	Chronic administration may be associated with intrauterine growth retardation
Phenytoin	Oral, parenteral	Digitalis toxicity; refractory ventricular tachyarrhythmias	10–18 μg/mL	0.8–1.0	<0.5	Not recommended for chronic use[e]	High risk of malformations ("fetal hydantoin syndrome")
Verapamil	Oral, parenteral	Paroxysmal supraventricular tachycardia; rate control in chronic atrial fibrillation	15–30 ng/mL	~0.4	?	Probably safe[d]	Rapid intravenous injection may occasionally cause maternal hypotension and fetal distress
Lidocaine	Parenteral	"Choice" in ventricular tachyarrhythmias; digitalis toxicity	2–4 μg/mL	0.5–0.6	~1.0	Safe	Toxic doses and fetal acidosis may cause central nervous system and cardiovascular depression in newborns

[a]Umbilical venous/maternal venous concentration ratio.
[b]Breast milk/maternal plasma concentration ratio.
[c]N-acetylprocainamide.
[d]These drugs have not been studied extensively enough in pregnant patients to establish safety, but no serious adverse effects to the fetus have been reported.
[e]Probably safe as acute therapy of digitalis-induced arrhythmia.

Table 14-5. Predisposing factors
for maternal venous thromboembolism

Bed rest

Obesity

Advanced maternal age

Previous thromboembolic disease

Operations involving dissection in the pelvis

Cesarean delivery

Congestive heart failure

the puerperium. Deep venous thrombosis (DVT) and its major sequela, pulmonary embolism, occur five to six times more frequently during pregnancy and the puerperium than in the general population. Although deaths from thromboembolism in pregnancy appear to be on the decline, pulmonary embolus is still a relatively common cause of maternal mortality [101]. Moreover, the sequelae of DVT often include chronic leg swelling, pain, and ulceration.

The relative risk of maternal thrombosis in pregnancy is enhanced by several factors (Table 14-5). These include multiparity, increased maternal age, obesity, prolonged bed rest during and after pregnancy, and suppression of lactation with estrogen compounds [102]. Cesarean delivery has a profound influence on maternal mortality, carrying a risk of fatal embolism seven times as high as that of vaginal delivery [101]. Postpartum surgical procedures such as tubal ligation enhance the risk, as does an association with congestive heart failure, pulmonary hypertension, and chronic atrial fibrillation. Finally, a history of previous DVT or pulmonary embolus places a woman at even greater risk. Although relatively less common, arterial embolization poses a special threat to women with prosthetic cardiac valves, uncorrected mitral stenosis, cardiomyopathy, and atrial fibrillation [103,104].

Pathophysiology

Postmortem studies strongly suggest that calf vein thrombosis occurs earlier and with greater frequency than involvement of the thigh veins. Most thrombi arise in the venous valve sinuses and probably in venous saccules or at vein junctions [105]. Virchow's triad (i.e., stasis, local vessel wall trauma, and hypercoagulability) continues to serve as the model for describing the etiology of venous thrombosis, although the interdependence of the three major features of the triad has yet to be fully understood.

In the latter half of pregnancy, the gravid uterus obstructs the venous outflow from the lower limbs especially in the standing and supine recumbent positions. Femoral venous pressure rises, and venous flow velocity decreases progressively. The venous pressure returns to normal within ten days post partum, and venous flow velocity also becomes normal.

Coagulation disturbances are more difficult to pinpoint. The elevated estrogen levels of pregnancy may predispose to clotting. Antithrombin III (AT III) levels are decreased in pregnant women, while other clotting factors and platelet adhesiveness are increased [106,107]. Further, estrogens lead to diminished smooth muscle tone in blood vessel walls [108,109]. Elastic tissue may become permanently impaired while intimal hyperplasia and fibrosis develop.

Deep venous thrombosis is the most common vascular complication during pregnancy. Only when iliofemoral occlusion has occurred can the diagnosis be made with confidence. Patients exhibit massive thigh and calf swelling, pain, and sometimes cyanosis. When DVT is confined to the calf, the clinical diagnosis is highly unreliable. Not only are there no clinical signs referable to the limbs in approximately half of patients with proved DVT, but 30% of patients with a positive clinical diagnosis have no radiographic evidence of thrombi [105]. Because of the unreliability of clinical diagnosis, the actual incidence of DVT in pregnancy is unknown. None of the recently introduced methods for noninvasive study (^{125}I fibrinogen scan, Doppler ultrasonography, plethysmography) has been studied prospectively. The incidence and course of DVT during pregnancy and the postpartum period rely largely on unsubstantiated clinical data.

The diagnosis of pulmonary embolism is just as difficult to make as that of DVT. When major and life-threatening embolism has occurred, the diagnosis is relatively straightforward. Massive embolism is characterized by severe dyspnea, cyanosis and circulatory collapse. Smaller (and by far more common) emboli produce dyspnea, chest pain, cough, apprehension, and palpitations, symptoms that are nonspecific [110]. In a majority of cases, chest roentgenograms and ECGs are of little value.

Unfortunately, the most precise diagnostic methods rely on radiographic contrast studies, which expose the fetus to unwanted levels of radiation. The risk of x-ray exposure must be weighed against the dangers of overlooking the diagnosis or the all too real hazards of inappropriate anticoagulant therapy.

Venography is the standard for establishing the diagnosis of DVT; accuracy in skilled hands exceeds 95% [111]. While radiation hazards limit the use of this procedure during pregnancy, proper shielding and reduction of field size permit its use in selected cases. As an alternative, impedance plethysmography and Doppler ultrasound scanning are procedures with no known risks to mother or fetus. In expert hands these techniques detect proximal thrombi (those involving popliteal, femoral, or iliac veins) in 95% of the cases. Since it is the proximal thrombi that are likely to detach and embolize, these techniques have significant clinical utility [112–115]. False readings are thought to occur in late gestation because of the effect of the gravid uterus on venous outflow from the legs. Venous thrombosis confined to the soleal plexus, the profunda femoris, or the hypogastric veins will not be detected by any noninvasive method.

When pulmonary embolism is suspected, lung scanning with macroaggregated albumin labeled with ^{99m}Tc (technetium) is the diagnostic method of choice. A normal scan effectively excludes the diagnosis. An abnormal scan cannot distinguish between perfusion disorders (emboli) and ventilatory problems (atelectasis, obstructive airways disease, pneumonia). The accuracy of lung scanning is enhanced by the use of ^{133}xenon washout, which will detect abnormal ventilatory patterns. A moderate or large ventilation-perfusion "mismatch" tends to support the diagnosis of pulmonary embolism [116].

The biologic half-life of ^{99m}Tc is approximately six hours, and the dosage required for lung scanning gives an extremely low radiation level to the fetus since the material tends to trap in the lung and very little passes to the placenta [101].

Angiography is the most sensitive and specific method for the diagnosis of pulmonary embolism [96]. The procedure is associated with the small maternal risk of right heart catheterization but a relatively high level of radiation exposure to the fetus. Angiography is to be avoided if at all possible during the first trimester and is reserved for situations in which a major therapeutic decision rests on the outcome of the study.

Therapy

Treatment with anticoagulant drugs is indicated for the duration of pregnancy in patients with iliofemoral venous thrombosis, pulmonary embolism, and prosthetic heart valves. The reason is that these patients are exposed to both local and general predisposing factors of further thromboembolic events throughout pregnancy. On the other hand, patients with a single episode of calf vein thrombosis are less vulnerable to recurrence, and in these cases it is reasonable to treat the acute episode with intravenous heparin and to follow

the patient carefully with noninvasive techniques for any signs of recurrence or extension of the thrombotic process.

There appears to be no ideal anticoagulant regimen for treating thromboembolism during pregnancy. A compromise approach is suggested, which is designed to offer maximal protection for the mother while minimizing risks to the fetus [129,130,132].

Warfarin

Oral anticoagulants, of which warfarin is the prototype, effectively prevent thromboembolism but pose special problems during pregnancy. These agents readily cross the placenta. The incidence of spontaneous abortion is estimated at 9%. A specific syndrome known as warfarin syndrome, or the fetal warfarin syndrome, results when the drug is used during the first trimester, and the critical period appears to be between six and nine weeks [117–119]. It is estimated that approximately 8% of infants exposed to the drug in utero will have malformations, including nasal hypoplasia, frontal bossing, and short stature with stippled epiphyses [118].

Fetal risk declines in the second and third trimester, but central nervous system abnormalities (mental retardation or blindness) occur in approximately 3% of infants [118]. Intracranial bleeding has been demonstrated in some but not all of these children, and the trauma of delivery produces further hazards.

Of 418 pregnancies reviewed by Hall et al. [118], in which coumarin derivatives had been used, one-sixth resulted in abnormal liveborn infants, one-sixth in abortion or stillbirth, and only approximately two-thirds in apparently normal infants [118]. Given that the literature tends to be biased toward reporting complicated cases, these retrospective estimates are likely to be the worst possible and in actual practice the risks are less. Nevertheless, it is recommended that warfarin be avoided during pregnancy if at all possible.

Heparin

Heparin is the only agent that has proved capable of arresting active thrombosis. It is therefore the drug of choice for an acute deep venous thrombosis or pulmonary embolism. Given by constant intravenous infusion, the heparin dosage is adjusted to prolong the partial thromboplastin time (PTT) 1.5 times the control level. Treatment is usually continued for seven to ten days to allow for organization and firm attachment of the thrombus to the vessel wall [124,125]. Recent evidence indicates that the risk of recurrent thromboembolism after cessation of intravenous therapy can be minimized by the use of heparin given subcutaneously every 12 hours in a dosage sufficient to prolong the PTT 1.5 times the control [126].

During the immediate postpartum period, the incidence of deep venous thrombosis increases sharply. The incidence is still too low to justify routine anticoagulant prophylaxis, yet in certain high-risk subgroups (see Table 14-5) use of a low-dose heparin regimen (5,000 units administered subcutaneously every 12 hours) may be indicated.

In a series by Spearing and associates, long-term subcutaneous heparin proved safe and effective throughout pregnancy. Nineteen women were followed through 22 pregnancies, each of which resulted in a healthy term infant. In this series there were no major complications from heparin therapy [120]. The potential hazard of heparin is maternal hemorrhage, which occurs in 5 to 10% of patients [101]. The risk of bleeding is particularly high if there has been recent trauma or surgery, in patients on platelet-inhibiting agents, or in patients receiving intramuscular injections. Less common but potentially serious complications include osteoporosis and thrombocytopenia. The former tends to occur in patients treated with moderate-to high-dose heparin for six months or longer. Thrombocytopenia is an especially serious complication [121–123]. An initial platelet count should be obtained before beginning heparin therapy and repeated within the first week.

The risk of thromboembolism in pregnant patients with prosthetic heart valves who are not anticoagulated is considerable [104]. In a recent review, no anticoagulant therapy was given in 29 pregnancies. All 29 infants were normal, but six maternal deaths occurred post partum, five from cerebral emboli. The risk of arterial embolization appears to be enhanced if any of the following are present: an enlarged left atrium, atrial fibrillation, congestive heart failure, or a history of past embolization [127].

The risk of embolization is lower in patients with porcine xenografts than with mechanical valves. In the absence of any additional risks, it may be possible to follow women with porcine xenografts during pregnancy without anticoagulation therapy, although there are little data at present to support this conclusion.

Breast-Feeding and Anticoagulant Therapy

The question of breast-feeding in mothers taking anticoagulants has been examined [131]. In women treated with full dosages of warfarin, no warfarin levels could be detected in either maternal milk or infant's plasma. Thus, warfarin appears to be a safe agent for breast-feeding mothers; heparin likewise is safe as it does not appear in breast milk and is ineffective when taken orally.

Platelet Antiaggregant Therapy

The importance of platelets in the formation of venous thrombi is uncertain. Several prospective clinical trials have evaluated antiplatelet agents for prevention of venous thrombosis. The results have not conclusively shown any benefit of these agents and do not support their use as the sole antithrombotic agent during pregnancy [104,128]. Further, little information is available regarding the teratogenic potential of the various antiplatelet drugs.

Thrombolytic Therapy

Case reports have described the relatively safe use of thrombolytic therapy during pregnancy. The drugs may prove lifesaving for the woman with a massive thromboembolism [133,134]. In this situation thrombolytic therapy appears preferable to pulmonary embolectomy. Placental transfer of ^{131}I streptokinase is minimal and insufficient to have fibrinolytic effects on the fetus [135].

Streptokinase or urokinase should be avoided at delivery because of the risk of hemorrhage. These drugs are not recommended except where life-threatening thromboembolism has occurred and the risk of severe hemorrhage is accepted. Local packing with an antifibrinolytic agent may reduce the risk of bleeding.

Surgery

Surgery occupies a minor place in the management of thromboembolism. The most successful application is removal of peripheral arterial emboli from a limb by means of a Fogarty catheter. Pulmonary embolectomy is reserved for those situations in which shock and hypoxemia persist after an attempt at nonoperative management. No patient should undergo embolectomy without prior confirmation of the diagnosis by pulmonary angiography [101].

Surgery for deep venous thrombosis involves either a thrombectomy for massive iliofemoral thrombosis or inferior vena caval interruption for recurrent pulmonary emboli. Results of thrombectomy have been generally unsatisfactory since there is a high incidence of recurrent thrombosis. Caval interruption is not without risk, nor does it always confer protection from pulmonary embolism. The newer "umbrella filters" can be implanted in the inferior vena cava via the jugular vein under fluoroscopic control. In the rare instances in which caval interruption is contemplated, the filter appears preferable to caval ligation during pregnancy [136,137].

REFERENCES

1. Metcalfe J, Ueland K. Maternal cardiovascular adjustments to pregnancy. Prog Cardiovasc Dis. 1974; 16:363–74.
2. Perloff JK. Pregnancy and cardiovascular disease. In: Braunwald E, ed. Heart disease. A textbook of cardiovascular medicine. Philadelphia: Saunders, 1980:1871–92.
3. Szekely P, Snaith L. Heart disease and pregnancy. Edinburgh: Churchill Livingstone, 1974.
4. Rubler S, Damani PM, Pinto ER. Cardiac size and performance during pregnancy estimated with echocardiography. Am J Cardiol. 1977; 40:534–40.
5. Burg JR, Dodek A, Kloster FE, Metcalfe J. Alterations of systolic time intervals during pregnancy. Circulation. 1974; 49:560–4.
6. Kerr MG. Cardiovascular dynamics in pregnancy and labour. Br Med Bull. 1968; 24:19–24.
7. Kerr MG, Scott DB, Samuel E. Studies of the inferior vena cava in late pregnancy. Br Med J. 1964; 1:532–3.
8. Ikard RW, Ueland K, Folse R. Lower limb venous dynamics in pregnant women. Surg Gynecol Obstet. 1971; 132:483–8.
9. Katz R, Karliner JS, Resnik R. Effects of a natural volume overload state (pregnancy) on left ventricular performance in normal human subjects. Circulation. 1978; 58:434–41.
10. Rovinsky JJ, Jaffin H. Cardiovascular hemodynamics in pregnancy. III. Cardiac rate, stroke volume, total peripheral resistance, and central blood volume in multiple pregnancy. Synthesis of results. Am J Obstet Gynecol. 1966; 95:787–94.
11. McAnulty JH, Metcalfe J, Ueland K. Heart disease and pregnancy. New York: McGraw-Hill, 1982.
12. King TM, Whitehorn WV, Reeves B, Kubota R. Effects of estrogen on composition and function of cardiac muscle. Am J Physiol. 1959; 196:1282–5.
13. Benedetti TJ, Cotton DB, Read JC, Miller FC. Hemodynamic observations in severe pre-eclampsia with a flow-directed pulmonary artery catheter. Am J Obstet Gynecol. 1980; 136:465–70.
14. Ueland K. Maternal cardiovascular dynamics. VII. Intrapartum blood volume changes. Am J Obstet Gynecol. 1976; 126:671–7.
15. Croall J, Sherrif S, Matthews J. Non-pregnant maternal plasma volume and fetal growth retardation. Br J Obstet Gynaecol. 1978; 85:90–5.
16. Ueland K, Hansen JM. Maternal cardiovascular dynamics. II. Posture and uterine contractions. Am J Obstet Gynecol. 1969; 103:1–7.
17. Ostheimer GW, Alper MH. Intrapartum anesthetic management of the pregnant patient with heart disease. Clin Obstet Gynecol. 1975; 18:81–97.
18. Ueland K, Novy MJ, Metcalfe J. Cardiorespiratory responses to pregnancy and exercise in normal women and patients with heart disease. Am J Obstet Gynecol. 1973; 115:4–10.
19. Longo LD, Hewitt CW, Lorijn RHW, Gilbert RD. To what extent does maternal exercise affect fetal oxygenation and uterine blood flow? Fed Proc. 1978; 37:905. abstract.
20. Knuttgen HG, Emerson K Jr. Physiological response to pregnancy at rest and during exercise. J Appl Physiol. 1974; 36:549–53.
21. Ravin A, Craddock LD, Wolf PS, Shander D. Auscultation of the heart. Chicago: Year Book, 1977.
22. Cutforth R, MacDonald CB. Heart sounds and murmurs in pregnancy. Am Heart J. 1966; 71:741–7.
23. Goldberg LM, Uhland H. Heart murmurs in pregnancy: a phonocardiographic study of their development, progression and regression. Dis Chest. 1967; 52:381–6.
24. Harvey WP. Alterations of the cardiac physical examination in normal pregnancy. Clin Obstet Gynecol. 1975; 18:51–63.
25. Schwartz DB, Schamroth L. The effect of pregnancy on the frontal plane QRS axis. J Electrocardiol. 1979; 12:279–81.
26. Bellet S. Clinical disorders of the heart beat. Philadelphia: Lea & Febiger, 1971. Pp. 701–707.
27. Turner AF. The chest radiograph in pregnancy. Clin Obstet Gynecol. 1975; 18:65–74.
28. Bresnahan DR, Askenazi J, Lesch M. Noninvasive assessment of cardiovascular function. Clin Obstet Gynecol. 1981; 24:711–42.
29. Meltzer RS, Serruys PW, McChie J, Hugenholtz PG, Roelandt J. Cardiac catheterization under echocardiographic control in a pregnant woman. Am J Med. 1981; 71:481–4.
30. Hibbard LT. Maternal mortality due to cardiac disease. Clin Obstet Gynecol. 1975; 18:27–36.
31. Chesley LC. Severe rheumatic cardiac disease and pregnancy: the ultimate prognosis. Am J Obstet Gynecol. 1980; 136:552–8.
32. Szekely P, Turner R, Snaith L. Pregnancy and the changing pattern of rheumatic heart disease. Br Heart J. 1973; 35:1293–303.
33. Burch GE. Heart disease and pregnancy. Am Heart J. 1977; 93:104–16.
34. Manning PR, Mestman JH, Lau FY. Management of the pregnant patient with mitral stenosis. Clin Obstet Gynecol. 1975; 18:99–106.
35. Wood P. An appreciation of mitral stenosis. Br Med J. 1954; 1:1051–63.
36. Marcus FI, Ewy GA, O'Rourke RA, Walsh B, Bleich AC. The effect of pregnancy on the murmurs of mitral and aortic regurgitation. Circulation. 1970; 41:795–805.
37. Rayburn WF, Fontana ME. Mitral valve prolapse and pregnancy. Am J Obstet Gynecol. 1981; 141:9–11.
38. Devereux RB, Perloff JK, Reichek N, Josephson ME. Mitral valve prolapse. Circulation. 1976; 54:3–14.
39. Haas JM. The effect of pregnancy on the midsystolic click and murmur of the prolapsing posterior

leaflet of the mitral valve. Am Heart J. 1976; 92:407–8.

40. Cannell DE, Vernon CP. Congenital heart disease and pregnancy. Am J Obstet Gynecol. 1963; 85:744–53.

41. Jones AM, Howitt G. Eisenmenger syndrome in pregnancy. Br Med J. 1965; 1:1627–31.

42. Pitts JA, Crosby WM, Basta LL. Eisenmenger's syndrome in pregnancy. Am Heart J. 1977; 93:321–6.

43. Neilson G, Galea EG, Blunt A. Eisenmenger's syndrome and pregnancy. Med J Aust. 1971; 1:431–4.

44. Midwall J, Jaffin H, Herman MV, Kupersmith J. Shunt flow and pulmonary hemodynamics during labor and delivery in the Eisenmenger syndrome. Am J Cardiol. 1978; 42:299–303.

45. Arias F, Pineda J. Aortic stenosis and pregnancy. J Reprod Med. 1978; 20:229–32.

46. Eilen B, Kaiser IH, Becker RM, Cohen MN. Aortic valve replacement in the third trimester of pregnancy: case report and review of the literature. Obstet Gynecol. 1981; 57:119–21.

47. Ross J Jr. Left ventricular function and the timing of surgical treatment in valvular heart disease. Ann Intern Med. 1981; 94:498–504.

48. Rosenthal MH. Intrapartum intensive care management of the cardiac patient. Clin Obstet Gynecol. 1981; 24:789–807.

49. Barash PG, Hobbins JC, Hook R, et al. Management of coarctation of the aorta during pregnancy. J Thorac Cardiovasc Surg. 1975; 69:781–4.

50. Deal K, Wooley CF. Coarctation of the aorta and pregnancy. Ann Intern Med. 1973; 78:706–10.

51. Hirst AE Jr, Johns VJ Jr, Kime SW Jr. Dissecting aneurysm of the aorta: a review of 505 cases. Medicine (Baltimore). 1958; 37:217–79.

52. Manalo-Estrella P, Barker AE. Histopathologic findings in human aortic media associated with pregnancy. Arch Pathol. 1967; 83:336–41.

53. McAnulty JH, Metcalfe J, Ueland K. General guidelines in the management of cardiac disease. Clin Obstet Gynecol. 1981; 24:773–88.

54. Ascuncion CM, Hyun J. Dissecting intramural hematoma of the coronary artery in pregnancy and the puerperium. Obstet Gynecol. 1972; 40:202–10.

55. Shaver PJ, Carrig TF, Baker WP. Postpartum coronary artery dissection. Br Heart J. 1978; 40:83–6.

56. Beary JF, Summer WR, Bulkley BH. Postpartum acute myocardial infarction: a rare occurrence of uncertain etiology. Am J Cardiol. 1979; 43:158–61.

57. Sasse L, Wagner R, Murray FE. Transmural myocardial infarction during pregnancy. Am J Cardiol. 1975; 35:448–52.

58. Ahronheim JH. Isolated coronary periarteritis: report of a case of unexpected death in a young pregnant woman. Am J Cardiol. 1977; 40:287–90.

59. Miller DC, Stinson EB, Oyer PE, Rossiter SJ, Reitz BA, Griepp RB, Shumway NE. Operative treatment of aortic dissections. Experience with 125 patients over a sixteen year period. J Thorac Cardiovasc Surg. 1979; 78:365–82.

60. Oakley GD, McGarry K, Limb DG, Oakley CM. Management of pregnancy in patients with hypertrophic cardiomyopathy. Br Med J. 1979; 1:1749–50.

61. Kolibash AJ, Ruiz DE, Lewis RP. Idiopathic hypertrophic subaortic stenosis in pregnancy. Ann Intern Med. 1975; 82:791–4.

62. Sugrue D, Blake S, Troy P, MacDonald D. Antibiotic prophylaxis against infective endocarditis after normal delivery—is it necessary? Br Heart J. 1980; 44:499–502.

63. Hirschmann JV. Rational antibiotic prophylaxis. Hosp Pract. 1981; 105–23.

64. Goodwin JF. Peripartal heart disease. Clin Obstet Gynecol. 1975; 18:125–31.

65. Demakis JG, Rahimtoola SH, Sutton GC, et al. Natural course of peripartum cardiomyopathy. Circulation. 1971; 44:1053–61.

66. Demakis JG, Rahimtoola SH. Peripartum cardiomyopathy. Circulation. 1971; 44:964–8.

67. Zitnik RS, Brandenburg RO, Sheldon R, Wallace RB. Pregnancy and open heart surgery. Circulation. 1969; 39(Suppl):257–62.

68. Ueland K. Cardiac surgery and pregnancy. Am J Obstet Gynecol. 1965; 92:148–62.

69. Ralstin JH, Dunn M. Pregnancies after surgical correction of tetralogy of Fallot. JAMA. 1976; 235:2627–8.

70. Harrison EC, Roschke EJ, Ferenczi G, Mitani GH. Managing the pregnant patient with a heart valve prosthesis. Contemp Ob Gyn. 1978; 11:82–90.

71. Selzer A. Risks of pregnancy in women with cardiac disease. JAMA. 1977; 238:892–3.

72. Bahary CM, Ninio A, Gorodesky IG, Neri A. Tococardiography in pregnancy during extracorporeal bypass for mitral valve replacement. Isr J Med Sci. 1980; 16:395–7.

73. Levy DL, Warriner RA III, Burgess GE III. Fetal response to cardiopulmonary bypass. Obstet Gynecol. 1980; 56:112–5.

74. Weber CE. Postmortem cesarean section: review of the literature and case report. Am J Obstet Gynecol. 1971; 110:15.

75. Metcalfe J, McAnulty JH, Ueland K. Cardiovascular physiology. Clin Obstet Gynecol. 1981; 24:693–710.

76. Pritchard JA, Barnes AC, Bright RH. The effect of the supine position on renal function in the near-term pregnant woman. J Clin Invest. 1955; 34:777–781.

77. Lund CJ, Donovan JC. Blood volume during pregnancy. Am J Obstet Gynecol. 1967; 98:393–403.

78. Ibarra-Perez C, Arevalo-Toledo N, Alvarez-de la Cadena O, Noriega-Guerra L. The course of pregnancy in patients with artificial heart valves. Am J Med. 1976; 61:504–12.

79. Gleicher N, Meller J, Sandler RZ, Sullum S. Wolff-Parkinson-White syndrome in pregnancy. Obstet Gynecol. 1981; 58:748–52.

80. Ueland K, McAnulty JH, Ueland FR, Metcalfe J. Special considerations in the use of cardiovascular drugs. Clin Obstet Gynecol. 1981; 24:809–23.

81. Hill LM, Malkasian GD Jr. The use of quinidine sulfate throughout pregnancy. Obstet Gynecol. 1979; 54:366–8.

82. Woosley RL, Shand DG. Pharmacokinetics of antiarrhythmic drugs. Am J Cardiol. 1978; 41:986–95.

83. Wolf PS. Arrhythmias in chronic pulmonary disease. Angiology. 1979; 30:676–82.

84. Brinkman CR III, Woods JR Jr. Effects of cardiovascular drugs during pregnancy. Cardiovasc Med. 1976; 1:231–51.

85. Curry JJ, Quintana FJ. Myocardial infarction with ventricular fibrillation during pregnancy treated by direct current defibrillation with fetal survival. Chest. 1970; 58:82–4.

86. Finlay AY, Edmunds V. D.C. cardioversion in pregnancy. Br J Clin Pract. 1979; 33:88–94.

87. Klepper I. Cardioversion in late pregnancy. Anaesthesia. 1981; 36:611–6.

88. Kenmure AC, Cameron AJ. Congenital complete heart block in pregnancy. Br Heart J. 1967; 29:910–2.

89. Rubin PC. Beta-blockers in pregnancy. N Engl J Med. 1981; 305:1323–6.

90. Habib A, McCarthy JS. Effects on the neonate of propranolol administered during pregnancy. J Pediatr. 1977; 91:808–11.

91. Cottrill CM, McAllister RG Jr, Gettes L, Noonan JA. Propranolol therapy during pregnancy, labor, and delivery: evidence for transplacental drug transfer and impaired neonatal drug disposition. J Pediatr. 1977; 91:812–4.

92. Gladstone GR, Hordof A, Gersony WM. Propranolol administration during pregnancy: effects on the fetus. J Pediatr. 1975; 86:962–4.

93. Pruyn SC, Phelan JP, Buchanan GC. Long-term propranolol therapy in pregnancy: maternal and fetal outcome. Am J Obstet Gynecol. 1979; 135:485–9.

94. Rogers MC, Willerson JT, Goldblatt A, Smith TW. Serum digoxin concentration in the human fetus, neonate and infant. N Engl J Med. 1972; 287:1010–3.

95. Leonard RF, Braun TE, Levy AM. Initiation of uterine contractions by disopyramide during pregnancy. N Engl J Med. 1978; 299:84–5.

96. Robin, ED. Overdiagnosis and overtreatment of pulmonary embolism: the emperor may have no clothes. Ann Intern Med. 1977; 87:775–81.

97. Kleinman CS, Donnerstein RL, DeVore GR, et al. Fetal echocardiography for evaluation of in utero congestive heart failure. N Engl J Med. 1982; 306:568–75.

98. Kerenyi TD, Meller J, Steinfeld L, Gleicher N, Brown E, Chitkara U, Raucher H, et al. Transplacental cardioversion of intrauterine supraventricular tachycardia with digitalis. Lancet. 1980; 2:393–4.

99. Harrigan JT, Kangos JJ, Sikka A, et al. Successful treatment of fetal congestive heart failure secondary to tachycardia. N Engl J Med. 1981; 304:1527–9.

100. Lindheimer MD, Katz AI. Sodium and diuretics in pregnancy. N Engl J Med. 1973; 288:891–4.

101. Bonnar J. Venous thromboembolism and pregnancy. Clin Obstet Gynaecol. 1981; 8:455–73.

102. Clagett GP, Salzman EW. Prevention of venous thromboembolism. Prog Cardiovasc Dis. 1975; 17:345–66.

103. Handin RI. Thromboembolic complications of pregnancy and oral contraceptives. Prog Cardiovasc Dis. 1974; 16:395–405.

104. Wessler S. Drug prophylaxis for arterial thromboembolism—1981. JAMA. 1981; 246:2484–7.

105. Fell G, Strandness DE Jr. Diagnosis and management of acute venous thrombosis. Clin Obstet Gynecol. 1981; 24:761–72.

106. Hirsh J. Hypercoagulability. Semin Hematol. 1977; 14:409–25.

107. Flessa HC, Glueck HI, Dritschilo A. Thromboembolic disorders in pregnancy: pathophysiology, diagnosis, and treatment, with emphasis on heparin. Clin Obstet Gynecol. 1974; 17:195–235.

108. Brenner PF, Mishell DR Jr. Contraception for the woman with significant cardiac disease. Clin Obstet Gynecol. 1975; 18:155–68.

109. Wood JE. The cardiovascular effects of oral contraceptives. Mod Concepts Cardiovasc Dis. 1972; 41:37–40.

110. Bell WR, Simon TL, DeMets DL. The clinical features of submassive and massive pulmonary emboli. Am J Med. 1977; 62:355–60.

111. Rabinov K, Paulin S. Roentgen diagnosis of venous thrombosis in the leg. Arch Surg. 1972; 104:134–44.

112. Hull R, Hirsh J, Sackett DL, Powers P, Turpie AG, Walker I. Combined use of leg scanning and impedance plethysmography in suspected venous thrombosis: an alternative to venography. N Engl J Med. 1977; 296:1497–1500.

113. Wheeler HB, O'Donnell JA, Anderson FA, et al. Occlusive impedance phlebography: a diagnostic procedure for venous thrombosis and pulmonary embolism. Prog Cardiovasc Dis. 1974; 17:199–205.

114. Sumner DS. Venous dynamics—varicosities. Clin Obstet Gynecol. 1981; 24:743–60.

115. Moser KM, LeMoine JR. Is embolic risk conditioned by location of deep venous thrombosis? Ann Intern Med. 1981; 94:439–44.

116. Wagner HN Jr, Strauss HW. Radioactive tracers in the differential diagnosis of pulmonary embolism. Prog Cardiovasc Dis. 1975; 17:271–82.

117. Pauli RM, Hall JG, Wilson KM. Risks of anticoagulation during pregnancy. Am Heart J. 1980; 100:761–2.

118. Hall JG, Pauli RM, Wilson KM. Maternal and fetal sequelae of anticoagulation during pregnancy. Am J Med. 1980; 68:122–40.

119. Stevenson RE, Burton OM, Ferlauto GJ, Taylor HA. Hazards of oral anticoagulants during pregnancy. JAMA. 1980; 243:1549–51.

120. Spearing G, Fraser I, Turner G, Dixon G. Long-term self-administered subcutaneous heparin in pregnancy. Br Med J. 1978; 1:1457–8.

121. Rhodes GR, Dixon RH, Silver D. Heparin induced thrombocytopenia. Ann Surg. 1977; 186:752–8.

122. White PW, Sadd JR, Nensel RE. Thrombotic complications of heparin therapy. Ann Surg. 1979; 190:595–608.

123. Bell WR, Royall RM. Heparin-associated thrombocytopenia: a comparison of three heparin preparations. N Engl J Med. 1980; 303:902–7.

124. Genton E, Hirsh J. Observations in anticoagulant and thrombolytic therapy in pulmonary embolism. Prog Cardiovasc Dis. 1975; 17:335–43.

125. Salzman EW, Deykin D, Shapiro RM, Rosenberg R. Management of heparin therapy: controlled prospective trial. N Engl J Med. 1975; 292:1046–50.

126. Hull R, Delmore T, Carter C, et al. Adjusted subcutaneous heparin versus warfarin sodium in the long-term treatment of venous thrombosis. N Engl J Med. 1982; 306:189–94.

127. Levine HJ. Which atrial fibrillation patients should be on chronic anticoagulation? J Cardiovasc Med. 1981; 6:483–7.

128. Genton E, Gent M, Hirsh J, Harker LA. Platelet-inhibiting drugs in the prevention of clinical thrombotic disease. N Engl J Med. 1975; 293:1296–1300.

129. Hirsh J, Cade JF, Gallus AS. Anticoagulants in pregnancy: a review of indications and complications. Am Heart J. 1972; 83:301–5.

130. Hirsh J, Cade JF, O'Sullivan EF. Clinical experience with anticoagulant therapy during pregnancy. Br Med J. 1970; 1:270–3.

131. Orme ML, Lewis PJ, de Swiet M, et al. May mothers given warfarin breast-feed their infants? Br Med J. 1977; 1:1564–5.

132. Merrill LK, VerBurg DJ. The choice of long-term anticoagulants for the pregnant patient. Obstet Gynecol. 1976; 47:711–4.

133. Pfeifer GW. The use of thrombolytic therapy in obstetrics and gynaecology. Australas Ann Med. 1970; 19(Suppl):28–31.

134. Hall RJ, Young C, Sutton GC, et al. Treatment of acute massive pulmonary embolism by streptokinase during labour and delivery. Br Med J. 1972; 4:647–9.

135. Pfeifer GW. Distribution and placental transfer of 131 I streptokinase. Australas Ann Med. 1970; 19(Suppl):17–8.

136. Crane C. Venous interruption for pulmonary embolism: present status. Prog Cardiovasc Dis. 1975; 17:329–33.

137. Mobin-Uddin K, Utley JR, Bryant LR. The inferior vena cava umbrella filter. Prog Cardiovasc Dis. 1975; 17:391–9.

138. Pyeritz RE. Maternal and fetal complications of pregnancy in the Marfan syndrome. Am J Med. 1981; 71:784–90.

139. Clemens JD, Horwitz RI, Jaffe CC, et al. A controlled evaluation of the risk of bacterial endocarditis in persons with mitral-valve prolapse. N Engl J Med. 1982; 307:776–81.

140. Rotmensch HH, Elkayam U, Frishman W. Antiarrhythmic drug therapy during pregnancy. Ann Intern Med. 1983; 98:487–97.

Nor does it matter a whit with what food the body is nourished, so long as you can digest what you take, and distribute it abroad through the limbs, and preserve the moisture of the stomach uninterrupted.
—Lucretius

15. GASTROINTESTINAL DISORDERS
Andrew Mallory, Steven J. Ayres, and Barry W. Frank

Digestive tract disorders during pregnancy range from relatively innocuous episodes of nausea to profound exacerbations of chronic inflammatory bowel disease. Likewise, hepatic abnormalities can vary from mild biochemical disturbances to fulminant hepatic failure. Management of the pregnant woman with disorders of the digestive system must first involve an understanding of the functional and anatomic alterations that accompany normal gestation. It is then possible to evaluate and manage digestive disorders resulting from pregnancy as well as disorders that are coincidental with pregnancy. A summary of physiologic changes occurring in the digestive system during pregnancy is presented in Table 15-1, and these changes are discussed in the appropriate sections of this chapter.

LIVER DISEASE
Hepatic Function During Normal Pregnancy
No distinct changes in liver size or histology by light microscopy have been demonstrated as a consequence of normal pregnancy, but increased smooth and rough endoplasmic reticulum and free ribosomes have been detected with electron microscopy. Several biochemical alterations accompany normal pregnancy, and several tests of liver function deviate from the normal values established for nonpregnant women. Changes in liver function tests during normal pregnancy are summarized in Table 15-2.

In nonpregnant women, serum alkaline phosphatase (SAP) includes isoenzymes derived from liver, bone, and small intestine. In the gravida the placenta contains an alkaline phosphatase isoenzyme that is resistant to denaturation at 65°C; it is referred to as the "heat stable fraction." During the first half of pregnancy, SAP activity of placental origin increases slowly, then sharply rises at about the seventh month, reaching its peak at term. Values average from two to four times those found in non-

pregnant women [1–6]. Approximately 40 to 65% of SAP activity found in the third trimester is of placental origin [4]. Levels usually return to normal shortly after parturition but may take as long as six weeks.

In about 2 to 6% of uncomplicated pregnancies, the serum bilirubin may be elevated to 1 to 2 mg/dL, and in about 20% of pregnant women with a normal total bilirubin the conjugated fraction may be increased [7,8].

Serum total protein is decreased during normal pregnancy. Values fall during the first trimester to 80% of nonpregnant levels. The decrease in serum albumin, which falls to 66% of nonpregnant values during the first trimester, is primarily responsible for the decline seen in total protein. Serum globulins are generally elevated, with increases in alpha and beta fractions and a small decrease in gamma globulins [8].

With the knowledge of these changes in liver function tests during pregnancy, the minor deviations from nonpregnant values should not greatly interfere with the interpretation of the basic patterns of cholestasis or hepatocellular injury. When the clinical and laboratory picture is unclear, and when therapeutic decisions are dependent on a specific diagnosis, a liver biopsy is indicated. Needle biopsy of the liver is reported to carry no increased risk during pregnancy [9].

Liver Disease Associated with Pregnancy
Acute Fatty Liver of Pregnancy (AFLP)
AFLP is a rare disease first recognized by Stander and Cadden in 1934 and characterized by Sheehan in 1940 as "obstetric acute yellow atrophy" [10,11]. With more than 118 cases in the world literature, it is one of the most common causes of fulminant hepatic failure in pregnancy, and it is associated with a maternal and fetal mortality of greater than 80% and 70% respectively [12].

AFLP ordinarily affects the young primagravida during the third trimester. Initial symptoms are

Table 15-1. Physiologic changes during pregnancy

Area	Change	Etiology
Digestion	Nausea and vomiting ("morning sickness")	Possibly estrogens, HCG, psychogenic components
Appetite, thirst	Increased food cravings and aversions; less commonly, pica	Unknown
Mouth	Increased caries; gingivitis	Unknown
Esophagus	Decreased lower esophageal sphincter tone; increased percentage of nonperistaltic contractions in distal esophagus	Possibly progesterone
Stomach	Decreased motility; increased incidence of hiatal hernia	Possibly progesterone; mechanical effects of enlarged uterus
Liver	Palmar erythema, spider nevi, liver function tests (see Table 15-2)	Probably estrogens
	Liver biopsy specimens show no significant change on light microscopy; increased smooth and rough endoplasmic reticulum and free ribosomes on electron microscopy	Unknown
Small intestine	Possible decreased motility	Possibly progesterone
Large intestine	Possible decreased motility	Possibly progesterone
Appendix	Displacement upward in counterclockwise direction as gestation advances	Mechanical effects of expanding uterus
Rectosigmoid and anus	Increased constipation and hemorrhoids	Pressure effects of gravid uterus; possibly progesterone; straining at stool

Table 15-2. Liver function tests during normal pregnancy

Increased
  Serum alkaline phosphatase
  Serum leucine aminopeptidase
  BSP retention
  Serum ornithine-carbamyl-transferase
  Ceruloplasmin
  Serum copper
  α_1-Antitrypsin
  Alpha and beta globulins
Decreased
  Total serum protein concentration
  Serum albumin
  Serum ferritin
  Serum gamma globulin
No changes
  Serum bilirubin
  Serum transaminases
  Serum gamma glutamyl transpeptidase
Conflicting data
  5'-Nucleotidase

subtle and nonspecific. The patient may present with nausea, vomiting, lethargy, depressive mood change, psychosis, fatigue, malaise, or headache. Pain is a prominent symptom and is characterized as "burning" usually located in the substernal or epigastric region with variable radiation to the right upper quadrant or back. Jaundice is nearly universal; however, it may not be recognized early in the course. The liver is usually not palpable. As the disorder progresses, oliguria and renal failure are characteristic. The exact nature of the renal failure is not well understood, but altered hemodynamic factors as in the hepatorenal syndrome have been incriminated, and disseminated intravascular coagulation (DIC) may play a role [13].

The differential diagnosis of acute hepatic failure in pregnancy includes viral hepatitis and drug- or toxin-induced hepatic injury. A history should be sought regarding tetracycline therapy, recent halothane exposure, isoniazid treatment, and possible acetaminophen overdose.

In AFLP, tests of liver function usually show a predominantly conjugated (direct) hyperbilirubinemia with elevated serum transaminases reflecting hepatocellular injury. The serum glutamic oxaloacetic transaminase (SGOT) is likely to be elevated to a greater degree than the serum glutamic pyruvic transaminase (SGPT), with both usually being less than 500 units. These findings help differentiate AFLP from viral hepatitis, in which SGPT is usually greater than SGOT, levels higher than 500 units being common. SAP activity is moderately elevated and may in part be of placental origin. Anemia and marked leukocytosis are common. Elevations in serum amylase activity may be secondary to renal failure or associated pancreatitis. Prolongation of the prothrombin time and partial thromboplastin time, thrombocytopenia, hypofibrinogenemia, and elevated fibrin split products indicate DIC. Liver biopsy is the most specific diagnostic test. The characteristic pathologic change is infiltration of all the hepatic cells by fine fatty droplets, without the necrosis that characterizes viral hepatitis [14].

Medical management does not differ from that of liver failure in nonpregnant patients. Immediate termination of pregnancy may improve maternal survival as well as survival of the mature fetus [7,12].

Intrahepatic Cholestasis of Pregnancy
Intrahepatic cholestasis of pregnancy (ICP) has been described under a variety of names, including *hepatosis of pregnancy, benign recurrent cholestasis of pregnancy, idiopathic jaundice of pregnancy,* and *pruritus gravidarum.* It is clinically characterized by either icterus, pruritus, or both. The major lesion is intrahepatic cholestasis with centrolobular bile staining without inflammatory cells or proliferation of mesenchymal cells. The pathogenesis of ICP is not known.

The patient characteristically presents with increasingly severe pruritus followed in one or two weeks by jaundice. Onset of pruritus is usually in the latter half of pregnancy but may be as early as six weeks [15]. Dark urine and acholic stools accompany the jaundice, but the patient feels well, without abdominal pain, fever, or malaise. Pruritus and jaundice persist until delivery and then uniformly disappear within several hours to several weeks.

Tests of liver function reflect cholestasis without prominent signs of hepatocellular injury. The predominantly conjugated (direct) hyperbilirubinemia is mild, with values generally ranging from 2 to 5 mg/dL. Higher values suggest another process. The serum alkaline phosphatase is moderately elevated above its normal minimally increased activity during the third trimester.

Liver histology shows only mild cholestasis with some intracellular bile and bile canalicular plugs. Inflammation and hepatocellular necrosis are absent or minimal, and the lack of these findings serves to distinguish ICP from viral hepatitis.

Management of ICP includes three general goals: (1) relief of pruritus, (2) prevention of secondary effects of malabsorption, and (3) assessment of fetal well-being.

Relief of pruritus can be achieved by reduction of serum bile acid levels. In ICP the efficiency of hepatic extraction of bile acids from blood is the principal derangement. After postprandial reabsorption of bile acids from the ileum, their rate of disappearance from the serum is prolonged. Bile salt-binding resins are capable of lowering serum bile acid levels but must mechanically mix with the bile acid pool in order to be effective. Timing their administration to coincide with gallbladder contraction is important. Javitt recommends giving 4 g of cholestyramine before a breakfast that includes fat or protein or both to stimulate gallbladder contraction, followed by 4 g after breakfast and 4 g before lunch [16].

ICP is a disease of relatively short duration; therefore, clinical effects of fat malabsorption are minimal. However, if maternal cholestasis is severe and prolonged, vitamin K deficiency may occur. Since the hepatic synthesis of coagulation factors II, VII, IX, and X requires adequate tissue levels of vitamin K, a deficiency may promote postpartum hemorrhage in these women. Prophylactic administration of parenteral vitamin K is recommended [15,16].

The influence of ICP on fetal prognosis is controversial. Recent studies have shown an increased incidence of prematurity, fetal distress, and stillbirth in patients with ICP [17]. The cause is unknown, but it has been suggested that ICP may permit unknown substances to cross the placenta and alter fetal steroid metabolism, thereby affecting placental function and the course of pregnancy. The individual fetus at risk for intrauterine death cannot be identified. Although interruption of pregnancy "cures" ICP, it is not indicated as the disease carries little risk for the mother.

The Liver in Preeclampsia and Eclampsia
The liver is not usually affected in preeclampsia and eclampsia. Jaundice occurs in approximately 10% of eclamptic patients but is usually related to hemolysis. Jaundice is occasionally related to hepatic dysfunction, in which case the prognosis is poor. Relatively minor increases in alkaline phosphatase and transaminases are more common. Increasing jaundice, anemia, and hepatomegaly should alert the physician to the possibility of an intrahepatic hematoma, which may rupture and require emergent surgical intervention. Histologic findings in preeclampsia are variable; focal areas of eosinophilic and fibrinoid necrosis are most common. In fatal eclampsia, periportal necrosis and extensive hemorrhagic necrosis are often seen.

There is no specific treatment for the acute liver abnormalities that accompany preeclampsia or eclampsia. Rather, management is directed at the underlying disorder. Termination of pregnancy is essential when severe hepatic dysfunction is evident.

Spontaneous Rupture of the Liver

Spontaneous rupture of the liver is a rare and potentially catastrophic complication of pregnancy. The correct preoperative diagnosis has been made in only 10% of reported cases. A review of 89 cases revealed a maternal mortality of 59% and a fetal mortality of 62% [18].

The exact etiology is not known. Although rupture of the liver in nonpregnant patients is almost always a direct result of trauma, a history of injury is absent or unremarkable with "spontaneous" rupture during pregnancy. More than 80% of reported cases are associated with preeclampsia or eclampsia [19].

Rupture of the liver usually occurs in the older multiparous patient late in the third trimester [20]. The initial symptom is abdominal pain located in the epigastrium or right upper quadrant, often with radiation to the back or right shoulder. The pattern of pain is not characteristic and has been mistakenly diagnosed as indicating peptic ulcer disease, biliary colic, pancreatitis, pulmonary embolus, and myocardial infarction. Associated symptoms may include nausea, vomiting, syncope, and abdominal swelling.

The presenting signs are variable and depend on the stage of the disease. Initially signs of preeclampsia or eclampsia may predominate; the liver may be enlarged and tender. With impending rupture or hemoperitoneum, the abdominal exam may reveal an ileus with distention, tympany, and hypoactive or absent bowel sounds. Purpuric lesions and bleeding from venipuncture sites suggest disseminated intravascular coagulation. Rupture and hemoperitoneum present with signs of hypovolemic shock.

The laboratory may be of minimal assistance in the diagnosis. A falling hematocrit without evidence of gastrointestinal bleeding or hemolysis may help in diagnosing hemoperitoneum, but initially the hematocrit may remain unchanged. Leukocytosis may be present but is nonspecific. Abnormalities of liver function tests are often observed but are not diagnostic.

Paracentesis or culdocentesis can yield valuable information; demonstration of intraperitoneal blood indicates the need for laparotomy.

Once the diagnosis is made, continuation of the pregnancy has been reported to worsen the prognosis for mother and fetus [21,22]. If the diagnosis of subcapsular hematoma is made prior to rupture, treatment should be directed toward management of preeclampsia or eclampsia, if present, and a cesarean delivery performed. Once the hematoma has ruptured, all patients require an operation.

Liver Disease Coincidental with Pregnancy

Acute Viral Hepatitis

Acute viral hepatitis is a common acute inflammatory disease of the liver caused by any of at least three strains of viruses. Type A hepatitis (formerly called infectious, short-incubation, or MS-1 hepatitis) is caused by hepatitis A virus (HAV), a 27-nm RNA virus. Type B hepatitis (formerly called serum, posttransfusion, long-incubation, MS-2, or Australia antigen hepatitis) is caused by hepatitis B virus (HBV), a 42-nm DNA virus. One or more additional virus(es) referred to as non-A, non-B virus(es) are responsible for approximately 90% of posttransfusion hepatitis and an unknown percentage of nontransfusion-associated cases. The nomenclature of hepatitis is summarized in Table 15-3, and the temporal sequence of serologic markers is depicted in Figures 15-1 and 15-2.

Reports from the United States and Europe indicate that the susceptibility, clinical course, abnormalities of liver function, and hepatic histology of viral hepatitis complicating pregnancy are the same as those found in the general nonpregnant population. Women in underdeveloped countries may suffer more often and more severely from viral hepatitis than the general population.

Pregnancies in women with acute viral hepatitis are generally uncomplicated. The incidence of preterm birth is approximately 20% [9]. Preterm delivery appears to be more common when acute viral hepatitis develops in the mother during the third trimester [23]. There is no correlation between preterm birth and the duration of jaundice, level of serum bilirubin, or severity of the course of hepatitis. Fetal survival depends on the degree of maturity of the infant and does not appear to be related to maternal health [7]. Spontaneous abortion is more frequent in mothers with acute viral hepatitis during the first trimester, or with hepatic coma. The incidence of fetal malformations is not increased [7]. Mothers who are carriers of hepatitis B surface antigen (HBsAg) have been shown to deliver a relative excess of male infants [24–26]. A selective increase in spontaneous abortions of female embryos has been postulated [24]. In mothers with viral hepatitis, in whom jaundice has resolved at the time of delivery, the amniotic fluid may still contain high levels of bilirubin. This finding may lead to the mistaken diagnosis of an Rh-immunized fetus [27].

Patients suspected of having viral hepatitis

Table 15-3. Hepatitis nomenclature

Term	Abbreviation	Comments
Hepatitis A virus	HAV	Causal agent of infectious hepatitis; probably an enterovirus; single serotype
Antibody to HAV	Anti-HAV	IgM detectable at onset of symptoms; lifetime persistence of IgG
Hepatitis B virus	HBV	Causal agent of serum or long-incubation hepatitis; also known as Dane particle
Hepatitis B surface antigen	HBsAg	Surface antigen(s) of HBV, detectable in large quantity in serum; several subtypes identified
Hepatitis Be antigen	HBeAg	Soluble antigen; correlates with HBV replication, high-titer HBV in serum, and infectivity of serum
Hepatitis B core antigen	HBcAg	No commercial test available
Antibody to HBsAg	Anti-HBs	Indicates past infection with and immunity to HBV, passive antibody from hepatitis B immune globulin, or immune response from HBV vaccine
Antibody to HBeAg	Anti-HBe	Presence in serum of HBsAg carrier suggests lower titer of HBV
Antibody to HBcAg	Anti-HBc	Indicates past infection with HBV at some undefined time
Non-A, non-B hepatitis	NANB	Diagnosis of exclusion; at least two candidate viruses; epidemiology parallels that of hepatitis B

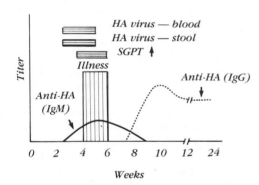

Fig. 15-1. Temporal sequence of serologic markers in acute hepatitis A.

Fig. 15-2. Temporal sequence of serologic markers in acute hepatitis B.

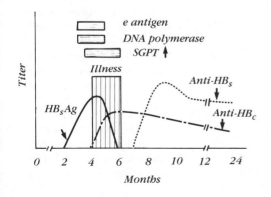

should have a baseline determination of the following laboratory tests: complete blood count (CBC), glucose, prothrombin time, SGOT or aspartate aminotransferase (AST), SGPT or alanine aminotransferase (ALT), serum alkaline phosphatase, serum bilirubin (total and direct), serum albumin and total protein, and viral serology including HBsAg, anti-HAV (IgM type), and anti-HBe (antibody to the e antigen). Early in the course of disease, serum transaminase values are elevated, often above 750 IU, reflecting hepatocellular damage. A cholestatic component may develop, when both conjugated and unconjugated bilirubin may be elevated. The serum alkaline phosphatase activity may be mildly increased. The height of elevation of serum transaminases has no prognostic significance. A prolonged prothrombin time, a low serum albumin level, or a bilirubin level greater than 15 mg/dL usually indicates severe disease. In 85% of patients laboratory abnormalities return to normal within 6 to 12 weeks. HBeAg and anti-HBe are not routinely determined but may be useful in patients with suspected chronic hepatitis.

Most patients with viral hepatitis can be managed as outpatients with close follow-up. There is no specific therapy for viral hepatitis. Patients should be advised to obtain adequate rest and caloric intake and to avoid ethanol consumption. Corticosteroids and antibiotics are not indicated. Antiemetics may be necessary in some patients, and metoclopramide may be a better choice than phenothiazines because it increases the rate of gastric emptying and has no deleterious effects on hepatic function. Phenothiazines can impair hepatic excretory function and may cause cholestasis.

Some pregnant women with viral hepatitis may require hospitalization. Women with intractable nausea and vomiting should be hospitalized for parenteral hydration and glucose administration. Patients with severe hepatitis have decreased hepatic glycogen stores, and in the presence of inadequate oral intake, hypoglycemia may occur. Women with severe anemia (e.g., G6PD deficiency) or diabetes mellitus may require hospitalization, since hepatitis complicates the management of these conditions.

Vertical transmission of maternal hepatitis B to the neonate can occur and correlates with the presence of maternal HBeAg. Okada et al. originally reported a series of HBsAg-positive mothers in which all ten infants of HBeAg-positive mothers became carriers of HBsAg. No infants of seven anti-HBe-positive mothers (HBeAg negative) became HBsAg carriers. Two of six infants of mothers who were negative for HBeAg and anti-HBe became HBsAg carriers [28]. Overall, approximately two-thirds of infants of mothers who have acute hepatitis B late in pregnancy or in the postpartum period can be expected to become positive for HBsAg [29]. When acute hepatitis B occurs early in pregnancy, HBsAg is detectable much less frequently in the neonates. In the United States the frequency of detectable infection in neonates when mothers are chronic carriers of HBsAg ranges from 5 to 35% [29,30].

In most infants who become carriers of HBsAg the antigenemia develops from six weeks to six months after delivery, suggesting viral transmission during the intrapartum or postpartum period. The long-term sequelae of antigenemia in these infants are unknown because of short follow-up periods, but, as in adults, they are assumed to be at risk for developing chronic active hepatitis, hepatoma, and possibly polyarteritis nodosa. Neonatal infection with HBV may take various forms. The most common picture is subclinical hepatitis with mild elevation of serum transaminases and development of the chronic HBsAg carrier state [9]. A less prevalent form of neonatal infection is clinical hepatitis manifested as "failure to thrive." Although rare, severe fatal hepatitis and chronic liver disease with cirrhosis and death may occur [31,32].

The route and timing of vertical transmission of HBV are controversial. As previously noted, the temporal occurrence of antigenemia in the infant suggests viral transmission during the latter part of pregnancy or early postpartum period. Fetal infection from oral contamination with maternal blood or feces during passage through the birth canal has been suggested. Lee et al. showed that 95% of in-fants had high-titer HBsAg in the gastric aspirate and considered this a possible portal of infection [33]. However, the fact that cesarean delivery is reported not to prevent transmission argues against this mode [34,35]. Transplacental transmission of HBV has been postulated, and HBsAg has been identified in umbilical cord blood [36,37]. Whether transmission occurs during pregnancy or by microscopic blood leaks across the placenta during labor and delivery is unclear.

HBsAg has been identified in maternal breast milk, but its role in vertical transmission is unproved [38]. Two studies found no correlation between breast-feeding and development of antigenemia in infants of HBsAg carrier mothers [39,40]. Breast-feeding in this situation is currently permitted, but the subject is controversial [41].

Immunoprophylaxis of the newborn with hepatitis B immunoglobulin (HBIG) has been studied by several investigators. A recent randomized, double-blind, placebo-controlled trial from Taiwan reported the efficacy of HBIG for the prevention of the vertically transmitted HBsAg carrier state [42]. Infants of mothers who were hepatitis BeAg positive, HBsAg carriers received either placebo, one dose of HBIG immediately after birth, or HBIG immediately after birth and at three and six months post partum; carrier rates in infants were 91%, 45%, and 23% for the three groups, respectively. The primary effect of HBIG in the newborn was prevention of HBsAg persistence, rather than actual prevention of HBV infection. The most common response to HBIG was development of the passive-active immunization although true passive immunity also occurred. The current recommendations from the Centers for Disease Control (CDC) regarding immunoprophylaxis of the newborn are that all infants born of HBsAg-positive mothers receive HBIG, a total dose of 0.5 mL intramuscularly, as soon after birth as possible (no later than 24 hours). The same dose should be repeated at three months and five months [43]. It is crucial that the HBIG be given as soon after birth as possible, as Beasley and Stevens found that persistent antigenemia developed in fewer infants who received HBIG at less than 48 hours of age than in those who received it at 48 hours or more [44]. Immune serum globulin (ISG) containing low-titer anti-HBs is not protective to infants born of HBsAg carrier mothers or to infants of mothers with acute hepatitis B during the delivery period [45].

A situation may arise in which a mother convalescing from acute hepatitis B, or a mother who has chronic liver disease does not have detectable HBsAg or anti-HBs, yet does have a positive test for anti-HBc. Studies of HBV transmission by blood transfusion suggest that in this situation the presence of anti-HBc indicates HBV virus infection and persistent viral replication with some detectable amounts of HBsAg in the circulation [46,47]. Although there are no studies addressing this situation, it would seem reasonable that infants born of mothers with this serology should receive HBIG under the same CDC guidelines recommended for infants of HBsAg-positive mothers.

Vertical transmission of hepatitis A or non-A, non-B, although uncommon, is possible [31,48, 49]. It has been recommended that infants born of mothers with acute hepatitis A or of mothers with chronic or acute non-A, non-B hepatitis should receive one dose of ISG (0.5 mL) intramuscularly immediately after delivery [50,51].

Chronic Hepatitis and Cirrhosis

Chronic hepatitis may be associated with viral disease, drugs, or various immune mechanisms. Clinically, cases can be characterized as chronic persistent hepatitis with a benign course requiring no therapy, or chronic active hepatitis, which can progress to cirrhosis and early death [52].

Women with chronic persistent hepatitis have been observed to have normal ovulatory cycles and no apparent problems with conception [53]. In contrast, anovulatory cycles are frequent in women with chronic active hepatitis [54]. However, conception is possible in all forms of chronic hepatitis and cirrhosis, even with previous manifestations of liver failure or previous portacaval shunts.

Pregnancy in chronic persistent hepatitis can be assumed to be safe for mother and child. It has been shown that pregnancy does not affect the clinical or biochemical course of the disease. In one series, pregnancies proceeded normally to term and all neonates were normal [53].

The effect of pregnancy in women with chronic active hepatitis is more controversial; while some authors report a significant maternal morbidity and mortality, others do not [54–57]. Nevertheless, the risk to the fetus is significant. The rate of abortion has been reported to be approximately 8%, stillbirth 10%, and preterm birth 15%. The varying reports from the literature may represent differences in the severity of the disease at the time of conception and the presence or absence of significant cirrhosis. One series reported no maternal deaths and four perinatal deaths from 30 pregnancies in women with chronic active hepatitis [54]. There was no apparent deterioration in maternal chronic active hepatitis during or after pregnancy, but the fetus was at risk from prematurity and low birth weight. Treatment with corticosteroids or azathioprine was continued safely throughout gestation [54,58].

Cirrhosis, from any cause, may often be associated with normal pregnancy and full-term delivery [54,56,59]. However, approximately 20% of pregnant women with cirrhosis decompensate with worsening liver function aggravated by the enlarging uterus, ascites, liver failure, or hemorrhage. The prognosis is poor for cirrhotics who decompensate during the first trimester, and therapeutic abortion should be considered.

During pregnancy, portal pressure increases along with venous return through the azygous system [60]. In the second stage of labor there is a dramatic increase in portal pressure. Hemorrhage from esophageal varices can occur at any time and should be treated as in the nonpregnant cirrhotic. If bleeding does not stop or recurs, the decision for portacaval shunt or therapeutic abortion must be considered. Splenorenal shunt has been advised for the pregnant patient [61].

Ascites should be treated as in the nonpregnant cirrhotic patient. Paracentesis is indicated for diagnostic reasons or for therapeutic indications if ascites is interfering with the normal progression of labor or causing maternal respiratory distress.

Postpartum hemorrhage can occur from defects in factors V and VII and less frequently from true prothrombin deficiency or thrombocytopenia due to hypersplenism. Treatment includes fresh whole blood and fresh frozen plasma.

Drug-Induced Jaundice

Drugs known to cause jaundice may do so in the gravida as well as the nonpregnant woman [62]. Pregnancy bestows neither resistance nor susceptibility to drug-induced jaundice, and each patient must be carefully questioned regarding medications taken. The mechanism may be due to (1) interference of the drug with biliary secretion, (2) liver cell toxicity, or (3) drug-induced hemolysis [9]. Cases of drug-induced jaundice do not differ in their course or severity during pregnancy. Sedatives, tranquilizers, antibiotics, antiemetics, anesthetics, diuretics, antihypertensives, and anti-inflammatory agents are medications used during pregnancy and are potentially associated with jaundice [63]. Withdrawal of the medication usually leads to prompt and complete resolution of the clinical and biochemical problem.

Wilson's Disease

Wilson's disease or hepatolenticular degeneration is an inborn error of copper metabolism transmitted by an autosomal recessive gene. The effect of Wilson's disease and its treatment on pregnancy has been reviewed by Toaff et al. [64]. Prior to the use of D-penicillamine for treatment of the disorder, infertility or spontaneous abortion was common. Walshe, however, reported 15 pregnancies in 11 women with Wilson's disease treated with D-penicillamine. Fourteen of the pregnancies reached term and the progeny were normal. One child was preterm and died [65].

Treatment of Wilson's disease is based on the assumption that high tissue and organ copper concentrations bring about the histologic and physiologic damage. During pregnancy there is a continuous slow rise of both free copper and copper bound to ceruloplasmin [66]. The elevated plasma copper of pregnancy may thereby provide a concentration gradient that permits transfer of free copper across the placenta for fetal storage.

Principles of management of Wilson's disease during pregnancy include minimizing dietary absorption of copper and enhancing excretion of absorbed copper. A copper-poor diet should be combined with D-penicillamine, the most effective available promoter of copper excretion.

Primary Biliary Cirrhosis

Pregnancy is uncommon in this progressive, severe liver disease of unknown etiology, because the disease usually occurs in women beyond the childbearing years [67]. When pregnancy has occurred in younger patients, it has been tolerated well. Pregnancy does not seem to alter the course of the disease, but the risk of spontaneous abortion may be increased [68]. Increasingly, patients with primary biliary cirrhosis are being recognized at a presymptomatic stage. Early in the course of the disorder during pregnancy it may be confused with cholestatic jaundice of pregnancy. The overall poor prognosis of the disease necessitates careful family counseling.

Familial Nonhemolytic Hyperbilirubinemia

The three forms of nonhemolytic hyperbilirubinemia most commonly encountered are Gilbert's syndrome (idiopathic unconjugated hyperbilirubinemia), Dubin-Johnson syndrome (chronic idiopathic jaundice), and Rotor syndrome [69]. An increase in jaundice during pregnancy has been noted in the Dubin-Johnson syndrome and tends to continue throughout the gestational period [7]. In icteric patients there appears to be an association with spontaneous abortion and stillbirth [70]. The biochemical and clinical course of Gilbert's and Rotor syndromes

seems to be unaffected by pregnancy. All are benign forms of jaundice and need no therapy during or after pregnancy.

BILIARY TRACT DISEASE
Biliary Tract Alterations in Normal Pregnancy

The study of bile and gallbladder function in pregnancy is important because of the well-documented increased prevalence of cholesterol gallstones in association with pregnancy [71,72]. Bennion and others have studied biliary lipid composition in males and females before and during puberty and in women influenced by sex hormone administration [73,74]. They found that the bile acid pool is smaller in women than in men. During puberty in the female and following contraceptive steroids bile becomes more saturated with cholesterol. Collection of bile from the duodenum in pregnant women has also demonstrated a bile more saturated with cholesterol [75].

The normal gallbladder distends with bile, with only small increases of pressure until full distention causes pressure to rise sharply. Gallbladder emptying is regulated by neural and hormonal factors, the most important of which is the hormone cholecystokinin. Released from the small intestine during ingestion of a meal, cholecystokinin contracts the gallbladder by means of a direct effect on smooth muscle. Other gastrointestinal hormones, such as secretin or vasoactive intestinal peptide, inhibit the effect of cholecystokinin. Thus, gallbladder contraction and subsequent refilling are regulated by hormones that interact with cholecystokinin. Studies of gallbladder function in pregnancy suggest that the female hormones also impair gallbladder contraction in response to cholecystokinin. Everson et al. showed that in pregnancy fasting gallbladder volume is increased and emptying after a small-volume liquid meal is incomplete [76].

Essential prerequisites for cholesterol gallstone formation during pregnancy have been identified. There is a hepatic excretion of lithogenic bile, and the lithogenic bile is retained in the gallbladder in the fasting and postprandial state. Lithogenic bile retention would allow for nucleation, crystal formation, and adherence of crystals necessary to generate gallstones.

Gallstones: Clinical Course and Diagnosis

A pregnant patient with gallstones may be entirely asymptomatic, have minimal complaints associated with a chronic form of cholecystitis, or present with an acute, sometimes life-threatening event. Although often thought to be diagnostically significant, symptoms of excessive flatulence, heartburn, postprandial bloating, and intolerance to fatty foods have not been shown to be more common in patients with gallstones [77].

Asymptomatic calculi occasionally have been observed with diagnostic ultrasound in pregnant patients undergoing evaluation for other abdominal or renal complaints, or there may be a history of preexisting stone disease found by other diagnostic modalities prior to the pregnancy. If the patient is asymptomatic, no therapy is indicated, particularly elective cholecystectomy because of the unnecessary risk to the fetus.

Gallstones can produce biliary colic, acute cholecystitis, or chronic cholecystitis. All are usually a consequence of cystic duct obstruction by a gallstone. The pain of biliary colic usually begins in the right upper quadrant or epigastrium, is abrupt in onset, and may radiate to the back. It may last for several minutes to several hours, during which time the patient moves about with great discomfort. There may be associated nausea, vomiting, anorexia, diaphoresis. The attacks are frequently recurrent. Between attacks, patients are usually asymptomatic. Acute cholecystitis usually begins with biliary colic but is longer in duration and associated with increasing signs of inflammation such as fever, tachycardia, and marked right upper quadrant tenderness. Jaundice may occur. Passage of the stone into the common bile duct may initiate pancreatitis. When the disease becomes chronic, there may be repeated attacks in which the above symptoms vary from attack to attack.

Physical examination in the pregnant patient with any one of these conditions may reveal exquisite tenderness in the right upper abdomen and epigastrium. A distended gallbladder is rarely palpated. Rebound tenderness may be present. When the examiner's hand is lightly pressed in the right upper quadrant, the patient may be unable to take a deep breath. Bowel sounds are not disturbed. When there is associated sepsis, involuntary guarding or rigidity may be present.

These symptoms and physical findings in the pregnant patient must be differentiated from those in other conditions. Appendicitis, acute hepatitis, primary pancreatitis, perforated peptic ulcer, bowel obstruction, renal colic, pyelonephritis, pulmonary embolus, and pneumonia must be considered in the differential diagnosis.

Clinical laboratory information may be difficult to interpret because of the normal elevations of leukocytes and alkaline phosphatase in pregnancy. However, the findings of an elevated gamma glutamyl transpeptidase (GGT), SGOT, amylase, or bilirubin in the serum should focus the clinician's attention on the gallbladder.

In the pregnant patient it is inadvisable to expose the fetus to radiation unless absolutely necessary. Fortunately, diagnostic ultrasound has proved to be quite helpful in the diagnosis of gallstones during pregnancy, with an accuracy rate of about 95% [78].

Patients with biliary colic can usually be treated with pain medication alone. Management of the patient with acute cholecystitis should begin with hospitalization and strict periodic observation with physical examination and serial blood chemistries. Initial therapy should take the form of intravenous fluids and colloid while oral intake is restricted. Meperidine is the drug of choice to control pain because it has less effect than morphine on the sphincter of Oddi. If there is vomiting, abdominal distention, or absent bowel sounds, intermittent nasogastric suction is indicated. Antibiotics should not be used unless there is evidence of sepsis, the patient is diabetic, or surgery is imminent. Only occasionally is there need for emergency surgical intervention. The most common indication for cholecystectomy in pregnancy is exacerbation of chronic cholecystitis that cannot be controlled medically. If at all possible, elective cholecystectomy should be performed in the late second trimester, when the incidence of spontaneous abortion is decreased [79,80].

DIGESTIVE TRACT DISEASE
Digestive Tract Alterations in Normal Pregnancy

A summary of digestive tract alterations is given in Table 15-1. The esophagus is probably the best-studied organ in the digestive tract, and the changes listed are well documented. Evidence regarding gastric acid secretion is conflicting; various authors have reported decreased, normal, or increased acid output. The weight of evidence currently suggests little change in fasting or stimulated acid output. Studies of serum amylase are likewise conflicting, with reports of increased, normal, and decreased levels. Although it is commonly written that bowel motility is decreased during pregnancy, evidence for this finding comes largely from in vitro studies of the effect of progesterone on human colonic smooth muscle.

Gastroesophageal Reflux

Gastroesophageal reflux with symptomatic heartburn is a common clinical problem in pregnancy. It occurs in 40 to 50% of all pregnant women and tends to be worse in the third trimester [81–83]. Studies of lower esophageal sphincter pressures have shown a progressive pressure reduction during pregnancy in association with gastroesophageal reflux [83]. Factors such as hiatal hernia and increase in abdominal pressure do not correlate with the presence of reflux or symptomatic heartburn.

Recent studies have shown that hormonal events associated with and specific for pregnancy are responsible for the decrease in lower esophageal sphincter pressure and the symptom of heartburn. Van Thiel et al. demonstrated that the lower esophageal sphincter pressure is reduced at all times during pregnancy [83]. The reduction is due to a progressive increase in plasma progesterone, alone or in combination with estrogens, that occurs during pregnancy.

Treatment of heartburn should consist in avoidance of large meals, caffeine, alcohol, tobacco, mints, and chocolate. The head of the bed should be elevated 4 to 6 inches on blocks. Liquid antacids should be used one hour after meals and at bedtime. Antacids should be selected according to the patient's preference, the need for sodium restriction, and the side effects of diarrhea or constipation. Alginic acid-containing antacids may provide additional benefit. Other medications helpful in this disease (e.g., cimetidine, metoclopramide, and bethanechol chloride) have had only limited use during pregnancy and should not be ordinarily employed.

Nausea and Vomiting

Nausea and vomiting are common complaints occurring in 50 to 80% of pregnant women [84,85]. Symptoms generally begin soon after the first missed menstrual period and usually last less than 12 weeks. Nutritional status is not likely to be impaired, but various metabolic abnormalities can occur if vomiting is protracted or caloric intake is significantly reduced.

In the majority of cases symptoms can be managed by avoidance of known noxious foods or odors, frequent small carbohydrate-rich meals, and reassurance that the condition is self-limited. In some cases antiemetic drugs are necessary. Several antiemetics are effective in nonpregnant patients, but none has been certified as safe for use during pregnancy.

Hyperemesis Gravidarum

This condition is characterized by severe nausea and intractable vomiting, beginning before the twentieth week of gestation and of such severity as to require hospital admission. There may be associated abdominal pain, which is usually poorly localized. The patients lose weight, become dehydrated, and can develop severe electrolyte alterations, ketosis, and neurologic disturbances. Death can occur in untreated patients.

Examination may show physical evidence of dehydration, orthostatic changes in blood pressure and pulse, and generalized abdominal tenderness. Bowel sounds may be diminished. The liver may be slightly enlarged if weight loss has been significant.

Laboratory examination should include a CBC, urinalysis, and assessment of electrolytes and liver and thyroid function. Because of the association of severe nausea and vomiting in women with hydatidiform moles, an abdominal ultrasound is indicated if symptoms occur in the first few weeks of pregnancy. Hospitalization and prompt correction of fluid and electrolyte disturbances are essential.

Peptic Ulcer Disease

Virtually all authors agree that the incidence of peptic ulcer and its complications decreases during pregnancy. There are virtually no convincing data to confirm this impression. Most authors also state that symptoms of preexisting ulcer disease diminish during pregnancy. Seeking support of this assumption, Clark interviewed women with preexisting ulcer disease who became pregnant [86]. In 313 pregnancies, 45% of women became symptom free; 43% had persistent symptoms but were improved. No complications developed during pregnancy. Improvement was short-lived; symptoms recurred within six months of parturition in 75% of women. Indirect support for a favorable effect of pregnancy on the course of ulcer disease comes from studies showing benefits of estrogens in promoting ulcer healing [87].

The incidence of peptic ulcer may be high in women with eclampsia and preeclampsia [88].

The diagnosis of ulcer disease is usually strongly suggested by the history. Barium studies and endoscopy should rarely be necessary except perhaps in the presence of complications. In doubtful cases, it is probably wiser to treat for peptic disease and defer diagnostic studies until after delivery.

Management of peptic ulcer disease includes attention to diet, antacids, and drugs capable of decreasing gastric acid secretion. Diet should consist of three meals a day of the patient's own choosing. Patients should be instructed to avoid coffee and alcohol during the acute episode and to abstain from any food that exacerbates symptoms. Bedtime snacks may cause unbuffered nocturnal acid secretion and should be avoided. The value of frequent small meals has not been adequately studied, but a theoretical disadvantage is that continuous secretion of acid may result. At least four studies have shown no benefit from a bland diet.

Cigarette smoking should be proscribed because of evidence that smoking may delay healing of peptic ulcers [89].

Antacids are generally considered safe in pregnancy although one study has demonstrated an increased use of antacids in the first trimester in a group of women giving birth to infants with anomalies [90]. Antacids vary in potency. In general, enough antacid should be given to neutralize 80 mEq of acid. Because of slowed gastric emptying following meals, antacids should be given one and three hours postprandially. A dose at bedtime, although not totally effective in neutralizing nocturnal acid secretion, is probably also useful.

Cimetidine has been shown to be effective in healing duodenal and probably gastric ulcers. Its safety in pregnancy has not been established, however. Its use should therefore be restricted to the rare instance of antacid failure.

Sucralfate, an aluminum salt of sucrose octasulfate, has been shown to be as effective as cimetidine in healing duodenal ulcers. Although less than 5% is absorbed, its safety in pregnancy has not been demonstrated.

Anticholinergics, although apparently safe in pregnancy, are probably ineffective in promoting healing of peptic ulcer when used alone. They may have a role as adjunctive therapy in combination with antacids or cimetidine in patients refractory to conventional therapy.

Management of complications of peptic ulcer (bleeding, perforation, obstruction) is in general similar in the pregnant and nonpregnant patient. In the patient with refractory symptoms, every effort should be made to postpone surgery until after delivery.

Constipation

Constipation is generally thought to be a common complication of pregnancy although a study by Levy et al. [91] could not confirm this claim. Extrinsic pressure on the rectum by the enlarged uterus, inefficiency of levator ani muscles, decreased exercise, decreased fluid intake, and decreased contractility of bowel have been held responsible.

Organic etiologies (e.g., anal fissure, fecal impaction, hypothyroidism) should be ruled out by history, physical exam, and appropriate laboratory tests. If no cause is found, initial therapy should consist in reviewing with the patient the value of exercise, regularity of meals, and adequate dietary roughage. A hot beverage with breakfast coupled

with allowance of enough time after breakfast to permit an unhurried visit to the bathroom may take useful advantage of the gastrocolic reflex. Use of psyllium preparations in increasing dosages will often be helpful. For hard stools, stool softeners (dioctyl sodium sulfosuccinate, mineral oil) by mouth or enema are indicated. Osmotic diuretics (magnesium hydroxide, phosphates, magnesium citrate) are considered safe in the absence of renal failure. Lactulose is often effective, but its safety in pregnancy has not yet been established. Finally, if the above fail, bowel stimulants (e.g., bisacodyl, senna, cascara) may be necessary and are generally considered safe for the pregnant woman.

Hemorrhoids

The incidence of symptomatic hemorrhoids appears to be increased in pregnancy, presumably as a result of increased intraabdominal pressure transmitted to the pelvic veins. Symptoms include bleeding, presence of a mass, mucoid discharge, itching, and pain. Bleeding usually appears as a red streak or spot on the surface of the stool or toilet paper. It may present as a jet of blood during straining or may drip into the toilet water after defecation. Prolapsing hemorrhoids may at first appear only during defecation; later, they may persist and require manual reduction. Rarely they may become irreducible. Pain is usually a result of thrombosis or associated inflammation.

External hemorrhoids are visible in the subcutaneous tissue distal to the dentate line and are covered by skin. Internal hemorrhoids are not visible externally unless they are prolapsed and cannot be palpated on rectal exam unless thrombosed. With the anoscope they appear as blue masses covered by rectal mucosa. When they are prolapsing, moist red mucosa is seen to cover at least the upper portions of the mass.

Measures thought to be helpful in preventing symptomatic hemorrhoids in the pregnant patient include intake of a high-roughage diet and stool softeners to prevent constipation, avoidance of straining at stool, avoidance of prolonged sitting on the toilet, and prompt response to the urge to defecate.

If symptomatic hemorrhoids develop, medical therapy will usually suffice. Stool softeners (e.g., psyllium preparations, dioctyl sodium sulfosuccinate, mineral oil enemas) should be administered. Warm sitz baths one to three times a day are often helpful. Local anesthetic ointments (e.g., dibucaine, benzoate) may provide symptomatic relief.

Surgery should be deferred as long as possible, because most hemorrhoids will regress after parturition. If symptoms are severe and fail to respond to medical therapy, local surgery may be required. For a thrombosed external hemorrhoid, excision of the clot usually provides prompt relief. For internal hemorrhoids, therapy is controversial. Rubber band ligation or local sclerosing injections are probably most applicable during pregnancy.

Ulcerative Colitis

Most studies agree that ulcerative colitis has little if any effect on fertility [92]. There is also general agreement that ulcerative colitis has no effect on the course of the pregnancy [93]. The incidence of normal live births, congenital anomalies, spontaneous abortions, and stillbirths is similar to that in pregnancies without associated ulcerative colitis. Exceptions to this conclusion are pregnant women with severe ulcerative colitis requiring surgery. McEwan reported a 44% incidence of abortion in this group [94].

The effects of pregnancy on ulcerative colitis have traditionally been discussed in the four clinical situations that follow [92,95–97].

1. *Quiescent colitis at onset of pregnancy.* About 70% of the patients will remain free of symptoms throughout pregnancy. Of the 30% who relapse, approximately half will do so in the first trimester. Approximately equal numbers of the remainder will relapse in the second or third trimester or early postpartum period.
2. *Active colitis at onset of pregnancy.* These patients generally do less well. In pooled series, approximately 67% show no change in activity or become worse during pregnancy.
3. *Onset of colitis during pregnancy.* Onsets are more often seen in the first trimester. Most reports indicate a higher frequency of severe attacks together with a higher maternal mortality although nonpregnant control patients have generally not been included in the studies. A recent study was unable to confirm this finding, however [92].
4. *Onset of colitis in the puerperium.* Most studies demonstrate an increase in severity of attacks and maternal mortality when onset is in the puerperium. Again, however, the study by Willoughby and Truelove found that even in this setting attacks are usually mild [92].

Management

In general the treatment of ulcerative colitis in the pregnant patient is the same as in the nonpregnant patient. A close physician-patient relationship is important. Women with ulcerative colitis have justifiable concerns about their pregnancy, their disease, and their ability to manage at home after delivery. Frequent office visits to monitor disease activity, to alter therapy, and to provide support are indicated.

Diet restriction plays little role in managing ulcerative colitis. Patients should be instructed to avoid foods that might worsen symptoms. Although it is not clear that lactase deficiency is more prevalent in ulcerative colitis, a trial of a lactose-free diet should be carried out to determine its effect on diarrhea. An occasional patient may do better on a low-roughage diet. Careful attention to good nutritional intake is essential.

Patients with severe ulcerative colitis are frequently dehydrated and may require hospitalization and parenteral fluids. Patients with significant hypoalbuminemia may benefit from parenteral administration of protein. Severely anemic patients may require transfusions. With anemia of a lesser degree, oral iron therapy may suffice although many patients will not respond.

Parenteral hyperalimentation may be useful in the markedly debilitated patient, in the patient with refractory diarrhea, or in the severely malnourished patient requiring surgery.

Diarrhea may demand use of antidiarrheal agents until a response to sulfasalazine or corticosteroids is achieved (see below). Narcotics (e.g., loperamide, diphenoxylate, paregoric) are frequently called for in nonpregnant patients. Because of uncertainty about their safety in pregnant patients and the possibility of fetal drug dependency, attempts with nonnarcotic antidiarrheal agents should be made first. If narcotic agents are employed, patients must be followed closely in view of the possibility that these agents may induce toxic dilatation of the colon.

Sulfasalazine has proved effective in this disease. Its major role is in maintaining remissions, but it can also be useful in treating mild to moderate attacks. Doses of 2 to 8 g per day are usually used. Side effects are common—most frequently nausea, vomiting, abdominal discomfort, headache, and skin rash. Hemolytic anemia and aplastic anemia can occur. The safety of this drug in pregnancy has not been conclusively demonstrated. Because sulfonamides can displace bilirubin from albumin, there is a theoretical risk of kernicterus in the fetus. This complication has not yet been reported. A recent survey demonstrated no increased risk of fetal abnormalities in 102 patients with inflammatory bowel disease treated with sulfasalazine alone [93]. The conclusion that this drug may be used just as in the nonpregnant patient appears justified.

There is little information regarding the safety of sulfasalazine during breast-feeding. The concentration of this drug in breast milk is approximately 45% of that in the mother's serum [98]. It is likely that sulfasalazine can be given safely during breast-feeding, but more data are needed.

CORTICOSTEROIDS. The major role for corticosteroids in chronic ulcerative colitis is in treatment of active disease rather than in prevention of exacerbations. The dosage and route of administration vary with the location and activity of the disease. In patients with primarily left-sided colitis, rectal administration of cortisone or prednisolone once or twice each day may be useful and may result in lower serum levels than an equivalently effective oral dosage. In patients with more widespread colon involvement, especially if symptoms are moderate to severe or extraintestinal complications are present, oral prednisone in doses of 20 to 80 mg daily is required. In the most severely ill patient, requiring hospitalization, continuous IV administration of 100 mg of prednisolone per day is indicated.

Following control of symptoms, corticosteroids should be tapered gradually, the objective being to discontinue them completely if symptoms do not recur.

Available evidence from human studies indicates that risks of corticosteroid therapy to the human fetus are probably minimal [93]. Just as in the nonpregnant patient, however, attempts to taper corticosteroid dosage should be made when disease becomes quiescent.

OTHER DRUGS. A number of other drugs have been used in patients with chronic ulcerative colitis, but none has been ascertained to be effective in controlled studies. Azathioprine and 6-mercaptopurine should probably not be used because of established teratogenic effects in animal studies and because of the lack of verified efficacy in patients with chronic ulcerative colitis.

SURGERY. The indications for emergency colectomy in the critically ill pregnant patient with chronic ulcerative colitis are the same as in the nonpregnant patient. The reader is referred to standard textbooks of gastroenterology for complete discussion.

Information regarding pregnancy in the patient with an ileostomy comes mostly from studies of chronic ulcerative colitis [99]. Minor stomal complications (e.g., mild bleeding, skin breaks, ileal prolapse) are common. Intestinal obstruction may occur in as many as 10% of cases.

Crohn's Disease

Most studies have found evidence of decreased fertility in women with Crohn's disease [100–102]. The reason for this is unclear. Some studies implicate small bowel disease; others, large bowel involvement. Prevalence of infertility has ranged from 30 to 60% in different studies.

The effect of Crohn's disease on pregnancy has been extensively studied. A few series have reported an increased risk of stillbirth or fetal abnormalities but this increase, if real, is probably small [102]. Most series report no increased risk [97]. In the unusual situation in which Crohn's disease first appears during pregnancy, risks of fetal death may be increased [103].

The effects of pregnancy on Crohn's disease are in general similar to the effects on patients with chronic ulcerative colitis [104,105]. If disease is quiescent at conception, it will remain so in 80 to 90% of patients. If disease is active, most patients will continue to experience a similar degree of activity throughout pregnancy. Between 10 and 35% will get worse. There are few reports of patients with onset of Crohn's disease during pregnancy, but of those patients reported many had severe disease [104]. All series report a high incidence of disease exacerbation post partum (15–43%) [100,101,104].

In general the treatment of Crohn's disease in the pregnant patient is the same as in the nonpregnant patient and closely parallels the treatment of chronic ulcerative colitis (see above). Several differences with regard to the latter should be noted. Because Crohn's disease frequently results in a narrowed intestinal lumen (especially with small bowel involvement), a low-roughage diet should be routine. Sulfasalazine has been shown to be effective in treating Crohn's disease, especially in Crohn's colitis. The value of this drug in preventing relapses in patients with quiescent disease, however, is less well established than with chronic ulcerative colitis [106].

Metronidazole has been used in the treatment of Crohn's disease. The fact that this drug has caused chromosomal changes in animals, together with its lack of proven efficacy, makes its use during pregnancy inadvisable.

Acute Diarrheal Illness

Pregnant women are obviously subject to the same diarrheal illnesses as nonpregnant women. Since most of these illnesses are mild and self-limited, diagnostic evaluation is usually not necessary. Indications for diagnostic evaluation include fever, bloody stools, illness lasting more than three or four days, and recent travel to areas where bacterial or parasitic diarrheal illness is common. If any of these indications exist, a fresh liquid stool should be submitted for culture and for microscopic exam for ova, parasites, and white blood cells. Moderate to large numbers of the latter generally indicate mucosal disruption (e.g., inflammatory bowel disease, bacterial diarrheas—as with *Salmonella, Shigella, Campylobacter*). If colitis is suspected, gentle sigmoidoscopy (unless late in pregnancy when the fetal head is fixed) is safe and may be indicated.

Management

General supportive measures include maintenance of hydration (oral fluids, especially carbohydrate-electrolyte mixtures), low-lactose diet, antidiarrheal agents (kaolin, pectin). Antidiarrheal agents that slow motility (e.g., loperamide, diphenoxylate) are relatively contraindicated in the presence of fever or rectal bleeding in view of evidence that certain bacterial diarrheal illnesses may be prolonged by these drugs. Furthermore, the safety of loperamide and diphenoxylate has not been established in pregnancy.

The usual *Salmonella* gastroenteritis should not be treated; there is evidence that symptoms and intestinal shedding of organisms may be prolonged with treatment. In the presence of severe symptoms or if bacteremia or the enteric fever syndrome is present, antibiotics are indicated. Ampicillin is the drug of choice if the organisms are sensitive. Trimethoprim-sulfamethoxazole is also effective for resistant organisms although it should not be used in the first or third trimester. Chloramphenicol is sometimes used in nonpregnant patients whose bacteria are resistant to both the above. However, its use should generally be avoided during pregnancy.

Shigellosis is usually a self-limited illness and need not be treated. With severe or prolonged symptoms, the same drugs used for salmonellosis are usually effective. Again, bacterial sensitivity studies should be used to guide choice of antibiotics.

Campylobacter infections are also usually self-limited. Erythromycin appears to be the drug of choice in severe or resistant cases [107].

The treatment of giardiasis during pregnancy is controversial. If symptoms are mild, treatment should be deferred until after parturition. If symptoms are severe, quinacrine (100 mg orally t.i.d. for 5 days) is effective, although its safety in pregnancy has not been established. In years past, its use for treatment of malaria did not result in recognizable problems in pregnancy. Nonetheless,

quinacrine does cross the placenta and should be used with caution in pregnancy. Metronidazole is equally effective but, for reasons discussed above, is also relatively contraindicated. A recent report demonstrated that paromomycin (25–30 mg/kg/day for 5–10 days) may be effective in this disease and, because it is poorly absorbed when given orally, may be safe in pregnancy [108]. More data are needed before safety can be established.

In intestinal amebiasis, numerous drugs have been used but none has been proved to be safe in pregnancy. With asymptomatic infection, treatment should probably be deferred until after parturition. For mild to severe intestinal disease, metronidazole (750 mg three times daily for 5–10 days) or diiodohydroxyquin (650 mg three times daily for 20 days) plus paromomycin (25 to 35 mg/kg/day in three doses for 5–10 days) is effective.

Pancreatitis

It is not clear that the incidence of pancreatitis is increased in pregnancy. Nonetheless, a large number of reports and reviews have been written detailing the features of this entity [109–113]. Its incidence has ranged in different reports from 1 per 1,000 to 1 per 10,000 births. Most reports describe the highest incidence in the third trimester or immediate postpartum period. Multiparous women are more commonly affected—55 to 82% of patients described in selected series [109–111].

The frequency of different etiologies varies from series to series. Corlett and Mishell reported 52 patients of whom 34 (65%) were classified as "idiopathic" [113]. In most series, however, more than 50% of patients had gallstones. In a recent report in which rigorous attempts were made to diagnose biliary tract disease (including ultrasound in many cases), 90% of patients had gallstones [111]. Alcoholism appears to be a far less common etiology than in the nonpregnant patient with pancreatitis. Serum lipids tend to increase during pregnancy, and in women with preexisting hyperlipidemia (especially Types I and V), severe hypertriglyceridemia and secondary pancreatitis are likely to develop. Drug-induced pancreatitis is uncommon in pregnancy. Drugs for which an etiologic association appear to have been proved include tetracycline, azathioprine, thiazides, estrogens, furosemide, and sulfonamides [114].

Diagnosis is usually made by history, physical findings, and an elevated serum amylase. Interpretation of the latter may be difficult because of studies reporting increased, decreased, or no changes in serum amylase in normal pregnancy [112]. A recent report suggests that the finding of an elevated amylase-creatinine clearance ratio may be helpful in pregnancy [115].

Treatment of pancreatitis is similar in the pregnant and nonpregnant patient. Vigorous intravenous fluid administration is necessary because these patients often sequester large amounts of fluid in the retroperitoneum. Analgesia is usually required, and meperidine appears to be the most commonly used agent. Nasogastric suction is probably not necessary in patients with mild to moderate pancreatitis but should be used in severe cases. Antibiotics and anticholinergics are not helpful in most patients [116]. The value of prophylactic antibiotics in hemorrhagic pancreatitis is controversial. The value of inducing labor in patients with severe pancreatitis has not been established.

Although mortality as high as 37% has been reported for both mother and fetus, more recent studies report lower rates. For example, in 20 patients reported by McKay et al. there were no maternal deaths and only one infant death [111].

REFERENCES

1. Romslo I, Sagen N, Haram K. Serum alkaline phosphatase in pregnancy. Acta Obstet Gynecol Scand. 1975; 54:437–42.
2. Hunter RJ, Pinkerton JH, Johnston H. Serum placental alkaline phosphatase in normal pregnancy and preeclampsia. Obstet Gynecol. 1970; 36:536–46.
3. Zuckerman H, Sadovsky E, Kallner B. Serum alkaline phosphatase in pregnancy and puerperium. Obstet Gynecol. 1965; 25:819–24.
4. Sadovsky E, Zuckerman H. An alkaline phosphatase specific to normal pregnancy. Obstet Gynecol. 1965; 26:211–4.
5. McMaster Y, Tennant R, Clubb JFS, Neale FC, Posen S. The mechanism of the elevation of serum alkaline phosphatase in pregnancy. J Obstet Gynaecol Br Comm. 1964; 71:735–9.
6. Boyer SH. Alkaline phosphatase in human sera and placentae. Science. 1961; 134:1002–4.
7. Haemmerli UP. Jaundice during pregnancy with special emphasis on recurrent jaundice during pregnancy and its differential diagnosis. Acta Med Scand. 1966; 179 (Suppl 444):1–111.
8. Lind T. Clinical chemistry of pregnancy. Adv Clin Chem. 1980; 21:1–24.
9. Krejs GJ, Haemmerli UP. Jaundice during pregnancy. In: Schiff L, Schiff ER, eds. Diseases of the liver. 5th ed. Philadelphia: Lippincott, 1982:1561–80.
10. Stander HF, Cadden JF. Blood chemistry in preeclampsia and eclampsia. Am J Obstet Gynecol. 1934; 28:856–71.
11. Sheehan HL. Pathology of acute yellow atrophy and delayed chloroform poisoning. J Obstet Gynaecol Br Emp. 1940; 47:49–62.
12. Riely CA. Acute hepatic failure at term. Diagnostic problems posed by broad clinical spectrum. Postgrad Med. 1980; 68:118–27.
13. Lindheimer MD, Katz AI. The renal response to pregnancy. In: Brenner BM, Rector FC, eds. The kidney. 2nd ed. Philadelphia: Saunders, 1981: 1762–1815.
14. Kunelis CT, Peters JL, Edmondson HA. Fatty liver of pregnancy and its relationship to tetracycline therapy. Am J Med. 1965; 38:359–77.
15. Reyes H. The enigma of intrahepatic cholestasis of pregnancy: lessons from Chile. Hepatology. 1982; 2:87–96.
16. Javitt NB. Cholestatic liver disease: mechanisms, diagnosis and therapy. Adv Intern Med. 1980; 25:147–68.
17. Laatikainen TJ, Peltonen JI, Nylander PL. Effect of maternal intrahepatic cholestasis on fetal steroid metabolism. J Clin Invest. 1974; 53:1709–15.
18. Bis KA, Waxman B. Rupture of the liver associated with pregnancy: a review of the literature and report of 2 cases. Obstet Gynecol Surv. 1976; 31:763–73.
19. Golan A, White RG. Spontaneous rupture of the liver associated with pregnancy. S Afr Med J. 1979; 56:133–6.
20. Hibbard LT. Spontaneous rupture of the liver in pregnancy: a report of eight cases. Am J Obstet Gynecol. 1976; 126:334–8.
21. Westergaard. Spontaneous rupture of the liver in pregnancy. Acta Obstet Gynecol Scand. 1980; 59:559–61.
22. Baumwol M, Park W. An acute abdomen: spontaneous rupture of liver during pregnancy. Br J Surg. 1976; 63:718–20.
23. Hieber JP, Dalton D, Shorey J, Combes B. Hepatitis and pregnancy. J Pediatr. 1977; 91:545–9.
24. Livadas D, Koutras DA, Economidou J, Hadziyannis S, Hesser JE. Fertility and sex ratio of offspring of female HBsAg carriers. J R Soc Med. 1979; 72:509–12.
25. Robertson JS, Sheard AV. Altered sex ratio after an outbreak of hepatitis. Lancet. 1973; 1:532–4.
26. Wilson AS, Pickworth KH. Sex ratio after outbreak of hepatitis. Lancet. 1973; 1:945.
27. Aickin DR, Campbell DG. Anomalous amniotic fluid bilirubin after hepatitis in an Rh immunized patient. Obstet Gynecol. 1971; 37:687–8.
28. Okada K, Kamiyama I, Inomata M, Imai M, Miyakawa Y, Mayumi M. e antigen and anti-e in the serum of asymptomatic carrier mothers as indicators of positive and negative transmission of hepatitis B virus to their infants. N Engl J Med. 1976; 294:746–9.
29. Wands JR. Viral hepatitis and its effect on pregnancy. Clin Obstet Gynecol. 1979; 22:301–11.
30. Gerety RJ, Schweitzer IL. Viral hepatitis type B during pregnancy, the neonatal period, and infancy. J Pediatr. 1977; 90:368–74.
31. Kattamis CA, Demetrios D, Matsaniotis NS. Australia antigen and neonatal hepatitis syndrome. Pediatrics. 1974; 54:157–64.
32. Wright R, Perkins JR, Bower BD, Jerrome DW. Cirrhosis associated with the Australia antigen in an in-

fant who acquired hepatitis from her mother. Br Med J. 1970; 4:719–21.

33. Lee AK, Ip HM, Wong VC. Mechanisms of maternal-fetal transmission of hepatitis B virus. J Infect Dis. 1978; 138:668–71.

34. Buchholz HM, Frosner GG, Ziegler GB. HBAg carrier state in an infant delivered by caesarean section. Lancet. 1974; 2:343.

35. Giraud P, Drouet J, Dupuy JM. Hepatitis-B virus infection of children born to mothers with severe hepatitis. Lancet. 1975; 2:1088–9.

36. Boxall EH, Davies H. Dane particles in cord blood. Lancet. 1974; 2:1513.

37. Khudr G, Benirschke K. Placental lesion in viral hepatitis. Obstet Gynecol. 1972; 40:381–4.

38. Linnemann CC, Goldberg S. HBsAg antigens in breast milk. Lancet. 1974; 2:155.

39. Beasley RP, Stevens CE, Shiao IS, Meng HC. Evidence against breast-feeding as a mechanism for vertical transmission of hepatitis B. Lancet. 1975; 2:740–1.

40. Derso A, Boxall EH, Tarlow MJ, Flewett TH. Transmission of HBsAg from mother to infant in four ethnic groups. Br Med J. 1978; 1:949–52.

41. Wong VC, Lee AJ, Ip HM. Transmission of hepatitis B antigens from symptom free carrier mothers to the fetus and the infant. Br J Obstet Gynaecol. 1980; 87:958–65.

42. Beasley RP, Hwang LY, Lin CC, et al. Hepatitis B immune globulin (HBIG) efficacy in the interruption of perinatal transmission of hepatitis B virus carrier state. Lancet. 1981; 2:388–93.

43. Immune globulins for protection against viral hepatitis. Recommendations of the Immunization Practices Advisory Committee. Center for Disease Control, Department of Health and Human Services, Atlanta, Georgia. Ann Intern Med. 1982; 96:193–7.

44. Beasley RP, Stevens CE. Vertical transmission of HBV and interruption with globulin. In: Vyas GN, Cohen SN, Schmid R, eds. Viral hepatitis. Philadelphia: Franklin Institute Press, 1978: 333–45.

45. Tong MJ, McPeak CM, Thursby MW, Schweitzer IL, Henneman CE, Ledger WJ. Failure of immune serum globulin to prevent hepatitis B virus infection in infants born to HBsAg-positive mothers. Gastroenterology. 1978; 76:535–9.

46. Hoofnagle JH, Gerety RJ, Ni LY, Barket LF. Antibody to hepatitis B core antigen sensitive indicator of hepatitis B virus replication. N Engl J Med. 1974; 290:1336–40.

47. Hoofnagle JH, Seeff LB, Bales ZB, Zimmerman JH, Veterans Administration Hepatitis Cooperative Study Group. Type B hepatitis after transfusion with blood containing antibody to hepatitis B core antigen. N Engl J Med. 1978; 298:1379–83.

48. Shwer M, Moosa A. The effects of hepatitis A and B in pregnancy on mother and fetus. S Afr Med J. 1978; 54:1092–5.

49. Tong MJ, Rakela J, McPeak CM, Thursby MW, Edwards VM, Mosley JW. Studies in infants born to mothers with type A hepatitis and acute non-A non-

B hepatitis during pregnancy. Gastroenterology. 1978; 75:991. abstract.

50. Seeff LB, Hoofnagle JH. Immunoprophylaxis of viral hepatitis. Gastroenterology. 1979; 77:161–82.

51. Joosten R, Sturner KH. Hepatitis and pregnancy. Risks for the newborn. Immunoprophylaxis of vertically transmitted hepatitis. J Perinat Med. 1981; 9:115–23.

52. Summerskill WHJ. Chronic active liver disease reexamined: prognosis hopeful. Gastroenterology. 1974; 66:450–64.

53. Infeld, DS, Borkowf HI, Varma RR. Chronic-persistent hepatitis and pregnancy. Gastroenterology. 1979; 77:524–7.

54. Steven MM, Buckley JD, Mackay IR. Pregnancy in chronic active hepatitis. Q J Med. 1979; 48:519–31.

55. Schweitzer IL, Peters RL. Pregnancy in hepatitis B antigen positive cirrhosis. Obstet Gynecol. 1976; 48 (Suppl):53S–56S.

56. Varma RR, Michelson NH, Borkowf HI, Lewis JD. Pregnancy in cirrhotic and noncirrhotic portal hypertension. Obstet Gynecol. 1977; 50:217–22.

57. Cheng YS. Pregnancy in liver cirrhosis and/or portal hypertension. Am J Obstet Gynecol. 1977; 128:812–22.

58. Powell D. Pregnancy in active chronic hepatitis on immunosuppressive therapy. Postgrad Med J. 1969; 45:292–4.

59. Borhanmanesh F, Haghighi P. Pregnancy in patients with cirrhosis of the liver. Obstet Gynecol. 1970; 36:315–24.

60. Kerr MG. The mechanical effects of the gravid uterus in late pregnancy. J Obstet Gynaecol Br Comm. 1963; 72:513–29.

61. Brown HJ. Splenorenal shunt during pregnancy. Am Surg. 1971; 37:441–3.

62. Steven MM. Pregnancy and liver disease. Gut. 1981; 22:592–614.

63. Clugg LE, Caranasos GJ, Stewart RB. Clinical problems with drugs. Vol. 5, Major problems in internal medicine. Philadelphia: Saunders, 1975:131–41.

64. Toaff R, Toaff ME, Peyser MR, Streifler M. Hepatolenticular degeneration (Wilson's disease) and pregnancy. Obstet Gynecol Surv. 1977; 32:497–507.

65. Walshe JM. Pregnancy in Wilson's disease. Q J Med. 1977; 46:73–83.

66. O'Reilly S, Loncin M. Ceruloplasmin and 5-hydroxyindole metabolism in pregnancy. Am J Obstet Gynecol. 1967; 97:8–12.

67. Sherlock S, Scheuer PJ. The presentation and diagnosis of 100 patients with primary biliary cirrhosis. N Engl J Med. 1973; 289:674–8.

68. Sherlock S. Jaundice in pregnancy. Br Med Bull. 1968; 24:39–43.

69. Billing BH. Bilirubin metabolism. In: Schiff L, Schiff ER, eds. Diseases of the liver. 5th ed. Philadelphia: Lippincott, 1982:349–78.

70. Friedlaender P, Osler M. Icterus and pregnancy. Am J Obstet Gynecol. 1967; 97:894–900.

71. Horn G. Observations on aetiology of cholelithiasis. Br Med J. 1956; 2:732–7.

72. Friedman GD, Kannel WB, Dawber TR. The epidemiology of gallbladder disease: observations in the Framingham Study. J Chronic Dis. 1966; 19:273–92.

73. Bennion LG, Drobny E, Knowler WC, et al. Sex differences in the size of bile acid pools. Metabolism. 1978; 27:961–9.

74. Bennion LG, Ginsberg RL, Gernick MB. Effects of oral contraceptives on the gallbladder bile of normal women. N Engl J Med. 1976; 294:189–92.

75. Kern F. Why more women than men have cholesterol gallstones: studies of biliary lipids in pregnancy. Trans Am Clin Climatol Assoc. 1978; 90:71–5.

76. Everson GT, McKinley C, Lawson M, Johnson M, Kern F. Gallbladder function in the human female: effect of the ovulatory cycle, pregnancy, and oral contraceptive steroids. Gastroenterology. 1982; 82:711–9.

77. Bainton D, Davies GT, Evans KT, et al. Gallbladder disease: prevalence in a South Wales industrial town. N Engl J Med. 1976; 294:1147–9.

78. Ferrucci JT Jr. Body ultrasonography. N Engl J Med. 1979; 300:538–42.

79. McCorriston CC. Nonobstetrical abdominal surgery during pregnancy. Am J Obstet Gynecol. 1963; 86:593–9.

80. Hill LM, Johnson CE, Lee RA. Cholecystectomy in pregnancy. Obstet Gynecol. 1975; 46:291–3.

81. Spiro HM. Clinical gastroenterology. New York: Macmillan, 1970:16.

82. Seymour CA, Chadwick VS. Liver and gastrointestinal function in pregnancy. Postgrad Med J. 1979; 55:343–52.

83. Van Thiel DH, Gavaler JS, Joshi SN, et al. Heartburn of pregnancy. Gastroenterology. 1977; 72:666–8.

84. Fairweather, DV. Nausea and vomiting in pregnancy. Am J Obstet Gynecol. 1968; 102:135–75.

85. Taylor HP. Nausea and vomiting of pregnancy. In: Kroger WS, ed. Psychosomatic obstetrics, gynecology, and endocrinology. Springfield, Ill: Thomas, 1962:117–26.

86. Clark DH. Peptic ulcer in women. Br Med J. 1953; 1:1254–7.

87. Truelove SC. Stilboestrol, phenobarbitone, and diet in chronic duodenal ulcer. Br Med J. 1960; 2:559–66.

88. Langmade CF. Epigastric pain in pregnancy toxemias. West J Surg Obstet Gynecol. 1956; 64:540–4.

89. Sonnenberg A, Muller-Lissner SA, Vogel E, et al. Predictors of duodenal ulcer healing and relapse. Gastroenterology. 1981; 81:1061–7.

90. Nelson MM, Forfar JO. Associations between drugs administered during pregnancy and congenital abnormalities of the fetus. Br Med J. 1971; 1:523–7.

91. Levy N, Lemberg E, Sharf M. Bowel habit in pregnancy. Digestion. 1971; 4:216–22.

92. Willoughby CP, Truelove SC. Ulcerative colitis and pregnancy. Gut. 1980; 21:469–74.

93. Mogadam M, Dobbins WO, Korelitz BI, Ahmed SW. Pregnancy in inflammatory bowel disease: effect of sulfasalazine and corticosteroids on fetal outcome. Gastroenterology. 1981; 80:72–6.

94. McEwan HP. Ulcerative colitis in pregnancy. Proc R Soc Med. 1972; 65:279–81.

95. Crohn BB, Yarnis H, Crohn EB, Walter RI, Gabrilove LJ. Ulcerative colitis and pregnancy. Gastroenterology. 1956; 30:391–403.

96. De Dombal FT, Watts JM, Watkinson G, Goligher JC. Ulcerative colitis and pregnancy. Lancet. 1965; 2:599–602.

97. Fielding JF. Inflammatory bowel disease and pregnancy. Br J Hosp Med. 1976; 15:345–52.

98. Jarnerot G, Into-Malmberg MB. Sulphasalazine treatment during breast feeding. Scand J Gastroenterol. 1979; 14:869–71.

99. Hudson CN. Ileostomy in pregnancy. Proc R Soc Med. 1972; 65:281–3.

100. Fielding JF, Cooke WT. Pregnancy and Crohn's disease. Br Med J. 1970; 2:76–7.

101. De Dombal FT, Burton IL, Goligher JC. Crohn's disease and pregnancy. Br Med J. 1972; 3:550–3.

102. Schofield PF, Turnbull RB, Hawk WA. Crohn's disease and pregnancy. Br Med J. 1970; 2:364.

103. Martimbeau PW, Welch JS, Weiland LH. Crohn's disease and pregnancy. Am J Obstet Gynecol. 1975; 122:746–9.

104. Crohn BB, Yarnis H, Korelitz BI. Regional ileitis complicating pregnancy. Gastroenterology. 1956; 31:615–28.

105. Homan WP, Thorbjarnarson B. Crohn disease and pregnancy. Arch Surg. 1976; 111:545–7.

106. Summers RW, Switz DM, Sessions JT, et al. National Cooperative Crohn's Disease Study: results of treatment. Gastroenterology. 1979; 77:847–69.

107. Gribble MJ, Salit IE, Isaac-Renton J, Chow AW. Campylobacter infections in pregnancy. Am J Obstet Gynecol. 1981; 140:423–6.

108. Kreutner AK, Del Bene VE, Amstey MS. Giardiasis in pregnancy. Am J Obstet Gynecol. 1981; 140:895–901.

109. Wilkinson EJ. Acute pancreatitis in pregnancy: a review of 98 cases and a report of 8 new cases. Obstet Gynecol Surv. 1973; 28:281–303.

110. Berk JE, Smith BH, Akrawi MM. Pregnancy pancreatitis. Am J Gastroenterol. 1971; 56:216–26.

111. McKay AJ, O'Neill J, Imrie CW. Pancreatitis, pregnancy and gallstones. Br J Obstet Gynaecol. 1980; 87:47–50.

112. Kaiser R, Berk JE, Fridhandler L. Serum amylase changes during pregnancy. Am J Obstet Gynecol. 1975; 122:283–6.

113. Corlett RC, Mishell DR. Pancreatitis in pregnancy. Am J Obstet Gynecol. 1972; 113:281–90.

114. Mallory A, Kern F. Drug-induced pancreatitis: a critical review. Gastroenterology. 1980; 78:813–20.

115. DeVore GR, Bracken M, Berkowitz RL. The amylase/creatinine clearance ratio in normal pregnancy and pregnancies complicated by pancreatitis, hyperemesis gravidarum, and toxemia. Am J Obstet Gynecol. 1980; 136:747–54.

116. Craig RM, Dordal E, Myles L. The use of ampicillin in acute pancreatitis. Ann Intern Med. 1975; 83: 831–2. letter.

16. NONOBSTETRIC ABDOMINAL SURGERY

Gilbert Hermann and John S. Simon

ABDOMINAL SURGICAL DISORDERS

Since an acute nonobstetric intraabdominal surgical emergency in a gravid female occurs but once in every 1,000 to 2,000 pregnancies, it is unlikely that a general surgeon or obstetrician will accumulate a large personal clinical experience [1,2,3]. Physiologic and anatomic changes associated with an enlarging uterus modify the usual physical findings associated with intraabdominal pathology. Also, some of our most useful laboratory and diagnostic aids, particularly those involving the use of x-rays and radioactive isotopes, may need to be limited. The general surgeon may hesitate to perform surgery unless the clinical situation appears critical. The obstetrician, on the other hand, may overlook subtle intraabdominal signs or symptoms that may herald the beginnings of a potentially serious intraabdominal problem. All of the aforementioned combine to make the appropriate diagnosis and management of the pregnant patient with a surgical problem unique and difficult.

Current surgical and anesthetic techniques, combined with excellent preoperative, intraoperative, and postoperative care, have reduced perioperative maternal mortality to that associated with the underlying intraabdominal problem [1,5]. Fetal morbidity or mortality following laparotomy alone is difficult to evaluate. Since approximately 15% of all pregnancies abort spontaneously, any increased risk to the fetus from surgery during pregnancy must be compared with that percentage. The underlying condition itself may increase the risk to the fetus. Nevertheless, the major risk to the fetus from surgery appears to be preterm labor and delivery.

Laparoscopy or diagnostic laparotomy can be performed with minimal risk, regardless of gestational age, as long as the gravid uterus is manipulated little or not at all. This is a fortunate situation since the difficulty in establishing a preoperative diagnosis frequently results in a "negative" laparotomy during pregnancy [1,2,4,5].

Appendicitis

Appendicitis is the most common nonobstetric surgical emergency during pregnancy. Incidence figures vary from 1 in 550 to 1 in 2,700 pregnant women [6–8]. A reasonable estimate is that appendicitis occurs in approximately 1 in 1,600 pregnancies. This is roughly the same incidence as in the general population [9]. There appears to be an equal occurrence in all three trimesters [10,11], although some smaller series have indicated a slightly increased frequency during the first and second trimesters [6,8].

The maternal and fetal mortality from appendicitis has steadily decreased in the past 20 years (Table 16-1). Improved preoperative and postoperative care, antibiotics, and better anesthetic techniques have all played a significant role.

Severe complications (e.g., perforation with peritonitis or abscess formation) increase with increasing gestational age. Finch and Lee and Babaknia et al., in separate studies, showed a 50% and 43% incidence of ruptured appendix in the second half of pregnancy compared with 0% and 10% incidence in the first half of pregnancy [6,10].

If perforation and peritonitis supervene, fetal mortality is approximately 30% [10,11]. Several factors have been advanced to explain the increased risk of peritonitis during late pregnancy. Dissemination of the infection appears to progress more rapidly during pregnancy. Localization of the infection is impeded by the elevation of the appendix from the confines of the pelvis into the general abdominal cavity. Also, the large uterus prevents the omentum from reaching and enclosing the inflamed organ. The increased vascularity associated with pregnancy may lead to early spread of the infection [18]. By far the principal cause for the increased incidence of peritonitis, with its associated increased fetal loss, is delayed diagnosis, and consequently delayed surgery.

Many of the subjective symptoms occurring early in the natural history of appendicitis (i.e.,

Table 16-1. Maternal and fetal mortality from perforated appendix in pregnancy

Author	Number of cases	Maternal mortality (%)	Fetal mortality (%)
Babler (1908) [12]	207	24.0	40.0
McDonald (1929) [13]	274	14.0	37.0
Black (1960) [11]	273	4.6	17.0
Brant (1967) [14]	286	2.0	17.0
Townsend and Greiss (1976) [8]	451	0.4	8.5
Babaknia et al. (1977) [10]	333	0.01	8.7
Gomez and Wood (1979) [15]	35	0	0

Adapted from Gomez and Wood [15].

nausea, anorexia, and abdominal discomfort) are very common, particularly early in gestation [17]. If they occur later in pregnancy, the diagnosis is often easier to establish.

During labor, pain associated with uterine contractions may obscure an inflammatory intraabdominal process. Signs and symptoms of appendicitis in the puerperium may be more typical, but the location of the appendix may vary and cause some confusion. With the increased incidence of cesarean delivery, postpartum diagnosis in the early postoperative period may be very difficult.

Persistent abdominal pain is present in all cases of appendicitis and is the single most reliable symptom [16]. In early pregnancy, the pain is usually localized to the right lower quadrant. As the uterus enlarges and the cecum and appendix are elevated out of the pelvis, the pain may occur in the right flank or even in the right upper quadrant [19]. In one series, 30% of patients with appendicitis in the third trimester complained of pain in the right lower quadrant as compared with 90% of patients with appendicitis occurring in the first and second trimesters [15].

Physical findings also become less reliable as pregnancy progresses, because of laxity of the abdominal wall musculature and upward and outward displacement of the appendix. Rebound tenderness and spasm, a response of the overlying somatic abdominal wall musculature to the underlying intraabdominal inflammatory process, may be absent in as many as 30 to 40% of patients in the third trimester [9, 15].

As in the nongravid female, the temperature is often of little aid in establishing a diagnosis. It is normal in 25%, low in 63%, and significantly elevated in only 12% of cases [6]. Because of a physiologic leukocytosis associated with pregnancy, the white blood count (WBC) associated with appendicitis during pregnancy may not be a helpful sign (Table 16-2). However, white counts greater than 12,000/mm^3 should be considered elevated.

Pyelonephritis is one of the more common conditions that may be confused with appendicitis.

Table 16-2. Range of white blood cell counts in patients with appendicitis in pregnancy

WBC (mm^3)	Cases with proved appendicitis (%)
<10,000	25
10,000–15,000	50
>15,000	25

Source: Babaknia et al. [10].

Because of the irritation to the adjacent renal pelvis and ureter by the pyelonephritic process, the patient may complain of bilateral or right lower abdominal pain and manifest acute abdominal signs. It is necessary to obtain a clean-catch or catheterized urine specimen if the diagnosis is to be made. Both pyuria and bacteriuria should be present in cases of acute pyelonephritis. Pain and tenderness in the right flank, particularly later in gestation, may be associated with pyuria in up to 24% of patients with proved appendicitis [8].

Because of the difficulty in diagnosis, the high risk to the fetus (especially should perforation occur), and the small risk to the mother and fetus from laparotomy, appendectomy should be performed, regardless of the stage of pregnancy, if appendicitis cannot be clinically ruled out. If a normal appendix is found at surgery, as may occur in 30 to 50% of cases, it should be removed [9,14].

A patient who is in labor when the diagnosis is made, with delivery imminent, should be delivered vaginally followed by an appendectomy. Should an obstetric problem necessitate a cesarean delivery, a low-segment transverse delivery should be performed followed by an appendectomy.

An adequate muscle-splitting incision, centered over the point of maximum tenderness, with minimal manipulation of the gravid uterus, will be satisfactory in most instances. Elevating the right side of the patient about 30 degrees allows the uterus to fall away from the operative field without additional traction.

Cholecystitis

Cholesterol gallstones are particularly common during pregnancy. The increased incidence during pregnancy is attributed to decreased motility of the gallbladder wall and increased residual gallbladder volume, related to the effect of progesterone on muscle contractility [20]. In addition to the increased residual volume there are changes in cholesterol saturation and a decreased bile salt pool [21].

While the incidence of cholelithiasis is increased, the incidence of cholecystitis during pregnancy (0.02%) is no greater than that in nonpregnant matched controls [16,23].

The symptoms and physical findings in patients with cholecystitis are the same in the pregnant and nonpregnant patient. Nausea and vomiting, associated with colicky right upper quadrant or epigastric pain, are the most common symptoms. The occurrence of the disease is equally distributed among all trimesters [22]. The differential diagnosis of right upper quadrant pain and tenderness must include appendicitis, particularly in the second or third trimester.

The diagnosis of cholelithiasis may be confirmed with ultrasonography. If essential, the diagnosis of acute cholecystitis can be documented by a nuclear isotope scan (see Chap. 8, Risks of Radiation Exposure). The laboratory is of no special aid. Alkaline phosphatase may be elevated, but it rises normally during pregnancy, reaching levels of 1.5 to 2.0 times normal, by the third trimester.

Initial therapy for cholecystitis during pregnancy is medical. Nasogastric suction, intravenous support, and analgesics will usually control the symptoms. Elective cholecystectomy can then be performed following delivery. However, should the attacks of biliary colic become increasingly frequent, or not responsive to medical measures, cholecystectomy should be carried out. This is necessary in approximately 25 to 30% of all patients with symptomatic gallstones [24,28]. In a small percentage of cases, cholecystectomy is indicated for complications associated with common duct stones, such as pancreatitis or cholangitis. The surgical technique is the same as in a non-

gravid patient. It is a safe operation for both mother and fetus. Table 16-3 summarizes the mortality risks from cholecystectomy.

Operative cholangiography is not routinely recommended but has been reported with no apparent injury to the fetus [27].

In summary, while cholelithiasis is common during pregnancy, chronic cholecystitis is unusual and acute cholecystitis and pancreatitis are rare. The large majority of patients with chronic cholecystitis can be treated medically until delivery. If a cholecystectomy does become necessary, it can be performed with minimal additional risk.

Bowel Obstruction

The incidence of bowel obstruction during pregnancy has increased dramatically in recent decades. This undoubtedly reflects the increasing incidence of prior intraabdominal surgery. The incidence may be as great as 1 in 1,500 pregnancies [20]. Adhesions are by far the most common cause, followed by volvulus, hernia, and tumor [29,30]. Shaxted and Jukes have described a "pseudo-obstruction" of the large and small bowel caused by compression of the intestines against the pelvic brim by the gravid uterus [32]. Others have reported an increased likelihood of volvulus of the small and large bowel due to an increased tendency of the mesentery to twist from upward displacement by the gravid uterus [31]. Acting in concert with intraabdominal adhesions, the moving uterus may act to entrap a piece of bowel.

Certain periods of gestation appear to be more favorable for bowel entrapment. At 12 to 16 weeks' gestation the uterus rises out of the pelvis into the abdomen; at 36 to 40 weeks the fetal head and uterus moves downward into the pelvis, and at delivery there is a sudden decrease in the size of the uterus [31]. Therefore, it is not surprising that bowel obstruction is most common in the third trimester and the puerperium [32]. Bowel obstruction has also been reported from the "violin string" adhesions formed as a result of the Fitz-Hugh–Curtis syndrome [33]. Intestinal obstruction can occur even if there has been no prior surgery, although it is rare.

Table 16-3. Maternal and fetal mortality secondary to cholecystectomy

Author	Number of cases	Maternal mortality	Fetal mortality
Greene et al. (1963) [25]	17	0	4 (23.5%)
Friley and Douglas (1972) [22]	8	0	0 (0%)
Hill et al. (1975) [26]	20	0	1 (.05%)
Printen and Ott (1978) [27]	26	0	0 (0%)

Many of the symptoms of bowel obstruction (cramps, constipation, bloating, indigestion, and vomiting) may occur, intermittently, in normal pregnancy. The presence of persistent pain or profound or fecal vomiting should alert the physician to the possibility of a bowel obstruction. Sometimes, however, the evolution of a bowel obstruction in the pregnant patient is insidious.

It is not unusual for pregnant women to have mild prodromal symptoms such as nausea or bloating prior to complete bowel obstruction, possibly because a gradual increase in the uterine size acts on a fixed loop of bowel. Because bowel obstruction may present atypically in pregnancy, these patients must be followed closely to avoid complications secondary to delayed surgery.

An abdominal roentgenogram is sometimes interpreted as normal for pregnancy even with a complete bowel obstruction [34]. The reason may be that the gravid uterus supports the bowel in the upper abdomen and does not allow dependent loops to descend or demonstrate the typical air-fluid levels.

The treatment of bowel obstruction for pregnant and nonpregnant women is the same: *early surgery*. Pregnant patients almost always proceed to have normal deliveries following relief of their obstruction. Occasionally, a cesarean delivery may be required at the time of bowel surgery if access to the surgical field is impossible. A simple lysis of adhesions, however, adds little risk to pregnancy. The severity of disease, rather than the surgery performed, determines the greatest risk to the mother and infant. Delaying surgery until the bowel has become gangrenous and subject to attendant peritonitis poses a very dangerous situation for the mother and fetus. If the diagnosis is in doubt, it is best to err on the side of early surgery.

Peptic Ulcer Disease

Most women with active ulcer disease experience significant remission during pregnancy. The incidence of exacerbation during pregnancy is reduced, and symptoms usually improve [35].

Of 118 women with previous duodenal ulcer disease, Clark found an 88% remission rate during pregnancy [36]. This suggests a relationship between the hormones of pregnancy and acid-pepsin secretion [36]. Progesterone tends to lower gastric acid secretion and stimulate gastric mucus production. Plasma histaminase from the placenta blocks the histamine effect on the parietal cell and hence lowers acid production [37].

Like so many diseases complicating pregnancy, peptic disease may be difficult to diagnose. The symptoms of peptic disease may appear to be simply an accentuation of the usual symptoms of pregnancy. More aggressive methods of study of peptic disease (e.g., endoscopy or upper GI series) tend to be avoided during pregnancy, making the absolute diagnosis less secure.

Becker-Andersen and Husfeldt reported 33 gastric perforations and 28 upper gastrointestinal hemorrhages [38]. Perforation occurs almost exclusively during the third trimester. The event is usually catastrophic, and the patient presents with a rigid, quiet abdomen. Because of the relaxed musculature of the abdominal wall during pregnancy, the rigidity may be less marked. Upright abdominal films usually show free air under the diaphragm but, as in the nonpregnant state, this may not be present. The management of perforation is surgical. Medical approaches to this condition should be abandoned [39].

After rapid stabilization of vital signs, the patient must undergo exploratory laparotomy. General lavage of the peritoneal cavity with saline is recommended. The management of the perforation is based on the findings at surgery. The authors prefer a simple Graham closure in pregnancy. Massive upper gastrointestinal hemorrhage from a duodenal ulcer during pregnancy poses an even greater fetal danger than perforation. The development of shock may compromise the uteroplacental circulation and is associated with a high risk of preterm labor.

Management of upper intestinal hemorrhage includes rapid fluid replacement, saline gastric lavage, and transfusion. Endoscopy, when possible, should be done early in the course of the disease. If the bleeding is not easily controlled, or if the patient cannot be stabilized, surgery is in order. More mothers and fetuses will be saved with early surgical intervention than with prolonged or unsuccessful medical approaches. Although cesarean delivery has been suggested at the time of ulcer surgery in the third trimester, the present authors, among others, would not support that approach as necessary in all cases.

Pancreatitis

Pancreatitis is rare during pregnancy, occurring in approximately 1 in 10,000 to 12,000 patients [42]. The mortality and morbidity are increased primarily because of delay in diagnosis [36].

New methods for evaluation of the gallbladder suggest that a correlation exists between pancreatitis in pregnancy and the presence of gallstones. As a result, fewer cases of pancreatitis will be called idiopathic [36,40–42]. The clinician should be aware that a mild elevation of serum amylase may be seen during normal pregnancy [43]. Also, during the third trimester, a mild acidosis may be present [34]. Except for these changes associated with pregnancy, diagnostic criteria for pancreatitis are not changed during pregnancy.

The treatment of pancreatitis is nasogastric suction and intravenous fluids. Surgery should be reserved for complications such as hemorrhagic necrosis or abscess [35]. Serious deterioration in the patient is an indication for termination of pregnancy or induction of labor. The course of the pregnancy is usually unaffected by pancreatitis unless complicated by abscess, acidosis, or shock. These complications reduce the chances for a successful pregnancy outcome. A history of previous episodes of pancreatitis is not a contraindication to pregnancy nor does it usually require termination of pregnancy. Any surgery on the biliary tree for pancreatitis performed during pregnancy should include a common duct exploration. X-ray cholangiography should be avoided.

INTRAABDOMINAL HEMORRHAGE
Hepatic Rupture and Splenic Artery Aneurysm
Spontaneous hepatic rupture and rupture of a splenic artery aneurysm are rare, life-threatening conditions that occur almost exclusively in pregnancy and can cause massive intraabdominal hemorrhage.

Fewer than 50 cases of hepatic rupture have been reported in the literature [44]. Most cases have occurred in association with eclampsia. It is believed that a coagulopathy secondary to the eclampsia results in hemorrhages beneath the capsule of the liver. The hemorrhages coalesce, with subsequent rupture through Glisson's capsule [45].

Clinically, the triad of preeclampsia, right upper quadrant pain, and shock should alert the physician to the possibility of spontaneous hepatic rupture. Immediate operative treatment may avoid fetal and maternal mortality. A cesarean delivery may be necessary to gain adequate exposure to explore the entire liver surface and to oversew bleeding sites.

Splenic artery aneurysm occurs in women four times as often as in men [45], is usually asymptomatic, and is most common in multiparous patients. The diagnosis may be made preoperatively by the identification of a calcified splenic vessel wall on a plain roentgenogram of the abdomen. Otherwise, the diagnosis is made at the time of surgery for shock. The reason for the aneurysm's appearing during pregnancy is unclear. It has been speculated that there is some hormonal effect on the

vessel wall or perhaps increased arteriovenous shunting in the spleen during pregnancy with increased flow through the splenic artery.

Rupture almost always occurs during the third trimester. The fetal mortality is extremely high. Treatment is immediate laparotomy, ligation of the splenic artery, and splenectomy. Should a splenic artery aneurysm be found in a woman in the child-bearing years or during pregnancy, elective surgery should be strongly considered.

Ectopic Pregnancy
Approximately 1 in 100 to 200 pregnancies will have an extrauterine site. Rupture of an ectopic pregnancy is responsible for 6 to 9% of all obstetric deaths [46]. The fallopian tube is the most common ectopic site, although rarely ovarian, omental, or peritoneal pregnancies can occur.

Prior to rupture, the patient will have the usual symptoms of early pregnancy. Any woman who misses a menstrual period, then has abnormal vaginal bleeding, especially with vague abdominal pain and symptoms of pregnancy, should be suspected of having an ectopic pregnancy.

A blood test for human chorionic gonadotropin should establish the presence of a pregnancy, if the gestation is still viable. Standard urine pregnancy tests will be positive in only approximately 50% of ectopic gestations (Table 16-4). Ultrasonography may be very helpful in establishing the intrauterine or extrauterine site of a gestational sac.

If surgery is not performed promptly after the diagnosis has been established from the vague symptoms discussed above, rupture may ensue, particularly if the pregnancy is implanted in a narrow portion of the fallopian tube. The rupture will usually occur before the twelfth gestational week. The torn uteroovarian vessels may bleed profusely, and profound pain, often followed rapidly by shock, results. A suggestive history, the presence of vasomotor instability, and pain with signs of acute peritonitis suggest the need for a culdocentesis. If a 20-gauge spinal needle is placed in the posterior cul-se-sac of the vagina with the patient's back slightly elevated, free-flowing, nonclotting blood is often returned. In the presence of profound shock, the time lost by performance of culdocentesis should be avoided and large intravenous lines placed and the patient taken immediately to surgery. The severity of the hemorrhage may be so great as not to allow for the delay entailed in waiting for cross-matched blood.

If emergency surgery for ruptured tubal pregnancy is necessary, only essential surgery should be performed. Only life-threatening pelvic pathology should be managed at the time. Other pathol-

Table 16-4. Expected time for positive pregnancy tests

Test	Source	Detection limit (mIU/mL)	Days after fertilization
Nuclear-Medical Chorio-Shure (RIA)	Serum	40	8–12
Wampole Biocept-G (RRA)	Serum	200	10
Organon Neocept (AIT)	Urine	200	14
Roche Pregnosis (LAI)	Urine	1,500	19
Ortho Gravindex (LAI)	Urine	3,500	28
Warner-Lambert e.p.t. (AIT)	Urine	750–1,000	23

mIU = milli-International Units; RIA = radioimmunoassay; RRA = radioreceptor assay; AIT = agglutination inhibition test; LAI = latex agglutination inhibition.
Source: Courtesy of Terri F. Rosenbaum, M.D., Rose Medical Center, Denver.

Table 16-5. Results of conservative surgery in ectopic pregnancy

Author	No. of cases	Follow-up (yr)	Follow-up (%)	Intrauterine pregnancies (%)	Repeat ectopic rate (%)
Ploman and Wicksell (1960)[47]	31[a] 69[b]	3–15	99	60[a] 40[b]	8
Timonen and Nieminen (1967)[48]	240	2–10	69	27	16
Stromme (1973)[49]	55		56		13
Stangel et al. (1976)[50]	2	1	100	100	0
Bukovsky et al. (1979)[51]	24			55	4
DeCherney and Kase (1979)[52]	48	1–4	73	39	19
Bruhat et al. (1980)[53]	60	½	42	72	12
DeCherney et al. (1980)[54]	9	2	100	55	0
DeCherney et al. (1981)[55]	16	1		50	0

[a]Conservative.
[b]Semiconservative.
Source: Courtesy of Terri F. Rosenbaum, M.D., Rose Medical Center, Denver.

ogy should be noted. Salpingostomy (removal of the products of conception through an incision in the tube), salpingectomy (removal of a tube), or salpingo-oophorectomy (removal of tube and ovary) may be required to control the bleeding. The results of conservative surgery and subsequent risk of repeat ectopic pregnancy are given in Table 16-5. In the unstable patient, elective hysterectomy or tubal ligation is not indicated.

Laparoscopy may be indicated for the patient who presents early in gestation with a confusing clinical picture. In the unstable patient, laparoscopy should be bypassed in favor of laparotomy.

Diagnostic dilatation and curettage may be done at the time of laparoscopy, if the pregnancy test is negative and laparoscopy fails to determine the cause for abnormal uterine bleeding and abdominal pain.

Abdominal Trauma

Six to seven percent of all pregnancies are complicated by accidental injury, mostly abdominal trauma [56]. The modern pregnant woman drives her own car, participates in athletics, and may be the victim of a violent act. Approximately 90% of female deaths from penetrating wounds, and 50% of female auto fatalities occur in women in the childbearing age [57]. Depending on the nature and severity of the trauma, a decision to terminate the pregnancy or to deliver the infant may be required. Prompt stabilization of the mother is critical. Early assessment of the fetal condition must also be part of initial resuscitative efforts.

The pregnancy itself may alter the severity or the pattern of the injury. Many of the signs and symptoms of trauma are changed or camouflaged by the pregnancy. During the first trimester the fetus is well protected by the bony pelvis. As the pregnancy advances and the uterus rises out of the pelvis, it becomes more accessible to blunt and penetrating injuries. The uterus and the amniotic fluid provide a cushion for the fetus against direct trauma. However, the position and mobility of the enlarging uterus may allow for acceleration-deceleration injuries seen in high-speed automobile accidents. Placental separation or uterine laceration may result.

Maternal and fetal morbidity and mortality are both dependent on the maternal condition, but there may be direct injury to the uterus, cord, placenta, or fetus. The fetus will usually tolerate maternal surgery very well, if it is required. If the mother becomes hypotensive, septic, or hypoxic, the prognosis for the fetus becomes grave. The mother may maintain her own hemestasis by markedly reducing placental blood flow, resulting in hypoxia in the fetus. For this reason, blood loss should be carefully monitored in the mother and replaced on a unit-to-unit basis. Continuous electronic fetal monitoring should be instituted, if feasible, for at least 24 hours following any major abdominal trauma to a pregnant patient [58].

In the case of fetal death, the mother should be stabilized, her coagulation profile evaluated, amniotomy performed, and labor induced if it does not begin spontaneously within 48 hours. Cesarean delivery of a fetus fatally injured by trauma is rarely required. If the mother shows evidence of disseminated intravascular coagulopathy or amniotic fluid emboli, delivery should be effected as soon as possible. Amniotomy, if it can be done, and oxytocin stimulation for a short time (2–8 hours), depending on the clinical condition of the patient, may achieve a less traumatic vaginal delivery. However, if delivery does not appear imminent or if the patient is unstable, cesarean delivery should be done.

Certain injuries dictate the need for cesarean delivery. If the risk of fetal injury or hypoxia outweighs the risk of preterm birth, or if the fetus demonstrates evidence of distress, or if a gunshot or stab wound has penetrated the uterus, surgical delivery is advisable.

If the uterus is severely contused or lacerated at abdominal exploration for other reasons or if the pregnant uterus interferes with the surgical approach to the maternal injuries, cesarean delivery is in order. Finally, if maternal death is imminent and the fetus has a chance for viability, cesarean delivery is indicated.

The physician must consult with the family to weigh the risk of a fetal death in utero against the risk of delivering a preterm infant. Electronic fetal monitoring, ultrasonography, x-rays, amniocentesis, or other modalities will be helpful in making this assessment, but often it falls to the clinician's judgment at the time of surgery.

GYNECOLOGIC DISORDERS
Ovarian Cysts
An ovarian cyst may be found in the first trimester of pregnancy before the adnexa have been elevated out of the pelvis by the enlarging uterus. Since clinical evaluation may become increasingly difficult as gestation proceeds, ultrasonography may be used to follow the progress of the mass. Prior to the clinical establishment of the intrauterine location of a pregnancy, ultrasonography may also help to distinguish intrauterine and ectopic pregnancy.

Ovarian cysts may rupture, with or without intraperitoneal hemorrhage, or they may twist. Most corpus luteum cysts are small (<5 cm). More than 90% will regress by early in the second trimester. The incidence of ovarian cysts is approximately 1 in 80 to 100 pregnancies. In approximately 1 case in 328 the cyst will be large or symptomatic and require surgical intervention [59]. Ovarian cancer in pregnancy occurs but is rare.

Once a cyst is identified, certain factors dictate the need for surgical intervention. Increasing symptoms or signs of rupture or torsion (pain, nausea and vomiting, and peritoneal signs), increasing size, evidence on ultrasonogram or clinical examination of mixed solid and cystic areas, bilaterality, irregularity or multicystic changes should suggest the need for surgery. If the mass does not disappear by 14 to 16 weeks' gestation, or if the patient is an older gravida, the mass is fixed, or there are suggestive signs of tumor elsewhere with metastatic disease to the ovary (e.g., ascites, hydrothorax), then exploratory surgery must be undertaken. If no signs of malignancy are present, yet surgery is required, it is best performed in the second trimester. If surgery is performed electively, ovarian cysts can usually be excised, conserving the remainder of the ovary. Rarely, the location, local reaction, or nature of the mass will require extirpation of the entire ovary.

Occasionally, the presence of an ovarian cyst in the pelvis will act as a barrier to vaginal delivery and first be discovered at cesarean delivery for failure of the presenting part to descend into the pelvis. Also, rupture of the ovarian cyst can occur and present with acute abdominal signs suggesting rupture of the uterus, abruptio placentae, or intraabdominal hemorrhage.

Torsion of the Adnexa

Since the broad ligaments usually shorten with increasing uterine size in pregnancy, torsion of the adnexa in pregnancy is infrequent. It may occur, however, in up to 10 to 15% of patients with ovarian cysts in pregnancy.

Symptoms of torsion include constant or colicky pain with waves of increased severity. Nausea and vomiting are frequent. Laboratory evidence of acute intraabdominal pathology may be lacking since the elevated values seen in the disease may not be incompatible with the changes seen in pregnancy alone (see Chap. 9, Clinical Chemistry). Because torsion is more likely to occur when the size of the uterus is changing rapidly, it is more commonly encountered early in pregnancy (6–16 weeks' gestation) or post partum.

As with other intraabdominal disease (e.g., appendicitis), the laxity of the abdominal wall and the unpredictability of the adnexal location at different times in gestation may make the diagnosis difficult. Preterm labor, abruptio placentae, degenerated leiomyomas, intermittent bowel obstruction or other bowel disease, ruptured ovarian cyst, and pyelitis are some of the conditions that must be differentiated from torsion of the adnexa. Torsion may involve the tube and ovary or the ovary or fallopian tube alone.

Ultrasonography may help to identify an enlarged cystic ovary that may have initiated the torsion. If the patient's symptoms persist and abdominal findings worsen, surgery is indicated. A verticle midline or paramedian incision is usually adequate in the first two trimesters of pregnancy. Later, the imposition of the uterus into the operative site might make resection difficult, and a high transverse incision should be considered.

If the vascular supply to the adnexa has been severely compromised, salpingectomy (or salpingo-oophorectomy, if the ovary is involved) is recommended.

With the present availability of tocolytic agents of moderate effectiveness, patients should be observed closely in the immediate perioperative period for premature labor. Tocolytic medication, particularly the beta-adrenergic agents, may further complicate the venous stasis seen postoperatively or increase the risk of postoperative phlebitis. Statistical risks of such medications in the postoperative pregnant patient are not available.

Salpingitis

The coincident occurrence of salpingitis with pregnancy is rare enough to make the diagnosis suspect. Because of the atypical location of the appendix, early appendicitis may present with physical findings suggestive of unilateral or bilateral salpingitis. Because of the limited number of cases reported and a reluctance to intervene with surgery prematurely, antibiotics are often used empirically. Whether the diagnosis was incorrect or symptoms subsided on account of the treatment is difficult to determine.

Surgery is always undertaken with caution, particularly when the patient is pregnant. However, any delay in surgical intervention during pregnancy jeopardizes both the mother and her fetus. Early diagnosis and prompt performance of necessary surgery ensure the best chance for a favorable outcome for the pregnant patient.

REFERENCES

1. McCorriston CC. Nonobstetrical abdominal surgery during pregnancy. Am J Obstet Gynecol. 1963; 86:593–9.
2. Radman HM. Pregnancy complicated by nonobstetric surgical disease. Arch Surg. 1964; 88:279–86.
3. Griffen WO, Dilts PV, Roddick JW. Non-obstetric surgery during pregnancy. (Curr Probl Surg. November, 1969.) Chicago: Year Book, 1969.
4. Saunders P, Milton PJ. Laparotomy during pregnancy: an assessment of diagnostic accuracy and fetal wastage. Br Med J. 1973; 3:165–7.
5. Shnider SM, Webster, GM. Maternal and fetal hazards of surgery during pregnancy. Am J Obstet Gynecol. 1965; 92:891–900.
6. Finch, DR, Lee E. Acute appendicitis complicating pregnancy in the Oxford region. Br J Surg. 1974; 61:129–32.
7. O'Neill JP. Surgical conditions complicating pregnancy. I. Acute appendicitis—real and simulated. Aust NZ J Obstet Gynaecol. 1969; 9:94–9.
8. Townsend JM, Greiss FC. Appendicitis in pregnancy. South Med J. 1976; 69:1161–3.
9. Cunningham FG, McCubbin JH. Appendicitis complicating pregnancy. Obstet Gynecol. 1975; 45:415–20.
10. Babaknia A, Parsa H, Woodruff JD. Appendicitis during pregnancy. Obstet Gynecol. 1977; 50:40–4.
11. Black WP. Acute appendicitis in pregnancy. Br Med J. 1960; 1:1938–41.
12. Babler EA. Perforative appendicitis complicating pregnancy. JAMA. 1908; 51:1310–4.
13. McDonald AL. Appendicitis in pregnancy. Am J Obstet Gynecol. 1929; 18:110–5.

14. Brant HA. Acute appendicitis in pregnancy. Obstet Gynecol. 1967; 29:130–8.

15. Gomez A, Wood M. Acute appendicitis during pregnancy. Am J Surg. 1979; 137:180–3.

16. Hamlin E, Bartlett MK, Smith JA. Acute surgical emergencies of the abdomen in pregnancy. N Engl J Med. 1951; 244:128–31.

17. Mersheimer WL, Kazarian KK. The acute abdomen in pregnancy. In: Barber HRK, Graber EA, eds. Surgical disease in pregnancy. Philadelphia: Saunders, 1974:99–111.

18. Taylor JD. Acute appendicitis in pregnancy and the puerperium. Aust NZ Obstet Gynaecol. 1972; 12:202–3.

19. Baer JL, Reis RA, Arens RA. Appendicitis in pregnancy. JAMA. 1932; 98:1359–64.

20. Braverman DZ, Johnson ML, Kern F Jr. Effects of pregnancy and contraceptive steroids on gallbladder function. N Engl J Med. 1980; 302:362–4.

21. Cohen S. The sluggish gallbladder of pregnancy. N Engl J Med. 1980; 302:397–9.

22. Friley MD, Douglas G. Acute cholecystitis in pregnancy and the puerperium. Am Surg. 1972; 38:314–7.

23. Aufses AH Jr. Biliary tract disease. In: Rovinsky JJ, Guttmacher AF, eds. Medical, surgical, and gynecologic complications of pregnancy. 2nd ed. Baltimore: Williams & Wilkins, 1965:251–3.

24. Sparkman RS. Gallstones in young women. Ann Surg. 1957; 145:813–24.

25. Greene J, Rogers A, Rubin L. Fetal loss after cholecystectomy during pregnancy. Can Med Assoc J. 1963; 88:576–7.

26. Hill LM, Johnson CE, Lee RA. Cholecystectomy in pregnancy. Obstet Gynecol. 1975; 46:291–3.

27. Printen KJ, Ott RA. Cholecystectomy during pregnancy. Am Surg. 1978; 44:432–4.

28. Stone ML, Folsome CE. Nonobstetric surgical complications of pregnancy. Surg Clin North Am. 1955; 35:487–96.

29. Coughlan BM, O'Herlihy CO. Acute intestinal obstruction during pregnancy. J R Coll Surg Edinb. 1978; 23:175–7.

30. Hill LM, Symmonds RE. Small bowel obstruction in pregnancy. Obstet Gynecol. 1977; 49:170–3.

31. Stavorovsky M, Iellin A, David M, Weintraub S. Midgut volvulus with secondary thrombosis of superior mesenteric vessels in a pregnant woman. Surgery. 1977; 81:353–6.

32. Shaxted EJ, Jukes R. Pseudo-obstruction of the bowel in pregnancy. Br J Obstet Gynaecol. 1979; 86:411–3.

33. Milne B, Johnstone MS. Intestinal obstruction in pregnancy. Scott Med J. 1979; 24:80–2.

34. Kammerer WS. Nonobstetric surgery during pregnancy. Med Clin North Am. 1979; 63:1157–64.

35. Burrow GN. Medical complications during pregnancy. Philadelphia: Saunders, 1975.

36. Clark DH. Peptic ulcer in women. Br Med J. 1953; 1:1254–7.

37. DeVore GR. Acute abdominal pain in the pregnant patient due to pancreatitis, acute appendicitis, cholecystitis, or peptic ulcer disease. Clin Perinatol. 1980; 7:349–69.

38. Becker-Andersen H, Husfeldt V. Peptic ulcer in pregnancy. Acta Obstet Gynecol Scand. 1971; 50:391–5.

39. Horwich M. Perforated duodenal ulcer during pregnancy. Br Med J. 1958; 1:145.

40. Wengert PA, Metzger PP, Ecker HA, Patterson LT. The use of ultrasonography in the diagnosis of calculous gallbladder disease. Am Surg. 1979; 45:439–43.

41. Parish FM, Richardson JB. Acute pancreatitis during pregnancy. Am J Obstet Gynecol. 1956; 72:906–9.

42. McKay AJ, O'Neill J, Imrie CW. Pancreatitis, pregnancy and gallstones. Br J Obstet Gynaecol. 1980; 87:47–50.

43. Hasselgren PO. Acute pancreatitis in pregnancy. Acta Chir Scand. 1980; 146:297–9.

44. Nelson EW, Archibald L, Albo D. Spontaneous hepatic rupture in pregnancy. Am J Surg. 1977; 134:817–20.

45. Stanley JC. Splanchnic artery aneurysms. In: Rutherford RB, ed. Vascular surgery. Philadelphia: Saunders, 1977:673–85.

46. Schiffer MA. A review of 268 ectopic pregnancies. Am J Obstet Gynecol. 1963; 86:264–70.

47. Ploman L, Wicksell F. Fertility after conservative surgery in tubal pregnancy. Acta Obstet Gynecol Scand. 1960; 39:143–52.

48. Timonen S, Nieminen U. Tubal pregnancy, choice of operative method of treatment. Acta Obstet Gynecol Scand. 1967; 46:327–39.

49. Stromme WB. Conservative surgery for ectopic pregnancy. A twenty-year review. Obstet Gynecol. 1973; 41:215–23.

50. Stangel JJ, Reyniak JV, Stone ML. Conservative surgical management of tubal pregnancy. Obstet Gynecol. 1976; 48:241–4.

51. Bukovsky I, Langer R, Herman A, Caspi E. Conservative surgery for tubal pregnancy. Obstet Gynecol. 1979; 53:709–11.

52. DeCherney A, Kase N. The conservative surgical management of unruptured ectopic pregnancy. Obstet Gynecol. 1979; 54:451–5.

53. Bruhat MA, Manhes H, Mage G, Pouly JL. Treatment of ectopic pregnancy by means of laparoscopy. Fertil Steril. 1980; 33:411–4.

54. DeCherney AH, Polan ML, Kort H, Kase N. Microsurgical technique in the management of tubal ectopic pregnancy. Fertil Steril. 1980; 34:324–7.

55. DeCherney AH, Romero R, Naftolin F. Surgical management of unruptured ectopic pregnancy. Fertil Steril. 1981; 35:21–4.

56. Baker NA. Trauma in the pregnant patient. Surg Clin North Am. 1982; 62:175–89.

57. Buchsbaum HJ. Trauma in pregnancy. Philadelphia: Saunders, 1979.

58. Stuart GCE, Harding TJR, Davies EM. Blunt abdominal trauma in pregnancy. Can Med Assoc J. 1980; 122:901–5.

59. Grimes WH, Bartholomew R, Calvin ED, Fish JS, Lester WM. Ovarian cyst complicating pregnancy. Am J Obstet Gynecol. 1954; 68:594–605.

17. ALLERGIC DISORDERS

David S. Pearlman

The concept of *allergy* arose at the turn of this century with the realization that contact with a foreign substance altered the way in which the host subsequently responded to that substance. Although the term encompassed any state of altered specific host reactivity, whether beneficial or unfavorable, allergy has come to refer principally to the adverse consequences of contact with foreign agents. The recognition that certain kinds of antibody-like substances often were associated with particular constellations of signs and symptoms led to a concept of "allergic disorders" with the implication that there was an immune basis to these disorders. Although in many instances the disorders are due to antigen-antibody interaction, nonimmune factors frequently play major precipitating or aggravating roles. Moreover, mediators involved in allergic reactions can be released also by nonimmune mechanisms, and so-called allergic disorders (e.g., some forms of asthma and urticaria) do not always have an "allergic" basis.

Allergic reactions and disorders observed in nonpregnant individuals all can occur during pregnancy. Signs, symptoms, and the course of the disorder are not substantially different from those in nonpregnant women. Diagnostic and therapeutic considerations of allergic disorders are also similar regardless of whether or not pregnancy is involved. Because of physiologic changes that occur during pregnancy, and the presence of a fetus, therapeutic considerations require judgment different from that which is applicable to the nonpregnant female. The major allergic syndromes of concern include upper respiratory tract manifestations of allergy, specifically perennial and seasonal allergic rhinitis, associated sinusitis, eustachian tube dysfunction and middle ear disease, asthma (discussed in Chap. 19), food hypersensitivity, particularly with gastrointestinal manifestations, atopic dermatitis, urticaria (discussed in Chap. 21), and anaphylactic reactions due mainly to drugs, foods, and insect stings.

RELATIONSHIP BETWEEN PHYSIOLOGIC CHANGES OF PREGNANCY AND ALLERGIC DISORDERS

Various physiologic alterations in pregnancy have an impact on the course, severity, and symptoms of allergic disorders. Vascular changes with resulting tissue engorgement, especially in the nasal passages, for example, may complicate or masquerade as allergic rhinitis [1]. Similar hormone-induced changes in the lungs [2], skin, and possibly gastrointestinal tract may cause an intensification of tissue responses to irritants and allergens in these organs. Although there is no evidence of marked changes in metabolism of or tolerance to the chemical mediators of allergic reactions, the discomfort of pregnancy accompanied by maternal concern for the well-being of the fetus can lead to decreased tolerance of allergic manifestations with exaggerated discomfort. Thus, itching may be more intense, nasal mucosal engorgement may intensify upper respiratory tract problems of allergic origin, and the physiologic dyspnea that occurs in pregnancy may complicate assessment and treatment of asthma (see Chap. 19).

IMMUNE ADAPTATIONS TO PREGNANCY

Various immune changes have been observed in pregnancy, but such changes are not found universally [3,4]. There is a tendency toward decreased IgE levels as well as a slight diminution in serum IgG. A decrease in the germinal centers of the pelvic and paraaortic lymph nodes has also been observed. The clinical significance of these observations is not clear, however, since maternal antibody responses appear to be substantially normal. On the other hand, there is evidence for decreased cell-mediated immunity in pregnancy in general, with suggestions of diminished ability to reject allografts, a lessening of the tuberculin response, a tendency toward regression of autoimmune diseases with decreased requirement for immunosuppressive drugs to maintain clinical well-being, and some increase in susceptibility to viral infections in which cell-mediated immune mechanisms are thought to have a role in host resistance. Variable and inconsistent changes in T and B cell function and numbers also have been described [3,4]. Fetal T cell suppressor activity increases during pregnancy and has been related to changes in maternal cellular immune function [5].

The immune changes observed probably represent physiologic adaptations that help maintain pregnancy. Previously, the ability of the mother to maintain a fetal graft possessing foreign (paternal) antigens was attributed to the development of an immunologically privileged site in utero, with sequestration of antigen for the maternal lymphoid system through the protection of nonimmunogenic trophoblast barrier. Transplacental passage of both maternal and fetal antigens into the alternative circulations occurs, however, with resultant maternal sensitization to fetal antigens. Paradoxically, an active maternal immune response appears important in maintaining normal pregnancy. Whereas maternal lymphocytes sensitized to fetal trophoblastic antigens presumably have the capacity for cytotoxic destruction of the trophoblast and fetus, a vigorous humoral response to similar or related antigens seems to provide noncytotoxic antibodies, which react with these antigens and serve to coat the trophoblast with maternal protein. As a result, antigen becomes unavailable to react with sensitized maternal lymphocytes. This process of immune enhancement is probably analogous to that which prolongs tumor survival. Immune enhancement may be aided by immunosuppressive serum factors, which have been found in the circulation of some pregnant women as well as in cord blood but are present in highest concentration in the vicinity of the trophoblast-decidua. This immunosuppressive activity has been related to numerous humoral substances including progesterone, estrogen, cortisol, human chorionic gondatropin, human somatotropin, human placental lactogen, prolactin, pregnancy zone protein, $alpha_2$-macroglobulin, and alpha-fetoprotein [4]. In the latter instance, estrogen bound to the fetoprotein may be the active immunosuppressive agent [6]. Thus, maternal immune changes observed may be "spillover" effects of local mechanisms that have survival advantage for the fetus and maintenance of pregnancy.

FETAL IMMUNITY

At birth, the major part of serologic immunity enjoyed by the newborn is maternally derived, con-

sisting of IgG antibody [7,8]. All subfractions of IgG (IgG_{1-4}) traverse the placenta, but passage of IgG_2 may be relatively less efficient. There are two mechanisms for transplacental passage of immunoglobulins: (1) simple diffusion, beginning early in pregnancy, probably as early as the first trimester, which results in low fetal IgG levels, and (2) an active secretory mechanism that comes into play in the last half of pregnancy [9]. The secretory process is responsible for the gradual and substantial increase in fetal IgG after about 20 weeks' gestation so that in full-term births IgG concentrations are equal to or slightly greater than those of maternal blood IgG. Preterm infants have less IgG in proportion to the relative degree of prematurity. Under normal circumstances there is no transplacental passage of immunoglobulins A, D, M, and E. Thus, passive allergic sensitization by maternally derived IgE antibody is virtually nonexistent. IgG_4, reported to have skin-sensitizing antibody activity somewhat similar to that of IgE antibody in some individuals [10], is acquired by the fetus. Presumably, therefore, transient passive sensitization due to maternally derived IgG_4 from a sensitized mother could lead to reactivity of the newborn to corresponding allergens. To the author's knowledge, this has not been documented, however. Cord blood may contain lower levels of immunoglobulins A and M, and possibly D of fetal origin, but in the absence of intrauterine infection the level of antibody produced by the fetus is negligible.

Immunoglobulin formation and the capacity to respond to antigenic stimulation occur early in fetal life [11]. For example, cells that form immunoglobulins M, G, and E have been found by 10 to 12 weeks of fetal life. The lack of fetal antibody formation consequently appears to reflect in utero protection of the fetus from immunogenic concentrations of foreign materials. Nevertheless, transplacental passage of antigen does occur, and instances of fetal sensitization to food allergens ingested by the mother, with subsequent allergic disease in the newborn period, have been reported [12]. Implications of this observation concerning prophylaxis of allergic disease will be discussed at a later point in this chapter.

EFFECTS OF ALLERGIC DISORDERS ON PREGNANCY

The effects of allergic disorders on pregnancy are variable, and, other than to generally increase the discomfort of pregnancy, there is no consistent pattern. Relationships between asthma and pregnancy are discussed in Chapter 19. Allergic upper respiratory tract disease and other allergic disorders probably increase the risk of upper respiratory tract complications such as sinusitis, eustachian tube dysfunction, and perhaps otitis media; and food hypersensitivity may compound gastrointestinal problems of pregnancy, but there is little documentation of such effects. Extreme allergic sensitivity to drugs, insect stings, foods, or other materials poses the same risk as in nonpregnant women, with the additional potential that anaphylactic reactions can interfere with the successful outcome of pregnancy. However, reports of abortion or fetal death associated with severe allergic reactions in pregnancy are extremely rare, and the survivability of the fetus in the face of severe allergic reactions is remarkably good [13]. With the additional possible exception of asthma, there is meager evidence to suggest that allergic disorders play a significant role in either preventing or interfering with the normal maintenance of pregnancy, labor, and delivery.

EFFECTS OF TREATMENT ON MOTHER AND FETUS

Pregnancy may complicate therapy for allergic disorders through occasional increased intolerance of pregnant women to side effects of antiallergic medications as well as through concern for possible effects of medications used in therapy on the fetus (see below). In general, however, there is little evidence that allergy therapy, including pharmacotherapy, increases the risk of teratogenesis or affects the outcome of pregnancy in any other way. In addition, since anaphylactic reactions and respiratory compromise in asthma can also lead to fetal damage, fetal risk from allergic disease itself must be weighed against possible risks to the fetus that may be associated with the use of therapeutic agents. Women who are known or thought to be hypersensitive to foods and who employ highly restrictive diets run the risk of nutritional deprivation both to themselves and to the fetus, and the nutritional adequacy of diet during pregnancy must be ensured. Because of evidence for active in utero sensitization to foods ingested by the mother in children with a propensity to become allergic, the intake of large amounts of commonly allergenic food by mothers who have a strong family history of allergic sensitivity, particularly to foods, may carry an increased risk of sensitization of the fetus to such foods.

CLINICAL EVALUATION OF ALLERGIC DISORDERS

Pregnancy does not alter the general principles of clinical evaluation of allergic disorders. As implied previously, the ability to become sensitized to allergens and to express such sensitivity is not substantially different in pregnancy and in the nonpregnant state. Pregnancy may complicate evaluation of signs and symptoms of allergy because of the intensified discomfort exhibited by many pregnant patients and the physiologic changes in nasal and other tissues commonly associated with allergy. In addition to history and physical examination, laboratory procedures can be of immense help in evaluating allergy and generally carry little risk of insulting mother or fetus. The possible exception is allergy skin testing in the extraordinarily sensitive patient.

Allergy Testing

Skin testing is the classic method of acquiring evidence of allergic sensitization. The general principles of allergy skin testing and the significance of findings can be found in allergy texts. Tests are correlative with historical and physical findings and are not diagnostic by themselves. Specifically, allergy tests are used to determine whether a patient has "allergic" antibody and therefore may be "allergic" in the first place, and by inference to implicate specific allergens which *may* play an etiologic role in the patient's disease. Identification of possible causative disease factors thus is used to provide a basis for some therapeutic action. Generally, prick or scratch tests are more correlative and are safer than intradermal tests, but systemic reactions from all forms of testing can occur. If a decision has been made prior to testing not to use immunotherapy (hyposensitization) during pregnancy to pollens and other nonavoidable allergens, allergy tests for such allergens can be postponed until after delivery. Tests for environmental allergens to which exposure can be manipulated, however, should be considered. There is no evidence that maternal allergy skin tests risk sensitization of the fetus or of the infant who is breast-feeding.

The radioallergosorbent test (RAST) is an alternative approach to allergy skin testing. In this test, IgE antibody to possible allergens is measured serologically. RAST is slightly less sensitive than skin testing in identifying problematic allergens and tends to be considerably more expensive than allergy skin tests. Moreover, allergens available for testing are relatively few in number [14]. In addition, allergic sensitivity in a small proportion of patients appears to be related to IgG_4 skin-sensitizing antibody, not measured by RAST [10]. Consequently, skin testing generally is more advantageous than RAST in evaluating the allergic patient.

However, in patients with histories of extreme allergic sensitivity to suspected allergens (e.g., the venom of stinging insects, or foods), a serologic test obviously eliminates any possible risk to mother and fetus. As with skin tests, serologic tests are correlative only.

The level of immunoglobulin E is often elevated in allergic individuals, and serologic measurement of IgE by the radioimmunosorbent test (RIST) or paper RIST (PRIST) is available in many laboratories. However, allergic hypersensitivity often exists in the presence of normal or low IgE levels, and the presence of a high IgE level does not establish a diagnosis of allergy or a so-called allergic disorder such as asthma. Consequently, this test for allergy is of extremely limited usefulness. Measurement of other immunoglobulins (G, A, M, and D) is of little benefit in evaluating individuals with allergic disorders, with the possible exception of disorders in which recurrent symptoms masquerade as allergy but may be due to immunodeficiency—for example, in some diarrheal states, or in recurrent upper and lower respiratory tract inflammation with an infectious component. If any question of immunodeficiency exists, it is important to determine immunoglobulin levels with particular attention to IgG, not only because of a question pertinent to maternal health, but also because of the maternal derivation of the infant's complement of antibodies at birth.

Eosinophilia

Because of the frequent association between the accumulation of eosinophils and allergic reactions, the finding of tissue and blood eosinophilia is often considered circumstantial evidence of allergy. But chemical mediators released by immune reactions are also liberated by nonimmune mechanisms, and the accumulation of eosinophils is not specific for allergy. Tissue and peripheral blood eosinophilia often occurs in asthma, for instance, regardless of whether allergic mechanims can be implicated, and nasal eosinophilia occurs in a small proportion of individuals who have nonallergic, noninfectious rhinitis [15]. There is little information on possible alterations of tissue or peripheral blood eosinophilia due to pregnancy per se and the relationship to allergic disorders in pregnancy, but there is no reason to believe that eosinophilia has any other significance than in the nonpregnant state, namely, circumstantial evidence suggestive of an allergic tissue reaction. The accumulation of eosinophils in nasal and other tissues in the newborn period to approximately three months of age may reflect the normal inflammatory response at this age [16].

Other Laboratory Tests

The laboratory tests mentioned seek to provide direct or indirect information for immune reactants possibly involved in an allergic disorder, or markers of allergic tissue inflammation. Since allergic disorders are associated with dysfunction in the organ or tissue involved, laboratory evaluation of such disorders obviously should include appropriate measures of organ function. These are of particular importance with regard to asthma, in which measurement of pulmonary function is an essential part of the evaluation of this disorder.

MANAGEMENT OF ALLERGIC DISORDERS
General Considerations in the Pregnant Woman

Principles of management of allergic disorders include elimination of allergens or irritants involved in precipitating or aggravating the disease, attempts to decrease hypersensitivity to nonavoidable allergens (hyposensitization), and the use of pharmacologic agents to prevent or reverse the pathologic changes of allergic disease. As with the evaluation of allergic disease, pregnancy does not alter the general principles of management of allergic disorders. There are obvious additional considerations relative to fetal risk and maternal comfort, however. Vigorous appropriate allergen and irritant control and elimination are the mainstay of therapy. They are of particular importance in the pregnancy allergic patient since they may diminish the need for other forms of therapy with which there may be potential added risk to the outcome of pregnancy. Thus, elimination of domestic animals from the environment in an individual who is animal sensitive, creating a dust- and mold-poor environment in individuals sensitive to these substances, keeping the bedroom windows closed at night and the house closed, providing an air-conditioning unit if necessary to filter out outside pollens and seasonal molds for pollen- or mold-sensitive persons, and avoiding foods to which a woman may be hypersensitive are all of special importance in managing allergic diseases in the pregnant woman [17,18].

Immunotherapy

Immunotherapy (hyposensitization, allergy injection therapy) is employed when the responsible allergens cannot be avoided and the degree of pathology they induce cannot be ameliorated satisfactorily with the use of palliative measures unassociated with significant side effects. There is a great deal of information on the use of immunotherapy during pregnancy, and recent reports suggest that with the proper precautions this procedure can be safe for mother and fetus throughout pregnancy [19,20]. Nonetheless, severe allergic reactions to allergy injections, including anaphylaxis, rarely with abortion, have been reported [21]. Consequently, it is wise to be particularly cautious when utilizing this therapeutic modality during pregnancy. As a general rule, women on immunotherapy prior to conception can be maintained on it throughout pregnancy, employing previous safely tolerated maintenance dosage and diminishing dosage during problematic allergy season (a decrease in dosage by one-third is recommended). Increments in dosage for individuals who are not yet on maintenance dosage should be conservative, with more gradual increments than usual. Dosage should not be maximized in the face of any local or possibly mild systemic manifestations until after delivery. Hyposensitization can be instituted in pregnancy, but it is the author's practice to defer institution of immunotherapy whenever possible until after delivery. There is no evidence that immunotherapy produces teratogenesis or any other harmful effects in the fetus. On the other hand, some recent evidence suggests that immunotherapy for the mother may diminish the likelihood of subsequent sensitization of the infant and young child to the allergens employed [22].

Pharmacotherapy

The use of any drug in pregnancy must be considered to carry with it the potential for teratogenesis and other adverse fetal effects. Some of the drugs employed in treatment of allergic disorders, in particular antihistamines, have been used very commonly by pregnant women (10–50% of all pregnancies in various series [23,24]). Considering the frequency of usage of such drugs, adverse effects on the fetus from their use should be readily apparent, yet there is little evidence to suggest significant detrimental effects of these drugs or of other antiallergic drugs, even corticosteroids, on outcomes of pregnancy, including fetal abnormalities or the course of pregnancy, labor, and delivery [23–26]. Nevertheless, the absence of documented adverse effects does not establish safety for such medications, and it is wise to adopt a relatively conservative attitude in prescribing drugs, particularly during the first trimester of pregnancy. This approach must be tempered by the possible risks to mother and fetus from the allergic disease itself. Unfortunately, the physician is often placed in a position of weighing undocumented and unknown possible risks especially to the fetus from the use of a pharmacotherapeutic agent against the obvious discomfort and potential risk to both mother and fetus from the consequences of cardiovascular or respiratory compromise, which can be associated with severe allergic disease. Table 17-1 summarizes information on adverse effects on the fetus of pharmacotherapeutic agents used in allergic disorders.

Many allergic disorders (e.g., disorders of the upper and lower respiratory tract, or the skin) respond to the actions of topical agents, which can induce maximal local therapeutic effect while associated with relatively little drug absorption in active form. These agents offer the opportunity of therapeutic benefits with predictably minimal systemic hazards to both mother and fetus. In the author's opinion, therefore, it makes most sense to maximize use of topically active agents whenever possible in place of comparable systemically active therapeutic agents. For example, inhalation of beta-adrenergic agents seems a preferable therapeutic approach to asthma as compared to administration of oral adrenergic agents. An argument can also be made for the use of topical corticosteroids in upper and lower respiratory tract disease and for inhaled cromolyn to help control respiratory tract inflammation, none of which is "approved for use" during pregnancy.

MANAGEMENT OF SPECIFIC DISORDERS
Allergic Rhinitis and Conjunctivitis

Allergic rhinitis is the most common of allergic conditions and is encountered frequently in pregnant women. Rhinitis is more likely to intensify during pregnancy, although occasionally it may ameliorate. Other noninfectious forms of rhinitis also occur frequently (see below) and may aggravate an underlying allergic condition or masquerade as allergic rhinitis. Treatment consists of maximizing control over allergens and other nonallergenic environmental factors that may aggravate symptoms, immunotherapy, and the use of palliative drugs.

Antihistamines classically are the drugs of choice in control of allergic rhinitis. Pharmaceutical manufacturers vary in their recommendations concerning the use of antihistamines in pregnancy, but most list their drugs as contraindicated in pregnancy or for use with the caution that "safety has not been established." As indicated previously, however, evidence for teratogenicity or other ad-

Table 17-1. Effects of drugs used to treat allergic disorders on the fetus and newborn

Drug	Teratogenicity	Comments
Antihistamines	No evidence of overall effect; questionable association with brompheniramine, some phenothiazines, and hydroxyzine	Extrapyramidal signs in newborn lasting for months may be associated with maternal phenothiazine use around time of delivery
Sympathomimetics	Suggestions that minor malformations may be associated with use of common ingredients in nose drops, inhalants, and preparations taken orally to relieve URIs	Beta receptor agonists can increase fetal heart rate; a few instances of cardiac arrhythmia reported
Parasympathomimetics	Suggestions that minor malformations occur more frequently in women who use atropine-like preparations	Transplacental passage occurs
Methylxanthines	No evidence for association	Toxicity in newborn can occur from transplacental transfer; cord blood levels of drug approximate maternal blood levels; half-life of theophylline 3–4 times longer in full-term newborns than in older children and more prolonged in prematures
Cromolyn sodium	No evidence for association	No adverse effects documented
Corticosteroids	No evidence for association	Rare hypoadrenalism in newborn in mothers taking corticosteroids; suggestions of slightly increased risk of retardation of intrauterine growth and fetal wastage
Expectorants (iodides)	Little information	Can cause hypothyroidism in newborn and respiratory tract obstruction from goiter; *use contraindicated in pregnancy*
Cough medications	No evidence	Abuse may lead to fetal distress syndrome from alcoholic content of preparations
Antibiotics (various)		
Tetracyclines	Suggestive evidence for association with tetracycline use *or* infection for which drug used (?)	Deposited in fetal bones; causes permanent staining of teeth; *should not be used in pregnancy*
Sulfonamides	No evidence	Readily cross placenta
Erythromycin	Little data	Concentrations in fetal plasma = 5–20% of maternal concentrations; can interfere with theophylline metabolism
Penicillins	No evidence	
Foods	No effects reported	Small amounts can traverse placenta and sensitize fetus
Immunotherapy (hyposensitization, allergy injection therapy)	No effects reported	Generally safe; can cause anaphylaxis and possibly abortion (rare report)

Source: Adapted from various sources. In particular, see references 20, 23–27, 36, 45, 62, 63.

verse effects on the fetus of these and other antihistamines is lacking [23,24]. Antihistamines tend to be more effective in controlling the rhinorrhea and itching and associated sneezing of allergic rhinitis than nasal congestion. Adrenergic agents, particularly pseudoephedrine and phenylpropanolamine, are used alone or as an adjunct to antihistamines to help control nasal congestion and "stuffiness." Topical adrenergic agents also are useful for short periods of time, but much caution has to be exercised to prevent overuse and congestive rebound. Profound nasal obstruction may interfere with sleep at night, and the temptation to overuse topical adrenergic agents is difficult to resist. Although topical steroids used over a prolonged period of time sometimes obviate the need for adrenergic agents, in some patients topical adrenergic agents may be required nightly for prolonged periods in order to permit a reasonable period of sleep.

As indicated, despite the potential teratogenicity of corticosteroids reported in experimental animals and the possible adrenal suppressive effects in the mother and fetus, the risk of such effects appears to be extraordinarily small. Topical steroids can be used alone, or as adjuncts to antihistamine/decongestants. Three topical nasal steroids are available in the United States: dexamethasone sodium phosphate (Turbinaire Decadron Phosphate nasal spray), beclomethasone dipropionate (Vancenase and Beconase) and flunisolide (Nasalide). Dexamethasone is readily absorbed in active form, and although the major part of the effect is topical, systemic effects from its use can occur and are dose related. Consequently, unless used in minimum dosage (e.g., one spray in each nostril once or twice a day), adrenal suppression conceivably can occur. The clinical significance of the degree of suppression that occurs with usually recommended dosages is unclear. Overuse can also lead to septal perforation. The other topical nasal steroid preparations mentioned exhibit insignificant systemic activity in the usual recommended therapeutic dosage but do not appear to be as potent as dexamethasone in relieving nasal symptoms.

Cromolyn sodium has been used with some success in the treatment of allergic rhinitis. It ordinarily is employed for this purpose every four to six hours, but its effectiveness is not as impressive as that of the topical steroids. It has also been used as a 4% solution in treating allergic conjunctivitis. Experience with it in pregnancy is limited, but available information points to a lack of untoward effects on the fetus [27].

Allergic conjunctivitis may be controlled by systemic antihistamines, or topical antihistamine/decongestant preparations, or simple vasoconstrictor eye drops with or without antihistamines. Corticosteroid eye drops may also be used for short periods of time to aid in controlling severe symptoms. Steroid preparations of mild potency (e.g., HMS Medrysone) are generally preferred, utilized for a few days at a time. Contraindications to the use of steroid eye drops in pregnancy are the same as in nonpregnant women, namely, herpes simplex eye infection or corneal ulceration. A short course of systemic steroid therapy may be necessary on occasion to limit side effects. Short-acting oral steroids such as prednisone should be employed for the briefest periods possible and are preferred to parenteral therapy for control of symptoms and steroids side effects. Intranasal steroid inoculation carries with it the added risk of inducing blindness in an occasional patient [28].

Immunotherapy is used as an adjunct in the treatment of allergic rhinitis when symptoms warrant and allergens cannot be eliminated (see above).

Other Forms of Noninfectious Rhinitis

A nonallergic, noninfectious rhinitis (sometimes called vasomotor rhinitis), which takes variable forms, occurs commonly and presents mainly as rhinorrhea, nasal congestion, or both. This form of rhinitis too may be intensified by the physiologic changes of pregnancy [1]. In addition, many women without a prior history of chronic nasal symptomatology develop bothersome and sometimes extensive nasal congestion with rhinorrhea to the point of complete nasal obstruction during pregnancy [1]. This so-called physiologic rhinitis of pregnancy usually begins in the latter part of the first trimester and continues for most of pregnancy. Considering the fact that a major portion of the problem is nasal mucosal hyperemia, oral or topical nasal decongestants constitute the most rational therapeutic agents, and there is little reason to believe that antihistamines should be of major therapeutic benefit in this disorder. Nevertheless, some individuals with nonallergic rhinitis, particularly those with accompanying eosinophilia, respond extremely well to antihistamine therapy, and a therapeutic trial with antihistamines in a woman not responsive adequately to oral decongestants can be worthwhile. Treatment for this form of rhinitis may also require topical decongestant agents and topical steroids. Under rare circumstances, a short course of systemic steroid therapy may be necessary to control symptoms, but it is by no means universally effective. Atropine and related drugs may help control serious rhinorrhea but should be used particularly cautiously in pregnancy (see Table 17-1).

Nonpharmacologic treatment of allergic and other noninfectious rhinitis includes the use of hot steam vapor and normal saline nasal douches and gargle, both to thin nasal mucosal secretions and to soothe irritated nasopharyngeal mucous membranes.

Associated Upper Respiratory Conditions

Along with the increased nasal congestion, epistaxis from increased nasal congestion can be encountered during pregnancy. Sinusitis and eustachian tube dysfunction with secretory or infectious otitis media may occur more commonly than in the nonpregnant state [29,30].

Sinusitis is more likely to be a complication of

perennial than of seasonal rhinitis and should be suspected when purulent nasal discharge, purulent pharyngeal drainage, headaches, and fever occur. Not all patients with this clinical constellation, however, have sinus involvement. On the other hand, purulent sinusitis can occur in the absence of these signs or symptoms as a concomitant of rhinitis during pregnancy [30]. Transillumination is an unreliable diagnostic indicator, but roentgenograms of the paranasal sinuses and sinus irrigation are extremely useful diagnostic tools [30,31]. *Hemophilus influenzae* and *Streptococcus pneumoniae* are the most common pathogenic organisms involved [32]. Thus, the antibiotic of choice would seem to be ampicillin or amoxicillin, considering the organisms involved as well as the relative lack of adverse effects of these drugs on the mother and fetus. Sinus ostia patency should be maximized with the short-term use of topical nasal decongestants; longer-term use of topical nasal steroids may help promote and maintain patency of the ostia. The correlation between bacteriologic findings from nasal or pharyngeal culture and organisms present in the sinuses is poor [32,33], and such cultures do not provide helpful information for therapy, therefore. Obstruction of the sinus ostia without sinusitis, with secondary vacuum headaches may occur, as may thickening of the sinus mucosa presumably as an extension or reflection of the same noninfectious process that involves the nose.

Nasal polyposis occurs in pregnancy as in the nonpregnant state, but there is little information indicating any significant change in its incidence or severity in pregnancy. Most commonly, nasal polyposis is either a reflection of infectious sinusitis or a concomitant of aspirin idiosyncrasy. It is a surprisingly uncommon complication of allergic rhinitis [34]. Treatment includes surgical removal of the polyps when obstructive, antibiotic treatment when associated with infectious sinusitis, and topical nasal steroids. With any question of aspirin hypersensitivity, aspirin and aspirin-containing products should not be used. There is an increased risk of idiosyncrasy to other nonsteroidal antiinflammatory agents, such as indomethacin, as well, in aspirin-sensitive patients. Tartrazine (FD&C Yellow No. 5) presents a similar problem in a small proportion of aspirin-sensitive individuals. Aspirin idiosyncrasy may also be associated with asthma (usually nonallergic) and with urticaria [35].

Eustachian tube dysfunction with tubal occlusion or patulous eustachian tubes also appear to occur more commonly in the pregnant than nonpregnant state [29]. In the case of patulous eustachian tubes, the major problem seems to be symptomatic. Symptoms are intermittent and commonly include a feeling of fullness in the middle ear, sometimes to the point of being extremely disconcerting. Symptoms occur mainly in the upright position—may be relieved temporarily by forceful sniffling—or during upper respiratory tract infections and often are aggravated by exercise and the use of nasal decongestants. Many women with this condition are asymptomatic. The condition is more likely to occur in the mid and later stages of pregnancy and tends to disappear after delivery. There is a correlation between this form of eustachian tube dysfunction and elevated serum estrogen levels.

Tubal occlusion with annoying symptoms and secondary secretory otitis media with or without infection also occurs. Treatment includes the use of antibiotics with evidence of otitis media, and oral or nasal decongestants and topical steroidal antiinflammatory agents (although evidence for the effectiveness of these therapeutic agents is meager).

Atopic Dermatitis

Atopic dermatitis is predominantly a disorder of childhood but may persist through adulthood in variable forms. It is a relatively uncommon problem in pregnancy, and there is little evidence for any predictable effect of pregnancy on this disease [37]. A characteristic feature of atopic dermatitis is pruritus. Pruritus occurs in the last trimester of pregnancy in many women without dermatitis, probably in relation to hormonal changes and hepatobiliary stasis. The latter may intensify the pruritus of atopic dermatitis and conceivably may make control more difficult.

Treatment of atopic dermatitis centers on attempts to minimize contact with factors that provoke or aggravate skin irritation and itching (e.g., detergents, rough contact materials, sweating), to ensure adequate skin hydration, and to control inflammation with appropriate skin care measures and topical corticosteroids. Clinically significant systemic absorption of topical corticosteroids can occur, particularly if they are used extensively over inflamed skin for prolonged periods of time. The more potent fluorinated corticosteroids are more likely to produce evidence of systemic effects, and absorption of all steroids is intensified by occlusion therapy [38]. As indicated previously, despite concerns about adverse effects of maternal steroid use on the fetus, there appears to be remarkably little fetal effect. Nevertheless, it is wise to be particularly cautious in the pregnant woman with the extensive use of topical corticosteroids.

The least potent steroids needed on a chronic basis to control eczema should be employed. A short course of systemic corticosteroids is required on rare occasions to control dermatitis. Antihistamines are used for their antipruritic effects, but the major antipruritic effect is achieved by control of inflammation.

Severe Allergic Reactions

Severe allergic reactions, including life-threatening ones, occur mainly in relation to extreme sensitivity to the inhalation or ingestion of food allergens, the ingestion or injection of drugs, or hypersensitivity to stinging insects of the order Hymenoptera (bees, wasps, hornets, and fire ants) [39]. Allergens known to induce or suspected of inducing reactions should be avoided scrupulously. Pharmacotherapy includes the use of epinephrine 1:1,000 (adrenaline) by injection as the drug of first choice with severe allergic reactions, followed by antihistamines given intramuscularly, slowly intravenously, or orally. Inhalation of epinephrine from metered-dose aerosols (e.g., Medihaler-Epi, Primatene), which can be carried easily in a pocketbook or pocket, is convenient and can be effective in relieving pharyngeal and laryngeal angioedema and bronchospasm. Corticosteroids should be added with severe reactions, although their onset of action is slow (hours) and it is uncertain whether they are necessary or effective in acute severe allergic reactions.

The major pathologic changes in anaphylactic reactions of importance include angioedema of the airway, bronchial obstruction, cardiovascular collapse, and cardiac arrhythmia. Hypotension due to vascular collapse and loss of intravascular fluid through increased capillary permeability may require the use of intravenous fluid, arterial vasopressor agents, and oxygen. An adequate airway must be ensured.

Treatment of severe sensitivity to the venom of stinging insects requires special consideration. Individuals who have had systemic and potentially life-threatening reactions to the stings of bees, wasps, hornets, or fire ants should be hyposensitized with venom extracts, assuming that the venom allergens to which the person is hypersensitive can be identified. Therapy with whole-body extracts does not appear to be efficacious. Pregnancy is not considered a contraindication to such therapy [40]. Patients on immunotherapy prior to conception should be maintained on such therapy, either continued on the previous maintenance dose or increased cautiously to recommended dosage if not yet at maintenance level. Pregnant women who are considered at risk for life-

threatening reactions from stinging insects and who have not yet been placed on therapy probably should be started on immunotherapy to identified venom allergens if substantial exposure to stinging insects is likely during the course of pregnancy. Instructions should be given in techniques for avoidance of stinging insects (for example, refraining from wearing perfumes or other odoriferous materials, wearing noncolorful clothing outside in areas where such insects reside; nests and other sources of insects should be eliminated from the environment) [41]. The pregnant woman at risk should have an Anakit or similar convenient therapeutic kit available for treatment of anaphylaxis should a sting occur, and should be properly instructed on its use.

EFFECTS OF DRUG THERAPY ON THE OUTCOME OF PREGNANCY
Effects on the Fetus
Because of the high incidence of allergic disorders in the population, and the incorporation of antihistamines and decongestants in cough medicines and other preparations for the treatment of various upper respiratory tract conditions, the use of antiallergic drugs in pregnancy is extremely common. In the few instances in which suspicions of teratogenicity in particular have arisen, further examination of the effects of the use of such drugs in pregnancy have not borne out a predictable relationship between drug use and teratogenicity or other significant adverse effects. Table 17-1 lists the classes of drugs generally used to treat allergic disorders and summarizes information concerning each class of drugs. Drugs of major concern for their effects on the fetus are iodide expectorants and certain antibiotics. *The use of iodides is contraindicated* in pregnancy because of their propensity to produce goiter in the fetus and newborn [42,43]. Tetracyclines in particular inhibit protein synthesis and can affect fetal growth including development of teeth with permanent staining of teeth [36]. The abuse of alcohol-based cough syrups and other preparations used to treat both allergic and nonallergic respiratory conditions may lead to the fetal alcohol syndrome [44].

There is no evidence that immunotherapy for allergic disorders is teratogenic or has any other adverse effect upon the fetus. The induction of anaphylaxis by immunotherapy, however, carries with it possible risk to the fetus as well as the mother.

Effects on Labor and Delivery
With the possible exception of drugs used for treatment of asthma (see Chap. 19), there is little

Table 17-2. Effects of drugs used to treat allergic disorders on breast-feeding

Drug	Excretion (secretion) in breast milk	Comments
Antihistamines	In low concentrations	Side effects rarely reported; may cause sleepiness and poor feeding of infant; cyproheptadine may inhibit lactation
Sympathomimetics	Some excreted, low concentration (?)	Probably safe (infant irritability and crying have been attributed to use of antihistamine/decongestant combination drugs)
Parasympathomimetics	Yes	Rarely significant effects in newborn; however, not recommended for use in lactating mother
Methylxanthines	Concentration of theophylline $\cong$ 70% of maternal blood level	Mild toxic effects in infant reported (vomiting, irritability, poor sleeping pattern)
Cromolyn sodium	No data	Probably safe
Corticosteroids	In low concentration	No significant effects reported; probably safe
Expectorants		
Iodides	Yes	May affect thyroid function
Other	Little data	
Antibiotics		
Tetracyclines	Low concentration	Potential for inhibiting protein synthesis and for permanent staining of teeth
Sulfonamides	Yes	May increase risk of prolonged jaundice in newborn
Penicillins	Semisynthetic penicillins probably not excreted; penicillin, ampicillin excreted in low concentration	Diarrhea in infants has been attributed to maternal use of ampicillin
Foods	Some in small amounts (e.g., eggs, wheat, peanuts)	May cause allergic symptoms; some foods claimed to cause colic through nonallergic mechanisms (e.g., cabbage, turnips, broccoli, beans, rhubarb, apricots, prunes, heavy diet of melons, peaches, and other fresh fruits)
Immunotherapy (hyposensitization, allergy injection therapy)	Small amounts may be excreted	No adverse effects reported

Source: Adapted from various sources. In particular, see references 42, 47–50.

evidence of significant untoward effects of antiallergic drugs on the process of labor or delivery. Some preparations used either for asthma or for other disorders may contain barbiturates, however, which may cause central nervous system and respiratory depression in the newborn. Chronic use of such preparations may also cause barbiturate addiction in the newborn. There are concerns that epinephrine or terbutaline given parenterally may impede the progress of labor [26], but vigorous treatment of asthma during labor with adrenergic drugs does not appear to do so.

Effects on the Breast-Feeding Infant

Secretion of drugs in breast milk is highly variable and depends on numerous factors, including the size and physical state of the drug taken and drug concentration (see Chap. 6). Information on secretion of antiallergic drugs in breast milk and the effect on the infant is summarized in Table 17-2. With the exception of iodides and possibly atropine [45], there is relatively little evidence for adverse effects of most drugs used by the lactating mother for therapy of allergic disorders. Antihistamines tend to be secreted in small concentrations, and, although ordinarily not problematic for the feeding infant, maternal ingestion of large amounts of antihistamines conceivably may have soporific or other central nervous system effects on the infant and interfere with feeding. Unfortunately, pharmaceutical manufacturers apparently are required by the FDA to take the position that antihistamine therapy is contraindicated in nursing mothers, perhaps raising a legal issue if prescribed.

In the presence of high concentrations of theophylline in maternal blood, sufficient drug may be transmitted through breast milk to produce at least minor central nervous system stimulation in the infant [46]. Tetracyclines are secreted in low concentrations [47,48] and should not be employed in lactating women. It is recommended that erythromycin and sulfonamides not be used in the first month after delivery because of their effects on bilirubin-binding to protein and increased risk of jaundice in the newborn period [49]. Semisynthetic penicillins and penicillin G are considered relatively safe [49].

Foods ingested by the mother also may be transmitted through breast milk with sufficient antigenic integrity to provoke symptoms in the already sensitized infant. Conceivably, the infant may be sensitized in this way [49]. It is probable that small quantities of antigen from allergy immunotherapy of the mother are transmitted via breast milk to the infant, but the effects of allergy injections in the mother on the breast-fed infant appear to be inconsequential (see reference 50 for more extensive review).

PREVENTION OF ALLERGIC DISEASE IN OFFSPRING OF ALLERGIC MOTHERS

The familial occurrence of allergic disease has long been known and was one of the bases of the term *atopy*, coined by Coca and Cooke 60 years ago. Although a genetic basis for allergic disorders is implied by this pattern of inheritance, the genetics of allergic disease are still poorly defined [51,52]. It is clear that the propensity to make IgE antibody is heritable and that there is some linkage between the ability to manufacture IgE antibody and the likelihood of developing atopic disease (asthma, allergic rhinitis, and atopic dermatitis). To what extent the expression of the familial tendency for atopic disease is genetic or rather a product of environmental influence remains to be determined, for even in studies of identical twins, concordance for such diseases as asthma is less than 50% [53]. It is generally accepted that there is a "polygenic inheritance" of allergic diseases, and that environmental factors can play a strong role in determining whether or not disease will develop. There is reason to believe, therefore, that control of environmental factors can alter the development of allergic disease.

In 1936, Grulee and Sanford [54] reported that more eczema developed in artificially fed babies than in breast-fed babies. Since that time numerous studies have indicated that breast-feeding, with exclusion of beef, eggs, and wheat for the first nine months of life [55], or with control of the environment to minimize contact with common inhalant allergens [56], is associated with a decreased likelihood of eczema, although this has not been a universal finding [57]. There is also suggestive evidence that avoidance of cow's milk early in life is associated with a diminished incidence of upper and lower allergic respiratory disease in potentially allergic children [55,58,59].

Although evidence for the prevention of allergic disease by avoiding certain highly allergenic foods and controlling inhalant allergens in the environment early in life can only be considered suggestive, it is reasonable to encourage such procedures in highly allergic families, particularly for offspring of allergic mothers. Thus, breast-feeding is recommended for at least the first three months of life without feeding supplements other than glucose and water [60]. Alternatively, soy formulas can be used in place of cow's milk, but soy too is potentially allergenic. It is recommended that all cow's milk products, beef and veal, eggs and wheat be avoided for the first nine months of life. These foods should also be avoided by the lactating mother during this time. Nutritional adequacy for both maternal and infant diets should be ensured, however. In addition, every attempt should be made to minimize contact with domestic animals and to maximize dust and mold control, especially in the bedroom. There is suggestive evidence that children exposed to smoke frequently in their households may have more respiratory tract infections and respiratory disease in general. Further, asthmatic children subject to passive smoking appear to have a higher incidence of chronic obstructive pulmonary disease in adult life [61].

In summary, allergic diseases in pregnant women are treated in a substantially similar manner to the way they are treated in women who are not pregnant. Changes in allergic disease in pregnancy are not predictable, with some diseases such as asthma ameliorating, worsening, or staying the same. Therapeutic decisions in pregnant women are somewhat more difficult than in nonpregnant patients because of the potential of adverse fetal effects either by the disease or by therapy or both. Evidence indicates, however, that classic therapeutic approaches to the treatment of allergic disease are associated with relatively little increased risk to the mother and fetus.

REFERENCES

1. Mabry RL. Intranasal steroid injection during pregnancy. South Med J. 1980; 73:1176–9.

2. Weinberger SE, Weiss ST, Cohen WR, Weiss JW, Johnson TS. Pregnancy and the lung. Am Rev Respir Dis. 1980; 121:559–81.

3. Sridama V, Pacini F, Yang S, Moawad A, Reilly M, De-Groot LJ. Decreased levels of helper T cells: a possible cause of immunodeficiency in pregnancy. N Engl J Med. 1982; 307:352–6.

4. Scott HS, Jenkins DM. Immunology of human reproduction. In: Parker CW, ed. Clinical immunology. Philadelphia: Saunders, 1980:982–1008.

5. Froelich CJ, Goodwin JS, Bankhurst AD, Williams RC Jr. Pregnancy, a temporary fetal graft of suppressor cells in autoimmune disease? Am J Med. 1980; 69:329–31. editorial.

6. Clemens LE, Siiteri PK, Stites DP. Mechanism of immunosuppression of progesterone on maternal lymphocyte activation during pregnancy. J Immunol. 1979; 122:1978–85.

7. Miller MD. Developmental immunity. In: Bierman CW, Pearlman DS, eds. Allergic diseases of infancy, childhood and adolescence. Philadelphia: Saunders, 1980:27–35.

8. Stiehm ER. The B-lymphocyte system. In: Stiehm ER, Fulginiti VA, eds. Immunologic disorders in infants and children. 2nd ed. Philadelphia: Saunders, 1980:52–81.

9. Gitlin D. Development and metabolism of the immune globulins. In: Kagan BM, Stiehm ER, eds. Immunologic incompetence. Chicago: Year Book, 1971:3–16.

10. Gywnn CM, Smith JM, Leon GL, Stanworth DR. Role of IgG$_4$ subclass in childhood allergy. Lancet. 1978; 1:910–1.

11. Lawton AR, Cooper MD. Ontogeny of immunity. In: Stiehm ER, Fulginiti VA, eds. Immunologic disorders in infants and children. 2nd ed. Philadelphia: Saunders, 1980:36–51.

12. Kurome T, Oguri M, Matsumura T, et al. Milk sensitivity and soybean sensitivity in the production of eczematous manifestations in breast-fed infants with particular reference to intrauterine sensitization. Ann Allergy. 1976; 37:41–6.

13. Baraka A, Sfeir S. Anaphylactic cardiac arrest in a parturient. Response of the newborn. JAMA. 1980; 243:1745–6.

14. Adkinson NF Jr. The radioallergosorbent test in 1981—limitations and refinements. J Allergy Clin Immunol. 1981; 67:87–9. editorial.

15. Mullarkey MF, Hill JS, Webb DR. Allergic and nonallergic rhinitis: their characterization with attention to the meaning of nasal eosinophilia. J Allergy Clin Immunol. 1980; 65:122–6.

16. Matheson A, Rosenblum A, Glazer R, Dacanay E. Local tissue and blood eosinophils in newborn infants. J Pediatr. 1957; 51:502–9.

17. Buckley JM, Pearlman DS. Controlling the environment. In: Bierman CW, Pearlman DS, eds. Allergic diseases of infancy, childhood and adolescence. Philadelphia: Saunders, 1980:300–10.

18. Lockey SD III. Environmental control of allergic disease. In: Lockey RF, ed. Allergy and clinical immunology. Garden City, N.Y.: Medical Examination Publishing Co., 1979:1163–75.

19. Fein BT, Kamin PB. Management of allergy in pregnancy. Ann Allergy. 1964; 22:341–8.

20. Metzger WJ, Turner E, Patterson R. The safety of immunotherapy during pregnancy. J Allergy Clin Immunol. 1978; 61:268–72.

21. Francis N. Abortion after grass pollen injection. J Allergy. 1941; 12:559–63.

22. Glovsky MM, Rejzek E, Ghekiere L. Can tolerance be induced in utero in children by immunotherapy of atopic pregnant mothers? J Allergy Clin Immunol. 1982; 69:100.

23. Heinonen OP, Slone D, Shapiro S, eds. Birth defects and drugs in pregnancy. Littleton, Mass.: Publishing Sciences Group, 1977.

24. Hill RM, Stern L: Drugs in pregnancy: effects on the fetus and newborn. Drugs. 1979; 17:182–97.

25. Greenberger R, Patterson R. Safety of therapy for allergic symptoms during pregnancy. Ann Intern Med. 1978; 89:234–7.

26. Schatz M, Patterson R, Zeitz S, O'Rourke J, Melam H. Corticosteroid therapy for the pregnant asthmatic patient. JAMA. 1975; 233:804–7.

27. Dykes MH. Evaluation of an antiasthmatic agent cromolyn sodium (Aarene, Intal). JAMA. 1974; 227:1061–2.

28. Mabry RL. Visual loss after intranasal corticosteroid injection: incidence, causes, and prevention. Arch Otolaryngol. 1981; 107:484–6.

29. Plate S, Johnsen NJ, Nødskov Pedersen S, Thomsen KA. The frequency of patulous eustachian tubes in pregnancy. Clin Otolaryngol. 1979; 4:393–400.

30. Sorri M, Hartikaiene-Sorri AL, Kärjä J. Rhinitis during pregnancy. Rhinology. 1980; 18:83–6.

31. Spector SL, Lotan A, English G, Philpot I. Comparison between transillumination and the roentgenogram in diagnosing paranasal sinus disease. J Allergy Clin Immunol. 1981; 67:22–6.

32. Evans FO Jr, Sydnor JB, Moore WE, et al. Sinusitis of the maxillary antrum. N Engl J Med. 1975; 293:735–9.

33. Wald ER, Milmoe GJ, Bowen A, Ledesma-Medina J, Salamon N, Bluestone CD. Acute maxillary sinusitis in children. N Engl J Med. 1981; 304:749–54.

34. Settipane GA, Chafee FH. Nasal polyps in asthma and rhinitis: a review of 6,037 patients. J Allergy Clin Immunol. 1977; 59:17–21.

35. Harnett JC, Spector SL, Farr RS. Aspirin idiosyncrasy, asthma and urticaria. In: Middleton E Jr, Reed CE, Ellis EF, eds. Allergy—principles and practice. St. Louis: Mosby, 1978:1002–22.

36. Shirkey HC. Adverse reactions to drugs: their relation to growth and development. In: Shirkey HC, ed. Pediatric therapy. 4th ed. St. Louis: Mosby, 1972:138–69.

37. Rajka G. Atopic dermatitis. Philadelphia: Saunders, 1975.

38. Baden HP. Hydrocortisone vs high-potency corticosteroid ointments. Arch Dermatol. 1978; 114:798–9. letter.

39. Lockey RF, Bukantz SC. Allergic emergencies. In: Lockey RF, ed. Allergy and clinical immunology. Garden City, N.Y.: Medical Examination Publishing Co., 1979:906–18.

40. Valentine MD, Golden DBK. Immunotherapy for hymenoptera allergy. In: Levine MI, Lockey RF, eds. Monograph on insect allergy. American Academy of Allergy Committee on Insects. Pittsburgh: Typecraft Press, 1981:47–52.

41. Mueller HL. Protective measures against insect stings. In: Levine MI, Lockey RF, eds. Monograph on insect allergy. American Academy of Allergy Committee on Insects. Pittsburgh: Typecraft Press, 1981:59–60.

42. APP Committee on Drugs. Adverse reactions to iodide therapy of asthma and other pulmonary diseases. Pediatrics. 1976; 57:272–4.

43. Galina MP, Avnet NL, Einhorn A. Iodides during pregnancy: an apparent cause of neonatal death. N Engl J Med. 1962; 267:1124–7.

44. Chasnoff IJ, Diggs G, Schnoll SH. Fetal alcohol effects and maternal cough syrup abuse. Am J Dis Child. 1981; 135:968.

45. AMA drug evaluations. 4th ed. New York: Wiley, 1980.

46. Yurchak AM, Jusko WJ. Theophylline secretion into breast milk. Pediatrics. 1976; 57:518–20.

47. Anderson PO. Drugs and breast feeding—a review. Drug Intell Clin Pharmacol. 1977; 11:208–23.

48. O'Brien TE. Excretion of drugs in human milk. Am J Hosp Pharm. 1974; 31:844–54.

49. Lawrence RA. Breast-feeding: a guide for the medical profession. St. Louis: Mosby, 1980.

50. Pratt WR. Allergic diseases in pregnancy and breast feeding. Ann Allergy. 1981; 47:355–60.

51. deWeck AL, Blumenthal MN, eds. HLA and allergy. Vol. II, Monographs in allergy. New York: Karger, 1977.

52. Marsh DG, Bias WB. The genetics of atopic allergy. In: Samter M, ed. Immunological diseases. 3rd ed. Boston: Little, Brown, 1978:819–31.

53. Lubs ML. Allergy in 7000 twin pairs. Acta Allergol. 1971; 26:249–85.

54. Grulee CG, Sanford HN. Influence of breast and artificial feeding on infantile eczema. J Pediatr. 1936; 9:223–5.

55. Glaser J, Johnstone DE. Prophylaxis of allergic disease in newborn. JAMA. 1953; 153:620–2.

56. Matthew DJ, Taylor B, Norman AP, Turner MW, Soothill J. Prevention of eczema. Lancet. 1977; 1:321–4.

57. Halpern SR, Sellars WA, Johnson RD, Anderson D, Saperstein S, Reich JS. Development of childhood allergy in infants fed breast, soy or cow milk. J Allergy Clin Immunol. 1973; 51:139–51.

58. Johnstone DE, Dutton AM. Dietary prophylaxis of allergic disease in children. N Engl J Med. 1966; 274:715–9.

59. Kaufman HS, Frick OL. Prevention of asthma. Clin Allergy. 1981; 11:549–53.

60. Johnstone DE, Soothill JF. Prevention of allergic disease. In: Bierman CW, Pearlman DS, eds. Allergic diseases of infancy, childhood and adolescence. Philadelphia: Saunders, 1980:346–52.

61. Woodcock AJ, Leeder SR, Peat JK, Blackburn CR. The influence of lower respiratory illness in infancy and childhood and subsequent cigarette smoking on lung function in Sydney school children. Am Rev Respir Dis. 1979; 120:5–14.

62. Dukes MN, ed. Meyler's side effects of drugs. Amsterdam: Excerpta Medica, 1980.

63. Martin EW, ed. Hazards of medication. 2nd ed. Philadelphia: Lippincott, 1978.

18. PULMONARY DISORDERS

Charles H. Scoggin

Pregnancy influences two organs of respiration: the maternal lungs and the placenta. Physiologic changes of breathing during pregnancy are well recognized and well tolerated by mother and fetus. However, disease may jeopardize respiration of both. This chapter considers the specific pulmonary medical problems of pregnancy, first by discussing normal physiologic alterations of breathing during gestation.

PHYSIOLOGIC ALTERATIONS DURING PREGNANCY

Mechanical and physiologic alterations of the lung occur as a result of pregnancy. Biochemical influences are present throughout the entirety of gestation. Mechanical alterations increase as the pregnancy progresses and become maximal during the last week before delivery. Both have normal physiologic as well as potential pathophysiologic consequences.

Biochemical Changes

The continued increase in serum progesterone concentration seen in pregnancy results in stimulation of respiration [1]. While the exact mechanism is unknown, it would appear that progesterone acts as a primary respiratory center stimulant. In addition, increased sensitivity to carbon dioxide stimulation of breathing can be experimentally demonstrated [1]. The observation that progesterone increases breathing has been of clinical importance beyond its role in pregnancy. It is now felt that, in part, the hyperventilation seen in other circumstances such as cirrhosis of the liver, luteal phase of the menstrual cycle, and use of oral contraceptives is a consequence of progestational stimulation [2]. The ventilatory stimulant effect of progesterone has been used clinically to treat disorders of hypoventilation such as the obesity-hypoventilation-hypersomnolence (pickwickian) syndrome [3], the "blue and bloated" patient with chronic obstructive pulmonary disease, and excess erythrocytosis of high altitude [4].

The influence of estrogen is less clear [5]. It has been suggested that estrogen may stimulate breathing by increasing the respiratory center's "irritability," but whether or not this is an effect over and above that of progesterone is as yet unclear.

Other biochemical alterations associated with pregnancy may impact on pulmonary function. Unlike progesterone and estrogen, which influence ventilatory control, other biochemical substances appear to have their effect on the mechanical function of the airways. For example, alterations in cyclic nucleotide levels are thought to play an important role in mediating bronchiole tone. Increased cyclic adenosine monophosphate (cyclic AMP) appears to cause bronchiole dilatation while cyclic guanosine monophosphate (cyclic GMP) has the converse effect of bronchoconstriction. Cyclic AMP has been found to vary predictably during the months of pregnancy [6]. Initially it increases during the first 14 weeks and then decreases until week 18, when it rises again, peaking during week 34. Cyclic GMP rises rapidly during the first trimester and then maintains a stable plateau. It is unknown whether these changes in cyclic nucleotide levels have any clinical consequence in pregnant patients regardless of the presence or absence of lung disease.

Corticosteroids are altered in pregnancy [5].

Levels of both free and bound steroid are elevated; however, this rise is apparently of no consequence in patients with normal lungs. Whether or not it has a beneficial effect in steroid-responsive lung disease such as asthma has been the subject of speculation and remains unknown. The clinical consequence of prostaglandin alteration in pregnancy is also not clear [7]. Certainly the pharmacologic introduction of bronchoconstrictor prostaglandin F_2-alpha for purposes of interruption of pregnancy will provoke acute asthma in patients with reactive airways dysfunction [8]. This prostaglandin appears in the plasma during pregnancy and is particularly elevated at the time of labor. Prostaglandins of the E category have the effect of bronchodilatation. They have been found to be increased during the third trimester [9]. As mentioned, it is unknown whether these elevations are of any pulmonary consequence.

Mechanical Changes

The pulmonary effect of the biochemical alterations attending pregnancy are subtle at best, but the mechanical consequences are well recognized. Air flow in the large airways, which is customarily measured by spirometry, is normal. Neither the absolute value for forced expiratory volume in the first second (FEV_1) nor its ratio to forced vital capacity (FVC) is decreased. In fact, one study has even suggested that air flow may be increased during pregnancy [10]. Hormone-induced decrease in bronchiole smooth muscle tone has been postulated as the mechanism. Studies of small airways function by closing volume technique have suggested small airway closure at high lung volumes in pregnancy as compared to the nonpregnant state [11]. Such a phenomenon would lead to decrease in ventilation of involved airways with resultant mismatching of ventilation of the lungs with air and perfusion with blood. This would cause arterial hypoxemia. The phenomenon would increase with progressive elevation of the diaphragm, the chest wall being deformed by both diaphragmatic enlargement and breast engorgement as pregnancy proceeds. Premature airway closure should be interpreted with caution since the technique used to demonstrate it is imperfect. Another measure of small airways function, the flow-volume loop, is unable to confirm the finding [12].

Pregnancy does result in decreased lung volumes [13], caused by two major mechanisms: elevation of the diaphragm as the gravid uterus enlarges and distortion of the chest wall. Physiologic consequences of these changes do not become apparent until the second half of pregnancy. The residual volume of air decreases both at the end of tidal respiration and at forced expiration. The former is termed the expiratory reserve volume (ERV) and the latter the residual volume (RV). It is unlikely that any of these changes are of clinical significance. Likewise, although alterations in diffusing capacity have been described, it is not clear what, if any, clinical consequence they may have [14].

CLINICAL SEQUELAE OF BIOCHEMICAL AND MECHANICAL ALTERATIONS DURING PREGNANCY

A consistent respiratory finding in normal pregnancy is an increase in resting ventilation. In addition, both metabolic rate and oxygen consumption rise [15]. However, somewhat curiously, the increase in ventilation is disproportionally higher than that of either of these two other parameters. It is currently thought that the increased ventilation is due to ventilatory stimulation by progesterone. The increase in ventilation is accomplished primarily by larger tidal volumes, with respiratory rate remaining more or less constant.

Hyperventilation decreases arterial PCO_2. Renal compensation leads to a loss of serum bicarbonate. The result is a combined respiratory alkalosis and compensatory metabolic acidosis. The changes in arterial blood gases and acid-base status are reflected in clinical determinations of their values [16]. PaO_2 is increased to the range of 101 to 108 torr. Some decrease may occur from first trimester to third, perhaps due to decline in functional residual capacity leading to small airways premature closure. $PaCO_2$ remains low (27–32 torr). pH is generally 7.40 to 7.47. Renal compensation for the respiratory alkalosis decreases serum bicarbonate to 18 to 21 mEq per liter, leading to a base deficit of 3 to 4 mEq per liter. Blood gases may change with position. PaO_2 may fall when a patient changes from a sitting to lying position. In the absence of disease it is unlikely that the change is of clinical importance.

NORMAL PULMONARY COMPLAINTS AND PREGNANCY

A frequent, but not totally understood, respiratory complaint during pregnancy is dyspnea. As many as 60 to 75% of women may note this symptom at some time during the course of gestation [15]. It does not appear to be a consequence of mechanical alterations since it often emerges during the first trimester when mechanical effects are at a relative minimum. It has been found that 15% of normal women will note dyspnea during the first trimester, 50% during the second, and up to 75% during the thirty-first week [17]. Thereafter, even though mechanical effects become more prominent, the severity of the dyspnea remains unchanged.

The mechanism by which dyspnea arises is not clear. Positional dyspnea may relate to pulmonary mechanical and hemodynamic factors. Thus, some women may feel more discomfort when lying supine. This position leads to diaphragmatic pressure and airways closure. In addition, caval compression, particularly when the pregnant woman is in the supine position, may result in hemodynamic alterations that lead to discomfort. The symptoms of dyspnea seem to be related to the increased ventilation that occurs with pregnancy. Women with higher ventilatory responses to carbon dioxide have been found to complain more of pregnancy-associated dyspnea [18]. Thus chemosensitivity may be a marker of susceptibility to the complaint. As mentioned, progesterone has been recognized as a potent ventilatory stimulant. It may well be that women with high respiratory chemosensitivity are more aware of the increased ventilation of pregnancy and thus complain of shortness of breath. The importance of this symptom for both patient and practitioner is that it is appropriate for the situation and represents a normal physiologic change. In most cases it should not be regarded as suggesting a pathologic pulmonary process.

PHYSIOLOGIC CONSEQUENCES OF RESPIRATORY DISEASE IN PREGNANCY

Obviously, the most serious consequence of respiratory disease during pregnancy is death of mother, fetus, or both. Specific incidences for particular diseases are discussed in their respective sections. Likewise, other possible adverse outcomes such as fetal malformations or worsening of maternal respiratory disease will also be discussed. Unfortunately, in many cases there are surprisingly few data, especially for the patient with preexisting respiratory insufficiency who desires to become pregnant. The lower limit of mechanical function that can be tolerated during pregnancy is unknown. A favorable outcome of pregnancy has been reported in a woman with a vital capacity of only 800 mL [19]. While carbon dioxide retention secondary to respiratory insufficiency would be expected to be associated with increased risk, this factor has not been scientifically investigated. Primary pulmonary hypertension has been described

as carrying a 50% maternal mortality [20,21]. It should be emphasized, however, that the degree of pulmonary hypertension seen in this disorder is usually higher than that seen in more common disorders of obstruction and restriction of pulmonary function. Similarly, the effect of maternal respiratory distress on the fetus is not predictable. Placental compensatory mechanisms may serve to give some protection. What can best be said in this rather difficult situation is that lacking thorough study each case must be dealt with on an individual basis. The decision to embark on pregnancy, and in certain circumstances continue it, must consider all factors including maternal motivation and the expected clinical course and outcome of the patient's pulmonary disease.

CLINICAL EVALUATION
Symptoms

As mentioned above, dyspnea is a very frequent normal complaint of pregnancy. The clinical challenge is to determine when it is something more serious. Other respiratory complaints, physical findings, and laboratory studies should be used to decide whether further investigation is warranted. Cough is not a normal complaint of pregnancy. It suggests infection or the irritable airway of asthma. Much less commonly it may be the result of interstitial pneumonitis or an intrabronchial lesion such as a bronchial adenoma. Hemoptysis is always a serious symptom and demands investigation. Causes include bronchitis, tumor, and cardiovascular abnormalities such as mitral stenosis and pulmonary embolism. Like dyspnea, fatigue is nonspecific and may be a normal consequence of pregnancy itself; however, other causes (anemia, heart failure, or pulmonary insufficiency) should be considered.

Physical Examination

If symptoms are thought to be something more than the normal result of pregnancy, the next step in the evaluation should be the physical examination. Important areas to concentrate on are the cardiovascular and pulmonary systems. Cardiovascular examination is discussed in Chapter 14. In the pulmonary examination, cyanosis is an ominous finding. It may be a result of severe respiratory insufficiency or congenital heart disease with a right-to-left intracardiac shunt. Tachypnea is also an important abnormality. As mentioned previously, the hyperventilation of pregnancy is a result not of increased respiratory rate but rather of an increase in respiratory volume. Auscultatory findings are helpful. Rales may be heard with either congestive heart failure, infection, or fibrosing alveolitis. Wheezing usually denotes asthma. The mechanical changes that accompany pregnancy in the normal woman are not of a magnitude to account for these findings.

If pulmonary disease is suspected, the next step beyond physical examination is to consider obtaining a chest roentgenogram.

Chest Roentgenogram

Chapter 8 discusses in detail the risk of radiation exposure in the setting of pregnancy. The diagnosis and evaluation of pulmonary disease often require the use of chest radiography. Potential adverse effect of x-rays on the fetus is a concern. With the fall in incidence of tuberculosis in the United States and other developed countries routine radiographic screening is no longer indicated in the pregnancy population [22]. Chest radiography should be performed only when there is a suspicion of either pulmonary or cardiac disease. Ideally, x-ray exposure should be avoided during the first trimester of gestation [23,24], when the teratogenic effect of irradiation is greatest. Beyond that period, limited exposure is acceptable; however, care must be used to ensure adequate lead shielding of the fetus. The limitations and usefulness of other chest radiographic diagnostic tests such as ventilation—perfusion lung scanning and pulmonary arteriography are discussed in Chapter 14.

Arterial Blood Gases and Pulmonary Function Testing

These tests are used to confirm suspicions of pulmonary impairment. They are useful diagnostic procedures for quantitating the degree of functional lung abnormality. Normal changes in these measurements during pregnancy are discussed above.

Bronchoscopy

Bronchoscopy, particularly flexible fiberoptic bronchoscopy, probably imparts no greater risk during pregnancy than in the nonpregnant state. Flexible fiberoptic bronchoscopy can be easily performed using local anesthesia. Supplemental oxygen should be administered via nasal cannula or other suitable device at a flow rate of 2 to 5 liters per minute. If transbronchial biopsy is necessary, it should be delayed if possible until at least the second trimester because the procedure requires fluoroscopy. In general, the same indications for bronchoscopy should be used in pregnancy as are used in the nonpregnant condition.

Lung Biopsy and Other Forms of Lung Surgery

Data on the outcome of pulmonary surgery during gestation are scant. Reason would dictate that biopsy be undertaken only if the information obtained is critical for the management of a life-threatening illness, such as rapidly progressive undiagnosed pulmonary infection. Similarly, other forms of surgery should be reserved for situations in which there is no alternative. Massive hemoptysis from an endobronchial adenoma is a circumstance that has been successfully dealt with.

SPECIFIC DISORDERS
Reversible Airways Dysfunction (Asthma)
See Chapter 19, Asthma.

Pulmonary Embolism
See Chapter 14, Cardiovascular Disorders.

Bacterial Pneumonia
Bacterial pneumonia is also discussed in Chapter 24, Infectious Diseases. A few points are important to emphasize. The advent of antimicrobial therapy has greatly reduced the risk of pneumonia to the mother [25]. The major adverse effect is on the fetus. Fetal abnormalities and abortion are increased by maternal fever in the first stages of pregnancy. Preterm labor is a complication of the last weeks. It follows that fever as well as the infection itself should be treated aggressively. *Streptococcus pneumoniae* remains the most common causative organism of bacterial pneumonia; however, in the setting of hospital-acquired pneumonia, gram-negative organisms must be considered. Pleural effusions may also complicate pneumonia. If the pleural fluid pH is less than 7.3, chest tube drainage must be initiated in order to adequately cure the infection and prevent the complication of pleural adhesion and possible persistence of infection in the pleural space [26].

Viral Pneumonia
In contrast to the positive effect of antibiotic therapy on bacterial pneumonia, viral pneumonia, particularly influenza, still represents a source of high maternal mortality. The overall virulence of the viral agent correlates with maternal mortality. During the 1958 Asian flu outbreak 50% of deaths from influenza in females of childbearing age were associated with pregnancy [27]. More recent influenza outbreaks have not been associated with increases in maternal mortality—probably be-

cause they have been caused by less virulent organisms. Influenza infection not only leads to acute respiratory failure but may also be complicated by disseminated intravascular coagulation and renal failure.

Whether or not pregnant women should receive vaccination during influenzal outbreaks is still debated by some physicians. As yet, no teratogenic effect of killed vaccine has been demonstrated [28].

Bronchitis

Bronchitis usually results from a viral upper respiratory tract infection. Two important complications that may occur are secondary bacterial infection with or without pneumonia and exacerbations of asthma. Pregnancy itself leads to a physiologic mucosal edema, which may aggravate the condition [29]. Treatment is directed at promoting expectoration of bronchial secretions. The methods used include steam inhalation and postural drainage with chest percussion. Antibiotics may be necessary when bacterial infection is suspected. When pneumonia is present, choice of antimicrobial agent should be ruled by sputum Gram stain and culture. Broad-spectrum antibiotics may be employed when persistent purulent sputum raises clinical suspicion of bacterial bronchitis. Neither tetracycline nor chloramphenicol should be used. Supersaturated iodide solutions should be avoided as expectorants because of effects on the fetal thyroid. Persistent cough is a sign of an irritable airway, and inhaled bronchodilators are more effective than narcotic cough suppressants in treating the cough. The chronic bronchitis associated with cystic fibrosis represents a special problem and will be considered later.

Fungal Infection

Fungal diseases are considered in detail in Chapter 24, Infectious Diseases. It is important to remember that coccidioidomycosis may disseminate during pregnancy. In women with coccidioidomycosis prior to conception, the risk of dissemination during pregnancy increases to 20% from the 0.2% incidence otherwise expected [30]. This risk is even higher when infection is contracted during pregnancy. Untreated disseminated coccidioidomycosis imparts a mortality approaching 100% [30]. Amphotericin B is the treatment of choice [31]. Experience is limited; however, as yet no adverse effects of such treatment on the fetus have been reported. Treatment improves not only the chances of survival of the mother but also the likelihood of successful pregnancy. Coccidioido-

mycosis does not cross the placental barrier, but dissemination in the mother is associated with risk of preterm birth as well as death of the fetus.

While other fungal infections have been reported in pregnancy, coccidioidomycosis is the most common. Other infections occur primarily in women who have compromised immune defenses.

Tuberculosis

The management of tuberculosis is also discussed in Chapter 24. Basically the same principles are followed in the pregnant as in the nonpregnant patient with tuberculosis [5].

One interesting problem of tuberculosis and pregnancy is the patient whose intermediate-strength tuberculosis skin test is positive. The author adopted the following approach to this problem. When a positive test is discovered in the first trimester and there is no indication from history or physical examination of active disease, chest roentgenography may be delayed until the start of the second trimester. If clinical suspicion of tuberculosis is high, a chest roentgenogram should be performed in any trimester. If the chest roentgenogram shows changes consistent with pulmonary tuberculosis, then three sputums for tuberculosis smear and culture are collected. If active tuberculosis is found, treatment is undertaken as outlined in Chapter 24. If the chest roentgenogram is normal or sputum smears and cultures are negative, prophylactic therapy with isoniazid, 300 mg daily for 12 months, may be delayed until after delivery. Finally, the risk of development of active disease in the child of a mother with active tuberculosis is approximately 50% [32]. Newborns of such mothers should be treated with isoniazid. An alternative approach is to administer bacille Calmette-Guerin (BCG) vaccination [32]. The advantage of the latter approach is that only a single injection is necessary rather than daily administration of isoniazid. The disadvantage of BCG vaccination is that the value of future tuberculin testing is lost.

Cystic Fibrosis

Cystic fibrosis is a disease of young adults as well as children [33]. While males with cystic fibrosis are usually infertile, females may conceive. Pregnancy in such a condition represents a challenging management problem.

Cystic fibrosis leads to air flow obstruction, pulmonary restriction, or a combined obstructive and restrictive pulmonary defect. Air flow impairment leads to a decreased forced expiratory volume in the first second (FEV_1), and lower lung volumes are reflected in a reduced forced vital capacity

(FVC) and total lung capacity (TLC). Patients are troubled by respiratory problems of chronic bronchitis, recurrent respiratory tract infections, and sinusitis. Complications include hemoptysis, pneumothorax, and acute respiratory failure. Patients almost invariably have clubbing of the fingers and toes. The chest roentgenogram shows fibrous scarring with small cysts throughout all lung fields.

The effect of the disease on the mother appears to relate to the severity of clinical involvement prior to pregnancy [34]. In general it is felt that pregnancy should be avoided in the setting of cystic fibrosis. As many as 50% of patients with cystic fibrosis may deteriorate during the course of pregnancy. The rest remain stable but do not improve. In a recent series, shortened gestation and increased maternal and perinatal mortality were related to the severity of infectious complications during the course of pregnancy with cystic fibrosis [34]. Cor pulmonale, carbon dioxide retention, and pulmonary hypertension are particularly bad prognostic signs. Pulmonary hypertension may be increased by the hypervolemia that occurs during pregnancy. The children of cystic fibrosis patients have in general been normal. In a recent national survey of cystic fibrosis and pregnancy in the United States and Canada, 100 patients were studied and 97 of 129 pregnancies were completed, resulting in 86 viable infants [34]. In spite of such statistics it is important to realize that overall experience with the circumstance of cystic fibrosis in pregnancy is limited. Therefore, it is difficult to make specific associations between severity of the disease and risk to the mother and fetus.

No definitive therapy of cystic fibrosis exists. Cystic fibrosis during pregnancy is managed in the same fashion as in the nonpregnant individual. Oral and inhaled bronchodilators are administered as they are in other forms of chronic obstructive pulmonary disease. Patients who do not yet have severe enough impairment to lead to respiratory insufficiency need not be given such therapy. Corticosteroids have not been shown to be of benefit in cystic fibrosis, although they have been employed as a last resort measure when all other measures have failed to improve respiratory function. Cultures of sputum from patients with cystic fibrosis usually disclose mucoid *Pseudomonas* or *Staphylococcus* organisms. Occasionally, *Hemophilus influenzae* may be the prominent organism. The exact pathogenic significance of these organisms in this condition is still debated. Broad-spectrum antibiotics, often on an alternating basis, are usually employed. Tetracycline and chloramphenicol are to be avoided during pregnancy. Postural drainage and chest percussion are useful techniques for sputum clearance. Early hospitalization of cystic fibrosis patients who show acute deterioration of pulmonary function and increased respiratory complaints is in order. This allows parenteral use of antibiotics such as aminoglycosides and intense pulmonary hygiene. With increasing resistance of mucoid *Pseudomonas* to aminoglycosides and carbenicillin, sputum culture and in vitro antibiotic sensitivity testing may be necessary to determine proper antibiotic selection. Hypoxemia and carbon dioxide retention are inevitable pulmonary complications of cystic fibrosis. When arterial blood gases disclose hypoxemia, home oxygen therapy should be instituted. Criteria include oxygen arterial saturations less than 90%, cor pulmonale, and disabling dyspnea. Many patients will require 1 to 2 liters per minute on a continuous basis. Higher oxygen flow rates will be required in some to obtain an oxygen saturation greater than 90%. Other complications of cystic fibrosis such as intestinal obstruction, pancreatic insufficiency, and cirrhosis of the liver relate primarily to the gastrointestinal tract and will not be discussed in this chapter.

Sarcoidosis

Sarcoidosis is a disorder of unknown cause that results in multisystem granuloma. The organ most likely to manifest involvement is the lungs. While most cases are probably asymptomatic and may go undetected, pulmonary fibrosis and hilar lymphadenitis are the usual findings. Diagnosis is customarily made by biopsy of skin, liver, lymph nodes, or lungs that show noncaseating epithelioid granulomas. No pulmonary impairment may be appreciable; however, restrictive lung disease from fibrosis may result in decreased vital capacity, lung volumes, and diffusion capacity, and in hypoxemia. Endobronchial sarcoidosis may cause airway obstruction. There is no evidence that sarcoidosis has an adverse effect on fertility or pregnancy.

The effect of pregnancy on sarcoidosis has been investigated a number of times, with general agreement of findings. It has been found that abnormalities due to sarcoidosis frequently improve spontaneously. Rarely does sarcoidosis become worse during gestation. In one small series 80% of patients improved during the course of pregnancy; however, one-half of the patients had deterioration of their disease within several months of delivery [35]. A possible explanation for improvement may be the increased level of corticosteroids during gestation, although this is only speculation.

The indications for corticosteroid therapy for sarcoidosis are the same as in nonpregnant patients. Deteriorating pulmonary function, central nervous system involvement, and cardiac involvement may respond to oral corticosteroids. Topical prednisolone eye drops should be administered for iridocyclitis. Oral corticosteroids will usually control hypercalcemia resulting from increased intestinal absorption of calcium. Likewise, hypercalcuria of sarcoidosis will respond to oral corticosteroids. Both local and oral steroids may improve disfiguring skin lesions such as lupus pernio.

Immunosuppressive therapy with azathioprine, chlorambucil, and methotrexate is an unproved therapeutic modality in sarcoidosis and should be avoided during pregnancy.

Fibrosing Alveolitis (Idiopathic Pulmonary Fibrosis)

Fibrosing alveolitis is characterized by cellular infiltration of the lung interstitium with increase in fibrosis of the areas surrounding the alveoli [36]. Such changes may also be seen in association with extrinsic allergic alveolitis, as in pigeon breeder's disease, lupus erythematosus, drug reactions, idiopathic pulmonary hemosiderosis, and eosinophilic granuloma. Where a distinct pathologic condition of this kind cannot be identified, the disorder is said to be idiopathic.

All the diseases that involve the lung interstitium may lead to restrictive lung dysfunction. Definitive diagnosis is usually made by lung biopsy. Severe cases are associated with progressive hypoxemia and cor pulmonale with eventual fatality. Treatment with corticosteroids and other immunosuppressive agents has variable results.

Since the disorder is often relentlessly progressive in spite of therapy, decision to undertake the burden of pregnancy should probably be discouraged. In the setting of hypoxemia with or without cor pulmonale, conception or continuation of pregnancy will appreciably jeopardize the survival of the mother. Chapter 20, Rheumatic Diseases, discusses autoimmune diseases and pregnancy.

Spontaneous Pneumothorax

Pneumothorax rarely occurs during pregnancy [37]. Iatrogenic pneumothorax may stem from diagnostic or therapeutic misadventures such as thoracentesis or intercostal nerve block. Most reported cases of spontaneous pneumothorax have occurred at term. Pneumomediastinum may coexist [38]. Spontaneous pneumothorax has been associated with other contributory illnesses such as tuberculosis and histoplasmosis. Pneumothorax should be considered in any patient complaining of chest pain and shortness of breath. Hypoxemia may accompany the complaint. While certain patients with small (less than 10%) pneumothoraxes

may be managed without chest tube, insertion of a chest tube under water seal is the most effective treatment. The use of a trocar for chest tube insertion somewhat decreases the pain of this procedure.

Kyphoscoliosis

Kyphoscoliosis causes restriction of ventilation and leads to respiratory impairment by thoracic skeletal encroachment on the lungs. Pregnancy may worsen such restriction because of diaphragmatic elevation and thoracic cage deformity. One lung becomes compromised and atelectatic. The overall consequence is reduction of vital capacity, hypoxemia, and cor pulmonale. Pulmonary abnormalities become particularly severe late in pregnancy. Maternal hypoxemia is reflected in an increased occurrence of stillbirth, prematurity, and perinatal mortality. A perinatal death rate of 102 per 1,000 pregnancies has been reported [34]. However, successful delivery of normal infants has been described in patients with vital capacities less than 1 liter [40]. Arterial blood gases should be monitored and oxygen therapy begun if hypoxemia is noted. Maternal death may occur. In one series of 50 patients with kyphoscoliosis, two maternal deaths were reported [39].

Kyphoscoliosis is often associated with anthropoid pelvic inlet and pelvic deformities. Cesarean rates of 50% have been described [39].

Amniotic Fluid Embolism

Amniotic fluid embolism may be a devastating pulmonary complication of pregnancy. It is one of the more common causes of maternal death, accounting for 10% of maternal deaths associated with pregnancy [41,42].

Amniotic fluid embolism results when amniotic fluid enters the maternal circulation, causing acute respiratory distress, disseminated intravascular coagulation, and cardiovascular collapse. Pulmonary edema, pulmonary hypertension, and bronchospasm are all clinical features. Patients are dyspneic and cyanotic. Shock, seizures, and cardiac arrest also occur.

The mechanism by which these events occur is unknown. Experimental injection of purified amniotic fluid does not result in the clinical syndrome [43]. It is thought that contaminants of fetal or placental origin are responsible. Three main causes have been postulated [41]: (1) mechanical occlusion of the pulmonary vasculature by particulate matter in amniotic fluid (fetal squames, meconium, mucin, bile, lanugo hairs, and fat have all been recovered from pulmonary circulation of victims); (2) intravascular coagulation initiated by introduction of procoagulants into the maternal circulation; (3) a hypersensitivity reaction to particulate matter or fetal antigens.

A number of risk factors have been noted, including (1) tumultuous labor, (2) induction of labor with uterine stimulants, (3) multiparity, (4) intrauterine fetal death, (5) meconium amniotic fluid. Amniotic fluid has been postulated to enter the maternal circulation by a variety of mechanisms. A uterine rupture, incision into the placenta during cesarean delivery, and placenta previa can allow fluid to gain access to the maternal circulation through the placenta. Likewise, with uterine trauma or vigorous uterine contraction, fluid could enter via the uterine veins. Finally, laceration of endocervical veins could lead to fluid embolism by this route.

Management is generally aimed at support as no definitive therapy exists. The pulmonary picture is much like that of other forms of the adult respiratory distress syndrome [44]. Oxygenation is critical. Mechanical ventilation, often with positive end-expiratory pressure, is likely to be necessary. Fluids and cardiovascular pressor agents will be necessary if shock occurs. Decision as to their proper use may require hemodynamic monitoring with a right heart flow-directed balloon catheter. Corticosteroid use in this situation is of unproved value. Heparinization has been proposed as therapeutic for the disseminated intravascular coagulation that may accompany this syndrome. Fluid administration should be closely monitored to prevent volume overload. Packed red blood cells will improve oxygen-carrying capacity. When hematocrit is normal, saline is preferred for volume replacement.

REFERENCES

1. Lyons HA, Antonio R. The sensitivity of the respiratory center in pregnancy and after the administration of progesterone. Trans Assoc Am Physicians. 1959; 72:173–80.
2. Skatrud JB, Dempsey JA, Kaiser DG. Ventilatory response to medroxyprogesterone acetate in normal subjects: time course and mechanism. J Appl Physiol. 1978; 44:939–44.
3. Sutton FD Jr, Zwillich CW, Creagh CE, Pierson DJ, Weil JV. Progesterone for outpatient treatment of Pickwickian syndrome. Ann Intern Med. 1975; 83:476–9.
4. Kryger M, Glas R, Jackson D, et al. Impaired oxygenation during sleep in excessive polycythemia of high altitude: improvement with respiratory stimulation. Sleep. 1978; 1:3–17.
5. Weinberger SE, Weiss ST, Cohen WR, Weiss JW, Johnson TS. Pregnancy and the lung. Am Rev Respir Dis. 1980; 121:559–81.
6. Scoggin CH, Petty TL. Clinical strategies in adult asthma. Philadelphia: Lea & Febiger, 1982.
7. Whalen JB, Clancy CJ, Farley DB, Van Orden DE. Plasma prostaglandins in pregnancy. Obstet Gynecol. 1978; 51:52–5.
8. Fishburne JI Jr, Brenner WE, Braaksma JT, Hendricks CH. Bronchospasm complicating intravenous prostaglandin $F_2\alpha$ for therapeutic abortion. Obstet Gynecol. 1972; 39:892–6.
9. Karim SM. Appearance of prostaglandin F_2 alpha in human blood during labour. Br Med J. 1968; 1:618–21.
10. Rubin A, Russo N, Goucher D. The effect of pregnancy upon pulmonary function in normal women. Am J Obstet Gynecol. 1956; 72:963–9.
11. Garrard GS, Littler WA, Redman CW. Closing volume during normal pregnancy. Thorax. 1978; 33:488–92.
12. Baldwin GR, Moorthi DS, Whelton JA, MacDonnell KF. New lung functions and pregnancy. Am J Obstet Gynecol. 1977; 127:235–9.
13. Cugell DW, Frank NR, Gaensler EA, Badger TL. Pulmonary function in pregnancy. I. Serial observations in normal women. Am Rev Tuberc. 1953; 67:568–97.
14. Gazioglu K, Kaltreider NL, Rosen M, Yu PN. Pulmonary function during pregnancy in normal women and in patients with cardiopulmonary disease. Thorax. 1970; 25:445–50.
15. Prowse CM, Gaensler EA. Respiratory and acid base changes during pregnancy. Anesthesiology. 1965; 26:381–92.
16. Lim VS, Katz AI, Lindheimer MD. Acid-base regulation in pregnancy. Am J Physiol. 1976; 231:1764–9.
17. Milne JA, Howie AD, Pack AI. Dyspnoea during normal pregnancy. Br J Obstet Gynaecol. 1978; 85:260–3.
18. Gilbert R, Auchincloss JH Jr. Dyspnea of pregnancy: clinical and physiological observations. Am J Med Sci. 1966; 252:270–6.
19. Hung CT, Pelosi M, Langer A, Harrigan JT. Blood gas measurements in the kyphoscoliotic gravida and her fetus: report of a case. Am J Obstet Gynecol. 1975; 121:287–9.
20. McCaffrey RM, Dunn LJ. Primary pulmonary hypertension in pregnancy. Obstet Gynecol Surv. 1964; 19:567–91.
21. Demas NW. Maternal death due to primary pulmonary hypertension. Trans Pac Coast Obstet Gynecol Soc. 1973; 40:64–7.
22. de March AP. Tuberculosis and pregnancy. Five-to-ten-year review of 215 patients in their fertile age. Chest. 1975; 68:880–4.
23. Bonebrake CR, Noller KL, Loehnen CP, Muhm JR, Fish CR. Routine chest roentgenography in pregnancy. JAMA. 1978; 240:2747–8.
24. Swartz HM, Reichling BA. Hazards of radiation exposure for pregnant women. JAMA. 1978; 239:1907–8.
25. Hopwood HG Jr. Pneumonia in pregnancy. Obstet Gynecol. 1965; 25:875–9.
26. Potts DE, Levin DC, Sahn SA. Pleural fluid pH in parapneumonic effusions. Chest. 1976; 70:328–32.

27. Hopwood HG Jr. Pneumonia in pregnancy. Obstet Gynecol. 1965; 25:875–9.

28. Influenza vaccine: recommendation of the Public Health Service Advisory Committee on Immunization Practices. Ann Intern Med. 1978; 89:657–9.

29. Fishburne JI. Physiology and disease of the respiratory system in pregnancy. J Reprod Med. 1979; 22:177–89.

30. Harris RE. Coccidioidomycosis complicating pregnancy. Obstet Gynecol. 1966; 28:401–5.

31. Ellinoy BR. Amphotericin B usage in pregnancy complicated by cryptococcosis. Am J Obstet Gynecol. 1973; 115:285–6.

32. Kendig EL Jr. The place of BCG vaccine in the management of infants born of tuberculous mothers. N Engl J Med. 1969; 281:520–3.

33. Wood RE, Boat TF, Doershuk CF. Cystic fibrosis. Am Rev Respir Dis. 1976; 113:833–78.

34. Cohen LF, di Sant'Agnese PA, Friedlander J. Cystic fibrosis and pregnancy. Lancet. 1980; 2:842–4.

35. Mayock RL, Sullivan RD, Dreening RR, Jones R, Jr. Sarcoidosis and pregnancy JAMA. 1957; 164:158–63.

36. Crystal RG, Gadek JE, Ferrans VJ, Fulmer JD, Line BR, Hunninghake BW. Interstitial lung disease: current concepts of pathogenesis, staging and therapy. Am J Med. 1981; 70:542–68.

37. Stewart B. Spontaneous pneumothorax and pregnancy. Can Med Assoc J. 1979; 121:25.

38. Hague WM. Mediastinal and subcutaneous emphysema in a pregnant patient with asthma. Br J Obstet Gynaecol. 1980; 87:440–3.

39. Kopenhager T. A review of 50 pregnant patients with kyphoscoliosis. Br J Obstet Gynaecol. 1977; 84:585–7.

40. de Swiet M. Respiratory disease in pregnancy. Postgrad Med J. 1979; 55:325–8.

41. Courtney LD. Amniotic fluid embolism. Obstet Gynecol Surv. 1974; 29:169–77.

42. Peterson EP, Taylor HB. Amniotic fluid embolism. An analysis of 40 cases. Obstet Gynecol. 1970; 35:787–93.

43. Adamsons K, Mueller-Heubach E, Myers RE. The innocuousness of amniotic fluid infusion in the pregnant rhesus monkey. Am J Obstet Gynecol. 1971; 109:977–84.

44. Andersen HF, Lynch JP, Johnson TR. Adult respiratory distress syndrome in obstetrics and gynecology. Obstet Gynecol. 1980; 55:291–5.

All that wheezes is not asthma.
—Chevalier Jackson
Boston Medical Quarterly

All that is asthma does not wheeze.
—Richard Rosenthal
New England Journal of Medicine

19. ASTHMA

David S. Pearlman and Charles H. Scoggin

The incidence of asthma in pregnancy is estimated to be 0.4 to 1.3% [1,2], but considering the frequency of undiagnosed asthma in the general population [3], the incidence is probably higher. Pregnancy's effect on asthma is highly variable and unpredictable [4,5]. In the majority of instances, the course and severity of asthma are changed little by pregnancy [6]. In one large study, for example, well over 90% of women with asthma reported no change in asthma during pregnancy [7]. Of the remainder, improvement appears to be somewhat more likely than worsening [8], but this is not a consistent finding in other studies [4]. Discrepant results may relate to differences in severity of asthma prior to pregnancy in the populations studied [5,9], for mild asthma has a tendency to improve [8] whereas severe asthma tends to worsen during pregnancy [10]. If improvement occurs, it is more likely to do so beginning in the first trimester and may continue through the postpartum period so long as lactation continues [11]. Asthma that worsens during pregnancy is more likely to do so somewhat later—in the second or third trimester [10]. The pattern established in the first pregnancy is generally repeated in subsequent pregnancies [8,10,12]. In the vast majority of instances, even in the face of severe asthma, the outcome of pregnancy is successful with regard to both maternal and fetal health [13]; nevertheless, maternal and fetal deaths attributable to severe asthma have occurred [5,9].

The effect of asthma on the outcome of pregnancy has been the subject of numerous studies, with various conclusions [5]. Some have found no significant influence [13] whereas others have observed a slight increase in maternal and fetal mortality, an increase in rate of preterm birth, more frequent complications of pregnancy and labor, as well as subsequent neurologic impairment of infants born of severely asthmatic mothers [5,7,9, 14]. Evaluation of the relationship between asthma

or its treatment and these abnormalities, however, is difficult since in many instances there have been concomitant unrelated medical problems involved. Since the extensiveness of asthma therapy including the use of corticosteroids is a reflection of the severity of asthma, interpretation of a relationship between abnormalities in the fetus from asthma itself and the therapy used to ameliorate this process in the mother is also difficult. By and large, asthma therapy does not seem to be associated with significant adverse effects on the fetus, nor does it interfere substantially with labor and delivery. Untoward effects from the use of iodides, some antibiotics, and barbiturates, as well as the rare abuse of alcohol in cough mixtures and similar preparations, are exceptions to this rule.

EVALUATION OF ASTHMA

Subjective assessment of the severity of asthma cannot be relied on to determine degree of air flow limitation and of hypoxemia [15]. The degree of dyspnea exhibited by a patient can be a grossly inadequate indication of the degree of obstruction, depending on the patient's personality, coping style, and prior experience with acute asthma. Useful signs on physical examination, although imperfect, include assessment of extent of hyperinflation of the chest, retractions, degree of accessory respiratory muscle use, coloring (pallor and cyanosis), respiratory rate (relatively poor assessor of severity), and tachycardia, which tends to be related to the degree of hypoxemia [16]. Assessment of airflow limitation by simple spirometry, measuring FEV_1 or peak expiratory flow or both, is an indispensable aid to evaluation of air flow limitation. Most patients who present with acute severe asthma have a one-second forced expiratory volume (FEV_1) below 1 liter, averaging on presentation in emergency rooms 25 to 30% of predicted values

[17]. Peak expiratory flow rates less than 100 L/min are frequent, with rates less than 200 L/min being usual [17]. Assessment of the degree of hypoxemia can be made by measurement of arterial blood gases and pH, which should be obtained as early as possible.

Important historical points in assessing acute asthma include the dosage and time of administration of all drugs the patient has used for asthma, particularly in the previous 24 hours. Information on concomitant drug intake not necessarily related to asthma is also important. Information on fluid balance, including intake of fluid, urinary output, and gastrointestinal loss, is useful. It is common for patients to be dehydrated with acute severe asthma. However, dehydration is less likely to occur in patients who have been under appropriate chronic asthma care.

Laboratory evaluation includes assessment of arterial blood gases and pH. Hypoxemia is common, largely because of a ventilation-perfusion imbalance that is characteristic of asthma, and can be extreme. This condition has particularly important implications not only for maternal health but for the risk it imparts to the fetus from hypoxia [9]. Arterial CO_2 tension is usually diminished in asthma because of hyperventilation; a "normal" $PaCO_2$ in the presence of severe asthma and hyperpnea should be considered inappropriately high. An increased $PaCO_2$ is an ominous sign in asthma. Early in the course of acute severe asthma, respiratory alkalosis may occur from hyperventilation. Serum electrolytes should be assessed; early measurement is important, especially if the patient has been vomiting or is dehydrated.

Urinalysis is helpful in determining state of hydration, but it should be remembered that aminophylline and theophylline are diuretics, particularly with short-term use, and the diuresis may result in a lower specific gravity than is appropriate for the patient's state of hydration. A roentgenogram of the chest should be obtained if there is a question of any complications of asthma, including pneumothorax, evidence of subcutaneous emphysema (which generally is a reflection of mediastinal emphysema and may also be related to pneumothorax), suggestion of massive atelectasis, pulmonary embolism, or extensive pneumonitis. However, depending on the clinical condition of the patient, chest roentgenography does not need to be a routine procedure for acute severe asthma. Paranasal sinus roentgenography should be considered for patients when severe sinusitis is suspected of aggravating the acute or chronic asthmatic state in a major way.

MANAGEMENT: GENERAL CONSIDERATIONS

Asthma is characterized by extraordinary hypersensitivity to chemical mediators of inflammation as well as the autonomic mediator, acetylcholine, which modulates airway patency [18]. The list of environmental agents that activate or release these mediators is long. Accordingly, factors that precipitate or aggravate asthma are numerous. Classically, asthma is related to allergic reactivity, in particular to inhalant allergens, but foods and drugs may also precipitate asthma. However, reactions to allergens are rarely the only significant asthma precipitants, and as many as half of all women in the childbearing age who have asthma have no evidence of "allergy." Respiratory tract infection (mainly viral), irritants such as smoke, air pollutants, strong odors including perfumes, cold air, coughing itself, weather changes, exercise that causes panting, inhaled chemicals as in industrial exposures, aspirin and other nonsteroidal antiinflammatory agents in some asthmatics (not an allergy), and psychological factors all may affect the course and severity of asthma.

The goal of asthma control is avoidance of all factors that precipitate or aggravate asthma. Obviously, from the list of factors cited, the ability to avoid or control potential exacerbating factors is often limited. Nevertheless, manipulation of factors that are susceptible to influence can have a critically important effect on asthma control and is particularly important in controlling asthma during pregnancy. Any inhalant known to precipitate asthmatic symptoms—or even suspected of precipitating them—such as the fur of domestic animals, dust, molds, or any foods implicated in causing asthmatic symptoms should be scrupulously avoided. Strict rules for environmental contacts with asthmagenic agents should be considered during pregnancy. Thus, occasional contact with domestic animals at the home of a friend or relative that ordinarily provokes only mild and transient symptoms is to be firmly discouraged in the woman who is pregnant. Although exercise is generally to be encouraged in individuals with asthma, judicious restriction of exercise during pregnancy to avoid asthma sufficient to require treatment should be initiated. Further discussion of environmental control procedures can be found in Chapter 17 and in other references [19,20].

Inflammation of the upper respiratory tract and, in particular, acute and chronic sinusitis can act as important exacerbating factors in asthma. Chronic sinusitis may not be clinically apparent and should be considered in patients with chronic asthmatic symptoms not readily controlled by usual methods of asthma therapy. Vigorous treatment of allergic and infectious upper respiratory tract conditions is an important aspect of asthma therapy. Other less common contributors to chronic symptomatic asthma include bronchopulmonary aspergillosis [21] and gastroesophageal reflux [22]. The frequency of aspirin idiosyncrasy with reactivity to other nonsteroidal antiinflammatory agents and to tartrazine is unclear, but recent evidence suggests that aspirin may play a role in aggravating asthma in a substantial subpopulation of chronic asthmatics [23].

Immunotherapy

Immunotherapy (hyposensitization, allergy injection therapy) is employed for asthma or associated upper respiratory tract allergic problems when symptoms due to nonavoidable allergens are sufficient. The use of this mode of therapy during pregnancy is considered further in Chapter 17.

Drug Therapy

Drug therapy remains the mainstay of management for asthma both to reverse acute paroxysms and to maintain optimal airway patency on a chronic basis. Despite the potential toxicity of drugs used in the treatment of asthma, there have been remarkably few reports of significant adverse effects on mother or fetus when these drugs have been used appropriately. Localization of drug effect to the tissue or organ affected makes sense not only in the therapy of asthma in general but in pregnancy especially, in order to minimize possible systemic side effects on mother and fetus. Consequently, whenever possible, the authors strongly advocate the use of inhaled topical agents in place of their systemic alternatives. Administration of medication by this route has the additional advantage of being better tolerated than oral therapy in gravidas with nausea. Since there is at least suggestive evidence that maintenance of normal or near-normal pulmonary function minimizes the frequency and severity of asthmatic paroxysms, maintenance of optimal pulmonary function throughout the entire period of pregnancy is an important goal of drug therapy. This goal must be tempered with considerations of potential toxicity, striving for the best balance possible between optimizing pulmonary functions and avoiding excessive drug therapy. Obviously, the "optimal" balance will differ from patient to patient, and much time, effort, and judgment may be required to determine this balance.

The pregnant patient with asthma whose condition is stable presents somewhat of a dilemma. Most concern revolves around administration of bronchodilator medications. If the patient is asymptomatic, should medications be cautiously decreased or withdrawn or continued? As mentioned above, it is not possible to predict whether or not gestation will be complicated by an acute episode of asthma. Nevertheless, an adverse outcome of pregnancy in the setting of asthma has been associated not with the use of bronchodilator medications but with uncontrolled asthma. Therefore, it is our philosophy to continue the therapeutic regimen of a stable asthmatic. This carries little risk and avoids the medically unfortunate situation of an acute episode of asthma precipitated by the physician's discontinuing the patient's usual drug regimen.

Four classes of drugs form the nucleus of pharmacotherapy: methylxanthines, adrenergic agents, cromolyn sodium, and corticosteroids. In the United States, methylxanthines (theophylline and aminophylline) are used as principal round-the-clock bronchodilators, with adrenergic agents, particularly the inhaled forms, as adjuncts. Cromolyn sodium is an asthma preventative, used mainly outside the United States as a first-line chronic asthmatic medication instead of methylxanthines. Adrenal corticosteroids can be added to the regimens of patients in whom air flow limitation is not relieved sufficiently by nonsteroid bronchodilators. Each of these classes of drugs will be considered separately, along with other drug and drug-related therapy used in the treatment of asthma. Their possible adverse effects on the fetus or newborn are also considered in Chapters 17 and 18.

Methylxanthines

Methylxanthines (aminophylline and theophylline) are used on an acute basis, to treat acute asthmatic paroxysms, or as chronic round-the-clock bronchodilators. The average plasma half-life of theophylline in a nonsmoking adult is approximately eight hours (in women who smoke, the half-life is approximately four hours). Recent evidence indicates that pregnancy does not materially alter metabolism of this class of drugs [24]. Methylxanthines are purported to act predominantly as phosphodiesterase inhibitors and prolong the effective concentration of cyclic AMP in various cells. Their predominant therapeutic action is relief of bronchial smooth muscle spasm. Optimal therapeutic serum concentrations are considered to be between 10 and 20 μg/mL although higher levels may be tolerated by some patients and lower levels are often adequate. The incidence of drug toxicity, however, increases significantly with concentrations above 20 μg/mL [25].

Average daily total dosage in a nonsmoking adult required to bring the level into the so-called optimal therapeutic range is about 13 mg/kg body weight (the 95% confidence limits are 10–16 mg/kg). Initial dosage should be conservative until the patient's susceptibility to the potential side effects of the medication is established. Toxic effects include central nervous system hyperirritability to the point that convulsions can occur and gastrointestinal discomfort including nausea, vomiting, and occasionally diarrhea. *These side effects are related to the theophylline blood level and therefore can occur regardless of route of administration;* local gastrointestinal irritation may also occur from oral ingestion.

The drug is metabolized in the liver and excreted through the kidney, so that any hepatic or renal disease or cardiac decompensation may be associated with markedly prolonged biologic half-life of the drug. Sustained-release preparations are preferred for chronic treatment in order to minimize fluctuation of drug blood levels. In addition, because they may be administered as infrequently as every 12 hours, they are convenient for patients to use and probably increase compliance. If they are used in the treatment of status asthmaticus by intravenous infusion, a steady infusion is recommended, beginning with a loading dose of 6 mg/kg body weight and proceeding then with a constant infusion of 0.4 to 0.8 mg/kg/hr initially until a blood theophylline level can be obtained and the intravenous dosage adjusted accordingly. Caffeine is also a methylxanthine, and the intake of caffeine can prolong the metabolism of theophylline and possibly intensify theophylline side effects. Consequently, in individuals on methylxanthine drugs the intake of caffeine should be minimized. Interference with theophylline metabolism may occur too with the concomitant use of erythromycin, and possibly lincomycin. Moreover, the use of theophylline with diuretics can intensify the diuretic effect of these drugs.

Despite concerns for possible teratogenic effects of caffeine and, in turn, theophylline, an association between caffeine use and teratogenic or other adverse effects on the fetus has not been found [26,27]. Nor is there evidence that theophylline used in the treatment of asthma in the mother induces teratogenic effects in the fetus [28,29]. Temporary toxicity can occur in the fetus from placental transfer of theophylline if theophylline blood levels are sufficiently high [29,30, 31], but this has not been reported as a frequent problem. Cord blood theophylline levels are com-

parable to maternal blood levels [29]. Similarly, theophylline is secreted in breast milk in concentrations approximately 75% of the concentration in maternal serum. There have been a few reports suggesting at least minor side effects from caffeine or theophylline taken by the lactating mother [32]. If a mother notes infant irritability or tachycardia during breast-feeding, theophylline toxicity should be suspected. Timing of feedings to the point when theophylline levels are lowest (before the next dose) are of questionable help.

Adrenergic Agents

Adrenergic agents are effective bronchodilators used alone or in conjunction with theophylline. With the development of agents with highly selective activity for beta-receptors, bronchodilator effectiveness has been increased relative to side effects from the use of these drugs. Adrenergic agents administered by inhalation can achieve as much large and small airway bronchodilatation as can the same drugs given parenterally, often with more prolonged effect and fewer systemic side effects [33]. Oral adrenergic bronchodilators, although effective, tend to be relatively less potent than inhalant drugs. In the effort to maximize bronchodilatation with the use of oral agents, side effects such as tremor are encountered with some frequency. Consequently, in general, the authors prefer inhalation of adrenergic drugs to oral administration.

The newer, selective beta$_2$ inhalant drugs are recommended: albuterol (Proventil, Ventolin), metaproterenol (Alupent, Metaprel), and isoetharine (Bronkometer, Bronkosol). As with all drugs, abuse of these agents is possible, and patients must be warned against overuse. A dosage of two inhalations from a pressurized canister no more than every four hours is considered safe, but more frequent administration for short periods may be beneficial. Limitations of elective aerosol use *should* be imposed on the patient, with instructions to maintain contact with the prescribing physician if asthma is not under adequate control with recommended dosages and frequency of use. Overuse of aerosolized drugs suggests that asthma is out of control and other therapeutic measures are required. Bronchodilatation may be maximized by spacing the two inhalations ten minutes apart [34]. In women with severe asthma, there may be some advantage to purchasing a compressed-air device (e.g., Maximyst, DeVilbiss Pulmo-aide) for delivery of aerosol by nebulization. According to recent studies, inhalation of aerosolized adrenergic drugs is as effective as parenteral epinephrine or terbutaline in reversing acute severe asthmatic paroxysms [35,36]. Nevertheless, in patients who are not in a position to cooperate adequately to inhale aerosolized agents, prompt administration of epinephrine in acute severe asthma may be lifesaving.

Oral adrenergic drugs exert an additive bronchodilating effect to methylxanthines, and these drugs can be employed together with good advantage on a chronic or an acute basis. If oral adrenergic drugs are used, selective beta$_2$ agents, namely, metaproterenol, terbutaline, and albuterol, but *not* ephedrine, are recommended.

There is weak statistical association between the use of adrenergic agents of various kinds during pregnancy and developmental anomalies in the fetus [28]. Whether this association is in fact real and, if so, reflects the effects of drug use or effects of the conditions for which the drugs were used remains to be determined. This possible risk must be weighed against the necessity of producing adequate bronchodilatation to maintain blood oxygen levels for both the mother and the fetus. In acute severe asthmatic paroxysms, it must always be assumed that the risk of hypoxemia and associated fetal damage is significant. Consequently, *neither adrenergic agents nor other antiasthmatic bronchodilators that can aid in reversing the paroxysms should be withheld.*

Adrenergic drugs are known to have tocolytic activity. In the rare event that the onset of labor appears to be delayed by an oral or parenterally administered adrenergic drug such as terbutaline, the drug should be discontinued and an inhalant drug can be substituted.

Cromolyn Sodium

Cromolyn sodium (Intal) has been used extensively as an asthma preventative both on an acute and on a chronic basis for more than a decade, with variable therapeutic effectiveness. This drug is topically active inhaled as a powder. A small amount of the drug is absorbed but probably is not significantly transported across the placenta or excreted in breast milk. It is often effective as an acute asthma preventative taken immediately before anticipated contact with asthmagenic agents (e.g., an animal, or cigarette smoke). When it is used on a chronic basis, ordinarily three or four doses a day are recommended. Although it is not officially approved for use during pregnancy, there has been considerable experience with its use in pregnant women, with no significant adverse effects on mother or fetus [37]. Its toxicity is minimal, and assuming effectiveness, its use makes a great deal of sense in controlling asthma during pregnancy. It is not effective in reversing acute

paroxysms, and the slight irritant action of the powder when inhaled may aggravate bronchospasm under such circumstances.

Corticosteroids

Corticosteroids are extremely useful adjuncts to the nonsteroid bronchodilators mentioned for treating chronic or acute severe asthma. The same rules apply to the use of steroids in pregnant asthmatics as in the nonpregnant woman: On an acute basis, a "large" dosage should be used to maximize antiinflammatory effect as rapidly as possible; the medication should then be withdrawn as quickly as feasible, usually within a few days. On a chronic basis, to aid in asthma control, the lowest dosage necessary to control symptoms should be utilized. For the latter purpose, either alternate-day short-acting corticosteroid (prednisone or prednisolone) given early in the morning to minimize systemic side effects, or topical steroid aerosol (beclomethasone dipropionate—Beclovent, Vanceril), which has relatively little systemic activity if used in generally recommended dosages, should be utilized [51]. For reasons stated earlier, the authors strongly prefer topical to systemic drug use if the former is sufficiently effective.

Although maternal administration of corticosteroids has been shown to produce cleft palate in experimental animals [38], fears of the development of this or any other congenital anomaly from the use of steroids have not been borne out [13,28,29]. The rare reports of a possible association between the use of corticosteroids and adverse fetal effects cannot be ignored, but numerous studies have been unable to find a relationship between corticosteroid usage during pregnancy and adverse fetal effects [13,28,39]. Indeed, there has been a surprising infrequency of adrenal suppression in the newborn of mothers who have been on intermittent or constant systemic corticosteroid therapy. Nevertheless, the inability to find an association does not eliminate the possibility of adverse effects from maternal corticosteroid use on the fetus. For this reason and because of the usual concerns of side effects of corticosteroids on the asthmatic patient herself, they should be used particularly cautiously in the pregnant asthmatic patient. Corticosteroid usage required for asthma control in the latter part of pregnancy should be continued during labor and delivery and into the immediate postpartum period. Corticosteroids are secreted in low concentration in breast milk, but their use in a lactating woman does not appear to pose any significant risk to the infant.

Atropine

Cholinergic activity is thought to play a role in

asthmatic airway obstruction. Inhaled atropine has been demonstrated to be useful in treating asthma, particularly when cough is a prominent complaint. While its effect on pregnancy has not been rigorously examined, experience has not disclosed adverse effects in the setting of pregnancy. Administration must be by inhalation to attain the desired local effect (bronchodilatation) with a minimum of systemic anticholinergic side effects [40].

Expectorants

A frequent dominant feature of asthma is thick tenacious mucus that obstructs air flow and is difficult to expectorate. Consequently, expectorants have been used commonly in the treatment of asthma. The major expectorants include guaifenesin and iodides. The effectiveness of guaifenesin as an expectorant in asthma remains to be determined. Although iodides have been reported to be beneficial in asthma (whether this outcome is related to their expectorant action or some other activity), iodides traverse the placenta and can cause hypothyroidism resulting not only in goiter but in respiratory compromise in the newborn [41]. Consequently, *iodides are contraindicated during pregnancy.* Iodides can also be secreted in breast milk and for similar reasons should not be taken by lactating women.

Adequate hydration is an important aspect of expectoration, and proper fluid intake is important. Expectoration may be aided by chest-clapping techniques in the earlier stages of pregnancy; in the later stages, tolerance for this procedure may be minimal.

Antitussive Agents

A common and often prominent feature of asthma is cough. Asthma may present in fact with cough in the absence of wheezing [42]. The use of antitussive agents is common, therefore, in pregnant asthmatic women. The use of antitussives for the treatment of cough associated with asthma is to be discouraged. Rather, coughing may be a reflection of airway obstruction, which requires more optimal bronchodilator therapy, and such treatment should be pursued. Cough may also result from nasopharyngeal irritation, from allergic or noninfectious rhinitis, or from sinusitis, and treatment of these underlying conditions rather than the cough per se is more appropriate. In addition, many antitussive preparations contain alcohol, and the excessive use of such preparations has been reported to lead to the fetal alcohol syndrome from overuse of alcohol [43]. Overuse of narcotic ingredients in cough preparations is another risk, possibly depressing respiration of the newborn at delivery. If coughing is severe and prevents sleep, and all other therapeutic modalities have been maximized, antitussive agents can be used mainly at bedtime to help relieve cough to the point that sleep is possible. For this purpose, the simplest nonnarcotic agents (e.g., dextromethorphan) are advised.

Antibiotics

The major infectious agents that intensify asthma are viral in origin. Further, bacterial infections of the upper respiratory tract, including the sinuses and ears, as well as the lower respiratory tract occur in asthmatic patients and may aggravate bronchospasm. Because of adverse effects on protein synthesis and fetal development including staining of enamel, the tetracyclines should not be employed during pregnancy.

Sedatives

It is not unusual for the asthmatic patient to be anxious during an asthmatic paroxysm. Although this apprehension often provokes similar apprehension among physicians and nurses attending the patient, more often than not the patient's anxiety is a reflection of her respiratory status. Relief of anxiety is more likely to follow appropriate treatment of asthma than attempted suppression with tranquilizers, hypnotics, or sedatives. Barbiturates and other respiratory depressants are contraindicated in asthma. This is particularly the case in the pregnant female, and especially at the time of labor and delivery since respiratory depression of the newborn also may occur. Chronic use of barbiturates by the pregnant asthmatic may cause barbiturate addiction and withdrawal in the newborn.

Effects of Common Obstetric Drugs on Asthma

The multiplicity of mediators to which the asthmatic tracheobronchial tree is hypersensitive includes prostaglandins. Since prostaglandins can provoke severe asthma, they should not be used in the pregnant asthmatic patient [44]. Beta-adrenergic receptor agonists used to retard abortion and labor should have only salutary effects on asthma. Care should be taken, however, to ensure that the patient is not already receiving adrenergic drugs or high dosages of methylxanthines. Systemic adrenergic agents along with high-dosage methylxanthines increase the toxicity of both the methylxanthine and the adrenergic agent. Agents that block beta-receptors (e.g., propranolol) have a propensity to induce bronchoconstriction in asthmatic patients and should be avoided in patients with a history of asthma [45].

Anesthetics

Cyclopropane is *not* recommended for asthmatics because of its ability to induce bronchoconstriction. Ether, while having some bronchodilating activity, may also induce bronchoconstriction by irritant reflex mechanisms. Halothane has bronchodilating activity and is regarded as an appropriate general anesthetic for asthmatic patients [46]. Ethrane too has been recommended [46]. The use of terbutaline and other beta-agonists to stop premature labor reportedly increases the risk of pulmonary edema, dysrhythmia, tachycardia, and hypotension when general anesthesia is used [47]. The same risks may apply to asthmatic patients who use large amounts of oral beta-adrenergic agonists. When intravenous beta-agonists are utilized, it is recommended that halothane not be used as the anesthetic because of its myocardial depressant qualities. Since cold air can act as a tracheobronchial irritant in asthma, it is helpful also to warm inhaled anesthetic and other inhaled vapors. Nitrous oxide appears safe.

Because of the hyperirritability of the tracheobronchial tree in asthmatics, the mechanical irritation of intubation can likewise be responsible for bronchoconstriction. For this reason and in order to avoid respiratory depression in mother and newborn at the time of delivery, local anesthesia is preferred to general anesthesia in asthmatic patients.

MANAGEMENT OF ACUTE ASTHMA

Therapy begins with the administration of humidified oxygen, which should be maintained at a level sufficient to keep the patient's arterial blood oxygen at a normal level. Oxygen should be continued until the patient can maintain her own arterial levels at normal or near-normal levels.

Beta-adrenergic agents are the drugs of first choice in reversing the asthmatic paroxysm. In a patient who is in extremis, or who cannot cooperate sufficiently to inhale medication, parenteral epinephrine or terbutaline can be used initially. This can be repeated at 20-minute intervals, arbitrarily, for a total of three doses. A preferable alternative is the initial use of parenteral agents for no more than one or two doses, switching then to an inhalant for further therapy. Although, on hypothetical grounds, parenteral agents would seem to be more effective than inhalant drugs in severe asthma, administration of beta$_2$ agents by inhalation is, in fact, as effective in emergency care of acute severe asthma as their administration parenterally [35,36]. The inhalant route has the advantage of allowing maximum therapeutic effect

while minimizing systemic side effects. In the initial phase of therapy, aerosolized agents can be used every half hour if necessary to induce bronchodilatation. Intermittent positive pressure breathing (IPPB) has not been shown to offer any advantage over simple aerosolization through humidified oxygen and carries with it a small risk of inducing pneumothorax [15]. Consequently, *the use of IPPB is not recommended*. Toxicity of adrenergic agents is accentuated under conditions of hypoxemia and acidosis; conversely, ensuring oxygenation and correcting acidosis (pH less than 7.3) can minimize cardiotoxic effects of adrenergic agents. Although isoproterenol (Isuprel) is a potent adrenergic bronchodilator, and is effective in acute severe asthma, the authors prefer the use of more selective beta$_2$-agonists, namely, isoetharine, metaproterenol, and, where available, terbutaline, albuterol (salbutamol) or fenoterol.

Aminophylline and theophylline are important bronchodilators utilized in the treatment of acute severe as well as chronic asthma. A blood level in the so-called optimal therapeutic range (10–20 µg/mL) should be achieved as rapidly as possible and maintained during the course of treatment. Close monitoring of blood levels is desirable. A constant intravenous infusion is recommended, but aminophylline can be "pulsed" intravenously over a 15- to 20-minute period every four hours as an alternative. If constant intravenous infusion is used, a blood theophylline level should be obtained in approximately four hours for initial determination and the dosage regulated accordingly. If aminophylline is pulsed, the peak blood level is obtained immediately after the infusion, with the trough just prior to the next infusion. Initially, a level midway between peak and trough will serve as a useful guide for dosing. However, with both methods, a steady state will not be realized for many hours, and theophylline blood levels should be monitored every 12 to 24 hours until stabilization at the desired blood level is apparent. For patients already receiving theophylline, a level obtained at the onset of therapy can be helpful. When the patient is able to tolerate oral medications, oral theophylline using a total daily dosage comparable to the total daily intravenous dosage of theophylline (remember, aminophylline = approximately 85% theophylline) is a usual starting point for oral therapy. After at least three days of round-the-clock oral therapy, a determination of a theophylline blood level should again be made to evaluate the appropriateness of the dosage.

Acute severe asthma is an emergency, and corticosteroid therapy should be started. Dosage recommendations are somewhat arbitrary, but hydrocortisone (Solu-Cortef, 200 mg) or equivalent medication (e.g., methylprednisolone, 40 mg) intravenously over a 10- to 15-minute period is recommended as an initial dose, followed by similar doses every four or six hours for at least 24 to 48 hours, or until the patient has shown a consistent, beneficial response to therapy. Another approach is to use a relatively high dose (e.g., methylprednisolone, 125 mg) as initial therapy, which is doubled every four hours until asthma is controlled. Decrease of steroid dosage and subsequent withdrawal are dictated by the degree of therapeutic response and prior history of corticosteroid use. For example, the patient who has been on large doses of inhaled corticosteroids, or on an alternate-day corticosteroid regimen, may take longer to recover adrenal function than the patient who has not been on such therapy for many months. In the former instance, a decreasing dosage schedule and weaning over a period of a week or more may be appropriate, whereas in the latter case, as little as 72 hours of corticosteroid therapy may be adequate, without the need for further tapering before complete withdrawal. When the route of corticosteroid administration is changed from intravenous to oral, the use of short-acting steroids (e.g., prednisone or prednisolone) is recommended.

Inhaled atropine may also be useful in controlling acute asthma. It is usually employed in patients with cough as a prominent complaint. It may also be considered when patients have failed to respond to conventional treatment with methylxanthines, adrenergic agents, and even corticosteroids. Initial dosage is 1 mg of an atropine solution delivered via nebulization every three to four hours. Up to 3 mg per dose may be given. Care must be exercised to avoid spray of the solution into the eye. Although of theoretical concern, drying of tracheal or bronchial secretions does not appear to be a clinical problem.

An intravenous line, for the purpose of infusing fluids and electrolytes as well as to serve as a vehicle for the administration of medication, should be established early. Fluid therapy should be maintained at a level sufficient to keep the patient adequately hydrated, but excesses are to be avoided since the high negative intrapleural pressure may predispose to pulmonary edema [48]. Intravenous fluids should contain glucose, an appropriate amount of sodium, and, when urine output is adequate, potassium since the concomitant administration of corticosteroids is likely to encourage sodium retention and potassium excretion. Although the patient is allowed to have oral fluids, the use of cold beverages is discouraged because imbibing cold fluid may aggravate asthma.

Acidosis with a pH of less than 7.3 should be corrected if possible by means of bicarbonate. Bicarbonate dosage may be calculated with the following formula: mEq bicarbonate needed = negative base excess $\times$ 0.3 body weight in kilograms. The bicarbonate may be given rapidly by intravenous infusion. Arterial or venous pH can be redetermined 10 to 15 minutes later, and further correction of acidosis is considered at that time if necessary. It should be remembered that bicarbonate administration for respiratory acidosis is only a temporizing maneuver until respiratory acidosis is corrected by improving ventilation.

A major part of asthmatic obstruction is due to plugging of bronchi and bronchioles with thick tenacious mucus. Consequently, the use of agents that can encourage expectoration presumably should be beneficial in asthma. Unfortunately, there are few data to suggest that expectorants are in fact helpful, particularly in the treatment of acute asthma. In addition, iodides are contraindicated in pregnancy because of their potential effects on the fetal thyroid. On the other hand, chest physiotherapy (postural drainage) when tolerated by the patient can be a useful device to encourage coughing and expectoration. In the initial stages of acute severe asthma, however, this is poorly tolerated and should not be encouraged. When used, it should be preceded by the inhalation of an adrenergic bronchodilator to maximize bronchial patency and the beneficial effects of coughing.

Infectious agents are frequent precipitators of severe asthma. By and large, they are viral [49], and antibiotics are therefore of little use, at least initially. Patchy "infiltrates" (sometimes the result of viral infection) and atelectasis, which frequently accompany asthma, may be seen on chest roentgenogram and are not indications by themselves for antibiotic therapy. However, in acute asthma in which bacterial infection is suspected as a significant concomitant, broad-spectrum antibiotics (other than tetracycline) should be considered.

Sedatives, narcotics, and tranquilizers should not be used in treatment of acute asthma since they may depress respiration.

Rarely, severe asthma may require mechanical ventilation. Indications include cardiac arrest and clinical deterioration with progressive CO_2 retention in spite of vigorous medical management. It is a method of life support and not a direct treatment of asthma. Furthermore, it must be borne in mind that mechanical ventilation in the setting of acute asthma is associated with high morbidity and mortality [10]. Principles of mechanical ventilation are listed in Table 19-1.

Table 19-1. Principles of
mechanical ventilation in acute asthma

1. Intubate with 8 mm or greater endotracheal tube.
2. Use volume ventilation.
3. Sedate or paralyze patient if necessary to alow adequate time for exhalation; manage resistance to ventilation.
4. Ensure adequate humidification.
5. Be alert for pneumothorax.
6. Deliver inhaled bronchodilators via in-line nebulizer.
7. Use low-dose subcutaneous heparin as measure to decrease the risk of deep venous thrombophlebitis and pulmonary embolism.

MANAGEMENT OF ASTHMA DURING LABOR AND DELIVERY

When an attack of acute asthma coincides with labor, the most important goal is the prevention of maternal and fetal hypoxemia. Supplemental oxygen must be administered at whatever rate is necessary to keep the mother's arterial oxygen saturation greater than 90%. Arterial blood gases should be monitored to determine whether oxygenation and arterial acid-base balance are acceptable. Recall that a "normal" arterial CO_2 in the setting of acute asthma is usually a sign of increasing alveolar hypoventilation. Inability to adequately oxygenate the mother will lead to fetal distress and may necessitate cesarean delivery.

In addition to ensuring oxygenation, vigorous efforts must be made to reverse acute airways obstruction. In general, the same sequence of drug administration and dosage outlined in the section on treatment of acute asthma should be followed. However, a potential adverse effect of bronchodilator drugs is arrest of labor. This probably results from their action on smooth muscle relaxation. Since most concern is centered around beta-adrenergic agents, this class of drugs should be administered by inhalation. Intravenous aminophylline has the same potential adverse side effect, which does not represent a contraindication to its use but only a point of caution. Because of the adverse consequences of uncontrolled asthma, when patients do not respond within one or two hours of receiving adequate aminophylline and beta-adrenergic therapy, we believe intravenous corticosteroids should be started, as discussed in the section on treatment of acute asthma. Patients who have been on maintenance corticosteroids should also receive hydrocortisone, 100 mg every eight hours, at the time of delivery and 24 hours post partum.

Acute asthma is a misnomer, since the acute paroxysm is simply the "tip of the asthmatic iceberg" [3,50]. Adequate follow-up therapy to the point of complete resolution of the asthmatic paroxysm is an essential part of the therapeutic regimen. The best treatment for acute severe asthma is actually its prevention, through recognition and therapy of chronic asthma and anticipation of acute problems. It cannot be emphasized too strongly: Asthma is a chronic disorder that may surface acutely, and continued assessment of the status of the lower respiratory tract function in a patient with asthma is important, especially during pregnancy.

REFERENCES

1. Hernandez E, Angell CS, Johnson JW. Asthma in pregnancy: current concepts. Obstet Gynecol. 1980; 55:739–43.
2. Mintz S. Pregnancy and asthma. In: Weiss EB, Segal MS, eds. Bronchial asthma: mechanisms and therapeutics. Boston: Little, Brown, 1976:971–82.
3. Pearlman DS, Bierman CW. Asthma (bronchial asthma, reactive airways disorder). In: Bierman CW, Pearlman DS, eds. Allergic diseases of infancy, childhood, and adolescence. Philadelphia: Saunders, 1980:581–604.
4. Weinstein AM, Dubin BD, Podleski WK, Spector SL, Farr RS. Asthma and pregnancy. JAMA. 1979; 241: 1161–5.
5. Turner ES, Greenberger PA, Patterson R. Management of the pregnant asthmatic patient. Ann Intern Med. 1980; 93:905–18.
6. Fein BT, Kamin PB. Management of allergy in pregnancy. Ann Allergy. 1964; 22:341–8.
7. Sahaefer G, Silverman F. Pregnancy complicated by asthma. Am J Obstet Gynecol. 1961; 82:182–91.
8. Williams DA. Asthma and pregnancy. Acta Allergol (Copenh.). 1967; 22:311–23.
9. Gordon M, Niswander KR, Berendes H, Kantor AS. Fetal morbidity following potentially anoxygenic obstetric conditions. VII. Bronchial asthma. Am J Obstet Gynecol. 1970; 106:421–9.
10. Gluck JC, Gluck P. The effects of pregnancy on asthma: a prospective study. Ann Allergy. 1976; 37:164–8.
11. Williamson AC. Pregnancy concomitant with asthma or hay fever. Am J Obstet Gynecol. 1930; 20: 192–7.
12. Jensen K. Pregnancy and allergic diseases. Acta Allergol (Copenh.). 1953; 6:44–53.
13. Schatz M, Patterson R, Zeitz S, et al. Corticosteroid therapy for the pregnant asthmatic patient. JAMA. 1975; 233:804–7.
14. Bahna SL, Bjerkedal T. The course and outcome of pregnancy in women with bronchial asthma. Act Allergol (Copenh.). 1972; 27:397–406.
15. McCombs RP, Lowell FC, Ohman JL Jr. Myths, morbidity, and mortality in asthma. JAMA. 1979; 242: 1521–4.

16. Scoggin CH, Sahn SA, Petty TL. Status asthmaticus. A nine-year experience. JAMA. 1977; 238:1158–62.

17. Georg J. The treatment of status asthmaticus. Allergy. 1981; 36:219–32.

18. Boushey HA, Holtzman MJ, Sheller JR, Nadel JA. Bronchial hyperreactivity. Am Rev Respir Dis. 1980; 121:389–413.

19. Buckley JM, Pearlman DS. Controlling the environment. In: Bierman CW, Pearlman DS, eds. Allergic diseases of infancy, childhood, and adolescence. Philadelphia: Saunders, 1980:300–10.

20. Lockey SD III. Environmental control of allergic disease. In: Lockey RF, ed. Allergy and clinical immunology. Garden City, N.Y.: Medical Examination Publishing Co., 1979:1163–75.

21. Slavin RG. Allergic bronchopulmonary aspergillosis. In: Middleton E Jr, Reed CE, Ellis EF, eds. Allergy: principles and practice. St. Louis: Mosby, 1978:843–54.

22. Overholt RH, Voorhees RJ. Esophageal reflux as a trigger in asthma. Dis Chest. 1966; 49:464–6.

23. Rachelefsky GS, Coulson A, Siegel SC, Stiehm EK. Aspirin intolerance in chronic childhood asthma. Pediatrics. 1975; 56:443–8.

24. Sutton PL, Rose JQ, Goldstein S, Koup JR, Middleton E, Juske WJ. Theophylline pharmacokinetics during pregnancy and postpartum. J Allergy Clin Immunol. 1980; 65:177.

25. Weinberger M, Hendeles L. Pharmacologic management. In: Bierman CW, Pearlman DS, eds. Allergic diseases of infancy, childhood, and adolescence. Philadelphia: Saunders, 1980:311–32.

26. Linn S, Schoenbaum SC, Monson RR, Rosner B, Stubblefield PG, Ryan KJ. No association between coffee consumption and adverse outcomes of pregnancy. N Engl J Med. 1982; 306:141–5.

27. Rosenberg L, Mitchell AA, Shapiro S, Slone D. Selected birth defects in relation to caffeine-containing beverages. JAMA. 1982; 247:1429–32.

28. Heinonen OP, Slone D, Shapiro S. Birth defects and drugs in pregnancy. Littleton, Mass.: Publishing Sciences Group, 1977.

29. Schatz M, Harden K, Saunders B, Porreco R, Hoffman C, O'Patry D, Sperling W, Mellon M, Zieger RS. The placental transfer of theophylline at term and its effect on the infant. J Allergy Clin Immunol. 1983; 71:130.

30. Arwood LL, Dasta JF, Friedman C. Placental transfer of theophylline: two case reports. Pediatrics. 1979; 63:844–6.

31. Labovitz E, Spector S. Placental theophylline transfer in pregnant asthmatics. JAMA. 1982; 247:786–8.

32. Yurchak AM, Jusko WJ. Theophylline secretion into breast milk. Pediatrics. 1976; 57:518–20.

33. Hetzel MR, Clark TJ. Comparison of intravenous and aerosol salbutamol. Br Med J. 1976; 2:919.

34. Heimer D, Shim C, Williams MH Jr. The effect of sequential inhalations of metaproterenol aerosol in asthma. J Allergy Clin Immunol. 1980; 66:75–7.

35. Rossing TH, Fanta CH, Goldstein DH, Snapper JR,

McFadden ER Jr. Emergency therapy of asthma: comparison of the acute effects of parenteral and inhaled sympathomimetics and infused aminophylline. Am Rev Respir Dis. 1980; 122:365–71.

36. Schwartz AL, Lipton JM, Warburton D, Johnson LB, Twarog FJ. Management of acute asthma in childhood: a randomized evaluation of beta-adrenergic agents. Am J Dis Child. 1980; 134:474–8.

37. Dykes MHM. Evaluation of an antiasthmatic agent cromolyn sodium. JAMA. 1974; 227:1061–2.

38. Fainstat T. Cortisone-induced congenital cleft palate in rabbits. Endocrinology. 1954; 55:502–8.

39. Snyder RD, Snyder D. Corticosteroids for asthma during pregnancy. Ann Allergy. 1978; 41:340–1.

40. Paterson JW, Woolcock AJ, Shenfield GM. Bronchodilator drugs. Am Rev Respir Dis. 1979; 120:1149–88.

41. Galina MP, Avnet ML, Einhorn A. Iodides during pregnancy; an apparent cause of neonatal death. N Engl J Med. 1962; 267:1124–7.

42. Corrao WM, Braman SS, Irwin RS. Chronic cough as the sole presenting manifestation of bronchial asthma. N Engl J Med. 1979; 300:633–7.

43. Chasnoff IJ, Diggs G, Schnoll SH. Fetal alcohol effects and maternal cough syrup abuse. Am J Dis Child. 1981; 135:968.

44. Fishburne JI Jr, Brenner WE, Braaksma JT, Hendricks CH. Bronchospasm complicating intravenous prostaglandin $F_{2\alpha}$ for therapeutic abortion. Obstet Gynecol. 1972; 39:892–6.

45. Richardson PS, Sterling GM. Effects of beta-adrenergic receptor blockade on airway conductance and lung volume in normal and asthmatic subjects. Br Med J. 1969; 3:143–5.

46. Benatar SR. Anaesthesia for the asthmatic. S Afr Med J. 1981; 59:409–12.

47. Ravindran R, Viegas OJ, Padilla LM, LaBlonde P. Anesthetic considerations in pregnant patients receiving terbutaline therapy. Anesth Analg (Cleve.). 1980; 59:391–2.

48. Stalcup SA, Mellins RB. Mechanical forces producing pulmonary edema in acute asthma. N Engl J Med. 1977; 297:592–6.

49. Berman SZ, Mathison DA, Stevenson DD, et al. Transtracheal aspiration studies in asthmatic patients in relapse with "infective" asthma and in subjects without respiratory disease. J Allergy Clin Immunol. 1975; 56:206–14.

50. McFadden ER. The chronicity of acute attacks of asthma—mechanical and therapeutic implications. J Allergy Clin Immunol. 1975; 56:18–26.

51. Greenberger PA, Patterson R. Beclomethasone diproprionate for severe asthma during pregnancy. Ann Intern Med. 1983; 98:478–80.

20. RHEUMATIC DISEASES

Herbert Kaplan

Rheumatologist and Nobel laureate (for his discovery of cortisone) Philip Hench was the first physician to publish his observation of the "ameliorating effect of pregnancy on chronic atrophic (infectious rheumatoid) arthritis, fibrositis, and intermittent hydrarthrosis" [1]. Certainly the same observation had been made by pregnant women themselves prior to this 1938 report, and it is not unusual for a patient with rheumatoid arthritis (RA) to comment that she "ought to keep pregnant all the time." Hench chose not to discuss the hypotheses concerning the agent responsible for this remission in the rheumatic process. The simple and obvious explanation of increased concentrations of blood cortisol during pregnancy has not withstood experimental study [2]. Efforts to treat RA by producing the "pseudopregnant state" with a combination of a 19-norprogestational compound and a small amount of estrogen have not been beneficial [3].

Not until the past decade were physiologic and immunologic changes occurring during pregnancy and the puerperium found that may explain the amelioration and, in other instances, the exacerbation of rheumatic disease by pregnancy. In a series of elegant experiments, Persellin has demonstrated that serum from pregnant women has an inhibitory effect on both the phagocytic function and the migration of neutrophils [4]. Since normally functioning leukocytes are necessary for the development of rheumatoid synovium, the suppression of these cells may be in part responsible for a remission in the synovitis. This inhibitory effect was shown to persist in serum for one month post partum. It is also at this time that the pregnancy-related remission of RA frequently ends. In more recent studies, a pregnancy-associated alpha$_2$-glycoprotein has been suggested as being associated with the suppression of inflammation [5].

Others, searching for immunologic changes occurring during pregnancy, have found evidence that the fetus comes to the aid of the mother in an effort to ensure its own survival. Froelich et al. [6], reviewed the evidence to date that the fetus has a hypertrophied suppressor system producing factors that inhibit the already decreased activity of suppressor cells of mothers with RA and systemic lupus erythematosus (SLE). This "fetal suppressor cell graft" may not only ensure the fetus's survival but also be in part responsible for the temporary break in the mother's immunologic disease and the observed clinical remission. Loss of the graft at parturition may explain the frequently observed postpartum exacerbation. Further evidence for a temporarily beneficial change in the immunologic climate during pregnancy is the recent demonstration of a fall in immune complexes in the sera of pregnant patients with RA that paralleled their clinical course [7]. Significant changes in immune complexes were not seen in normal pregnancies.

Further study of the physiologic and immunologic changes occurring in both mother and fetus will certainly be of more than academic interest to physicians caring for pregnant patients and for those treating rheumatic disease in general. The emergence of a therapeutic alternative to "keeping pregnant all the time" may result from the study of this experiment of nature.

RHEUMATOID ARTHRITIS
Natural History of Rheumatoid Arthritis During Pregnancy and Post Partum

It should be emphasized at the outset that the pessimism of former years with regard to the course and prognosis of the two major rheumatic diseases of childbearing years, RA and SLE [8], is no longer justified. With a more sophisticated medical community and a more informed laity, the early diagnosis and treatment of these diseases allows for a more optimistic outlook when considering the advisability and management of the pregnancy and puerperium. The natural remission during pregnancy of 75% of patients with rheumatoid arthritis [1,9] has already been noted. Additional reasons for optimism are the recent therapeutic advances in the use of nonsteroidal antiinflammatory drug (NSAID) therapy, the advent of true "remission-inducing drugs," and the proper use of allied health personnel in a team approach to the patient with rheumatic disease. The exciting and monumental studies made in the surgical correction and replacement of damaged joints, now extending to patients in the childbearing years, offer yet one more therapeutic alternative.

If one were to judge the frequency and the magnitude of the problems of the pregnant patient with rheumatoid arthritis and the pregnant patient with SLE using the space allotted to each in both the medical and obstetric literature as a criterion, one would conclude that RA is of relatively minor concern. The converse is true. This literature artifact is another example of the medical profession's intrigue with the exotic and the unusual. RA is the more common disease and a more frequently encountered management problem. There seems little justification, however, from a review of the original paper and the paucity of subsequent similar observations, for Oka's statement in 1953 that "the onset of RA during pregnancy or immediately after is so common that in certain circumstances pregnancy can be regarded as an etiological factor" [10,11]. In a comprehensive review of the effect of pregnancy on RA, Persellin confirmed Hench's 1930 observations and noted improvement in the symptoms of RA during pregnancy in 74% of 274 pregnancies [9]. Of those that improved, 74% improved in the first trimester, 20% during the second, and 6% after the 24th week. In the 126 cases suitable for analysis in this literature review of postpartum exacerbations, 9% occurred in the first two weeks after delivery, 17% between the second and fourth weeks, 27% between the fourth and sixth weeks, 12% between the sixth and eighth weeks, and 35% more than eight weeks after delivery. More than 90% of patients with clinical relief during pregnancy had a postpartum exacerbation.

Although the supporting data are sparse, given the frequent remission of RA during pregnancy, it is not surprising that no adverse effect of pregnancy has been noted in the patients with RA [12,13]. Indications for termination of pregnancy are chiefly social ones, except in the rare patient with advanced destructive disease in whom the mechanical stresses to involved joints may be deemed severe enough to consider abortion.

Even less information is available on the outcome of the pregnancy in patients with RA. From the few observations in the literature [8,13], and personal observation, it appears that RA does not increase the risk of delivering an abnormal fetus. The effect of the mother's medication during pregnancy may be considerable. This will be discussed below.

Clinical Evaluation

An extensive discussion of the clinical, laboratory, and radiographic criteria for the diagnosis of RA is beyond the scope of this chapter, and the reader is referred to standard rheumatology texts [14,15]. The patient does *not* have RA unless the criteria set up by the American Rheumatism Association (ARA) in 1958 [16], and now recognized throughout the world, are met (Table 20-1). The 20% spontaneous remission rate in RA [17], the lack of specificity of all of the laboratory and x-ray criteria used in the diagnosis of RA, and the absence of evidence that instantaneous diagnosis is beneficial to the patients who are eventually proved to have RA suggest extreme caution on the part of the physician before making or accepting a previously made diagnosis of RA. A recent modification of the ARA criteria, using data stored and analyzed with the American Rheumatism Association Medical Information System, has grouped common signs and symptoms into seven more meaningful RA clinical syndromes [18] (Table 20-2).

The following clinical observations should be of help to the physician who may use the occurrence of a pregnancy to review the validity of a previously made diagnosis of rheumatoid arthritis.

Symmetric small joint (wrist, metacarpophalangeal, metatarsophalangeal) arthritis, at first episodic, then persistent, is the hallmark of RA. An observation on the part of the patient of *swelling*, not just pain, is important in early diagnosis, especially in the common situation in which the swelling has subsided by the time the physician examines the patient. In a female of childbearing age, morning stiffness to the degree that the patient, on her own and *without* the benefit of medical advice, uses a morning hot bath or shower to alleviate generalized stiffness or soaks her hands in hot water for symptomatic relief is rarely if ever seen in any disease other than rheumatoid arthritis.

A warm boggy joint, tender to the point of causing the patient to wince when it is palpated, suggests true synovial inflammation. Finding a joint with this abnormality should prompt a careful examination of the symmetric contralateral joint, even if the patient has not mentioned her discomfort in that area. Special attention to the metatarsophalangeal joints, commonly involved early

Table 20-1. American rheumatism association diagnostic criteria for rheumatoid arthritis

1. Morning stiffness
2. Pain on motion or tenderness in at least one joint
3. Swelling (soft tissue thickening or fluid, not bony overgrowth alone) in at least one joint
4. Swelling of at least one other joint
5. Symmetric joint swelling with simultaneous involvement of the same joint on both sides of the body
6. Subcutaneous nodules
7. Roentgenographic changes typical of rheumatoid arthritis
8. Positive rheumatoid factor test
9. Poor mucin clot in synovial fluid
10. Positive synovial biopsy
11. Positive nodule biopsy

Criteria 2, 3, 4, 5, 6 must be observed by a physician
Classical RA = 7 criteria
Definite RA = 5 or 6 criteria
Probable RA = 3 or 4 criteria

Table 20-2. The major rheumatoid arthritis clinical syndromes

Classification		Syndrome
Equivocal	I	Seropositive arthralgia
	II	Gelling arthralgia
	III	Seronegative monarthritis
Probable	IV	Monarticular arthritis, seropositive or with morning stiffness
	V	Seronegative polyarthritis
Definite	VI	Polyarthritis with symmetry, sometimes with one of seropositivity, erosions, or nodules
Classic	VII	Symmetric seropositive polyarthritis with nodules and/or erosions

Source: Mitchell and Fries [18].

in RA, may detect a surprising degree of tenderness not spontaneously volunteered by the patient. A dramatic, and to the patient surprising, response to salicylates is yet another early but nonspecific sign in a young female who usually reports that ordinarily she doesn't like to take pills.

A "positive" test for the rheumatoid factor does *not* establish the diagnosis of RA, and the laboratory that reports this test as positive without reporting the *degree* of positivity (i.e., rheumatoid factor titer) should not be reimbursed for its labor! In most laboratories, a titer of 1:80 or greater has clinical significance, but this must be correlated with other historical, physical, and laboratory findings before it is of value in making a diagnosis of RA. The erythrocyte sedimentation rate remains a valuable and inexpensive diagnostic test in the nonpregnant patient. The normal tendency of sed rate to increase in uncomplicated pregnancy and with advancing age makes the test's interpretation difficult [19]. A low value in pregnancy does not rule out RA.

A positive antinuclear antibody (ANA) test does not rule out the diagnosis of RA, nor does it establish the diagnosis of SLE. The ANA must be titered and, if it is positive, a pattern of positivity reported. "Significant" titers and patterns vary with different laboratories using different substances to detect the presence of autoantibodies, and it is incumbent on the physician using this test to be familiar with the experience of the individual laboratory when applying the results to a patient. A positive ANA is not an unusual finding in early uncomplicated RA [20].

The presence of synovial fluid should be sought for in an undiagnosed patient, since it is the best "biopsy" available in the rheumatic diseases. Fluid of poor viscosity (dropping from the end of the aspiration syringe like water), with a white blood cell count of between 2,000 and 50,000/mm^3, no crystals on microscopic exam, and negative bacteriologic study, is consistent with a diagnosis of RA.

Rarely will radiographic evidence be necessary for the diagnosis or management of the pregnant patient with rheumatic disease. Periarticular osteoporosis, the earliest radiographic change in RA, is nonspecific and often difficult to detect. Appropriate management of the patient with known RA and previously demonstrated radiographic erosions will not be affected by evaluating these bone changes during pregnancy. A chest roentgenogram (with appropriate screening of the fetus) may be a valuable diagnostic tool in the pregnant patient with acute undiagnosed arthritis if the hilar adenopathy of sarcoidosis is seen or an unexpected pleural effusion warns of extraarticular RA or SLE. A flexion film of the cervical spine should be obtained in every pregnant patient with known RA prior to delivery. More than 3 mm of C1-2 subluxation indicates the need to send the patient to the delivery room wearing a soft cervical collar and to alert the anesthesiologist to the chances of cervical cord damage with excessive manipulation during intubation or other anesthetic maneuvers. The author's personal experience is consistent with that of others who have found 25% of unselected outpatients with RA who have abnormal C1-2 subluxation [21].

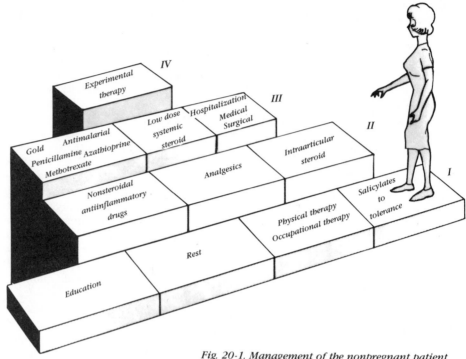

Fig. 20-1. Management of the nonpregnant patient
with rheumatoid arthritis.

Drug Therapy

The physician faced with a pregnant patient with
RA complaining of muscle and joint pain, who
searches the literature for a "safe" drug to relieve
the symptoms, may conclude that he or she does
not even have the traditional therapeutic option of
"take two aspirin and call me in the morning." If
only 650 mg of aspirin can prolong the bleeding
time for up to seven days, and its antiprostaglandin
effect can prolong gestation and possibly result in
premature closure of the ductus arteriosus [22],
what can be done to alleviate pain, possibly suppress synovitis, and maintain joint function during
gestation? Given the 75% or greater spontaneous
remission rate in RA during pregnancy, the primary and most difficult decision the physician and
the pregnant patient must make is whether the assistance of drug therapy is indicated during this
nine-month interval in a chronic disease such as
RA.

The traditional stepwise pyramidal approach to
the management of RA [23] (Fig. 20-1) must be
modified in pregnancy. The mother may be less
tolerant of "salicylates to tolerance," even if her
fetus is not, and the use of NSAIDs is rarely justified
because of their potential toxicity. When one considers the self-limited nature of the pregnant state
and the potential risk of drugs in pregnancy, a new
"pregnant pyramid" can be constructed (Fig. 20-

2). The basic program (level I) will have a greater
emphasis on measures such as education, rest,
physical and occupational therapy, and analgesic
doses of salicylates. The diagnosis of the pregnancy should stimulate a reevaluation of the validity of the diagnosis of RA and the efficacy of the
current treatment program.

Poor control of pain and inflammation is an indication to climb to level II. Considering the potential toxicity of other drug options, low-dose systemic corticosteroid therapy (5 mg/day) may be
used earlier than in the nonpregnant patient.
Analgesic dosages of salicylates can be increased to
antiinflammatory levels (3 g/day). As in the nonpregnant patient, intraarticular corticosteroids
offer symptomatic relief, although reinjection of
the same joint at intervals closer than every three
or four months is to be avoided. In the event of
constant and progressive disease, hospitalization
for supervised rest and regular use of physical
medicine modalities offers yet another therapeutic
option to the pregnant patient with unremitting
RA.

Salicylates

Two billion aspirin tablets are taken each year in
the United States, and 64% of gravid women admit
to the use of the drug during pregnancy [24]. The
majority of these women most certainly use aspi-

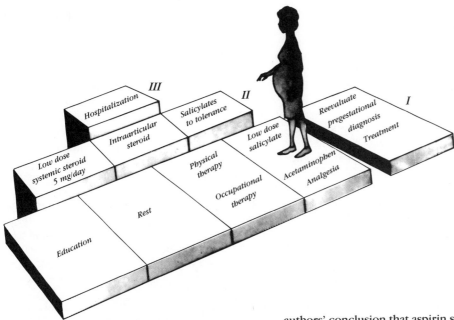

Fig. 20-2. Management of the pregnant patient with rheumatoid arthritis. Note that rest plays a noticeably larger role in the pregnant than in the nonpregnant patient; salicylates play a noticeably smaller role in the pregnant patient.

rin in analgesic dosages, rather than the antiinflammatory dosages required to suppress synovitis in RA. Four to six aspirin tablets daily may afford significant symptomatic relief (see Fig. 20-2, level I). An important question, not answered by recent studies on salicylate usage and toxicity, is whether aspirin in *antiinflammatory* dosages (i.e., more than 3 g/day) used *chronically* during a nine-month gestation results in higher neonatal morbidity or in increased teratogenicity. For analgesia during pregnancy, low-dose "as necessary" acetaminophen, without the gastric effects or platelet inhibitory capability of aspirin, is another option.

Aspirin has been reported to result in teratogenicity in animals but not in humans [25,26]. Increase in blood loss after delivery and increased perinatal mortality in one study were reported with heavy aspirin users [27]. Clotting defects and jaundice in the fetus have been found when mothers ingested large amounts of aspirin during gestation [28]. In a small controlled study, fetal hemostatic abnormalities including petechiae over the presenting part, hematuria, a cephalohematoma, conjunctival hemorrhage and bleeding from a circumcision were attributed to maternal use of aspirin. Infants of mothers using aspirin within five days of delivery had more complications than the offspring of mothers given the drug between six and ten days before delivery [34]. The

authors' conclusion that aspirin should be avoided during pregnancy is a medical and philosophical caveat that applies more to patients with mild aches and pains than to the mother with active polyarticular inflammation. Although other reports are more reassuring regarding the lack of significant aspirin toxicity for mother and child [24,29, 30], minimal use of salicylates during pregnancy, especially during the last month of gestation is most certainly recommended.

Despite the hazards, aspirin remains the drug of choice for the treatment of joint inflammation in pregnancy. Careful monitoring of the patient for other nonpregnancy-related manifestations of aspirin toxicity (i.e., gastrointestinal irritation and blood loss, ototoxicity, and lethargy) should also be done. Hepatotoxicity of salicylates, manifested by an elevation in SGOT, is rarely of clinical significance and, in the absence of symptoms, is not an indication for salicylate withdrawal. The use of nonacetylated salicylates in pregnancy has been studied even less than that of aspirin, but the reversible antiplatelet effect, a result of the absence of the acetyl component, may offer some therapeutic advantage. Enteric-coated salicylates are less reliably absorbed, especially in patients with rapid gastrointestinal motility, and their use mandates the use of serum salicylate levels when efficacy is questioned.

Nonsteroidal Antiinflammatory Drugs (NSAIDs)

In view of the general lack of superiority of NSAIDs when compared to aspirin in the treatment of RA, the paucity of data describing their use in pregnancy, and the uniform warning against their use in pregnancy [31], these drugs are rarely if ever justified during pregnancy. The physician considering the use of one of the rapidly burgeoning number of NSAIDs must remember that they do not offer an increase in antiinflammatory effect in the patient with RA when compared to that of aspirin.

Most rheumatologists believe that phenylbutazone and indomethacin have more potent analgesic and antiinflammatory effects than the other drugs in this group. This outcome may be due to a more potent inhibition of prostaglandin synthetase production, which in turn certainly increases the risk of using these drugs in the pregnant patient since prostaglandins are essential in maintaining normal uterine blood flow. The recent association between maternal indomethacin therapy and primary pulmonary hypertension of human newborns [32], oligohydramnios, and transient neonatal anuria [33] militates against the use of this class of drugs in the pregnant patient. The rare use of indomethacin in the pregnant patient with ankylosing spondylitis in a severe flare will be discussed below.

Antimalarial Drugs

Even the most ardent supporters of antimalarial drugs agree that they should not be used during pregnancy. Chromosome damage and selective concentration of antimalarials in the fetal uveal tract have been demonstrated.

Gold

In reviewing the *United States Pharmacopeia* or the *Physicians' Desk Reference,* one finds few drugs that have survived 50 years of clinical use. Gold salts, first employed in 1929 by Forestier in the treatment of RA, are still the mainstay of therapy in active progressive RA. The efficacy of gold has been demonstrated in well-controlled double-blind studies [35] and a favorable effect on the rate of development of bone erosions shown in patients given an adequate course [36]. The effect on bone erosion, inhibition of immunoglobulin synthesis and macrophage function has been justification for classifying gold as a "remission-inducing drug." To categorically state that this mode of therapy is contraindicated in pregnancy [37] is to deny an important therapeutic agent to the patient with RA who is not fortunate enough to have had a spontaneous remission with her pregnancy or who has not responded to salicylates. Since most rheumatologists would agree that a four- to six-month trial of aspirin and other conservative measures is indicated in RA before initiation of gold

therapy, the problem of gold usage in RA does not arise in a patient who develops RA during pregnancy but rather in the patient with established disease receiving gold who becomes pregnant.

Although effective in approximately 80% of patients with RA in whom it is used, the potential toxicity of gold to the patient is well recognized. In 20% of patients in whom gold therapy is initiated, it must be discontinued because of unacceptable toxicity. Another 20% will continue to use the drug in the face of minor skin, renal, or hematologic toxicity because the clinical benefit is deemed to outweigh the risk or discomfort of toxicity. A well-recognized clinical observation, only recently documented in a careful study, is that, once gold therapy is discontinued in a patient experiencing a remission, a repeat course may be less effective than was the original trial [38]. Hence the reluctance to discontinue gold once a remission has been achieved.

There are several reports that gold was used during pregnancy with no toxic effects on the mother or fetus [39,40–42]. Twenty-six patients with bronchial asthma received gold throughout pregnancy, and 43 others discontinued gold in early to mid pregnancy, with no gross deformities in the offspring save two hip abnormalities [43]. One study demonstrated the transplacental passage of gold in quantities sufficient to reach levels encountered in patients on gold therapy and then a normal decrement of gold levels over the first few weeks of life [42]. The potential exists, however, for the fetus to experience renal and hematologic toxicity seen in patients receiving gold therapy. There are no reports in humans implicating gold in neonatal mortality or teratogenicity. The reasons for the absence of a blinded control study are obvious and there is little likelihood of the appearance of other than anecdotal experience to support or discourage the use of gold during the pregnancy.

The decision to discontinue gold, a possibly irreplaceable therapeutic agent in a patient who by definition has had unremitting and probably destructive joint disease, must be made with full participation of the patient, husband, family physician, obstetrician, and perhaps a consulting rheumatologist. If the beneficial effect of gold has not yet been established, the decision will be an easier one; the loading phase of therapy can be reinstated post partum. It is in the patient who has had a partial or complete remission in RA as the result of gold that the real problem arises.

The dilemma is the same in a patient with a gold-induced remission who is contemplating pregnancy. Serum levels of gold will fall to presumably safe, nontoxic levels within one month after the last injection [44]. The safety of the fetus must be contrasted with the potential risk of a flare in the mother. The decision to continue therapy should be accompanied by a signed informed-consent document. It is not anticipated that the availability of an oral gold preparation will in any way affect this therapeutic dilemma in the near future.

Penicillamine

Although considered by some physicians to be as effective as gold in the treatment of rheumatoid arthritis [45], penicillamine seems scarcely justified in the pregnant patient. This drug is known to cross the placenta, to inhibit disulfide bridges, and to inhibit collagen cross-linking.

Corticosteroids

It is by intent that corticosteroid therapy is discussed at this point, after salicylates, NSAIDs and gold therapy, since in the nonpregnant patient only after unsatisfactory control of synovitis with the use of these agents are corticosteroids considered. An exception to this rule would be the patient with RA whose social or economic situation is such that rapid amelioration of symptoms is required at the possible expense of steroid toxicity or associated complications. The increased physical and psychological stress of pregnancy in a patient with RA, especially if there is an existing family, plus the potential for drug toxicity outlined above, presents a situation in which the cautious use of 5 mg of prednisone daily may be justified at a relatively early stage (Fig. 20-2, level II). It is essential that explaining the risks as well as the temporary benefits of corticosteroid therapy be a part of writing the steroid prescription.

The clinical benefit of corticosteroids in RA is presumably a result of their effect on the immune response as well as of their suppression of inflammation. There is no evidence, however, that these drugs have any long-term beneficial effect on the destructive course of RA, and they are therefore used as adjuvant rather than primary therapy in this disease. The primary practical clinical problem in their use is that the drug makes the patient (and doctor) feel "too good," and thus excessive, unnecessary, and dangerous use is encouraged. It is a rare patient with RA who cannot be kept comfortable with 7.5 mg of prednisone daily or less, and periodic attempts to taper the dosage below 7.5 mg daily, using decrements of 1 mg per day, at two- to four-week intervals should be made. Alternate-day therapy, often a useful technique in nonrheumatic diseases that respond to corticosteroids, is not effective in most patients with RA. The

symptoms on the "off" day are such that a return to daily therapy is soon requested. Supplementation of corticosteroid therapy during delivery in the adrenal-suppressed woman, by the parenteral route if necessary, is essential.

Hazards to the fetus of corticosteroid therapy are few, and in several large series congenital malformations were no greater than would be expected in pregnancies not complicated by steroid use [46,47]. Similarly, maternal use of corticosteroids does not seem to increase the risk of abortion, preterm labor, or stillbirth [48]. Routine use of supplemental corticosteroid in the infant born of a mother treated with corticosteroids is not necessary, but the infant should be observed for signs of adrenal insufficiency.

Intraarticular Corticosteroid Therapy

The judicious injection of insoluble corticosteroid preparations into the acutely inflamed joint of a patient with RA is a well-accepted form of therapy. This route should be used only if the standard basic salicylate regimen has not effected a significant remission. Intraarticular corticosteroid therapy can be used before systemic corticosteroids, especially in a patient with a degree of synovitis in one or two joints that is out of proportion to the disease elsewhere. Although the therapeutic goal is to achieve a "medical synovectomy" in the joint that is injected, the patient will frequently report a generalized improvement in other joints due to some systemic absorption of the injected material.

A general accepted rule of thumb is not to inject one joint more frequently than at three-month intervals, and only in the rare situation would one joint be injected more than once a year. There seems to be little evidence that one long-acting corticosteroid is better than any other. Large joints such as a knee or shoulder are injected with 1 mL, wrists and elbows with 0.5 mL, and metacarpophalangeal or interphalangeal joints with 0.25 mL. Injection of intraarticular corticosteroid into the hips of patients with RA is not recommended.

Immunosuppressive and Antimetabolite Drugs

As in the case of penicillamine, the potential toxicity and relative lack of experience with immunosuppressive drugs make their use extremely limited in a pregnant patient with a nonfatal disease such as RA. There are virtually no indications to initiate immunosuppressive drugs in a pregnant patient. In the extremely rare situation in which a pregnancy occurs in a patient with RA already taking immunosuppressive drugs, the risk of continued therapy may possibly be justified. The patient will often be well into the first trimester, the time when fetal damage is more likely to occur from chemotherapeutic agents, before she is aware of the pregnancy. If the beneficial response to immunosuppressive therapy has been established, usually in a patient with "malignant" arthritis and vasculitis, a decision to continue may be made. Since there is evidence for transplacental passage of some agents [49,50], the damage to the fetus may have already taken place by the time the pregnancy is detected. The fact that normal pregnancies have occurred in women taking cyclophosphamide and azathioprine [49,50] gives scanty comfort to the physician and patient faced with aggressive RA and failure to respond to more standard forms of therapy. The possible teratogenicity of these drugs must be recognized, and although possibly safer when used only during the second and third trimesters [51], and not in combination with radiation therapy, they are to be discouraged in a patient with RA in the childbearing years.

An analogous dilemma arises in the patient using immunosuppressive drugs who is *contemplating* pregnancy. The often irreversible ovarian failure associated with cyclophosphamide therapy should be recognized prior to its use. Methotrexate has recently been shown to have beneficial effects in patients with severe RA who have become refractory to standard therapy [52]. No fetal abnormalities were seen at birth in a small group of patients who had been treated with methotrexate in the past [53]. Measures to avoid conception during the use of methotrexate and for at least 12 weeks after discontinuing therapy have been recommended [54]. Methotrexate is an abortifacient and is teratogenic if taken during pregnancy.

Physical Therapy

The beneficial effects of symptomatic physical therapy in RA are often overlooked by the physicians trained to "cure" disease. Especially during the gestational period, when analgesic and antiinflammatory medications may be either reduced or withdrawn (see above), the diminution of pain afforded by locally applied cold or hot packs or a paraffin bath to the hands and feet may be appreciated. Maintenance of affected joint mobility by continuing (possibly initiating) a range-of-motion exercise program may result in a more mobile and effective mother post partum. An educational program, under the supervision of both a physical and an occupational therapist, aimed at protecting inflamed joints and recommending appropriate as-

sistive devices is therapy that should be offered to the pregnant patient with RA.

Indications for Termination of Pregnancy

Though data are scanty, there is no indication that RA per se calls for therapeutic abortion [11]. As has already been discussed, none of the standard analgesic and antiinflammatory drugs, including gold, have been incriminated in fetal morbidity or mortality so as to warrant termination of pregnancy as a result of their continued use. The risks associated with prior or concomitant use of immunosuppressive drugs have also been discussed. Gross normality at birth does not, however, assure the absence of a more remote drug-induced defect in a child whose mother (or father, as in the case of cyclophosphamide) was exposed to an immunosuppressive or antiinflammatory agent.

Obstetric Problems During Delivery

The excessive bleeding of a patient on salicylates will rarely be a problem. Supplemental parenteral corticosteroid should be given any woman who has used systemic corticosteroids in the preceding 12 months. The status of the atlantoaxial joint should be established by a roentgenogram of the cervical spine taken in flexion. More than 3 mm of separation of the anterior arch of the atlas from the odontoid suggests the potential for cervical cord compression during delivery or as a result of maneuvers by the anesthesiologist. In patients with this abnormal mobility it is appropriate to send the patient to the delivery suite wearing a soft cervical collar as a warning to the obstetrician and anesthesiologist of susceptibility to trauma in this area. In patients with rheumatoid involvement of one or both hips, vaginal delivery may be difficult. Adequacy of mobility should, of course, be established prior to parturition, and plans for cesarean delivery made when necessary.

Family Planning

Despite increasing evidence of a genetic predilection for the development of RA, the presence of this disease in parent or sibling is not alone a factor in deciding on the wisdom of conception [55]. The obvious increased physical stress imposed on a mother with multiple joint inflammation and possible deformity will certainly be the main factor in determining ultimate family size. Socioeconomic factors such as availability of assistance from family members or paid assistants are other variables to be considered.

The wide spectrum of the clinical manifestations of RA extends from those of spontaneous remission or mild nonerosive synovitis in a few joints to those of polyarticular destructive disease defying all forms of therapy. The advice of a consulting rheumatologist, schooled in the vicissitudes of the disease, may be invaluable when decisions regarding the long-term impact of this illness on the family are made.

SYSTEMIC LUPUS ERYTHEMATOSUS

It is incumbent on the physician treating a young female who has been diagnosed as having SLE not only to be aware of the improved diagnostic and therapeutic measures for this illness in recent years but also, when the clinical situation justifies it, to be more optimistic regarding the long-term prognosis than might have been possible just a few years ago. The 98% survival after five years and 90% survival after ten years (using the first symptom as the starting point) should be emphasized [56]. Specific reference must be made to the outdated and now incorrect information regarding this disease that may be found in various "family medical advisers" or given by well-meaning but uninformed friends. Educational material is available from local chapters of the Arthritis Foundation or the Lupus Foundation to assist the physician in this endeavor. The increased risk of an abnormal pregnancy must be discussed once the diagnosis of SLE has been established.

Pathophysiology

The normal decrease in suppressor cell function in pregnancy has already been referred to, and this may be exaggerated in SLE [57]. A demonstration of deficient suppressor function in healthy asymptomatic first-degree relatives of patients with SLE (the vast majority female) suggests a genetic predisposition as well [58]. Alterations in estrogen metabolism have been found in SLE, and this extended estrogen activity has been proposed as another explanation for the greater prevalence of SLE in women [59].

Effect of Pregnancy on SLE

Given a woman with SLE and apparently normal or minimally impaired renal function, there is no reason to proscribe pregnancy. The patient and her family should be apprised, however, of the possibility of an exacerbation of disease activity during pregnancy or post partum [60] and of the increased fetal wastage associated with maternal lupus nephritis. Corticosteroid therapy has proved to be a major therapeutic advance in the treatment

of the pregnant patient with SLE and will reduce the frequency and severity of exacerbations during pregnancy and after delivery. Even mild or moderate renal disease does not produce a major threat to maternal welfare, and a review of three retrospective studies of a total of 114 pregnancies shows that in only 15 did permanent deterioration of renal function occur [61]. In a still more optimistic review of 12 patients with diffuse glomerulonephritis, 10 patients had a completely uncomplicated pregnancy [62]. One authority is not convinced that "pregnancy per se has any permanent adverse effect upon the disease unless there is advanced cardiac or renal involvement" [63]. The fact that women with more than minimal renal disease probably have a decreased fertility is certain to influence these impressions.

A complete clinical remission for six months prior to conception can be considered the most favorable prognostic sign for an uncomplicated pregnancy in a patient with SLE [64,65]. A postpartum flare is seen in 25 to 40% of patients, but this can be effectively treated and possibly prevented with prophylactic corticosteroid therapy (see below) [66,67]. Unlike RA, in which a favorable course with one pregnancy may portend similar uncomplicated pregnancies in the future [1,68], in SLE the course of previous pregnancies has no prognostic value [69].

Effect of SLE on the Fetus

In the absence of severe renal, hematologic, or central nervous system manifestations of SLE, overall fertility and sterility rates in women with SLE do not differ significantly from those in the general population [70]. As would be expected, increased fetal wastage is directly proportional to the degree of renal disease in the mother. Proteinuria of greater than 300 mg per 24 hours in patients with SLE was associated with 38% fetal wastage, and creatinine clearance less than 100 mL per minute with a fetal wastage of 45%. A combination of these abnormalities in the same patient produced a fetal wastage of 80% [61]. It can be assumed that these renal abnormalities were manifestations of a more widespread small vessel involvement. In the same series, treatment during gestation with corticosteroids did not decrease fetal wastage, although other investigators have found a lower fetal mortality associated with corticosteroid therapy [70]. In one group of 35 pregnancies in 15 patients with "histological and/or biochemical and serological evidence of lupus nephritis" (type and amount not specified) the outcome was not different from that in patients without renal involvement [66]. Onset of SLE during gestation is a poor prognostic sign, fetal wastage reaching 43% in one series [65]. In a recent prospective study using the combined services of the obstetrician (urinary estriol and fetal monitoring), a rheumatologist (careful control of SLE activity), and a perinatologist (intensive care of newborn), fetal wastage was reduced to 19%, compared to 40% when a combined approach was not emphasized [70].

Multiple explanations have been offered to explain the increased fetal morbidity when the mother has SLE, including transplacental passage of antinuclear antibodies, the presence of lymphocytotoxic antibodies, and a decidual vasculopathy of the placenta [71]. Clinical manifestations in the newborn consistent with SLE, including butterfly rash, thrombocytopenia, and anemia, have been reported [72]. Intrauterine growth retardation is more common in children of mothers with SLE. A recently recognized neonatal complication is congenital heart block, one series noting that one in three mothers who deliver babies with congenital heart block has or will have SLE or other connective tissue disease [73]. This same review of 67 cases of congenital heart block associated with maternal connective tissue disease notes a significant incidence of sibling involvement, 22 of 67 children having affected brothers or sisters. Although the heart block is permanent, the pathology is not progressive, and the long-term prognosis is good.

A recent finding with great diagnostic and therapeutic implications is the presence of SS-A autoantibody in seven of eight infants with neonatal lupus, all of whom had mothers with the same autoantibody. Five of the infants had discoid lupus skin lesions, one had discoid lesions and congenital heart block, and two had congenital heart block alone. Four of the mothers had no clinical symptoms, two had xerostomia, one had Sjögren's syndrome, and one had SLE [74]. Since the SS-A autoantibody may not be found on the routine screening for antinuclear antibodies (ANA), this study should specifically be requested for all pregnant women with SLE or Sjögren's syndrome, as well as all infants with discoid LE or congenital heart block [75].

Clinical Evaluation

There is no one physical finding or single laboratory datum that establishes a diagnosis of SLE. The advent of the "LE prep" in 1948 and more recently the immunofluorescent test for ANA have been major diagnostic aids, but positive historical and physical evidence as well as laboratory studies are necessary before the physician can be reasonably confident in making this diagnosis. The ANA test may be positive in diseases other than SLE, and the physician using the test must be aware of the experience of the reference laboratory with regard to the significance of the titer and pattern of ANA.

In an effort to establish some uniformity among different research centers as well as to provide a guide for the clinician in making a diagnosis of SLE, the American Rheumatism Association in 1971 listed 14 clinical manifestations, the presence of four being strong evidence for SLE and a high specificity *against* RA and a variety of other nonrheumatic disorders. In its original presentation of the clinical criteria, the American Rheumatism Association committee stressed that these manifestations may be present *serially* or *simultaneously*. Early in the course of SLE, when the diagnosis may be in question, these findings are rarely present simultaneously, and only by careful probing during several examining sessions can the physician be reasonably certain of a diagnosis of SLE. A proposed revision of the criteria has been offered [76] (Table 20-3).

When the diagnosis is in doubt, the patient should be encouraged to contact the physician when the rash or Raynaud's phenomenon is actually present, or when the painful joint is visibly swollen. The fact that 20% of patients with SLE have a positive rheumatoid factor and that possibly 60% of patients with RA may have a positive ANA diminishes the value of these studies in establishing a firm diagnosis. The erythrocyte sedimentation rate, though frequently elevated in SLE, has lit-

Table 20-3. Criteria for the classification of SLE (proposed 1982 revision)

Diagnosis of SLE requires presence of four or more items.

1. Malar rash
2. Discoid lupus
3. Photosensitivity
4. Oral ulcers
5. Arthritis
6. Proteinuria (>0.5 g/day) or cellular casts
7. Seizures or psychosis
8. Pleuritis or pericarditis
9. Hemolytic anemia or leukopenia or lymphopenia or thrombocytopenia
10. Antibody to DNA or antibody to Sm or LE cells or false-positive STS
11. Positive FANA

tle value in differentiating between the various connective tissue diseases. Special attention to the urinary sediment by the physician, rather than submitting the specimen to "routine urinalysis," may detect a cast that would otherwise be missed. Proteinuria must be quantitated; a report of 1+ or more should be quantitated with a 24-hour urine protein. A value greater than 0.5 g per 24 hours has some diagnostic significance with regard to SLE. Though listed in the original ARA criteria as "arthritis without deformity," the joint disease of SLE may indeed produce joint deformity as a result of soft tissue damage if not from bony erosion. The roentgenogram can sometimes differentiate SLE from RA by the *absence* of erosive changes in SLE.

Increase in antibodies to native DNA, presence of cryoglobulins, and decrease in total hemolytic complement or C3 or C4 are other values that may be helpful in diagnosing and later in assessing the response to therapy of a patient with SLE. Synovial fluid is less inflammatory than that of RA, with a white blood cell count usually less than 2,000. Complement levels in synovial fluid may be low in both RA and SLE. Skin biopsy, the "lupus band test," is rarely indicated in view of the nonspecificity of the presence of immunoglobulins at the dermal-epidermal junction.

Management

The diagnosis of pregnancy in the patient with SLE, like the initial diagnosis of SLE, is *not* alone an indication to initiate corticosteroid therapy. Certainly the patient will be followed more closely, by several physicians, during her gestation than previously. Salicylates remain the drug of choice for arthralgias, arthritis, fever, and pleuritic and pericardial symptoms not associated with effusions that compromise function. The risks of adequate salicylate therapy have been discussed in the section on RA. From 12 to 16 aspirin tablets daily may be required to afford significant symptomatic relief and, used in a fashion as outlined in the section on RA, is the least hazardous drug available. Indomethacin is the most potent of the NSAIDs and is a valuable agent in the treatment of fever and polyserositis associated with SLE. In the pregnant patient, the benefit of this agent must be measured against the possible risks mentioned earlier. There is no experience with other NSAIDs to suggest that they offer any advantages, regarding either efficacy or toxicity, over salicylates, and they should be avoided if at all possible.

Hydroxychloroquine is considered an effective agent for treatment of the dermatologic and musculoskeletal manifestations of SLE but, as already discussed, is best avoided in the pregnant patient.

Whereas corticosteroids are used as adjunct therapy in RA, these drugs have been shown to play an important primary role in the treatment of SLE. In pregnancy not only can the more ominous renal, cardiopulmonary, central nervous system, hematopoietic, and vasculitic manifestations that arise be treated, but there is merit in initiating or increasing the dose of corticosteroids during labor and for two months after delivery to reduce the prevalence of postpartum exacerbations [61,65, 67,77]. Pregnancy constitutes a definite danger to the patient with SLE, as is not the case in the RA patient. Of 20 maternal deaths in four series of patients with SLE, 19 took place in the postpartum period [60].

A patient with SLE treated with corticosteroids who becomes pregnant should have her maintenance dose continued. A flare in systemic manifestations or a decrease in serum complement requires that the dosage of prednisone or its equivalent be increased to 40 to 60 mg daily. When a therapeutic response has been achieved, the dosage should be tapered by 5 to 10 mg at weekly intervals. There has been some evidence that monthly serum complement determinations may be of prognostic value, and a falling value of C3 (in contrast to the normal *increase* seen in uncomplicated pregnancy) should be an indication for initiating more aggressive steroid therapy [65,78]. Although the data to support its value are meager, intravenous hydrocortisone, 100 mg every eight hours at the time of delivery and continuing for the first day thereafter, has been considered to be of value in decreasing postpartum flares [67]. Oral corticosteroids should be continued for two months at a level slightly greater than that required ante partum.

The precise role of immunosuppressive therapy in the management of the nonpregnant patient with SLE has not been established [78]. Initiating immunosuppressive therapy during pregnancy should rarely if ever be necessary. The physician faced with managing a pregnant patient on immunosuppressive drugs derives little comfort from reports of successful pregnancies in mothers receiving azathioprine [80]. In a patient being successfully treated with azathioprine who becomes pregnant, the absence of data to demonstrate fetal injury, plus the concern of a flare of SLE upon discontinuance of azathioprine therapy, suggests that this drug be continued [81].

Renal Disease in SLE

Few would argue that SLE complicated by nephritis poses a significant hazard to the pregnant female. Lupus nephropathy does not, however, preclude a successful pregnancy. In a recent multi-center study reporting 65 pregnancies in 47 patients, 90% of whom had antecedent lupus nephropathy (12 with renal biopsy showing type III glomerulonephropathy), the activity of SLE was not influenced by pregnancy in two-thirds of the cases [82]. The consensus of those reporting the experience with lupus nephritis in pregnancy confirms optimistic reports [60,61,65,83,84] although opposing, more ominous opinions do exist [85,86]. As would be expected, a complete clinical remission of signs and symptoms of lupus nephritis for three to six months prior to the onset of pregnancy is certainly a favorable prognostic sign both for the course of the mother's disease during pregnancy and for fetal survival [65,84].

Early in pregnancy the urine should be examined carefully for casts, and proteinuria if present should be quantitated with a 24-hour urine specimen. Serum creatinine and creatinine clearance and a serum complement (C3) are obtained for baseline levels. These values should be repeated at monthly intervals. A falling C3 level has been suggested as being the most reliable serologic value to warn of renal deterioration [65,84]. Progressive hypocomplementemia signals the need for corticosteroid therapy in a dosage adequate to suppress the clinical and laboratory abnormalities being monitored. As disease activity is controlled, corticosteroid dosage should be tapered with caution, but the tendency for postpartum flare requires continuing therapy for at least two months post partum.

Indications for and Risks of Therapeutic Abortion

There is unanimity among students of the problem of the pregnant patient with SLE regarding therapeutic abortion. Not only does therapeutic abortion fail to accomplish its goal of terminating a disease flare [67,78,87] but it may in and of itself be responsible for an increase in disease activity. The common postpartum disease flare may only be hastened by the premature evacuation of the uterus performed during a therapeutic abortion. When indicated for psychosocial reasons, termination of pregnancy in the first trimester is relatively safe and not associated with a deleterious effect on the mother [61]. Vigorous corticosteroid therapy for complications, renal and otherwise, as in the nonpregnant patient, is preferred to a therapeutic abortion. There is no evidence that corticosteroids or cytotoxic drugs have resulted in developmental abnormalities in the fetus or mother so treated [70,78,83,84].

Oral Contraceptives and SLE

Although the precise relationship between oral contraceptives and SLE is not clear, there is no question that in some patients both clinical signs and serologic abnormalities consistent with SLE appear after their use [88]. Oral contraceptives may induce SLE or may merely "unmask" the as yet clinically quiescent diathesis [89]. Studies of patients with SLE and their families demonstrate genetic and hormonal factors predisposing to autoimmunity *before* autoantibodies or clinical symptoms appear [58]. It is not unreasonable to conclude that iatrogenic hormone manipulations, as with the use of oral contraceptives, may trigger the SLE syndrome in some individuals. The fact that prospective studies of healthy women attending birth control clinics have not shown a significant association between oral contraceptives and SLE [90] does not negate these findings.

The available evidence suggests that women with SLE should not use oral contraceptives. The appearance of clinical findings consistent with SLE after initiation of oral contraceptive therapy, especially if associated with the appearance of a positive ANA, certainly militates against their further use. A biologic false positive test for syphilis has been suggested as an early marker for patients in whom the lupus diathesis is likely to develop, and the appearance of SLE after oral contraceptive therapy in two patients with this marker suggests the use of other forms of birth control in these patients [88].

SERONEGATIVE SPONDYLOARTHROPATHIES

Included in this category are ankylosing spondylitis (AS), postenteric arthritis, Reiter's syndrome, and, when the spine and sacroiliac joints are involved, psoriatic arthritis and the arthritis associated with inflammatory bowel disease. Also affected are a group of children, previously thought to have juvenile RA, who are probably juvenile spondylitics, and who in adult life develop typical AS. In addition to being seronegative for the rheumatoid factor, these diseases share a propensity for involvement of the axial skeleton (spine and sacroiliac joints), a 20 to 30% incidence of peripheral joint arthritis, and, commonly, involvement of the skin and uveal tract of the eye, and inflammation of the large and small bowel. Most important, they also share a high incidence (70–90%) of bearing the HLA-B27 histocompatibility antigen [91]. Bearers of this antigen, and by implication having a common genetic makeup, are thought to be peculiarly susceptible to some as yet unidentified environmental agent that is responsible for their disease. In some cases of arthritis associated with enteric bacterial infection, the responsible agent has been identified [92].

A physician dealing with women in the childbearing age group must be aware that the previously taught dictum of the rarity of AS and Reiter's syndrome in the female is no longer accepted, and that there may be an equal incidence of AS in both sexes although the disease tends to run a slower and more benign course in women [93–95]. The insidious onset of unilateral or bilateral low back pain, most severe upon arising in the morning and improved (rather than aggravated) by activity, with frequent radiation to the buttocks, with or without peripheral synovitis, should arouse suspicion of this entity. The peripheral arthritis tends to be asymmetric and involves the lower extremities more than the upper. "Sausage-shaped" swelling of the toes and heel involvement are other clues of importance. Absence of rheumatoid factor and presence of the HLA-B27 antigen (in up to 90% of AS) further confirm the diagnosis. An elevated sedimentation rate is not necessary for the diagnosis nor is radiographic abnormality of the sacroiliac joint.

Since the importance of AS and these related diseases in women has only recently been recognized, systematic study of this problem during pregnancy has been rare. A retrospective review of 87 pregnancies in 50 patients with AS suggests that the disease is largely unaffected by pregnancy [96]. Approximately half of the pregnant AS patients experienced no change in disease activity during or immediately after pregnancy; exacerbation was noted in 24% but remission was noted in 20%, a variation that can be expected in the nonpregnant patient with AS. Approximately 50% of patients experienced aggravation of symptoms for a short time post partum, possibly in part due to the stress associated with parturition and increased physical demands of motherhood. Fetal morbidity was no different from what could be expected in a normal population.

Drug management during pregnancy is similar to that of RA, with salicylates used as necessary for pain relief and maintenance of function. Corticosteroid, antimalarial, and immunosuppressive therapy have not been used. In the series referred to above, "continuous use" of antiinflammatory drugs (type not specified) was reported during 12 pregnancies, all of which ran a normal course and concluded with normal babies [96]. The author has recently successfully followed a markedly

symptomatic spondylitic through pregnancy, using indomethacin after fetal heart sounds were heard and discontinuing it one month ante partum. Indomethacin remains the drug of choice for the flares of back pain seen with AS, with up to 250 to 300 mg daily often necessary. The concern regarding the use of this and other NSAIDs has already been discussed.

CARPAL TUNNEL SYNDROME

Fluid retention during pregnancy is presumably responsible for compression of the median nerve at the wrist as it passes beneath the transverse carpal ligament into the hand. Numbness and tingling, frequently more severe during the night, in the first, second, and third fingers, but occasionally in the fourth and fifth fingers as well, are typical complaints. Pain *proximal* to the wrist is also seen. Abnormal nerve conduction studies across the wrist are not necessary for the diagnosis. Although usually no primary disease will be found, in the pregnant patient with carpal tunnel syndrome the possibility of early RA or hypothyroidism should be considered.

Recognition and reassurance are usually the only therapy necessary in the patient with carpal tunnel syndrome. Wrist splints worn at night or rarely during the day may be of value, as may the empiric use of local steroid injected at the distal flexor wrist crease. Surgical release of the median nerve should be considered only if symptoms continue beyond pregnancy.

INFECTIOUS ARTHRITIS

Whereas the lack of urgency in making a diagnosis of RA and SLE has been emphasized, the converse is true when the question of sepsis in a joint arises. The appearance of acute arthritis in a pregnant patient, especially if associated with tenosynovitis, must be considered to be of gonococcal origin until proved otherwise. Arthritis is the most common manifestation of disseminated gonococcal infection, and in one ten-year review up to 25% of women with disseminated gonococcal infection were pregnant [97]. Infection can occur during any trimester, and the majority of patients have asymptomatic anogenital infections. In only 50% of patients are joint fluid bacteriologic studies positive for the gonococcus, and both monoarticular and polyarticular disease is seen [98].

Two clinical forms of arthritis occur, both probably representing successive stages of the same disease. Initially fever, chills, and papular or vesicular skin lesions accompany a polyarticular arthritis or tenosynovitis. Knees, wrists, small joints of the hands, elbows, and ankles are most frequently involved, usually without perceptible effusion. This has been considered to be the bacteremic stage of the disease, and it may evolve in two or three days to produce signs and symptoms in one joint, at which time the likelihood of a positive joint fluid culture increases. The peripheral white blood cell count is often normal. All sites of potential gonococcal infection must be cultured, including rectal, urethral, cervical, oropharyngeal, and blood. Cultures of skin lesions are rarely positive. An important contribution to the diagnosis of gonococcal infection has been the introduction of Thayer-Martin selective culture medium, which should be available at the bedside for immediate inoculation when material for culture is being obtained.

Aqueous penicillin G, 10,000,000 units IV per day for three days or until initial improvement occurs, followed by oral ampicillin, 0.5 g four times a day to complete a course of 14 days, has been considered adequate therapy for gonococcal arthritis. Penicillin G 2,500,000 units IV over 30-minute periods every six hours for three days has also proved to be effective [99]. In a recent trial, erythromycin stearate, 500 mg orally every six hours for five days, proved to be as effective in treating patients with gonococcal arthritis [100]. The instillation of penicillin into the joint is not necessary, but repeated aspiration is recommended both for follow-up of total white blood cell count as a measure of clinical efficacy of treatment and for removal of pus and metabolic breakdown products from the joint. The use of phenoxymethyl penicillin in the treatment of gonococcal arthritis is to be deplored since this antibiotic is inactive against *Neisseria gonorrhoeae.* All patients should be followed after therapy for a repeat culture of the endocervix and rectum to determine the efficacy of treatment.

In a pregnant patient who has an acute, unexplained arthritis or tenosynovitis and in whom a high index of suspicion of gonococcal arthritis exists, a therapeutic trial of parenteral penicillin can be considered justifiable "shotgun" therapy, once complete bacteriologic studies are obtained. Gonococcal disease should respond dramatically, within days or possibly overnight. Failure to respond should cause the diagnosis of gonococcal arthritis to be questioned.

CRYSTALLINE ARTHROPATHY
Gout is rare in premenopausal women. In view of the hyperuricemia seen with toxemia, acute arthritis in pregnancy cannot be considered secondary to gout until sodium monourate crystals are aspirated from an involved joint. Pseudogout, associated with the presence of calcium pyrophosphate crystals within a joint, is also not common in the childbearing age group. The presence of calcium pyrophosphate crystals in synovial fluid should stimulate a search for some other underlying illness such as hypothyroidism or diabetes.

Colchicine, which has generally been replaced by indomethacin and other NSAIDs in the treatment of acute gout and pseudogout in the nonpregnant patient, should certainly not be used during pregnancy. Colchicine's mode of action is to arrest cell division in the metaphase, and chromosomal abnormalities have been reported [101]. Aspiration of the involved joint and, once the diagnosis is made, intraarticular corticosteroid would seem to be the treatment of choice in the pregnant patient, avoiding the risks referred to above associated with the use of indomethacin and other NSAIDs. The use of prophylactic colchicine to prevent acute gout attacks mandates concomitant birth control at all times.

FIBROSITIS
Fibrositis is a controversial clinical diagnosis, with some experienced rheumatologists reporting that it constitutes a large part of their practice while others deny the existence of the malady [102]. Despite the first use of the term in 1904, only recently has an effort been made to establish criteria for the diagnosis [103]. Systematic study of a psychological disturbance in the patients, which might separate them from an even more nebulous group with psychogenic rheumatism, has been suggested [104]. Since the majority of patients with fibrositis are females of childbearing age, the physician dealing with pregnant patients should be aware of the entity and the controversies regarding its existence and management.

Fibrositis is a diagnosis of exclusion, made only in patients with persistent musculoskeletal pain for at least three months in three different anatomic sites, with no other rheumatoid or systemic disease being found. Some authorities require the presence of local "trigger" or "tender" points on physical examination. Objective measurements such as laboratory and radiographic studies are normal, and muscle biopsy has shown no abnormality. In a personal uncontrolled series, inflammatory changes have been seen in the fascia of two patients with fibrositis, but this finding certainly needs confirmation [105].

Fibrositis can be used as a convenient label to

explain otherwise nondefinable musculoskeletal aches and pains in the pregnant patient once the above exclusions and criteria are met. Ample reassurance that the illness will in no way affect the course or outcome of the pregnancy can be given, and at a time when all forms of drug therapy are best avoided, it is a comfort to know that none are indicated.

POLYARTERITIS NODOSA, PROGRESSIVE SYSTEMIC SCLEROSIS (SCLERODERMA), AND DERMATOMYOSITIS

The grouping of these three diseases does not suggest any common etiology or management regimen but rather their rarity when compared to RA, SLE, and the other rheumatic diseases already discussed.

Polyarteritis Nodosa (PN)

PN is a necrotizing vasculitis of small and medium-sized arteries. In the pregnant patient it may present with hypertension and renal insufficiency and thus may be confused with preeclampsia. Myalgias, arthralgias, fever, anorexia, sensory and motor neuropathy, and central nervous system signs and symptoms are all evidence of multisystem involvement. The presence of the hepatitis B surface antigen is seen in 30% of the patients. Despite an occasional response to corticosteroid therapy [106], the course in pregnancy has usually resulted in maternal death, although fetal survival may be normal [107,108]. Recently, combined therapy with several immunosuppressive agents suggests that a more optimistic outlook may be justified [109].

Progressive Systemic Sclerosis

Despite the fact that the peak age of onset of progressive systemic sclerosis (PSS) is in the 30- to 50-year age group, it is not uncommon for the first clinical signs to begin in a woman in her twenties. In a majority of patients, the initial clinical signs will be Raynaud's phenomenon, arthritis of the hands, or diffuse myalgias and arthralgias, associated with a symmetric painless insidious thickening of the skin of the fingers and, later, forearms. Despite relatively optimistic statements regarding PSS in pregnancy [110,111], an increased abortion rate [112] and increased incidence of premature labor and perinatal mortality [113] have been reported. Parturition in the patient with PSS may present problems with regard to perineal skin contractures and absence of relaxation of the pelvic structures, but not with regard to poor healing of abdominal incisions or episiotomy scars [111]. No

drug regimen has proved effective in the medical treatment of PSS. Corticosteroids offer only unpleasant side effects.

The patient who has only cutaneous involvement (scleroderma) and no overt evidence of visceral involvement may request advice regarding the risks of becoming pregnant. The unpredictable course must be stressed, including the 45% survival rate at seven years should visceral involvement occur [114]. Eclampsia will certainly present an added risk to the patient with PSS. A recent report of postpartum death from renal failure in a patient with PSS, and the similarity in renal pathologic changes seen in PSS and in the syndrome of irreversible postpartum renal failure attests to the risk of pregnancy in this disease [115].

Dermatomyositis (DM)

A 1973 literature review uncovered only 15 cases of pregnancy in patients with DM [116]. In nine the disease was unaffected by pregnancy, in three the patient deteriorated, and in three others there was a remission. A 46% fetal mortality was seen in this group. In three instances of DM developing during pregnancy, in one patient (not treated with corticosteroids) the pregnancy did not seem to adversely affect the mother's disease although the infant died 24 hours post partum [116]. In one mother who did receive corticosteroid therapy there was a dramatic postpartum remission in symptoms although muscle enzymes remained markedly elevated [117]. In the third case, mother and child did well, with a postpartum remission without benefit of corticosteroid therapy [118]. Since corticosteroid therapy may be curative in DM, the potential risk to a patient with DM who becomes pregnant would seem to be less than in the other connective tissue diseases. The high fetal mortality and the admittedly few case reports remain a cause for concern when counseling patients with this disease.

REFERENCES

1. Hench PS. The ameliorating effect of pregnancy on chronic atrophic (infectious rheumatoid) arthritis, fibrositis, and intermittent hydrarthrosis. Proc. Staff Meet Mayo Clin. 1938; 13:161–7.
2. Smith WD, West HF. Pregnancy and rheumatoid arthritis. Acta Rheumatol Scand. 1960; 6:189–201.
3. Gilbert M, Rotstein J, Cunningham C, Estrin I, Davidson A, Pincus G. Norethynodrel with mestranol in treatment of rheumatoid arthritis. JAMA. 1964; 190:235.
4. Takeuchi A, Persellin RH. The inhibitory effect of pregnancy serum on polymorphonuclear leukocyte chemotaxis. J Clin Lab Immunol. 1980; 3:121–4.

5. Thomson AW, Horne CH. Biological and clinical significance of pregnancy-associated alpha$_2$-glycoprotein—a review. Invest Cell Pathol. 1980; 3:295–309.

6. Froelich CJ, Goodwin JS, Bankhurst AD, Williams RC. Pregnancy, a temporary fetal graft of suppressor cells in autoimmune disease? Am J Med. 1980; 69:329–31.

7. Pope RM, Yoshinoya S, McChesney L, Persellin RH. Variations in immune complex concentrations during pregnancy in rheumatoid arthritis patients. Arthritis Rheum. 1981; 24:S80. abstract.

8. Morris WI. Pregnancy in rheumatoid arthritis and systemic lupus erythematosus. Aust NZ J Obstet Gynaecol. 1969; 9:136–44.

9. Persellin RH. The effect of pregnancy on rheumatoid arthritis. Bull Rheum Dis. 1976–1977; 27:922–7.

10. Oka M. Effect of pregnancy on the onset and course of rheumatoid arthritis. Ann Rheum Dis. 1953; 12:227–9.

11. Felbo M, Snorrason E. Pregnancy and the place of therapeutic abortion in rheumatoid arthritis. Acta Obstet Gynecol Scand. 1961; 40:116–26.

12. Oka M, Vainio U. Effect of pregnancy on the prognosis and serology of rheumatoid arthritis. Acta Rheumatol Scand. 1966; 12:47–52.

13. Kaplan D, Diamond H. Rheumatoid arthritis and pregnancy. Clin Obstet Gynecol. 1965; 8:286–303.

14. McCarty DJ, ed. Arthritis and allied conditions: a textbook of rheumatology. 9th ed. Philadelphia: Lea & Febiger, 1979.

15. Kelley WN, Harris ED, Ruddy S, Sledge CB. Textbook of rheumatology. Philadelphia: Saunders, 1980.

16. Ropes MW, Bennett GA, Cobb S, Jacox R, Jessar RA. 1958 revision of diagnostic criteria for rheumatoid arthritis. Bull Rheum Dis. 1958; 9:175–6.

17. Short CL, Bauer W, Reynolds WE. Rheumatoid arthritis. Cambridge, Mass.: Harvard University Press, 1957.

18. Mitchell DM, Fries JF. An analysis of the American Rheumatism Association criteria for rheumatoid arthritis. Arthritis Rheum. 1982; 25:481–7.

19. Pritchard JA, MacDonald PC. Williams obstetrics. 16th ed. New York: Appleton-Century-Crofts, 1980:236.

20. Aitcheson CT, Peebles C, Joslin F, Tan EM. Characteristics of antinuclear antibodies in rheumatoid arthritis. Arthritis Rheum. 1980; 23:528–38.

21. Mathews, JA. Atlanto-axial subluxation in rheumatoid arthritis. Ann Rheum Dis. 1969; 18:260–6.

22. Vane JR. Inhibition of prostaglandin synthesis as a mechanism of action for aspirin-like drugs. Nature. 1971; 231:232–5.

23. Smyth CJ. Therapy of rheumatoid arthritis. Postgrad Med. 1972; 51:31–9.

24. Rumack BH. Aspirin and acetaminophen. Clin Toxicol. 1979; 15:313–40.

25. Mills JA. Nonsteroidal anti-inflammatory drugs. N Engl J Med. 1974; 290:781–4.

26. Slone D, Heinonen OP, Kaufman DW, Siskind V, Monson RR, Shapiro S. Aspirin and congenital malformations. Lancet. 1976; 1:1373–5.

27. Collins E, Turner G. Maternal effects of regular salicylate ingestion in pregnancy. Lancet. 1975; 2:335–7.

28. Bleyer WA, Breckenridge RT. Studies on the detection of adverse drug reactions in the newborn. II. JAMA. 1970; 213:2049–53.

29. Neely NT, Persellin RH. Activity of rheumatoid arthritis during pregnancy. Tex Med. 1977; 73:59–63.

30. Shapiro S, Monson RR, Kaufman DW, Siskind V, Heinonen OP, Slone D. Perinatal mortality and birth-weight in relation to aspirin taken during pregnancy. Lancet. 1976; 1:1375–6.

31. Physicians' desk reference. 36th ed. Oradell N.J.: Medical Economics Company, 1982.

32. Levin DL, Fixler DE, Morriss FC, Tyson J. Morphologic analysis of the pulmonary vascular bed in infants exposed in utero to prostaglandin synthetase inhibitors. J Pediatr. 1978; 92:478–83.

33. Cantor B, Tyler T, Nelson RM, Stein GH. Oligohydramnios and transient neonatal anuria. J Reprod Med. 1980; 24:220–3.

34. Stuart MJ, Gross SJ, Elrad H, Graeby JE. Effects of acetysalicylic acid ingestion on maternal and neonatal hemostasis. N Engl J Med. 1982; 307:909–12.

35. The Cooperating Clinics Committee of the American Rheumatism Association. A controlled trial of gold salt therapy in rheumatoid arthritis. Arthritis Rheum. 1973; 16:353–8.

36. Sigler JW, Bluhm GB, Duncan H, Sharp JT, Ensign DC, McCrum WR. Gold salts in the treatment of rheumatoid arthritis. A double-blind study. Ann Intern Med. 1974; 80:21–6.

37. Bulmash JM. Rheumatoid arthritis and pregnancy. Obstet Gynecol Annu. 1979; 8:223–76.

38. Evers AE, Sundstrom WR. Second course gold therapy in rheumatoid arthritis. Arthritis Rheum. 1981; 24:S82. abstract.

39. Betson JR Jr, Dorn RV. Forty cases of arthritis and pregnancy. J Int Coll Surg. 1964; 42:521–6.

40. Plotz CM, Goldenberg A. Rheumatoid arthritis. In: Rovinsky JJ, Guttmacher AF, eds. Medical, surgical, and gynecologic complications of pregnancy. 2nd ed. Baltimore: Williams & Wilkins, 1965:720–8.

41. Freyberg RH. Gold therapy for rheumatoid arthritis. In: Hollander JL, ed. Arthritis and allied conditions. 8th ed. Philadelphia: Lea & Febiger, 1972:455–82.

42. Cohen DL, Orzel J, Taylor A. Infants of mothers receiving gold therapy. Arthritis Rheum. 1981; 24:104–5. letter.

43. Miyamoto T, Miyaji S, Horiuchi Y, Hara M, Ishihara K. Gold therapy in bronchial asthma with special emphasis upon blood level of gold and its

teratogenicity. J Jpn Soc Intern Med. 1974; 63:1190–7.

44. Gottlieb NL, Smith PM, Smith EM. Pharmacodynamics of [197]Au and [195]Au labeled aurothiomalate in blood. Arthritis Rheum. 1974; 17: 171–83.

45. Jaffe IA. D-Penicillamine. Bull Rheum Dis. 1977–1978; 28:948–52.

46. Barnes CG. Medical disorders in obstetric practice. 4th ed. Oxford: Blackwell Scientific Publications, 1974:324.

47. Serment H, Charpin J, Tessier G, Felce A. Corticothérapie et grossesse. Bull Fed Soc Gynecol Obstet Lang Fr. 1968; 20:159–61.

48. Sidhu RK, Hawkins DF. Prescribing in pregnancy. Corticosteroids. Clin Obstet Gynecol. 1981; 8:383–404.

49. Saarikoski S, Seppala M. Immunosuppression during pregnancy: transmission of azathioprine and its metabolites from the mother to the fetus. Am J Obstet Gynecol. 1973; 115:1100–6.

50. Krueger JA, Davis RB, Field C. Multiple-drug chemotherapy in the management of acute lymphocytic leukemia during pregnancy. Obstet Gynecol. 1976; 48:324–7.

51. Finkbeiner JA. Antineoplastic chemotherapy in pregnancy. In: Barber HRK, Graber EA, eds. Surgical disease in pregnancy. Philadelphia: Saunders, 1974:711–26.

52. Michaels RM, Nashel DJ, Leonard A, Sliwinski AJ, Derbes SJ. Weekly intravenous methotrexate in the treatment of rheumatoid arthritis. Arthritis Rheum. 1982; 25:339–41.

53. Cohen MM, Gerbie AB, Nadler HL. Chromosomal investigation in pregnancies following chemotherapy for choriocarcinoma. Lancet. 1971; 2:219. letter.

54. Roenigk HH, Auerbach R, Maibach HI, Weinstein GD. Methotrexate guidelines revised. J Am Acad Dermatol. 1982; 6:145–55.

55. Miller ML, Glass DN. The major histocompatibility complex antigens in rheumatoid arthritis and juvenile arthritis. Bull Rheum Dis. 1981; 31:21–5.

56. Grigor R, Edmonds J, Lewkonia R, Bresnihan B, Hughes GR. Systemic lupus erythematosus. A prospective analysis. Ann Rheum Dis. 1978; 37:121–8.

57. Sakane T, Steinberg AD, Green I. Studies of immune functions of patients with systemic lupus erythematosus. I. Dysfunction of suppressor T-cell activity related to impaired generation of, rather than response to, suppressor cells. Arthritis Rheum. 1978; 21:657–64.

58. Miller KB, Schwartz RS. Familial abnormalities of suppressor-cell function in systemic lupus erythematosus. N Engl J Med. 1979; 301:803–9.

59. Lahita RG, Bradlow HL, Kunkel HG, Fishman J. Alterations of estrogen metabolism in systemic lupus erythematosus. Arthritis Rheum. 1979; 22:1195–8.

60. Zulman JI, Talal N, Hoffman GS, Epstein WV. Problems associated with the management of pregnancies in patients with systemic lupus erythematosus. J Rheumatol. 1980; 7:37–49.

61. Fine LG, Barnett EV, Danovitch GM, Nissenson AR, Conolly ME, Lieb SM, Barrett CT. Systemic lupus erythematosus in pregnancy. Ann Intern Med. 1981; 94:667–77.

62. Fairley KF, Whitworth JA, Kincaid-Smith P. Glomerulonephritis and pregnancy. In: Kincaid-Smith P, Mathew TH, Becker EL, eds. Glomerulonephritis. New York: Wiley, 1973:997–1012.

63. Dubois EL. Management of discoid and systemic lupus erythematosus. In: Dubois EL, Lupus erythematosus. 2nd ed. Los Angeles: University of Southern California Press, 1974:585–612.

64. Tozman EC, Urowitz MB, Gladman DD. Systemic lupus erythematosus and pregnancy. J Rheumatol. 1980; 7:624–32.

65. Jungers P, Dougados M, Pelissier C, Kuttenn F, Tron F, Lesavre P, Bach JF. Lupus nephropathy and pregnancy. Arch Intern Med. 1982; 142:771–6.

66. Grigor RR, Shervington PC, Hughes GR, Hawkins DF. Outcome of pregnancy in systemic lupus erythematosus. Proc R Soc Med. 1977; 70:99–100.

67. McGee CD, Makowski EL. Systemic lupus erythematosus in pregnancy. Am J Obstet Gynecol. 1970; 107:1008–12.

68. Estes D, Larson DL. Systemic lupus erythematosus and pregnancy. Clin Obstet Gynecol. 1965; 8:307–21.

69. Fraga A, Mintz G, Orozco J, Orozco JH. Sterility and fertility rates, fetal wastage and maternal morbidity in systemic lupus erythematosus. J Rheumatol. 1974; 1:293–8.

70. Gutierrez G, Jiminez J, Mintz G. Results of a prospective multidisciplinary approach to pregnancy in systemic lupus erythematosus. Arthritis Rheum. 1981; 24:S107. abstract.

71. Abramowsky CR, Vegas ME, Swinehart G, Gyves MT. Decidual vasculopathy of the placenta in lupus erythematosus. N Engl J Med. 1980; 303:668–72.

72. Scott JS. Immunological diseases in pregnancy. In: Scott JS, Jones WR, eds. Immunology of human reproduction. New York: Grune & Stratton, 1976:229–95.

73. Esscher E, Scott JS. Congenital heart block and maternal systemic lupus erythematosus. Br Med J. 1979; 1:1235–8.

74. Tan EM. Autoantibodies to nuclear antigens (ANA). Their immunobiology and medicine. Adv immunol. 1982; 33:167–240.

75. Scott JS, Maddison PJ, Taylor PV, et al. Connective-tissue disease, antibodies to ribonucleoprotein, and congenital heart block. N Engl J Med. 1983; 309:209–12.

76. Tan EM, Cohen AS, Fries J, et al. Criteria for the classification of systemic lupus erythematosus (proposed 1982 revision). Arthritis Rheum. 1982; 25:S3.

77. Zurier RB, Argyros TG, Urman JD, Warren J, Rothfield NF. Systemic lupus erythematosus. Man-

agement during pregnancy. Obstet Gynecol. 1978; 51:178–80.

78. Decker JL, Steinberg AD, Reinertsen JL, Plotz PH, Balow JE, Klippel JF. NIH Conference. Systemic lupus erythematosus: evolving concepts. Ann Intern Med. 1979; 91:587–604.

79. Sztejnbok M, Stewart A, Diamond H, Kaplan D. Azathioprine in the treatment of systemic lupus erythematosus. Arthritis Rheum. 1971; 14:639–45.

80. Gillibrand PN. Systemic lupus erythematosus in pregnancy treated with azathioprine. Proc R Soc Med. 1966; 59:834.

81. Sharon E, Kaplan D, Diamond HS. Exacerbation of systemic lupus erythematosus after withdrawal of azathioprine therapy. N Engl J Med. 1973; 288:122–4.

82. Hayslett JP, Lynn RI. Effect of pregnancy in patients with lupus nephropathy. Kidney Int. 1980; 18:207–20.

83. Houser MT, Fish AJ, Tagatz GE, Williams PP, Michael AF. Pregnancy and systemic lupus erythematosus. Am J Obstet Gynecol. 1980; 138:409–13.

84. Devoe LD, Taylor RL. Systemic lupus erythematosus in pregnancy. Am J Obstet Gynecol. 1979; 135:473–9.

85. Bear R. Pregnancy and lupus nephritis. Obstet Gynecol. 1976; 47:715–8.

86. Garsenstein M, Pollak VE, Kark RM. Systemic lupus erythematosus and pregnancy. N Engl J Med. 1962; 267:165–9.

87. Zurier RB. Systemic lupus erythematosus and pregnancy. Clin Rheum Dis. 1975; 1:613–20.

88. Garovich M, Agudelo C, Pisko E. Oral contraceptives and systemic lupus erythematosus. Arthritis Rheum. 1980; 23:1396–8.

89. Travers RL, Hughes GR. Oral contraceptive therapy and systemic lupus erythematosus. J Rheumatol. 1978; 5:448–51.

90. McKenna CH, Wieman KC, Shulman LE. Oral contraceptives, rheumatic disease, and autoantibodies. Arthritis Rheum. 1969; 12:313–4. abstract.

91. Woodrow JC. Histocompatibility antigens and rheumatic diseases. Semin Arthritis Rheum. 1977; 6:257–76.

92. Julkunen H. Reactive arthritis. Bull Rheum Dis. 1978–1979; 29:1002–5.

93. Calin A, Fries JF. Striking prevalence of ankylosing spondylitis in "healthy" W27 positive males and females. N Engl J Med. 1975; 293:835–9.

94. Kidd KK, Bernoco D, Carbonara AO, Danco V, Steiger U, Ceppellini R. The "illness-susceptible" gene frequency and sex ratio in ankylosing spondylitis, HLA and disease. In: Dausse J, Svejgaard A, eds. Genetic analysis of HLA-associated diseases. Copenhagen: Munksgaard, 1977:72–80.

95. Smith DL, Bennett RM, Regan MG. Reiter's disease in women. Arthritis Rheum. 1980; 23:335–40.

96. Ostensen M, Romberg O, Husby G. Ankylosing spondylitis and motherhood. Arthritis Rheum. 1982; 25:140–3.

97. Chapman DR, Fernandez-Rocha L. Gonococcal ar-

thritis in pregnancy: a ten-year review. South Med J. 1975; 68:1333–6.

98. Holmes KK, Counts GW, Beaty HN. Disseminated gonococcal infection. Ann Intern Med. 1971; 74:979–93.

99. Blankenship RM, Holmes RK, Sanford JP. Treatment of disseminated gonococcal infection. N Engl J Med. 1974; 290:267–9.

100. Thompson SE, Jacobs NF, Zacarias F, Rein MF, Shulman JA. Gonococcal tenosynovitis-dermatitis and septic arthritis. JAMA. 1980; 244:1101–2.

101. Ferreira Frota-Pessoa O. Trisomy after colchicine therapy. Lancet. 1969; 1:1161–2.

102. A description of rheumatology practice. The American Rheumatism Association Committee on Rheumatologic Practice. Arthritis Rheum. 1977; 20:1278–81.

103. Yunus M, Masi AT, Calabro JJ, Miller KA, Feigenbaum SL. Primary fibromyalgia (fibrositis): clinical study of 50 patients with matched normal controls. Semin Arthritis Rheum. 1981; 11:151–71.

104. Payne TC, Leavitt F, Garron DC, Katz RS, Golden HE, Glickman PB, Vanderplate C. Fibrositis and psychologic disturbance. Arthritis Rheum. 1982; 25:213–7.

105. Kaplan H. Unpublished observations. 1980.

106. Debenkelaer MM, Travis LB, Roberts DK. Polyarteritis nodosa and pregnancy. Report of a successful outcome. South Med J. 1973; 613–5.

107. Burkett G, Richards R. Periarteritis nodosa and pregnancy. Obstet Gynecol. 1982; 59:252–4.

108. Reed N, Smith MT. Periarteritis nodosa in pregnancy. Report of a case and review of the literature. Obstet Gynecol. 1980; 55:381–4.

109. Fauci AS, Haynes B, Katz P. The spectrum of vasculitis. Ann Intern Med. 1978; 89:660–76.

110. Rodnan GP. Progressive systemic sclerosis. In: McCarty DJ, ed. Arthritis and allied conditions. 9th ed. Philadelphia: Lea & Febiger, 1979:762–809.

111. Winkelmann RK. Scleroderma and pregnancy. Clin Obstet Gynecol. 1965; 8:280–5.

112. Knupp MZ, O'Leary JA. Pregnancy and scleroderma. J Fla Med Assoc. 1971; 58:28–30.

113. Karlen JR, Cook WA. Renal scleroderma and pregnancy. Obstet Gynecol. 1974; 44:349–54.

114. Medsger TA, Masi AT, Rodnan GP, Benedek TG, Robinson H. Survival with systemic sclerosis (scleroderma). A life-table analysis of clinical and demographic factors in 309 patients. Ann Intern Med. 1971; 75:369–76.

115. Palma A, Sanchez-Palencia A, Armas JR, Milan JA, Fernandez-Sanz J, Llach F. Progressive systemic sclerosis and nephrotic syndrome. Arch Intern Med. 1981; 141:520–1.

116. Tsai A, Lindheimer MD, Lamberg SI. Dermatomyositis complicating pregnancy. Obstet Gynecol. 1973; 41:570–3.

117. Bauer KA, Siegler M, Lindheimer MA. Polymyositis complicating pregnancy. Arch Intern Med. 1979; 139:449.

118. Katz AL. Another case of polymyositis in pregnancy. Arch Intern Med. 1980; 140:1123. letter.

When nature's phenomena are elucidated, pay attention to all its phases. Nothing is inside, nor outside, because what is inside is also manifested outside.
—Goethe

21. DERMATOLOGIC DISORDERS
Marc J. Sorkin

The interaction of the pregnant state and the skin is conveniently categorized into the occurrence of physiologic changes in the skin, the effect of pregnancy on preexisting dermatologic problems, and those conditions that are peculiar to pregnancy. In addition, therapy of cutaneous problems in the gravid patient must often be altered for the benefit of the expectant mother and the expected offspring.

PHYSIOLOGIC CUTANEOUS CHANGES IN PREGNANCY
Vascular and hemodynamic changes that have manifestations in the skin are thought to be consequences of physiologic alterations in blood volume, hydrostatic pressure, and hormonal influences on the vasculature. The expectant mother may encounter spider angiomas, red palms, a peculiar form of pyogenic granuloma, urticaria (and its equivalent, dermatographism), or varicosities in the course of her normal pregnancy [7,26,31].

Spider angiomas are red, macular radiations of tiny blood vessels extending from a central flat or raised arteriole. Being identical to spiders seen with chronic liver diseases, these vascular malformations can be blanched in their entirety by pressure on the central arteriolar source. They are found mostly on the upper body and occur in about seven out of ten white pregnancies and one out of ten black pregnancies [33]. They are first seen in the second to fifth month. No therapy is usually required, and the lesions tend to regress after parturition. For persistent lesions, or lesions during gestation that are cosmetically unacceptable, treatment by light electrocoagulation of the center, without anesthesia, is the method of choice.

The palmar erythema of pregnancy is similar to the same condition seen with chronic hepatic disease, estrogen therapy, and hyperthyroidism [7]. Its incidence is similar to that of spider lesions, and it often occurs in patients with these spiders. The erythema is either a diffuse mottling of the palms or circumscribed areas of redness that are usually warmer than the normal appearing areas. This condition resolves spontaneously and requires no treatment.

Another vascular abnormality associated with pregnancy is the so-called pregnancy tumor or granuloma gravidarum. It is an oral lesion seen on the anterior interdental gingival papillae. It has a very similar histologic and clinical appearance to pyogenic granuloma. This lesion usually begins around the third month and enlarges continually until term. It appears as an oval, pedunculated, red nodule that bleeds easily. The cause is unknown. Occasionally the lesion requires excision, but it usually recedes spontaneously post partum [33, 35].

Urticaria, common in the second half of gestation, is marked by pinkish, pruritic plaques, which may occur anywhere on the skin and are, by definition, evanescent. An individual lesion lasts less than 24 hours, but often newer areas develop while existing lesions regress. Dermatographism, which is a form of urticaria, is produced by stroking the skin or by pressure. These manifestations of vasomotor instability (along with hot flashes and flushing) are most often encountered in the second half of pregnancy [34]. Vascular dilatation and leakage of vascular fluid into the extracellular space are the proximate causes of the clinical lesions. Although the idiopathic variety is common, other causes of acute urticaria should be sought. Infection (often respiratory, urinary, or dental), drug reaction, or allergy to food or inhalant must be ruled out. Treatment includes avoidance of the offending agent when possible, avoidance of tight garments, lubrication of the skin, oral antihistamines, and, in extreme cases, the use of systemic steroids. Corticosteroids are indicated when angioedema compromises respiration or makes the daily task of living excessively difficult.

If a woman has had difficulty with a preexisting Raynaud's phenomenon (a hyperreactivity constriction of the arteries to the hands upon exposure to cold), this often improves as pregnancy progresses [31]. Whether the amelioration is due to increased blood volume, relaxin, or other hormonal effects on blood vessels is not known.

Venous Change

Varicosities occur or are aggravated during pregnancy in the hemorrhoidal venous system and in the lower extremities. Increased blood volume, obstruction of flow in the inferior vena cava due to pressure from the enlarging uterus, and decreased physical activity contribute to this troubling problem. Treatment includes positioning to prevent caval obstruction when recumbent, frequent elevation of the legs during the day, and external support garments for the legs [7]. Obviously, constricting foundation garments and garter belts must be avoided. Chronic problems may include recurrent phlebitis, stasis dermatitis, and persistent varicose vein.

Striae

Striae distensae gravidarum (stretch marks) develop in about 90% of pregnant women and tend to be familial. These are commonly seen on the breasts, abdomen, and buttocks. Simple tension on the skin is not a full explanation of their genesis; hormonal, genetic, and biochemical forces contribute to the fraying of elastic fibers and disruption of collagen in the upper dermis. The orientation of these striae usually follows lines of tension, however. These lesions, when acute, are often purple or red and may itch [35]. They later fade to be paler than the adjacent skin. Although similar lesions are seen in hypercorticism [4], overactive adrenal cortical activity seems not to be involved in the development of the striae in pregnancy. Nevertheless, the use of topical corticosteroid compounds exaggerates the tendency toward striae formation and so must be prescribed judiciously. Despite a multitude of recommendations from the lay public, there is neither effective treatment nor any known preventive therapy for these unsightly marks. Soothing topical emollients may help if pruritus is a bothersome symptom. As always, topical antihistamines should be avoided because of the risk of contact allergy [5].

Pigmentary Alteration

Localized areas of hyperpigmentation are to be expected in pregnancy. The mechanism of these changes is probably hormonal, but the exact hormonal interaction resulting in the physiologic, but cosmetically troublesome, changes is not clear. Melanocyte-stimulating hormone elevation alone will not explain the phenomenon, which also depends on ACTH, estrogen, and progesterone.

Darkening of the areolae, linea nigra, axillae, perineum, and preexisting nevi is to be expected, even in a fair-complexioned female. This hyperpigmentation will rarely revert to the nulliparous shade and requires no treatment [33]. Any pigmented nevi showing enlargement or change other than darkening should be subjected to biopsy to rule out the development of melanoma.

Melasma (chloasma), the "masque of pregnancy," is the marginated, flat (macular) hyperpigmentation of the forehead and malar areas, common and more severe in darker-skinned women [2,40]. It is usually seen in the second half of pregnancy but may also be seen in nonpregnant females, those on oral contraceptives, males or females taking estrogens, and even some otherwise normal men on no medication [1]. This change is dependent on ultraviolet light acting on a susceptible pigmentary apparatus. Unfortunately, chloasma often persists after birth but can be treated with combinations of hydroquinone, retinoic acid, and mild topical steroid creams [3]. Because the pigmentation is mostly epidermal, repeated applications of mild peeling agents such as 10% and 25% trichloroacetic acid are helpful. Sunlight avoidance and strong (sun protection factor >15) sunscreens must be used for indefinite periods after treatment to prevent recurrence. Treatment should be delayed until after parturition.

Connective Tissue Alterations

Gingival hypertrophy, thought to be related to hormonal changes and increased vascularity of the gingival mucosa, is seen to some degree in 80% of gravid females. This occurs any time from the second month on and resolves post partum. Good oral hygiene is said to ameliorate the problem [33].

The so-called molluscum gravidarum is a condition in which benign skin tags develop at the base of the neck, in the axillary folds, and under the breasts during pregnancy [8]. These are also seen in men and women with obesity and hyperhidrosis. They do not resolve after pregnancy. They can be an unsightly nuisance and often become irritated. Treatment with liquid nitrogen, scissors excision, or light electrodesiccation with or without local anesthesia can be performed during pregnancy.

Alterations in Hair Growth

Although alterations in scalp hair growth is normal in pregnancy, patients rarely notice change until several months post partum [33,35]. Approximately 80% of hairs on a nonpregnant woman are in anagen (active phase of hair growth) and 20% are in telogen (resting phase of hair growth). During pregnancy an increasing proportion of follicles are recruited into the anagen phase, creating a thicker mane, but this seems to be rarely noticed. Soon after delivery, the proportion of hair in telogen increases even above the basal level. The telogen hairs persist in the resting follicle until pushed out by new anagen growth from beneath. In the consequent shedding, which is sometimes marked, the telogen (club) hairs are expelled with their loose fibrous "root." This whitish tissue clinging to the proximal hair is actually the involuted contents of the follicle, not a root, and its rounded, bulbous feature designates it a club hair. Between 50 and 100 such hairs are shed daily from a normal scalp. The increased shedding after pregnancy is called telogen effluvium and occurs two to four months post partum as new anagen growth is then replacing the loosened telogen hairs. It is not universally seen and is more common when there is hemorrhage, fever, or difficult delivery complicating the pregnancy [34]. The hair may become noticeably thinner as there had been increased thickness during pregnancy and it takes time for the new growth to lengthen and fill in. Density should return to normal 12 to 15 months after the end of the telogen effluvium period. Reassurance is the treatment of choice. Telogen effluvium can occur in anyone following significant stress of either physical or psychological nature [6].

Hirsutism or increased growth of body hair is a common problem, occurring in the second half of pregnancy [40]. When associated with the onset or worsening of acne or accompanied by male pattern hair loss (excessive thinning of hair on the top of the head leaving the forelock and parietal fringe, or temporal recession), this indicates an androgenic effect. Underlying ovarian or adrenal sources of sex hormone imbalance should be sought and treated [34]. However, hirsutism may be the response of genetically programmed follicles that convert normal circulating hormones of placental origin into dihydrotestosterone via 5-alpha-reductase enzyme activity within the cutaneous structure. In this case the excess hair growth will probably not revert after delivery and may require treatment by epilation, estrogen therapy, bleaching, or possibly spironolactone, when endocrine dysfunction has been ruled out [33].

Nail Changes

Several nonspecific nail changes can occur during pregnancy [40]. These include distal onycholysis, transverse grooving, and brittleness. Since these changes may not be pathologically related to pregnancy, other causes must be sought (e.g., thyroid alterations, recent febrile illness, and protein-calorie malnourishment).

MANAGEMENT OF SPECIFIC CUTANEOUS DISORDERS AFFECTED BY PREGNANCY

Pregnancy may have a beneficial or detrimental effect on any of several preexisting skin diseases. Therapy that patients had been receiving prior to conception may have to be altered, or at times withheld, to ensure a safe outcome of gestation.

Cutaneous Diseases That Usually Improve During Pregnancy
Psoriasis

Psoriasis [33,34,37], the red, scaly, chronic, unsightly cutaneous condition that affects about 2% of the general population, improves during pregnancy in about 50% of patients [26]. This disease, with its unpredictable course, can be treated with topical steroids, tars, ultraviolet light–B (sunburn spectrum), methotrexate, hydroxyurea, or 8-methoxypsoralen and ultraviolet light A (320–400 nm) (PUVA) therapy. Obviously, the antimetabolites methotrexate and hydroxyurea, with their impact on cellular growth, should be avoided in women at risk for conception, throughout gestation, and during lactation. PUVA therapy, which entails ingestion of 8-methoxypsoralen (a photosensitizer) followed in two hours by measured exposure to ultraviolet light–A (320–400 nm wavelength), is at this writing in its investigational stage and not recommended for pregnant patients. Topical steroid or tar preparations are probably safe when used on small areas, but for widespread disease the problem of systemic absorption must be considered. Tars used in the United States are petroleum based and consist of many different chemicals produced during petroleum distillation. Cutaneous tumors often develop in laboratory animals after chronic topical tar applications. Because of unknown potential risk to the fetus, tars should probably be withheld from therapy in pregnant or lactating females. Topical steroids are absorbed through the skin, especially if used under occlusive dressings. Changes in the function of a healthy patient's pituitary-adrenal axis can be demonstrated after widespread use. These drugs, applied topically, can aggravate the tendency toward striae distensae and so should be used with caution, if at all, in pregnancy. The safest therapy, then, during pregnancy, is an adequate course of ultraviolet light–B, which is preceded by lubrication of the skin. This therapy is effective and has few side effects.

Atopic Dermatitis

Pregnancy has a variable effect on atopic dermatitis [33], the chronic, annoyingly pruritic condition that often coexists with seasonal rhinitis or asthma [26]. The adult form of atopic dermatitis exists as thickened, scaly plaques of the antecubital areas or popliteal fossae. This dermatitis (eczema) may, however, be widespread or localized to other areas, often the ankles, nape of neck, groin, or perianal area. Its course is often complicated and the rash exacerbated by secondary infection. This infection is sometimes overlooked because it may exist only as small red papules within or separated from the areas of dermatitis. Standard therapy for the condition, which can be continued during pregnancy, includes avoidance of irritants to the skin (soaps, hot water, woolens, detergents, etc.), adequate lubrication of the skin, and ultraviolet light. Systemic antibiotics are often very beneficial during flare-ups of the rash, and selection should be guided by culture and sensitivity testing when possible. In general, antistaphylococcal antibiotics are used. The use of topical tar and steroid preparations, sometimes helpful in atopic dermatitis, was addressed under the section on psoriasis.

Hidradenitis Suppurativa

Hidradenitis suppurativa [26,34] is a chronic inflammation of apocrine glands, which occurs in the axillae, groin, and on the buttocks. Its cause is unknown. The disease is characterized by the development of tender, red nodules, which at first are firm and later become fluctuant and painful. Rupture of the lesion, suppuration, and formation of sinus tracts are distinctive for this process. As these lesions heal recurrent lesions form. Use of tetracycline should be avoided during pregnancy. Therapy includes careful surgical drainage with marsupialization of cysts and sinuses under local anesthesia and systemic antibiotics. Topical care includes warm moist packs and Vleminckx's solution compresses.

Fox-Fordyce Disease (Apocrine Miliaria)

Plugging of apocrine gland ducts, with subsequent inflammation and rupture of the duct leading to pruritic, pigmented papules in apocrine areas, is known as Fox-Fordyce disease [26,34]. It is most often seen in females soon after puberty when apocrine glands become functional. The annoying itching and chronicity require treatment. Fortuitously, apocrine function is hormonally related, being inhibited by estrogens. For this reason, pregnancy often brings a temporary reprieve from the condition, and oral contraceptive agents bring relief to patients who are not desirous of pregnancy.

Pemphigus

Pemphigus vulgaris [26,34], an uncommon, potentially fatal, blistering disease, is usually ameliorated by pregnancy. This severe disease is characterized by flaccid, often large bullae and denuded areas of skin occurring anywhere on the cutaneous surface and usually involving oral mucous membranes. If it is untreated, death can ensue from infection, malnourishment, or fluid and electrolyte disturbance. The newer diagnostic techniques of direct and indirect immunofluorescence indicate that immunoglobulin is deposited between epithelial cells. This immunoglobulin (IgG or IgM) both circulates and is fixed in the skin, with specificity for the "intercellular cement substance." Acantholysis, or separation of the epidermal cells, causes the blisters, which then erode, leaving denuded skin. Presumably, this process is mediated by an autoimmune mechanism, as the disease may coexist with other autoimmune conditions such as thymoma, myasthenia gravis, and lupus erythematosus. Treatment in nonpregnant patients may require very high doses of systemic corticosteroids, immunosuppressive drugs (Cytoxan, azathioprine), or gold therapy. The latter two therapies should not be used in pregnancy. Plasmapheresis has been effective in helping to manage some cases of pemphigus, but its effect on pregnancy is not known.

Skin Diseases That Usually Worsen During Pregnancy

Fibroneurocutaneous Diseases

Neurofibromatosis and tuberous sclerosis are diseases that can progress rapidly during pregnancy [26]. Neurofibromatosis, or von Recklinghausen's disease, manifests itself in the skin at birth as hyperpigmented oval macules (café au lait spots) that are more easily discerned by Wood's light exam. As the child ages, this dominantly inherited condition exhibits freckling of the axilla (Crowe's sign) and the growth of soft tumors in the skin (neurofibromas), which are growths of the neurilemma. Grotesque malformations may result from the large masses of external or internal tumors, which may cause bony deformity of the spine or intracranial growths commonly of the eighth cranial nerve. An increased occurrence of pheochromocytoma is noted. Pregnancy can accelerate the growth of the tumors and can precipitate severe arterial hypertension. Genetic counseling is mandatory. Pregnancy may have to be avoided or terminated if life-threatening complications arise.

Tuberous sclerosis is a neurocutaneous disease that may be accelerated by pregnancy. It is characterized by several skin lesions, epilepsy, and mental retardation. The severity of the cutaneous manifestations is independent of the severity of the nervous system involvements. At birth, examination of the skin under Wood's light may show the characteristic ash-leaf hypopigmented macules. Later, fibrous benign growths around the nails may occur. In adenoma sebaceum, angiofibromas of the central face are formed, which are neither adenomas nor related to sebaceous glands. These appear in childhood. Another cutaneous clue to the disease is the shagreen patch, a fibrous, soft plaque, usually in the lumbar area, which is a connective tissue hamartoma. The skin signs may precede the development of epilepsy by several years. Mental deficiency is not a universal finding. With this autosomal dominantly transmitted disease, genetic counseling is needed for females before pregnancy. Treatment of the adenoma sebaceum by electrosurgery or dermabrasion may bring cosmetic improvement.

Condylomata Acuminata

These venereal warts [33,34] are a nuisance to the afflicted pregnant patient, a therapeutic problem for the physician, and potentially lethal for the newborn if infected during passage through the birth canal. Virally induced, they are benign tumors that grow rapidly in pregnancy. This growth has been attributed to increased vascularity and secretions in the perineal area, but much is yet to be learned about the body's immune response to any variety of viral verruca. Moist condylomata acuminata must be differentiated from the condylomata lata of secondary syphilis. Syphilis serology should be obtained. Management of the lesions is required because of the potential threat to the newborn. An infected newborn may develop laryngeal papillomas that can cause respiratory obstruction. These laryngeal papillomas may require several operations throughout childhood. Podophyllin, the therapeutic agent of choice in the nonpregnant female, should not be used during pregnancy because of increased systemic absorption, its known neurotoxicity, and its cytotoxicity. Alternative treatment is available. Local fulguration and cryosurgery, both of which may have to be repeated several times, are the therapeutic mainstays during pregnancy. Conservative management recommends cesarean delivery if condylomata are present at the time of delivery.

Systemic Lupus Erythematosus

Systemic lupus erythematosus (SLE) [26,33,34], is discussed in detail in Chapter 20, Rheumatic Diseases, is mentioned here because of a certain subset known as subacute lupus erythematosus, which may be present in the mother as widespread discoid lupus-like skin lesions. The lesions are oval and scaly, with some epidermal atrophy and telangiectasia. Systemic manifestations may also be present. This subset of SLE patients is characterized serologically by the presence of the RO or SS-B antigen and poses several problems for the newborn. The newborn may demonstrate skin lesions for the first six months of life [38]. They usually resolve without sequelae. More important, some fetuses may develop heart block in utero. This is generally permanent and must be differentiated from an abnormal fetal heart rate in a pattern suggesting fetal distress. A pacemaker should be available at the time of birth [36].

Miscellaneous Disorders

Other skin problems that have been described as worsening during pregnancy include progressive systemic sclerosis, morphea, Ehlers-Danlos syndrome, leiomyomas, and leprosy [26].

Skin Conditions That Show Variable Changes During Pregnancy

Acne Vulgaris

Acne vulgaris [26,33] may improve if the mother's pilosebaceous apparatus responds to increased estrogen levels. If, however, the increased progesterone has an androgenic effect, acne will worsen. Treatment with tetracycline is to be avoided because of its effect on fetal bones and teeth. Erythromycin is safe and may be used if necessary. Vitamin A acid (tretinoin or Retin-A) is teratogenic if given systemically and so must be avoided because of possible percutaneous penetration. Clindamycin phosphate (Cleocin-T) produces no measurable blood levels when applied topically but has been implicated in production of pseudomembranous colitis in previously healthy adults and hence is not recommended during pregnancy. Topical benzoyl peroxides seem to be safe but often are not effective. Cryotherapy and ultraviolet light may be used with some benefit. The expectant mother may need to tolerate this unsightly problem until parturition, when therapy may resume if the mother is not nursing. The condition may ameliorate without treatment.

Dermatitis Herpetiformis

This exceptionally pruritic, chronic, vesicobullous disease usually presents on the extensor extremities, lumbar area, or scalp [26,34]. Skin pathology and direct immunofluorescent studies indicate deposition of IgA at the dermoepidermal junction, with collection of polymorphonuclear cells in the papillary dermis. There is often subepidermal separation between the dermis and the epidermis, which accounts for the vesicles and blisters. Sulfones, especially dapsone, remain the primary effective treatment. Treatment must often be continued during pregnancy. Common side effects include both dose-related and idiosyncratic hemolysis, reversible neuropathy, and, rarely, toxic hepatitis. Dapsone seems to be safe to use during pregnancy, but hematologic side effects must be carefully managed. This drug crosses the placenta and may cause methemoglobinemia in the fetus [19].

SKIN CONDITIONS MOSTLY UNIQUE TO PREGNANCY

Certain cutaneous problems described over the years are, for the most part, so limited to occurrence in pregnancy that they have been categorized into various syndromes (Table 21-1). Effects range from annoying to life threatening.

Pruritus Gravidarum and Idiopathic Jaundice of Pregnancy

These two problems are discussed together because of their apparently similar pathophysiology [26,31,33–35,40]. Pruritus gravidarum is the mild clinical manifestation of intrahepatic cholestasis; idiopathic jaundice of pregnancy is more severe.

The pruritus may be localized to the abdomen only, in which form its etiology is unknown and apparently unrelated to hepatic malfunction. This occurs in approximately 20% of pregnancies in the second or third trimester. Treatment is local and symptomatic: emollients, cool moist soaks, or topicals with 0.5% menthol or camphor. Phenol is avoided because of the risk of absorption and possible maternal or fetal nephrotoxicity or cardiotoxicity. Potent topical steroids are avoided so as not to increase striae distensae.

Generalized pruritus in pregnancy is less common than the localized form. Underlying pruritic dermatosis such as eczema, scabies, asteatosis, and contact dermatitis must be differentiated. Urticaria (and dermatographism) are common in the second and third trimesters but are separate clinical problems. As always, diabetes, thyroid abnormalities, and renal dysfunction should be looked for when pruritus occurs. The specific syndrome of generalized pruritus gravidarum, however, is due to intrahepatic cholestasis and is first seen in the third trimester. Bile salts regurgitated into the bloodstream are the cause of the itching. There are no primary skin lesions, but scratching may lead to excoriations and eventually lichenification. This problem often recurs in subsequent pregnancies or with use of oral contraceptives (refer to Chap. 15).

Treatment involves oral antihistamines. Judicious use of diphenhydramine, tripelennamine, pheniramine, or chlorpheniramine seems to be safe [28]. Cholestyramine, which is not absorbed from the gastrointestinal tract and has the ability to bind bile salts, may be helpful. After birth, affected mothers quickly recover.

Idiopathic jaundice of pregnancy [17,18,20–22, 26], which also occurs in the third trimester, consists of clinical jaundice and generalized pruritus with an incidence of 1 in 1,500. It is considered the more severe form of pruritus gravidarum, which has progressed to clinical liver dysfunction. Other causes of jaundice must be sought. When no other causes are found, treatment and prognosis are the same as for pruritus gravidarum.

Pruritic Urticarial Papules and Plaques of Pregnancy

This syndrome, only recently described, and more easily known by its acronym, PUPPP, has been said to be possibly the most common pruritic dermatosis of pregnancy [25,26,31,40]. As with idiopathic jaundice of pregnancy, it is most likely to be seen in the third trimester. The name describes the erythematous papules and hive-like swollen plaques, which are seen on the abdomen and proximal extremities but spare the face. Biopsies yield nonspecific histopathology. Direct immunofluorescent tests yield no specific findings. No significant chemical abnormalities of the blood are found. Fetal and maternal effects are not well described. Maternal symptoms can be relieved with mild topical steroids, soothing emollients, and oral antihistamines. Differential diagnosis includes infestation, contact dermatitis, drug reaction, erythema multiforme, toxemic rash, and papular dermatitis of pregnancy. It may be that the PUPPP syndrome includes one or more of the pruritic dermatoses that have been classified as separate entities in the past.

Prurigo Gestationis

This problem, which has been said to occur in 1 of 100 pregnancies, has an unknown etiology and a benign fetal and maternal prognosis [14,15,20,31,

Table 21-1. *Pruritic dermatoses of pregnancy*

Disorder	Onset	Clinical lesions	Maternal toxicity	Fetal mortality	Laboratory abnormalities
Herpes gestationis (HG)	2nd trimester or post partum	Grouped, erythematous papules, vesicles, or bullae; circinate; rarely mucosal blisters	Malaise, headache, nausea	20–30%	Eosinophilia, positive immunofluorescence, elevated HCG level
Impetigo herpetiformis	any trimester	Pustules with crusting, annular patterns in groin or trunk	Fever, toxicity, tetany	Up to 70%	Hypocalcemia, hyperphosphatemia
Papular dermatitis of pregnancy	any trimester	Trunk and limb papules; occur in crops; hyperpigmentation	None	Probably	Elevated urinary HCG levels
Prurigo gestationis	2nd–3rd trimester	Papules and nodules of extensor surfaces of limbs; atopic background	None	None	None
Toxemic rash of pregnancy	late 3rd trimester	Striae itch initially followed by wheals with crusts and spread to limbs	None	None	None
Pruritic urticarial papules and plaques of pregnancy (PUPPP)	3rd trimester	Erythematous papules and hives of abdomen and thighs	None	Possibility	None
Pruritus gravidarum	3rd trimester	Minimal primary lesions; excoriations; may be icteric	Nausea, anorexia	None	Elevated bilirubin (in idiopathic jaundice of pregnancy)
Autoimmune progesterone dermatitis of pregnancy	1st trimester	Acneform papules and pustules on arms, legs, and buttocks	Arthritis	Possibility	Elevated estriol, IgG, IgM

HCG = human chorionic gonadotropin; DHE = Dihydroepiandosterone.

33–35]. It is a condition of the last two trimesters and is seen as excoriated papules of the extensor extremities and trunk. The differential diagnosis is similar to that of PUPPP, and treatment is with topical and systemic antipruritics. Steroids are usually not needed.

Papular Dermatitis of Pregnancy

This condition [16,25,26,31,33,35,40], originally described by Spangler et al. in 1962, has not often been discussed in the literature in the last decade. Unfortunately, a fetal mortality of up to 30% has been attributed to it, but the condition can be ameliorated by treatment of the mother with systemic steroids. The increased incidence of preterm birth accounts for some of the high fetal mortality, and the 30% mortality figure was described before the great advances in newborn care since the 1960s. Papular dermatitis occurs in 1 of 2,000 pregnancies and may begin any time during gestation. The generalized 3- to 5-mm papules itch intensely and heal in seven to ten days, often with hyperpigmentation, while new lesions continue to arise. Clearing at delivery or shortly afterward is the rule, but recurrence with subsequent pregnancy is common. Laboratory evaluation of the mother may aid in diagnosis, as urinary human chorionic gonadotropin (HCG) is elevated in the last trimester while urinary estriol is decreased. Skin testing to human placental extract is positive, but not standardized as a diagnostic test. Skin histopathology is not specific.

Toxemic Rash of Pregnancy

This pruritic and urticarial rash [25,26,31,33,35, 40] was described in 1962 and may be a form of what is now known as PUPPP. Abdominal pruritus, beginning often in the striae, progresses to urticarial papules and plaques, extends peripherally, spares the face, clears at delivery, and is said to recur with subsequent pregnancies. Prognosis for the mother and fetus is uncertain. In spite of its name, this rash is apparently not clearly associated with preeclampsia/eclampsia. Symptomatic relief from topical and systemic antipruritics is the only known safe treatment.

Herpes Gestationis

This rare blistering disease of pregnancy [9–13,25, 26,29–31,33,35,40] appears to be similar to severe erythema multiforme or bullous pemphigoid. Direct immunofluorescence of the skin, however, has allowed a distinct categorization of this problem. IgG, C3, and C1q are found at the basement membrane zone. A circulating IgG, the "HG factor," is deposited and fixes complement. The problem may begin any time during pregnancy with papules, tense vesicles, or bullae. These start on the abdomen, buttocks, and proximal extremities and then generalize. In addition to erythema multiforme and bullous pemphigoid, dermatitis herpetiformis and drug eruption must be considered. Headache, fever, and malaise may be present. While immunofluorescence is diagnostic, routine skin pathology reveals subepidermal separation. The course of the disease is one of exacerbation and remission throughout pregnancy. Post partum there is a rapid resolution, usually within 30 days. Residual pigmentation can occur but is usually slight. Frequently herpes gestationis recurs during subsequent pregnancies. Fetal prognosis is not entirely clear. Some newborns have had lesions at birth that then resolve. Treatment of the disease is with systemic corticosteroids.

Impetigo Herpetiformis

This severe, life-threatening dermatosis [23,24,26, 31,33,35,40] seems to be associated with pregnancy in a more than casual correlation but has also been seen in males and nonpregnant females, and even children. It is a cutaneous-systemic disease similar to generalized pustular psoriasis. Occurring any time in pregnancy, the dramatic presentation of painful red plaques studded with sterile pustules, painful oral lesions, and lakes of sterile pus in the epidermis is associated with systemic signs and symptoms of fever, leukocytosis, hypocalcemia in excess of the associated hypoalbuminemia, arthralgias, and splenomegaly. The condition progresses rapidly after onset and may recur later, without pregnancy. The maternal mortality, which can reach 70 to 90%, demands treatment with systemic steroids or termination of pregnancy. Fetal prognosis is likewise poor.

Autoimmune Progesterone Dermatitis

Although only infrequently reported, cases of this acne-like papuloerosive skin condition [34,35] have resulted in fetal mortality. It is a disease of the first trimester with acneiform papules and pustules on arms, legs, and buttocks. Serum abnormalities that have been described include decreased progesterone but increased estriol, immunoglobulin, and eosinophils. This problem has been associated with arthritis. Administration of an oral contraceptive will exacerbate the disease, but estrogens reverse it. Intradermal skin testing with progesterone may produce a delayed hypersensitivity reaction with histopathologic features of the original disease. The disease can also occur post partum. Differential diagnosis includes acne fulminans, halogenoderma, and acneform drug eruptions. The pathology findings include intradermal abscesses with many eosinophils and a lobular panniculitis with lymphocytes, histiocytes, and eosinophils. No satisfactory treatment during gestation is known. For nonpregnant women effective treatment has been achieved with the use of estrogen to inhibit ovulation.

DRUG THERAPY DURING PREGNANCY FOR CUTANEOUS DISEASE

Certain topical or systemic medications are used almost exclusively in treatment of cutaneous disease and deserve some attention as regards their use in pregnancy [27,28,32,34,35]. Most drugs applied to the skin are absorbed systemically to some extent. Factors that affect absorption include lipid solubility, type of vehicle, site of applications, whether occlusion is used, and whether the normal barrier function of the skin has been disturbed.

Tretinoin (Retin-A) and Oral Retinoids

A derivative of vitamin A, tretinoin [36] is used topically in the treatment of acne and has been used for various keratinizing disorders. Oral retinoids, synthetic derivatives of vitamin A, have recently been introduced for use in the United States. These drugs are useful in treating cystic acne and show potential for treating many cutaneous diseases including psoriasis, uncommon keratinizing diseases, and certain malignancies [40]. Most retinoids studied so far are teratogenic and must be avoided during pregnancy.

Systemic Use of Corticosteroids

Systemic corticosteroids have not been shown to cause any fetal complications [27]. By inference, absorption of topical steroids should not present major problems, although local effects may increase the risk for or severity of striae gravidarum.

Antibiotics

Tetracycline, erythromycin, and clindamycin are used frequently as topical agents for acne. Tetracycline is well known to be deposited in fetal teeth and bone. Erythromycin is safe for use during pregnancy. Clindamycin phosphate in a hydroalcoholic vehicle (Cleocin-T, Upjohn) is said not to produce detectable blood levels after topical use but has been associated with several cases of pseudomembranous colitis after oral use. Erythromycin can be used when systemic antibiotic treatment is necessary.

Sulfone usage is, for the most part, limited to the domain of dermatology. Employed as primary treatment for dermatitis herpetiformis and leprosy, sulfone is also useful in subcorneal pustular dermatosis, pemphigus, pemphigoid, pyoderma gangrenosum, pustular psoriasis, acne, and some forms of vasculitis [19]. Although it is not approved for use during pregnancy, pregnant women have been safely treated with dapsone [19]. Maternal complications stemming from the use of dapsone are similar to those in the nonpregnant state: dose-related and idiopathic hemolysis leading to anemia, idiosyncratic hepatitis, peripheral neuropathy, and agranulocytosis. The hematologic status of the newborn should be checked at birth if the mother had been taking a sulfone.

Scabicides, gamma benzene hexachloride, crotamiton, and sulfur are pediculicides that have been used during pregnancy [32]. Gamma benzene hexachloride (Kwell) is the most effective agent, is potentially neurotoxic [32]. Crotamiton (Eurax), which also is an antipruritic, is slightly less effective as a scabicide-pediculicide and has had few adverse effects attributed to it, but patient exposure experience has not been as extensive as with Kwell. Sulfur in an ointment base is still less effective, but can be used safely during pregnancy.

Podophyllin, a cellular toxin, is very effective for condylomata acuminata but should not be used during pregnancy. The potential of neurotoxicity or teratogenicity and the likelihood of increased systemic absorption because of the moist, engorged genital skin and mucous membranes make its risk unacceptable.

REFERENCES

1. Snell RS, Turner R. Skin pigmentation in relation to the menstrual cycle. J. Invest Dermatol. 1966; 47: 147–55.
2. Newcomer VD, Lindberg MC, Sternberg TH. A melanosis of the face ("chloasma"). Arch Dermatol. 1961; 83:284–99.
3. Klingman AM, Willis I. A new formula for depigmenting human skin. Arch Dermatol. 1975; 111:40–8.
4. Poidevin LO, Sydney MB. Striae gravidarum. Their relation to adrenal cortical hyperfunction. Lancet. 1959; 2:436–9.
5. Li DT. Striae gravidarum. Lancet. 1974; 1:625. letter.
6. Schiff BL, Kern AB. Study of postpartum alopecia. Arch Dermatol. 1963; 87:609–11.
7. Bean WB, Cogswell RC, Dexter M, Embick JF. Vascular changes of skin in pregnancy. Surg Gynecol Obstet. 1949; 88:739–52.

8. Brickner SM. Fibroma molluscum gravidarum: a new clinical entity. Am J Obstet. 1906; 53:191–9.

9. Bushkell LL, Jordan RE, Goltz RW. Herpes gestationis. Arch Dermatol. 1974; 110:65–9.

10. Yaoita H, Hertz K, Katz S. Complement binding factor in herpes gestationis. J Invest Dermatol. 1975; 64:203–4.

11. Katz SI, Hertz KC, Yaoita H. Herpes gestationis. Immunopathology and characterization of the HG factor. J Clin Invest. 1976; 57:1434–41.

12. Jordon RE, Heine KG, Tappeiner G, Bushkell LL, Provost TT. The immunopathology of herpes gestationis. J Clin Invest. 1976; 57:1426–33.

13. Kolodny RC. Herpes gestationis: a new assessment of incidence, diagnosis, and fetal prognosis. Am J Obstet Gynecol. 1969; 104:39–45.

14. Pregnancy prurigo. Br Med J. 1969; 1:397–8.

15. Nurse DS. Prurigo of pregnancy. Aust J Dermatol. 1968; 9:258–67.

16. Spangler AS, Reddy W, Bardawil WA, Roby CC, Emerson K. Papular dermatitis of pregnancy. JAMA. 1962; 181:577–81.

17. Brown DG, Porta EA, Reder J. Idiopathic jaundice of pregnancy. Arch Intern Med. 1963; 111:592–606.

18. Adlercreutz H, Svanborg A, Anberg A. Recurrent jaundice in pregnancy. Am J Med. 1967; 42:335–47.

19. Lang PG. Sulfones and sulfonamides in dermatology today. J Am Acad Dermatol. 1979; 1:479–92.

20. Holzbach RT, Sanders JH. Recurrent intrahepatic cholestasis of pregnancy. JAMA. 1965; 193:542–4.

21. Larsson-Cohn U, Stenram U. Jaundice during treatment with oral contraceptive agents. JAMA. 1965; 193:422–6.

22. Eliakim M, Sadovsky E, Stein O, et al. Recurrent cholestatic jaundice of pregnancy. Arch Intern Med. 1966; 117:696–705.

23. Sauer GC, Geha BJ. Impetigo herpetiformis. Arch Dermatol. 1961; 83:119–26.

24. Katzenellenbogen I, Feuerman EJ. Psoriasis pustulosa and impetigo herpetiformis—single or dual entity? Acta Derm Venereol (Stockh.). 1966; 46:86–94.

25. Lawley TJ, Hertz KC, Wade TR, Ackerman AB, Katz SI. Pruritic urticarial papules and plaques of pregnancy. JAMA. 1979; 241:1696–9.

26. Sasseville D, Wilkinson RD, Schnader JY. Dermatoses of pregnancy. Int J Dermatol. 1981; 20:223–41.

27. Schatz M, Patterson R, Zeitz S, et al. Corticosteroid therapy for the pregnant asthmatic patient. JAMA. 1975; 233:804–7.

28. Greenberger P, Patterson R. Safety of therapy for allergic symptoms during pregnancy. Ann Intern Med. 1978; 89:234–7.

29. Lawley TJ, Stingl G, Katz SI. Fetal and maternal risk factors in herpes gestationis. Arch Dermatol. 1978; 114:552–5.

30. Katz A, Minto JO, Toole JW, Medwidsky W. Immunopathologic study of herpes gestationis in mother and infant. Arch Dermatol. 1977; 113:1069–72.

31. Winton GB. Dermatoses of pregnancy. J Assoc Milit Dermatol. 1981; 7:20–7.

32. Rasmussen JE. The problem of lindane. J Am Acad Dermatol. 1981; 5:507–16.

33. Kahn G. Skin problems of pregnancy. Consultant. Part I, 1976; 16:201–5. Part II, 1976; 16:190–2. Part III, 1977; 17:116–22.

34. Rook AJ, Wilkinson DS, Ebling FJG. Textbook of dermatology. Oxford: Blackwell, 1979.

35. Wade TR, Wade SL, Jones HE. Skin changes associated with pregnancy. Obstet Gynecol. 1978; 52:233–42.

36. Thomas JR, Doyle JA. The therapeutic uses of topical vitamin A acid. J Am Acad Dermatol. 1981; 4:505–13.

37. Cram DL. Psoriasis: current advances in etiology and treatment. J Am Acad Dermatol. 1981; 4:1–14.

38. Weston W. Personal communication, 1982.

39. Winton GB, Lewis CW. Dermatoses of pregnancy. J Am Acad Dermatol. 1982; 6:977–98.

40. Kamm JJ. Toxicology, carcinogenicity, and teratology of some orally administered retinoids. J Am Acad Dermatol. 1982; 6:652–9.

> *We can go wrong in our minds, but what our blood feels and believes and says is always true.*
> —D. H. Lawrence
> *The Letters of D. H. Lawrence*

22. HEMATOLOGIC DISORDERS

Alan S. Feiner

NORMAL PHYSIOLOGIC RESPONSE TO PREGNANCY

Alterations in Plasma and Red Cell Volumes

Both plasma and red cell volumes rise during pregnancy. The increase in plasma volume begins at the third month and peaks at the ninth month. The increase in red cell volume begins at the sixth month but is not proportionately as great as the plasma volume expansion [1]. The increase in total blood volume during a single pregnancy ranges from 1,500 to 2,000 mL, an average increase of 48% in blood volume over the nonpregnant state. Because plasma volume expansion exceeds the increase in red cell mass, pregnancy most often results in a dilution of the red cell mass (hydremia) rather than an actual decrease in the red cell mass (anemia) [2].

During the second trimester, plasma volume continues to increase at a rate greater than red blood cell (RBC) production; consequently, the hematocrit falls. During the second and early third trimesters, the hematocrit reaches a nadir near 35%. Transport of maternal iron to the fetus occurs primarily during the third trimester, and this might also contribute to the hematocrit decline. A rising hematocrit during weeks 24 to 32 is worrisome and suggests volume contraction. As the red cell mass increases toward the end of pregnancy, the hematocrit may rise. Without excessive blood loss at delivery, the hematocrit should return to pregravid levels by the third postpartum day.

Iron Metabolism

Pregnancy alters iron metabolism. The average menstruating woman loses 2 mg per day of iron. Since only 10% of dietary iron can be absorbed, a diet should contain 18 to 20 mg of iron each day to prevent iron deficiency. The average American woman consumes 10 to 12 mg per day of iron and is usually iron deficient as she begins pregnancy [3]. Loss of menses with pregnancy helps to conserve iron, but pregnancy places increased demand on body iron stores. Iron losses include 300 to 400 mg of iron to the fetus and 300 to 400 mg to blood in the placenta. An uncomplicated vaginal delivery of a single fetus results in the loss of an additional 190 mg of iron, and lactation requires 0.5 to 1.0 mg per day of iron. Thus, a normal pregnancy demands a total of approximately 1,100 mg of maternal iron [1,3].

As iron requirements increase during pregnancy, absorption from the duodenum increases. Interestingly, the fetus acquires sufficient iron stores despite iron deficiency in the mother [3]. Placental transport mechanisms trap maternal transferrin and transport iron to the fetus. Most fetal iron enters red cells, and the fetal liver stores the remainder as the storage protein ferritin. Since most iron transport occurs during the last trimester, preterm infants can have diminished total body iron stores.

Folate Metabolism

Pregnancy causes the daily folic acid requirement to increase from 50 to 100 mg per day to 150 to 300 mg per day. The higher requirement results from decreased gastrointestinal absorption, increased maternal need, and fetal parasitism [1]. Folate stores in the liver are usually adequate for six weeks. Most folate deficiency anemias in pregnancy are associated with concomitant iron deficiency. The appearance of folate deficiency usually occurs in the third trimester or in the puerperium, but folate deficiency may develop post partum because of folate need during lactation. Women at particular risk of acquiring folic acid deficiency include those with hemolytic anemia, those using phenytoin, and those with multiple or closely spaced pregnancies.

Vitamin B_{12} deficiency is extremely uncommon during pregnancy.

Platelets

Changes in platelet count have been variously reported during pregnancy. A recent investigation showed a decline in the platelet count in iron-supplemented women until weeks 31 to 34 of gestation. This pattern suggests a dilution effect from gestational increase in blood volume. However, the average count rarely drops below 250,000/mm^3 [6]. Thrombocytosis (platelet count greater than 400,000/mm^3) suggests either inflammation or concomitant iron deficiency. Platelet *function* does not change during pregnancy [7].

White Cells

The white cell count increases slightly during pregnancy. This increase begins around the 20th week and remains fairly constant during the remainder of the pregnancy. The leukocytosis results primarily from additional segmented neutrophils, with a decline in lymphocytes, eosinophils, and basophils. The total white count rarely exceeds 12,000 leukocytes/mm^3. It has been suggested that the white cell response in pregnancy results from increased levels of cortisol [6].

Coagulation Factors

Normal pregnancy is a mildly hypercoagulable state. Fibrinogen, prothrombin, and factors VII, VIII, X, and XII all increase in activity. Fibrin split products rise modestly during pregnancy, but there is no evidence of a generalized fibrinolysis [7]. Although patients with hereditary antithrombin III deficiency may be at increased risk of clotting when pregnant [7–9], the usual antithrombin III activity in pregnancy is normal or only slightly decreased.

ANEMIA

Anemia is present in pregnancy whenever the hemoglobin concentration is less than 11 g/dL [3,10,11]. Nonpregnant menstruating women are anemic at hemoglobin concentrations of less than 12 g/dL. The hemoglobin concentration most often declines between weeks 24 and 32 because of the increase in plasma volume. The incidence of anemia in a pregnant population varies from 21 to 81% depending on the population studied [10]. Most mild anemias do not constitute a serious risk to mother or fetus. However, hematocrits below 29% impart a significant risk of fetal death, preterm birth, and low birth weight [12].

Clinical Evaluation of the Anemic Patient

The symptoms of the pregnant woman with anemia are typically few. Pica, the ingestion of nonnutrients such as starch, dirt, and ice, can be a useful clue to iron-deficient erythropoiesis. In the history of a pregnant patient with anemia one should attempt to establish the duration of the problem. Documentation of a previously normal hemoglobin concentration would make a congenital anemia very unlikely. Family history as well as a careful history of any blood loss, chronic illness, or drug use is imperative.

Evaluation of any anemia must include a review of the peripheral blood smear (Fig. 22-1). This simple procedure is extremely useful and is underutilized. Review of the peripheral smear will distinguish between a pure red cell disorder and a disorder of several cell lines. In addition, the peripheral smear will often provide morphologic clues to the cause of an anemia. Most simple anemias can be classified according to the size of the peripheral blood RBCs. Although useful, automated laboratory cell counters can provide misleading information about complex anemias. A dimorphic population of RBCs will probably elude the automated cell counter. Patients with reticulocytosis will tend to have higher mean corpuscular volumes when the machine averages volumes of all RBCs.

Following review of the peripheral blood smear, several additional laboratory tests may prove useful. A reticulocyte count of greater than 3.5% usually signifies that the marrow is able to respond to the anemia [13]. As anemia becomes severe, the bone marrow may release red cells early. Thus, a reticulocyte may persist in the peripheral blood longer than the usual 24 hours. A correction factor for the patient's low hematocrit and for premature bone marrow release of reticulocytes yields a reasonable estimate of the bone marrow's response to anemia. The correction factor multiplied by the observed reticulocyte count produces the *corrected reticulocyte count.* The corrected count should be greater than 3.5% if the marrow is responding appropriately.

After clinical evaluation and supplemental laboratory tests, the cause of the anemia will usually become apparent. However, failure of the anemia to respond to seemingly appropriate treatment is an indication for bone marrow biopsy. This is particularly the case in complex anemias.

Bone marrow aspiration and biopsy from the posterior iliac crest are simple and often valuable diagnostic procedures. Both aspiration and biopsy

Fig. 22-1. Evaluation of anemia during pregnancy.

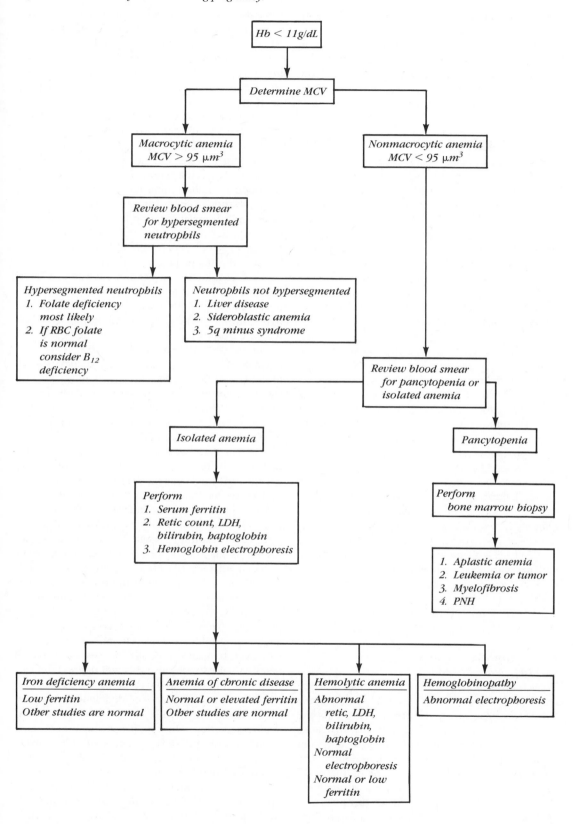

are usually indicated because they yield complementary information. Core biopsy specimens better reveal overall marrow cellularity; aspiration specimens better reveal individual cellular morphology. Serious complications from bone marrow aspiration and biopsy are rare; they include excessive bleeding and permanent bone, muscle, or nerve damage.

Macrocytic Anemia

In a pregnant woman, a macrocytic anemia (mean corpuscular volume [MCV] greater than 95 μm^3) usually reflects folate deficiency. A mild pancytopenia, hypersegmentation of the neutrophils, a low reticulocyte count, and response to oral folate supplementation support this diagnosis. The serum folate quantitation reveals only folate balance and *not* tissue deficiency. Tissue deficiency is reflected by a low *erythrocyte* folate concentration [15]. Vitamin B_{12} deficiency can occur but is extremely uncommon in pregnancy. Other possible causes of macrocytosis during pregnancy are listed in Figure 22-1.

Women at high risk of acquiring folate deficiency during pregnancy include phenytoin users, women with hemolytic anemias, and women with closely spaced or multiple pregnancies. Patients with proven folate deficiency anemia or patients at high risk should receive an additional 1 to 3 mg of oral folate each day. Several authors suggest that folate supplements are appropriate for *all* pregnant women [14].

Iron deficiency anemia frequently coexists with folate deficiency. The peripheral blood might show a dimorphic population of macrocytic and microcytic red cells. Occasionally, hypersegmentation of neutrophils alone without macroovalocytosis is a clue to a complex anemia [15]. In patients with hypersegmentation from folate deficiency, the average neutrophil lobe count will fall after 12 to 14 days of treatment, but the earliest sign of a response is a rise in the reticulocyte count after 48 to 72 hours [16].

Nonmacrocytic Anemias

Iron Deficiency Anemia

Total body iron stores must be evaluated in the diagnostic evaluation of a nonmacrocytic anemia (MCV less than 95 μm^3). Ferritin represents the major iron storage protein in humans; it resides primarily in liver, spleen, and bone marrow. Serum ferritin measurement by immunoradiometric assay provides an accurate reflection of total body iron in most patients [5,17,18]. A low serum ferritin is diagnostic of iron-deficient erythropoiesis in an anemic patient. Unfortunately, inflammation

can raise a serum ferritin in an iron-deficient patient. If there is no evidence of inflammation, the ferritin measurement is sufficient as a diagnostic test of iron stores. The total iron-binding capacity may be inaccurate in pregnancy because estrogen and progesterone can stimulate transferrin production [4,10].

Low body iron stores raise the question of blood loss from previous menses or from the gastrointestinal tract. Radiologic investigation of the gastrointestinal tract is seldom necessary unless active bleeding or occult blood in the stool is found. Impaired iron absorption rarely causes iron deficiency, although ingestion of tea has been implicated in iron malabsorption [19]. Vitamin C supplements can cause a false negative result in stool testing for occult blood [20]. Mild iron deficiency features normochromic normocytic red cells. As iron stores continue to decline, the red cells first become microcytic and then hypochromic. Fewer than 20% of patients progress to the microcytic hypochromic phase [21]. Indeed, not all gravidas who are iron deficient become anemic.

The most rapid method to correct severe anemia (Hb less than 7 g/dL) in pregnancy is with blood transfusions. Pregnancy does not preclude the transfusion of any donor-compatible blood product. However, transfusions should be reserved for definite and presumably serious problems. There are small risks of hepatitis and antibody formation associated with the use of blood products. If the patient is not volume depleted, packed red blood cells should be transfused to correct severe anemia. Prior to transfusion, appropriate diagnostic tests for anemia (serum ferritin, lactate dehydrogenase [LDH], haptoglobin, bilirubin, reticulocyte count) should be obtained. If the anemia is macrocytic or possibly complex, then red cell folate and serum B_{12} levels should be drawn before transfusion. If the patient is judged to be volume depleted, then the use of saline solutions, fresh frozen plasma or whole blood is appropriate. Transfusion should convert a severe anemia to a milder anemia (Hb more than 9 g/dL). However, transfusion should not reestablish a normal hemoglobin, because this will depress the patient's own bone marrow response to anemia.

The treatment of mild iron deficiency anemia is controversial. In Europe and Japan, routine iron supplementation during pregnancy does not occur. Some physicians feel that the lower hematocrit favorably affects blood viscosity and that diminished iron-binding proteins may protect against bacterial infection [22]. Some authors note that deleterious effects of mild anemia are difficult to demonstrate [10,23]. As discussed previously, infants of iron-deficient mothers are seldom iron deficient. Nevertheless, the frequency of iron deficiency in menstruating women and the increased demands of pregnancy clearly define a potentially debilitating situation. The problem could become quite serious in subsequent pregnancies or with heavy blood loss. One reasonable approach is to give 40 to 65 mg of elemental iron per day during the first 20 weeks of gestation. In anemic women or in women more than 20 weeks pregnant, 40 to 65 mg of elemental iron should be given twice a day [21]. Failure to improve within two weeks should prompt further investigation. Improvement should appear as a rise in reticulocyte count within two weeks and a rise in hemoglobin within four weeks. One should suspect beta-thalassemia trait if the ferritin becomes normal and the patient is still anemic or the red cells remain microcytic. Concomitant iron deficiency and beta-thalassemia trait may not demonstrate the characteristic hemoglobin A_2 elevation until the iron deficiency has been corrected. If the serum ferritin is normal and the hemoglobin concentration is low, the problem might be excessive plasma volume [16].

The most common cause of treatment failure in iron deficiency anemia is patient noncompliance [24]. Iron preparations are notoriously difficult to tolerate. To circumvent this problem, various iron salts are available. At least one study has failed to show an advantage to either ferrous fumarate or ferrous gluconate over ferrous sulfate. Although iron absorption may be impaired by using food or antacids, one author has made a cogent plea for giving small doses of iron in any acceptable way to improve patient compliance [25]. Prenatal multivitamin preparations with iron may not deliver the amount of iron anticipated [26]. The use of iron dextran (e.g., Imferon) infusions for iron deficiency is controversial. There is very little, if any, increase in the rapidity of response compared with oral iron preparations. The singular advantage of this form of therapy is the certainty that iron gets into the patient. Nevertheless, allergic (sometimes fatal) reactions have occurred with iron dextran; and it should not be used routinely for the treatment of mild anemia in pregnancy.

Anemia of Chronic Disease

Some pregnant women with anemia may have normal or increased iron stores as measured by serum ferritin or by bone marrow aspirate iron stain. The patients may have either normocytic or microcytic RBCs. The reticulocyte count is low, and there is no evidence of bleeding or hemolysis. The laboratory data in these patients resemble those seen in iron deficiency anemia except for the iron

Table 22-1. Laboratory tests in anemias of iron deficiency and chronic disease during pregnancy

Test	Iron deficiency anemia	Anemia of chronic disease
Serum iron	Low or normal	Low or normal
TIBC	Elevated	Normal or low
Serum ferritin	Low	Normal or high
Reticulocyte count	Low (unless patient is receiving iron)	Low
RBC size	Normal or microcytic	Normal or microcytic
Bone marrow iron	Low	Normal or high

studies (Table 22-1). The patients usually have a definable chronic illness (such as infection, collagen vascular disease, renal or liver disease) causing their anemia. The only effective treatment for the anemia of chronic disease is treatment of the underlying disorder.

Aplastic Anemia

Aplastic anemia is a rare cause of anemia during pregnancy. It usually presents as a pancytopenia rather than as a simple anemia. Bone marrow biopsy is essential for the diagnosis. Some patients may recover after delivery or premature termination of pregnancy [27].

Hemolytic Anemia

The incidence of hemolytic anemia in pregnancy is unclear. Hemolysis should be considered in any nonmacrocytic anemia. Symptoms of hemolysis are few; suspicion may first be aroused when the routine antibody screen of the mother shows a positive autocontrol. In reviewing the peripheral smear of a patient suspected of hemolyzing, one should look for RBC fragments and polychromasia. However, the absence of fragmented RBCs on peripheral smear *in no way* excludes hemolysis. Other screening tests for hemolysis include reticulocyte count, LDH, bilirubin, and haptoglobin. The Coombs test alone is difficult to interpret unless screening tests suggest that the patient is actively hemolyzing. If the patient is actively hemolyzing and the Coombs test is negative, one should consider hemoglobinopathies, RBC enzyme and structural defects, infections, and toxins.

Autoimmune Hemolytic Anemia (AIHA)

The diagnosis of AIHA is suggested by an elevated reticulocyte count, LDH, and bilirubin. The unbound serum haptoglobin should be undetectable in a significant hemolysis. The direct Coombs test should be positive in AIHA, indicating that antibody is present on red cells. The indirect Coombs test is often positive also, indicating the presence of antibody in the serum. The most sensitive test for the detection of hemolysis is the nuclear medicine RBC survival study; this test is potentially dangerous to the fetus and is probably never necessary to perform during pregnancy. The type of antibody mediating the hemolysis in AIHA is usually warm reacting.

When the mother has a Coombs-positive hemolytic anemia, an underlying cause should be sought. The clinical history may help guide further investigation into collagen vascular disease, neoplasm, and viral infection. If available, subclassification of the antibody may prove helpful. IgM-mediated AIHA poses no risk to the fetus. Subclasses IgG_1 and IgG_3 cross the placenta easily and may present problems for the fetus [28]. If the mother's indirect Coombs test is positive and antibody subclass IgG_1 or IgG_3 is detected, maternal antibody titers should be followed. Most patients with potential problems will be detected in Rh compatibility screening. Only 1 to 2% of obstetric patients will have a positive indirect Coombs test because of an irregular antibody [29].

If the antibody crosses the placenta, then hemolytic disease could develop in the fetus. The guidelines for following the fetus are those used in managing Rh isoimmunization. Serial sonograms can be used to monitor fetal development. Amniotic fluid analysis for optical density and bilirubin determination should be performed every two to four weeks during the last trimester [30]. Criteria for intervention have been described by Liley [31].

If the maternal hemoglobin drops below 8 g/dL or if the mother becomes symptomatic from the anemia, corticosteroid therapy should be started. The effective prednisone dosage ranges from 60 to 100 mg per day. A high dosage should be continued until the hemoglobin concentration becomes stable. When hemoglobin rises and the reticulocyte count falls, the prednisone dosage may be reduced to 30 to 45 mg daily. As long as the patient remains stable, dosage reduction can proceed by 5 mg per week. A daily dosage of 15 to 20 mg of prednisone should be continued for 8 to 12 weeks after the acute hemolysis has subsided; further dosage reductions should proceed gradually during the next four to eight weeks. In patients with idiopathic autoimmune hemolytic anemia, favorable response to corticosteroid therapy occurs in 50 to 65% of patients. No response to 100 to 200 mg prednisone after two weeks represents a therapeutic failure. Patients who require 15 mg

prednisone a day chronically or who fail to respond to high-dosage therapy should be considered for splenectomy. Unfortunately, splenectomy does not cure a high percentage of these patients, and may have a maternal mortality as high as 15% [32]. Splenectomy and corticosteroids are of little value in hemolytic anemia of the cold antibody type. Little information exists on the management of cryopathic hemolytic syndromes during pregnancy.

Patients with hemolytic anemia during pregnancy have an increased folate requirement and should receive 1 to 3 mg of folic acid supplement per day. These patients may be extremely difficult to cross-match for blood transfusion. Transfusion needs should be anticipated early and adequate blood bank support secured.

Hemoglobinopathies and Thalassemias in Pregnancy

The most common of these entities are sickle cell anemia (HbSS), sickle–β-thalassemia (HbS-thal), sickle cell hemoglobin with hemoglobin C (HbSC), hemoglobin C disease (HbCC), sickle cell trait (HbAS), and beta-thalassemia trait. The other hemoglobinopathies and thalassemias are rare and beyond the scope of this discussion. Hemoglobinopathy refers to a structural alteration in one or more of the globin polypeptide chains of the heme moiety. Thalassemia refers to a quantitative change in globin chain production; there is no change in the affected globin's structure.

The initial diagnostic test for the sickling disorders (HbSS, HbS-thal, HbSC, and HbAS) is the sodium metabisulfite test (Sickledex) or a turbidity test (Fig. 22-2). Since false negatives and false positives occur with these tests, all suspected individuals should have a hemoglobin electrophoresis on cellulose acetate at alkaline pH [33]. This electrophoresis does not distinguish among hemoglobins S, D, and G. Sometimes separation of hemoglobins F and S is not optimal either. Patients with a positive Sickledex and hemoglobin S on cellulose acetate need not be studied further. Patients with a negative Sickledex and possible hemoglobin S on cellulose acetate should have a subsequent electrophoresis on citrate agar at acid pH to distinguish hemoglobins S, D, F, and G. Quantitation of the hemoglobin A_2 concentration is useful in the detection of beta-thalassemia. Since a 10% falsely elevated quantitation of HbA_2 has been reported with the electrophoretic technique, quantitation of HbA_2 by column chromatography is preferred [34]. Special stains for fetal hemoglobin may help to distinguish hereditary persistence of fetal hemoglobin, a generally benign condition seen most com-

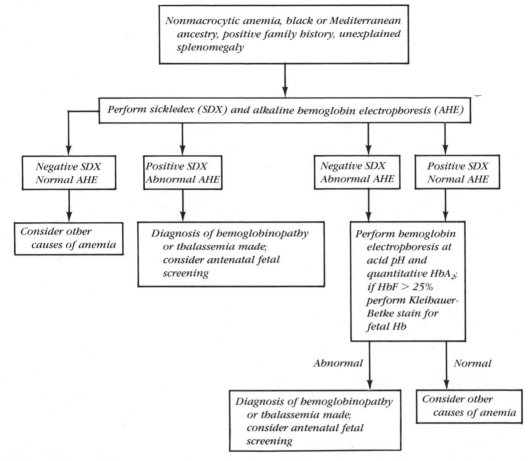

Fig. 22-2. Diagnostic approach to sickling disorders and thalassemias.

monly in blacks, from compensatory hemoglobin F production in a hemoglobinopathy.

The detection of a hemoglobinopathy or thalassemia in a pregnant woman raises several important questions. Concerns for complications in the mother and fetus are obvious. Other concerns about the kind of life that will develop if the pregnancy is successful are also real. The diagnosis of a hemoglobinopathy or thalassemia in a mother increases the risk of a severe disorder in the child. The father should have a Sickledex and a hemoglobin electrophoresis. If these tests indicate a significant chance that the fetus might have a severe hemoglobinopathy or thalassemia, then more complete antenatal diagnostic testing should be considered. Currently, the availability of an assay for sickle–beta-globin gene allows the direct study of amniotic fluid cells to establish the presence of the sickle cell gene [35,36].

Sickle Hemoglobinopathies
Variations in a single amino acid in a beta-globin side chain lead to the manifestations of the sickling

disorders. The information for globin chain synthesis is carried on four separate autosomal genetic loci. Individuals normally possess two alleles at each locus, one coming from each parent. When the alleles differ, dissimilar chains are produced and abnormal hemoglobins result. The substitution of valine for glutamic acid in the beta chain results in hemoglobin S (HbS) production. Substitution of lysine in this position results in hemoglobin C (HbC) production.

Sickle cell trait (HbAS) is a comparatively benign anomaly that occurs in approximately 1 out of 12 blacks [37]. Patients with sickle cell trait have an increased incidence of hyposthenuria, renal hematuria, and splenic infarction with hypoxia [38]. There also seems to be an increased incidence of bacteriuria and pyelonephritis in pregnant women with HbAS [39]. However, there is no increase in fetal wastage if infection does not develop in the patient. Patients with sickle cell trait should receive routine iron and folic acid supplementation. Additionally, cord blood should be checked for HbAS [40].

Approximately 0.3% of the black population in the United States (roughly 50,000 people) have sickle cell anemia (HbSS). Studies of pregnancy in sickle cell anemia are significantly biased toward groups of women who are healthy enough to become fertile. Interestingly, the pattern of sickling complications before pregnancy does *not* predict the actual complications of a patient during pregnancy. The concentration of hemoglobin F is not predictive of the severity or the type of problems encountered in women with sickle cell disease during pregnancy [41]; hereditary persistence of fetal hemoglobin should be considered in women with more than 25% HbF [42]. Patients with sickle cell disease are prone to anemia (100%), preeclampsia (13–33%), infection (55–65%), and painful crises (10–20%) during pregnancy [37]. In one series the abortion rate in women with sickle cell disease was 33% [39]. The maternal death rate ranges from 0 to 22%. Many of the severe clinical problems of these patients result from stagnation of oxygenated erythrocytes in viscera; stagnation leads to deoxygenation; deoxygenation leads to sickling, which leads to further stagnation and vaso-occlusive crises [43].

Hemoglobin C trait is rare and innocuous [44]. Hemoglobin C (HbC) is also seen in the black population, but the gene frequency (1 out of 40) is less than that of HbS. Homozygous HbCC is quite rare. It may be associated with a low-grade hemolysis, splenomegaly, and mild anemia. Patients may have occasional abdominal or bone pain, but the pain is not as severe as that seen with sickle cell disease. The risks of patients with HbCC during pregnancy are not well described [44].

Hemoglobin SC disease is fairly common in the black population (1 out of 480 blacks). Prior to pregnancy, these patients often have a very uneventful clinical course; consequently, as a group they are more likely to reach reproductive age fertile. Splenomegaly is common. For unclear reasons, patients with HbSC are more likely than patients with HbSS to have aseptic necrosis of the femoral heads and proliferative retinopathy. The incidence of spontaneous abortion, maternal death, and perinatal mortality has been reported to be less in patients with HbSC than in patients with HbSS [11]. Complications of preeclampsia, urinary tract infection, and painful crises during pregnancy are all reported to be approximately 20% in HbSC disease [37]. The complications of HbSC disease in late pregnancy can be particularly severe. There is a 5 to 10% chance of pulmonary infarction. This may result from a modest increase in sickling in patients with comparatively high hematocrits. The increased sickling could lead to bone marrow necrosis with subsequent fat embolization to the lungs [45].

The incidence of heterozygous thalassemia in the black population is 0.8%. The most commonly encountered thalassemic condition is sickle–beta-thalassemia (HbS-thal): sickle cell trait accompanied by an underproduction of normal beta chains. The result is a relative overproduction of HbS compared with HbA. At times, family studies may be necessary to distinguish sickle–beta-thal from sickle cell anemia, depending on the severity of the beta-thal component. Clinical manifestations of sickle–beta-thalassemia can be extremely variable because of the differing proportions of HbS and HbA. Mediterranean populations tend to have more HbS and more clinical problems than African populations. One study of pregnancy in sickle–beta-thalassemia reported no maternal deaths and an 8% abortion rate. Morbidity during the third trimester was common. Bone pain, infection, and symptoms of pulmonary infarction were as common as in HbSC disease [39].

Other than sickle–beta-thalassemia, there is little information about pregnancy in patients with clinically significant thalassemic syndromes. Beta-thalassemia trait usually appears as an asymptomatic microcytosis, with only an occasional anemia. The hemoglobin electrophoresis characteristically shows an elevation of HbA_2. With the exception of one published report, beta-thal trait is not usually associated with problems during pregnancy [11, 46]. If a pregnant woman has thalassemia trait, the father should be screened with a Sickledex, hemoglobin electrophoresis, and quantitative HbA_2. If the father has any hemoglobinopathy or thalassemic syndrome, prenatal examination of the fetus should be considered for the possible detection of a more serious hematologic problem.

Treatment of the Sickle
Hemoglobinopathies
Sickle cell disorders (HbSS, HbSC, HbS-thal) are not definite contraindications to pregnancy, although the risks during pregnancy are greater than normal. Initial assessment should accurately define the hemoglobinopathy with Sickledex and electrophoresis. The concentration of hemoglobin F (HbF) deserves special attention. If the HbF concentration is greater than 25%, the special Kleihauer-Betke stain for fetal hemoglobin should be ordered. This stain distinguishes between sickle cell disease with excessive HbF production and sickle cell disease with hereditary persistence of fetal hemoglobin (HPFH). Patients with HPFH have fetal hemoglobin in each RBC, which stabilizes the cell membrane; they seldom have complications during pregnancy. On the other hand, sickle cell disease patients with high fetal

hemoglobin have variable distributions of HbF. Such patients can have serious problems during pregnancy. A prior history of a benign course during pregnancy does not ensure the absence of complications during subsequent pregnancies [41].

The pregnant patient with a sickle cell disorder is very likely to be anemic. This condition should be evaluated as discussed previously with review of the peripheral smear, reticulocyte count, assessment of iron and folate stores as appropriate, and screening tests for hemolysis. Evaluation will usually reveal a Coombs-negative hemolytic anemia. If the patient has received multiple blood transfusions in the past, she will probably have a positive indirect Coombs test, in which case evaluation will be more difficult. If the reticulocyte count is low, one should consider iron and folate deficiency. The anemia of chronic illness is also possible if the patient has had repeated infections. A much less likely possibility is an aplastic crisis. Aplastic crises most commonly result from infection, but the overall incidence of these crises does not appear to be increased during pregnancy. Megaloblastic crisis from folate deficiency is most likely to occur during late pregnancy [47]. Zinc deficiencies have also been described in association with sickle cell anemia [48].

There is no contraindication to either spontaneous labor or cesarean delivery in patients with sickling disorders. The use of oxytocin for induction or augmentation of labor has not been shown to be harmful in this group of patients. Analgesics can be used with no unusual risk of respiratory depression. Some physicians have used exchange transfusions before a general anesthetic, but the data to support this practice are meager. Hypotension during any kind of anesthesia in a patient with a sickling disorder should be avoided. At least one authority recommends a segmental epidural block as optimal anesthesia [42].

Partial exchange transfusion of RBCs given prophylactically during pregnancy to prevent maternal and fetal complications remains controversial. Among the indications for transfusion during pregnancy are symptomatic anemia, prolonged painful crisis, and vaso-occlusive complications.

There are several different ways to administer partial exchange transfusions. Each technique results in a decreased concentration of HbS. One technique is presented in Table 22-2. Some patients transfused prophylactically have an increased sense of well-being and fewer crises. Disadvantages to exchange transfusions include the risk of hepatitis and isosensitization of the mother. Unfortunately, the mother's previous history of

Table 22-2. Protocol for partial exchange transfusions

1. Obtain baseline hemoglobin, hematocrit, hemoglobin A (HbA) quantitation. Proceed with transfusion when HbA is less than 35%.
2. Type and cross-match for 2 units of packed buffy coat–poor, washed red cells.
3. Infuse 200–400 mL of normal saline over 1 hour (assuming normal cardiac and renal function).
4. Phlebotomize 500 mL of blood into vacutainer over 15–30 min.
5. Repeat hemoglobin, hematocrit, and HbA quantitation.
6. Continue steps 2–5 until hemoglobin A quantitation is at least 35%. Patients with HbSC may be difficult to raise beyond this point.
7. For prophylactic transfusion therapy, repeat whenever HbA is 20% (usually every 4–8 weeks).

problems during pregnancy is not a reliable indicator for the use of prophylactic exchange transfusions. In 1979, a Consensus Development Conference on Transfusion Therapy in Pregnant Sickle Cell Disease Patients concluded that routine prophylatic transfusions were not indicated [49].

POLYCYTHEMIA RUBRA VERA
Very rarely, women with polycythemia rubra vera become pregnant. There is an increased incidence of infertility, preeclampsia, and fetal wastage. Hemorrhage and thrombosis do not seem to occur during pregnancy, but serious postpartum hemorrhages have been reported [50].

WHITE CELLS IN PREGNANCY
As noted earlier, the white blood cell count may be mildly elevated during pregnancy. Twenty percent of third-trimester women may have white counts of 10,000/mm³. Myelocytes and metamyelocytes can be seen in the peripheral smear occasionally during late pregnancy. In most patients with increased granulocytes during pregnancy, the white count becomes normal by the sixth postpartum day [2].

Total white blood cell counts in excess of 12,000/mm³ without infection are unusual; consequently, further investigation may be worthwhile. Additional indications for further workup during pregnancy include a rapidly rising white count or platelet count, anemia, fever, hyperuricemia, unexplained blast cells in the peripheral blood smear, eosinophilia, or basophilia. In such instances, a bone marrow aspirate for Philadelphia chromosome may prove helpful. Analysis of leukocyte alkaline phosphatase (LAP) activity in peripheral blood granulocytes may help distinguish a leukemoid reaction (normal or high LAP) from chronic granulocytic leukemia (low LAP).

Neutropenia (WBC less than 2000/mm^3) is uncommon during pregnancy. Some patients may chronically have mild granulocytopenia without any problems related to recurrent infection. However, if the patient has concomitant anemia or thrombocytopenia, one should consider performing a bone marrow biopsy and aspiration to distinguish underproduction from peripheral sequestration or destruction of white cells. Patients with neutropenia alone and recurrent infections should be evaluated by analysis of white cell enzymes and tests for humoral and cell-mediated immunity.

COAGULATION DISORDERS DURING PREGNANCY

History and physical exam are crucial in the evaluation of a potential coagulopathy. The history should elicit any previous problems with bleeding or easy bruising, family history of bleeding, and the use of any medication (including such nonprescription substances as aspirin and vitamin E). Physical exam should search for sites of bleeding, ecchymoses, petechiae, and telangiectasias. The history of easy bruising is heard often and is not always significant; further evaluation is indicated when bruises enlarge with time, appear spontaneously on the trunk, or are larger than 2.5 cm. Spontaneous bleeding from multiple sites strongly suggests a coagulopathy; severe, localized bleeding is less indicative of a systemic coagulopathy.

When history and physical exam suggest a possible bleeding diathesis, six simple screening tests are necessary: a quantitative platelet count, a template bleeding time (BT), a prothrombin time (PT), a partial thromboplastin time (PTT), a fibrin-ogen concentration (FIB), and a determination of the titer of fibrin split products (FSP). These six tests assess the major components of the coagulation cascade. Adequate numbers of platelets are necessary for clotting. The template bleeding time screens for platelet dysfunction and vascular disease. The prothrombin time measures the extrinsic clotting pathway while the partial thromboplastin time assays the intrinsic pathway. The fibrinogen concentration yields information about the end of the cascade. Fibrin split products indicate that clotting and clot lysis have occurred. A thrombin time in some instances may substitute for the FSP and fibrinogen assays. A normal thrombin time suggests an adequate concentration of fibrinogen and a low titer of fibrin split products.

The template bleeding time may not be helpful if the platelet count is less than 50,000/mm^3. The prothrombin and partial thromboplastin times may be prolonged by high titers of fibrin split products and by low concentrations of fibrinogen (less than 70 mg/dL). Table 22-3 displays the predicted results of coagulation screening tests for various coagulopathies.

Thrombocytopenia

Platelet counts fluctuate during pregnancy, with a slight decline (about 20%) in the average platelet count noted between the first and the third trimesters [6]. A platelet count of less than 150,000/mm^3 should prompt an evaluation (Fig. 22-3).

The history of a pregnant woman with thrombocytopenia should include information regarding drug use, toxin exposure (e.g., quinine), infection, and autoimmune disorders. A history of easy bleeding or bruising may give some idea of duration. Physical examination should include a search for ecchymoses, petechiae, lymphadenopathy, and splenomegaly. Documentation of fever or any neurologic impairment is imperative in any patient

Table 22-3. Screening tests for coagulopathies

Disorder	Platelet count	BT	PT	PTT	FIB	FSP
ITP	L	N or P	N	N	N	N
Aspirin use	N	SP	N	N	N	N
TTP	L	N or P	N	N	N	N
DIC	L	N or P	P	P	L	H
Vitamin K deficiency	N	N	P	P	N	N
Hemophilia A	N	N	N	P	N	N
Von Willebrand's disease	N	P	N	P	N	N

N = normal; L = low; H = high; P = prolonged; SP = slightly prolonged; BT = bleeding time; PT = prothrombin time; PTT = partial thromboplastin time; FIB = fibrinogen concentration; FSP = fibrin split products.

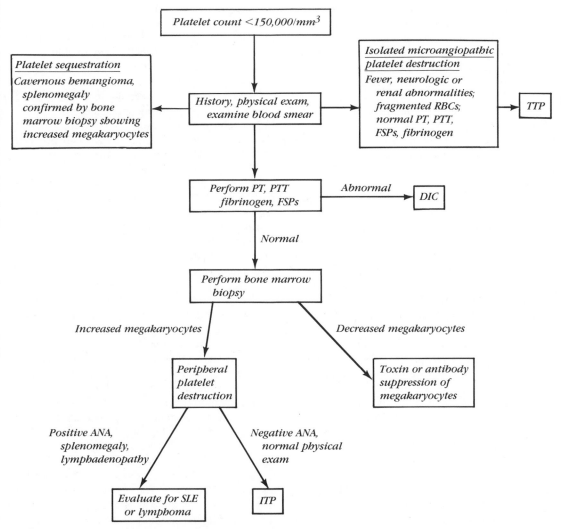

Fig. 22-3. Diagnostic approach to thrombocytopenia.

suspected of having thrombotic thrombocytopenia purpura (TTP).

The peripheral smear merits special attention. It can readily reveal platelet morphologic abnormalities as well as indicate the presence of polychromasia, neutropenia, blasts, spherocytosis, or fragmented RBCs (schistocytes).

Further evaluation of thrombocytopenia must establish whether there is decreased platelet production or increased peripheral destruction. This will often necessitate a bone marrow aspiration and biopsy.

Decreased Production of Platelets

This problem is extremely uncommon. Primary megakaryocytic failure can occur with toxin exposure. Specific therapy involves identification and removal of the toxin. Decreased platelet produc-

tion coupled with either granulocytopenia or anemia suggests a primary bone marrow process. The differential diagnosis should consider infection, aplastic anemia, bone marrow infiltration, paroxysmal nocturnal hemoglobinuria, and folate deficiency.

Sequestration of Platelets

This is another uncommon cause of thrombocytopenia in pregnancy. Sequestration occurs in hypersplenism or in association with a cavernous hemangioma. Optimal therapy for these conditions during pregnancy must be individualized.

Autoimmune Thrombocytopenia (ATP)

Antibody-mediated peripheral destruction of platelets is the most common autoimmune hematologic disorder encountered during pregnancy [52]. Diagnosis is established by documenting the presence of peripheral thrombocytopenia, increased bone marrow megakaryocytes, and no evidence of preeclampsia or any other coagulopathy. If an antibody-mediated thrombocytopenia is suspected, tests for systemic lupus erythematosus (SLE) should be performed, since this disorder can present as an immune thrombocytopenia. Lymphoma is a rare cause of ATP in pregnancy. If the patient has a normal-sized spleen and no obvious cause for the antibody, the condition is called idiopathic thrombocytopenia purpura (ITP).

The antibody usually involved in ATP is of the IgG$_3$ class, which can cross the placenta and produce thrombocytopenia in the fetus. This phenomenon in the fetus can occur despite splenectomy in the mother. Although many tests for antiplatelet antibodies exist, the accuracy of these assays is open to question. Patients with a history of ATP before pregnancy are not at increased risk of relapse during pregnancy [52].

The management of patients with ATP (Table 22-4) is not significantly altered by pregnancy. Patients with peripheral platelet counts of less than 50,000/mm^3 may bleed spontaneously and excessively. Intramuscular injections should be avoided. Venipuncture sites should be compressed for at least three minutes. Aspirin and other drugs known to cause gastrointestinal bleeding are relatively contraindicated. In addition, drugs that inhibit platelet function such as aspirin, vitamin E, and sulfinpyrazone should be avoided.

Corticosteroids should be instituted (0.5–2.0 mg/kg/day) for bleeding or for a platelet count of less than 50,000/mm^3. Permanent improvement occurs in 60% of patients; temporary remissions occur in 20%. Corticosteroids can reduce the production of antibody, inhibit the binding of antibody to the platelet surface, and retard the phagocytosis of opsonized platelets [53]. Some response to therapy is usually evident within two weeks. If corticosteroid therapy fails, splenectomy is indicated. It should be noted that a 31% fetal mortality has been reported following splenectomies performed during pregnancy [54]. When the platelet count exceeds 50,000/mm^3, gradual reduction in corticosteroid dosage can proceed. At least weekly, platelet counts are necessary while the dosage is being tapered.

Controversy surrounds management of mothers with active ATP. Some sources suggest 10 to 20 mg of prednisone a day beginning at least ten days before delivery in any woman with active ATP or with a previous history of ATP. Some data suggest that infants delivered after this treatment are at no risk of hemorrhage and may be delivered vaginally [55]. Fetal platelet counts can be checked immediately prior to vaginal delivery to minimize the risk of bleeding from thrombocytopenia. The scalp sampling technique appears relatively safe even in thrombocytopenic fetuses [51].

One recent report suggests that maternal platelet counts may be unreliable in assessing the risk of fetal thrombocytopenia [56]. Its authors advocate the monitoring of maternal circulating antiplatelet antibody titers to anticipate the extent of neonatal thrombocytopenia. Platelet transfusions for ATP are seldom necessary and may be ineffective because of circulating antibodies.

Hemostatic abnormalities occur in both mother and fetus with aspirin use. Aspirin use should be restricted to specific indications, particularly in the last three months [57].

Thrombotic Thrombocytopenia Purpura

Thrombotic thrombocytopenia purpura (TTP) is an incompletely understood clinical entity characterized by microangiopathic hemolytic anemia, thrombocytopenia, fluctuating neurologic signs, renal disease, and fever. It is an uncommon disorder occurring primarily in the third and fourth decades of life. The diagnosis is mainly clinical and is supported by finding schistocytes in the peripheral blood. A gingival biopsy may show characteristic histologic changes of subendothelial and intraluminal hyaline deposits and the lack of inflammatory change in vessels and stroma [58]. Except for the thrombocytopenia, most standard coagulation tests are normal in TTP. The pathogenesis of TTP is unclear; the characteristic hyaline thrombosis may be the result of disseminated intravascular platelet consumption or aggregation at sites of discontinuous endothelial cell in-

Table 22-4. Management of autoimmune thrombocytopenia purpura

Delivery

Vaginal, if platelet count is greater than 100,000/mm^3 and there has been no splenectomy

Cesarean, if splenectomy has been performed before delivery, or if maternal platelet count is less than 100,000/mm^3

Therapy for ATP

1. Corticosteroids. Give supplemental IV steroids during delivery if the patient received them during gestation.
2. Platelet transfusions may be given if hemostasis is a problem.
3. Consider splenectomy during cesarean delivery for patients who appear to have failed steroid therapy.

Source: Carloss et al. [54]

jury [59]. In late pregnancy, TTP may be difficult to distinguish from severe preeclampsia. At times it may be necessary to presume that the patient has preeclampsia and to proceed with delivery. Subsequent clinical remission of thrombocytopenia would suggest that preeclampsia was, indeed, the original problem.

Controversy surrounds the treatment of TTP. The disease is rare, and controlled trials of therapy are difficult to perform. Because platelets themselves have been implicated in the pathogenesis, platelet transfusions are usually discouraged. Various treatments have been used in TTP, including antiplatelet drugs [60], plasmapheresis [60,61], vincristine [62], exchange transfusions [63], and plasma infusions [64]. Optimal therapy for TTP remains to be defined.

Thrombocytopenia and Preeclampsia

Thrombocytopenia occurs in as many as 15% of patients with preeclampsia [55]. The mechanism causing this is unclear, but it may result from a selective intravascular consumption of platelets *without* a concurrent fibrinogen consumption. There is no specific therapy for the thrombocytopenia associated with preeclampsia other than early delivery. Interestingly, patients with preeclampsia and thrombocytopenia do not seem to have a worse prognosis than preeclamptic patients with a normal platelet count [65], although this observation is disputed by at least one author [53].

Acquired Bleeding Coagulopathies During Pregnancy

The coagulopathies acquired during pregnancy are not common; consequently, optimal management is usually not well defined. Often these problems present as catastrophes associated with delivery. Coagulopathies are present in half of maternal deaths due to hemorrhage [66]. The majority of acquired bleeding coagulopathies result from other conditions that induce a hemorrhagic diathesis. The diagnosis of a coagulopathy during pregnancy obligates the physician to look for a cause.

Preeclampsia and Eclampsia

In 2.6% of patients with preeclampsia and in 9.1% with eclampsia, there is evidence of disseminated intravascular coagulation (DIC) [67]. The clot-initiating site is the damaged vascular endothelium, especially on the arterial side. As discussed earlier, at times only a thrombocytopenia may be evident. Consumption of clotting factors may become apparent only by serial determinations of clotting factors such as factor VIII and fibrinogen. Isolated thrombocytopenia with preeclampsia or eclampsia may be difficult to distinguish from ITP or even TTP.

There is no proven benefit to the use of heparin for DIC or thrombocytopenia secondary to toxemia. The only effective treatment for the coagulopathy associated with preeclampsia or eclampsia is delivery. The contraction of the myometrium after delivery will help to control bleeding [68]. Excessive blood loss should be treated with red cells and plasma. If the patient is bleeding profusely and the platelet count is less than 50,000/mm^3, platelet transfusions are indicated.

Abruptio Placenta

In many obstetric practices, this is the most commonly encountered cause of severe coagulopathy. The fundamental coagulopathy is DIC, which is seen in 30 to 40% of patients with abruptio placenta [67]. The associated hemorrhage and often shock tend to propagate the coagulopathy. Treatment consists in restoration of blood volume and delivery. The administration of fibrinogen concentrates is not recommended. Oxytocin stimulation can be used to hasten delivery; however, when delivery is not imminent and the fetus is alive, cesarean delivery may be necessary to save the baby [68].

Amniotic Fluid Embolism

This is an uncommon but extremely serious problem encountered during labor, often presenting as sudden shock with cyanosis and respiratory distress. It appears that amniotic fluid entering the circulation triggers a consumptive coagulopathy. Stabilization of the blood volume should be accomplished with fresh whole blood or with packed cells, fresh frozen plasma, and, rarely, platelets. Some authors have also recommended the use of heparin [68]. Ventilatory support and careful central venous pressure monitoring are also necessary.

Prolonged Retention of a Dead Fetus

This is an uncommon consumptive coagulopathy that tends to develop over four to five weeks. Heparin may be useful in stopping coagulation and in allowing regeneration of clotting factors. Heparin can be given as an IV infusion of 1,000 units hourly for 24 to 48 hours until clotting factors are restored. After restoration of clotting factors, heparin can be stopped and oxytocin used to stimulate delivery of the dead fetus [68]. Delivery of the dead fetus is mandatory for definitive treatment of the coagulopathy.

Endotoxic Shock and Intrauterine Infection

The coagulopathy associated with endotoxic shock is DIC. Treatment of the underlying infection is the mainstay of therapy, but heparin may also be beneficial.

Congenital Coagulopathies During Pregnancy

Hemophilia A and B

These are sex-linked recessive hemorrhagic disorders. They rarely complicate pregnancy. Female carriers are virtually always asymptomatic. Recognition of the carrier state for hemophilia A is possible and is important for genetic counseling. The carrier state in hemophilia A can be defined by determining the ratio of factor VIII antigen to activity. Antenatal determination of fetal gender and fetal coagulation activity is available in some centers [69]. Recognition of the carrier state of hemophilia B is more difficult.

Von Willebrand's Disease

This disorder is transmitted as an autosomal dominant trait. Women may present with a pregestational history of excessive menstrual bleeding. Diagnosis in most patients is suggested by a prolonged bleeding time and a prolonged PTT. Further testing usually reveals a characteristic platelet aggregation defect to ristocetin and low factor VIII activity. Curiously, the hemorrhagic tendency in von Willebrand's disease may improve during pregnancy, as evidenced by rising factor VIII activity. Patients with von Willebrand's disease should be evaluated repeatedly during pregnancy. If factor VIII activity remains less than 50%, cryoprecipitate or fresh frozen plasma should be given at the onset of labor and should be repeated for four to five days post partum. Patients with von Willebrand's disease have an exaggerated and prolonged response to plasma transfusions, in contrast to hemophiliac patients. Factor VIII coagulant activity may increase for 24 to 48 hours after transfusion; the activity should be maintained at 50% during and immediately after delivery.

Since von Willebrand's disease is inherited in an autosomal dominant manner, there is a 50% chance that an affected mother will have an affected fetus. Antenatal detection of the disease has been described but it is not widely available. The authors of one report feel that vaginal delivery is contraindicated in von Willebrand's disease because of potential danger to the fetus [70]. No data were presented to support this concern, however. Other authors advocate vaginal delivery to minimize blood loss [68].

Hypercoagulability in Pregnancy

Acute venous thrombosis complicates 1 out of 70 pregnancies. The risk of thrombosis or embolism during pregnancy or the puerperium is 5.5 times greater than for the nonpregnant woman [71]. One author reported a 24% incidence of pulmonary embolism during the puerperium in untreated women with deep venous thrombosis; the incidence fell to 4.5% when anticoagulants were used. The incidence of thromboembolic death is ten times higher after cesarean delivery than after vaginal delivery. The risk of maternal death from pulmonary embolism is increased by age, multiparity, and obesity and in patients with blood groups other than type O. Pregnancy has also been associated with cerebral thrombophlebitis and the Budd-Chiari syndrome.

There are several possible factors to explain the increased risk of clotting during pregnancy. Increases have been reported in concentrations of fibrinogen and factors VII, VIII, X, and XII; and antithrombin III activity declines during the last trimester and post partum [72]. Other predisposing conditions to clotting in pregnancy include prolonged bed rest, sickle cell disease, and congestive heart failure [71].

For a complete discussion of the management of thromboembolic disease during pregnancy, the reader is referred to Chapter 14 as well as several other reviews [73–76].

REFERENCES

1. Levin J, Algazy KM. Hematologic disorders. In: Burrow GN, Ferris TF. Medical complications during pregnancy. Philadelphia: Saunders, 1975:689–737.
2. Peck TM, Arias F. Hematologic changes associated with pregnancy. Clin Obstet Gynecol. 1979; 22:785–98.
3. McFee JG. Iron metabolism and iron deficiency during pregnancy. Clin Obstet Gynecol. 1979; 22:799–808.
4. Cook JD, ed. Iron. New York: Churchill Livingstone, 1980:20.
5. Puolakka J, Janne O, Pakarinen A, Vihke R. Serum ferritin in the diagnosis of anemia during pregnancy. Acta Obstet Gynecol Scand [Suppl]. 1980; 95:57–63.
6. Pitkin RM, Witte DL. Platelet and leukocyte counts in pregnancy. JAMA. 1979; 242:2696–8.
7. Howie PW. Blood clotting and fibrinolysis in pregnancy. Postgrad Med J. 1979; 55:362–6.
8. Essien EM. Changes in antithrombin III levels in pregnancy, labour, and in women on the contraceptive pill. Afr J Med Sci. 1977; 6:109–13.
9. King PG, Huang AH, Palkuti HA, Farris VL. An evaluation of antithrombin III laboratory tests. Am J Clin Pathol. 1980; 73:537–40.
10. Puolakka J. Serum ferritin as a measure of iron stores

during pregnancy. Acta Obstet Gynecol Scand [Suppl]. 1980; 95:1–31.

11. Pritchard JA. Anemias complicating pregnancy and the puerperium. In: Maternal nutrition in the course of pregnancy. Washington, D.C.: National Academy of Sciences, 1970:74–109.

12. McFee JG. Anemia: A high risk complication of pregnancy. Clin Obstet Gynecol. 1973; 16:153–71.

13. Ward PC. Investigation of nonpoikilocytic normochromic normocytic anemia. Postgrad Med. 1979; 65:233–43.

14. Lillie EW. Obstetrical aspects of megaloblastic anaemia of pregnancy. J Obstet Gynaecol Br Comm. 1962; 69:736–8.

15. Herbert V. Diagnosing megaloblastic anemia. Med Times. 1982; 110:63–75.

16. Kitay DZ. Anemia. In: Queenan JT (ed). Management of high-risk pregnancy. Oradell N.J.: Medical Economics Co., 1980:245–54.

17. Jacobs A, Worwood M. Ferritin in serum. N Engl J Med. 1975; 292:951–6.

18. Ances IG, Granados J, Baltazar M. Serum ferritin as an early determinant of decreased iron stores in pregnant women. South Med J. 1979; 72:591–604.

19. De Alarcon PA, Donovan ME, Forbes GB, Landaw SA, Stockman JA. Iron absorption in the thalassemia syndromes and its inhibition by tea. N Engl J Med. 1979; 300:5–8.

20. Jaffe RM, Kasten B, Young DS, et al. False-negative stool occult blood tests caused by ingestion of ascorbic acid (vitamin C). Ann Intern Med. 1975; 83:824–6.

21. Carr MC. Iron deficiency. In: Queenan JT (ed). Management of high-risk pregnancy. Oradell N.J.: Medical Economics Co., 1980:255–61.

22. Goodlin RC. Perinatal report: is routine iron supplementation necessary during pregnancy? Nebr Med J. 1971; 66:3.

23. McCurdy PR. Anemia during pregnancy. Med Challenge. 1976; 8:66–75.

24. Taylor DJ. Prophylaxis and treatment of anaemia during pregnancy. Clin Obstet Gynecol. 1981; 8:297–314.

25. Crosby WH. Prescribing iron? Think small. Arch Intern Med. 1978; 138:616–7.

26. Seligman PA, Caskey JH, Frazier TL et al. Measurements of iron absorption from prenatal multi-mineral supplements. Obstet Gynecol. 1983; 61:356–62.

27. Gale RP, Champlin RE, Feig SA, Fitchen JH. Aplastic anemia: biology and treatment. Ann Intern Med. 1981; 95:477–94.

28. Sacks DA, Platt LD, Johnson CS. Autoimmune hemolytic disease during pregnancy. Am J Obstet Gynecol. 1981; 140:942–6.

29. Weinstein L. Irregular antibodies causing hemolytic disease of the newborn. Obstet Gynecol Surv. 1976; 31:581–91.

30. Bowman JM, Friesen RF. Rh isoimmunization. In: Goodwin JW, Godden JO, Chance GW, eds. Perinatal medicine. Baltimore: Williams & Wilkins, 1976:92–107.

31. Liley AW. Liquor amnii analysis in the management of the pregnancy complicated by rhesus sensitization. Am J Obstet Gynecol. 1961; 82:1359–70.

32. Swisher SN, Burka ER. Acquired hemolytic anemia due to warm-reacting autoantibodies. In: Williams WJ, Beutler E, Erslev AJ, Rundles RW, eds. Hematology. 2nd ed. New York: McGraw-Hill, 1977:585–96.

33. Scott RB, Castro O. Screening for sickle cell hemoglobinopathies. JAMA. 1979; 241:1145–7.

34. Zaino EC. Iatrogenic beta (β) thalassemia. JAMA. 1977; 238:342.

35. Seale TW, Rennert OM. Prenatal diagnosis of thalassemias and hemoglobinopathies. Ann Clin Lab Sci. 1980; 10:383–94.

36. Chang JC, Wai Kan Y. A sensitive new prenatal test for sickle-cell anemia. N Engl J Med. 1982; 307:30–2.

37. Jennings JC. Hemoglobinopathies in pregnancy. Am Fam Physician. 1977; 15:104–10.

38. Sears DA. The morbidity of sickle cell trait. Am J Med. 1978; 64:1021–36.

39. Pritchard JA, Scott DE, Whalley PH, et al. The effects of maternal sickle cell hemoglobinopathies and sickle cell trait on reproductive performance. Am J Obstet Gynecol. 1973; 117:662–70.

40. Blattner P, Dar H, Nitowsky HM. Pregnancy outcome in women with sickle cell trait. JAMA. 1977; 238:1392–4.

41. Morrison JC, Schneider JM, Whybrew WD, Bucovaz ET, Menzel DM. Prophylactic transfusions in pregnant patients with sickle hemoglobinopathies: benefit versus risk. Obstet Gynecol. 1980; 56:274–80.

42. Morrison JC, Propst MG, Blake PG. Sickle hemoglobin and the gravid patient: a management controversy. Clin Perinatol. 1980; 7:273–84.

43. Henderson AB, Potts EB, Burgess D, White F. Sickle-cell thalassemia disease and pregnancy: a case study. Am J Med Sci. 1962; 244:605–11.

44. Turner R. Hemoglobin C disease. Med Challenge. 1977; 9:28–35.

45. Davey RJ, Esposito DJ, Jacobson RJ, Corn M. Partial exchange transfusion as treatment for hemoglobin SC disease in pregnancy. Arch Intern Med. 1978; 138:937–9.

46. Alger LS, Golbus MS, Laros RK. Thalassemia and pregnancy: results of an antenatal screening program. Am J Obstet Gynecol. 1979; 134:662–73.

47. Lehmann H, Huntsman RS, Casey R, Lang A, Lorkin PA, Comings DE. Sickle cell disease and related disorders. In: Williams WJ, Beutler E, Erslev AJ, Rundles RW, eds. Hematology. 2nd ed. New York: McGraw-Hill, 1977:495–524.

48. Niell HB, Leach BE, Kraus AP. Zinc metabolism in sickle cell anemia. JAMA. 1979; 242:2686–7.

49. NIH consensus development conference summaries. Vol 2. 1979:17–20. Bethesda, Maryland.

50. Harris RE, Conrad FG. Polycythemia vera in the childbearing age. Arch Intern Med. 1967; 120:697–700.

51. Scott JR, Cruikshank DP, Kochenour NK, Pitkin RM, Warenski JC. Fetal platelet counts in the obstetric management of immunologic thrombocytopenic purpura. Am J Obstet Gynecol. 1980; 136:495–9.

52. Handin RI. Neonatal immune thrombocytopenia—the doctor's dilemma. N Engl J Med. 1981; 305:951–3.

53. Romero R, Duffy TP. Platelet disorders in pregnancy. Clin Perinatol. 1980; 7:327–8.

54. Carloss HW, McMillan R, Crosby WH. Management of pregnancy in women with immune thrombocytopenic purpura. JAMA. 1980; 244:2756–8.

55. Karpatkin M, Porges RF, Karpatkin S. Platelet counts in infants of women with autoimmune thrombocytopenia. N Engl J Med. 1981; 305:936–9.

56. Cines DB, Dusak B, Tomaski A, Mennuti M, Schreiber AD. Immune thrombocytopenic purpura and pregnancy. N Engl J Med. 1982; 306:826–31.

57. Rumack CM, Guggenheim MA, Rumack BH et al. Neonatal intracranial hemorrhage and maternal use of aspirin. Obstet and Gynecol [Suppl] 1981; 58: 52S–56S.

58. Goodman A, Ramos R, Petrelli M, Hirsch SA, Bukowski R, Harris JW. Gingival biopsy in thrombotic thrombocytopenic purpura. Ann Intern Med. 1978; 89:501–4.

59. Nalbandian RM, Henry RL, Bick RL. Thrombotic thrombocytopenic purpura. Semin Thromb Hemostas. 1979; 5:216–40.

60. Myers TJ, Wakem CJ, Ball ED, Tremont SJ. Thrombotic thrombocytopenic purpura: combined treatment with plasmapheresis and antiplatelet agents. Ann Intern Med. 1980; 92:149–55.

61. McLeod BC, Wu KK, Knospe WH. Plasmapheresis in thrombotic thrombocytopenic purpura. Arch Intern Med. 1980; 140:1059–60.

62. Gutterman LA, Stevenson TD. Treatment of thrombotic thrombocytopenic purpura with vincristine. JAMA. 1982; 247:1433–6.

63. Rossi EC, del Greco F, Kwaan HC, Lerman BC. Hemodialysis–exchange transfusion for treatment of thrombotic thrombocytopenic purpura. JAMA. 1980; 244:1466–8.

64. Walker BK, Ballas SK, Martinez J. Plasma infusion for thrombotic thrombocytopenic purpura during pregnancy. Arch Intern Med. 1980; 140:981–3.

65. Perkins RP. Thrombocytopenia in obstetric syndromes. A review. Obstet Gynecol Surv. 1979; 34:101–14.

66. Bonnar J. Haemostasis and coagulation disorders in pregnancy. In: Bloom AL, Thomas DP, eds. Haemostasis and thrombosis. New York: Churchill Livingstone, 1981:454–71.

67. Kuhn W, Graeff H. Coagulation problems in pregnancy. Contrib Nephrol. 1981; 25:78–84.

68. Hathaway WE, Bonnar J. Perinatal coagulation. In: Monographs in neonatology. New York: Grune & Stratton, 1978.

69. Hoyer LW, Carta CA, Mahoney MJ. Detection of hemophilia carriers during pregnancy. Blood. 1982; 60:1407–10.

70. Graeff H, Kuhn W. Coagulation disorders in obstetrics. Philadelphia: Saunders, 1980:104.

71. Kwaan HC, Gratkins LV. Thromboembolism in obstetrical patients. In: Kwaan HC, Bowie EJW. Thrombosis. Philadelphia: Saunders, 1982:158–74.

72. Conrad J. Inhibitors of blood coagulation. In: Thomson JM, ed. Blood coagulation and haemostasis. Edinburgh: Churchill Livingstone, 1980:220–1.

73. Hirsch J, Genton E, Hull R. Venous thromboembolism. New York: Grune & Stratton, 1981:145–51.

74. Stevenson RE, Burton OM, Ferlauto GJ, Taylor HA. Hazards of oral anticoagulants during pregnancy. JAMA. 1980; 243:1549–51.

75. Jespersen J. Termination of pregnancy in a woman with hereditary antithrombin deficiency under antithrombotic protection with subcutaneous heparin and infusion of plasma. Gynecol Obstet Invest. 1981; 12:267–71.

76. Pfeifer GW. The use of thrombolytic therapy in obstetrics and gynaecology. Australas Ann Med. 1970; 19 (Suppl):28–31.

In the final analysis, the question of why bad things happen to good people translates itself into some very different questions, no longer asking why something happened, but asking how we will respond, what we intend to do now that it has happened.
—Rabbi Harold Kushner
When Bad Things Happen to Good People

23. ONCOLOGIC DISEASE
William A. Robinson and Linda U. Krebs

Of all the complications of pregnancy, none can be more devastating to the expectant mother, her family, and her physician than the development of cancer. The very word conjures up visions of a cachectic, pain-racked, dying mother, a motherless child, and a grieving family. Although this is generally not a true picture, society and often various members of the health care team perceive the diagnosis of cancer as impending death, thus frustrating any rational approach to management. Cancer is the second leading cause of death in the United States. Most cancers occur in individuals over age 50 and therefore do not coincide with the childbearing years. Many cancers that do occur in young women (Hodgkin's disease, breast cancer, and the leukemias) are now curable or at least treatable. Skillful medical management of the pregnant woman with cancer can, in numerous cases, yield a healthy newborn and a mother in sufficiently good health to care for her child for years.

Equally important to medical management of a malignant disease is psychosocial support of the patient and her family. Many issues need to be addressed: treatment, prognosis, possible damage to the fetus, as well as physical limitations during the years of child rearing. Each of these issues requires much thought and will provoke all ranges of emotions from rage and anger to confusion and fear, and, it is hoped, in the end to acceptance and rational planning for the future.

If possible, a psychiatrist, psychologist, or social worker should be part of the health care team in order to provide emotional stability and support. If this is not a possibility, a physician or nurse should provide that focus and be available to answer questions with accurate information, anticipate problems, and comfort the family. Without strong emotional support neither the patient nor her family will be able to cope with the medical treatment and its potential side effects.

PATHOPHYSIOLOGY OF CANCER IN PREGNANCY
Effect of Pregnancy on Neoplastic Cell Growth
One might anticipate that the multiple physiologic changes occurring in the vascular, endocrine, and immune systems during pregnancy would have significant effects on the growth and development of neoplastic cells. It is clear that certain human neoplasms retain responsiveness to various physiologic influences. This is exemplified by the finding of estrogen- and progesterone-binding proteins in breast cancer tissue and by changes in the rate of neoplastic cell growth when estrogens are administered or withdrawn in patients with this malignant disease. To what extent the physiologic changes that occur during pregnancy alter neoplastic cell growth has not been fully determined. There is evidence, as will be seen under the discussion of specific neoplasms, that some cancers arising in pregnancy have a worse prognosis than similar cancers arising in nonpregnant women. Whether this finding simply represents delayed diagnosis, or that the changes occur in various body systems during pregnancy adversely affect the growth of neoplastic tissue is not entirely clear. Probably both factors are involved. Nevertheless, there is no evidence that termination of pregnancy in the presence of any neoplastic disease will stop or retard the growth of cancer once it has arisen.

Fetal Effects of Maternal Malignancy
The most dreadful complication that can occur in the pregnant woman with cancer is the concomitant development of cancer in the fetus [1–3]. Fortunately, this is a rare event. Rothman et al. reviewed 36 cases of placental and/or fetal involvement from maternal cancer [1]. Twenty-six of the cases had placental involvement. In 11 the fetus

had some evidence of neoplastic disease, and nine newborns died of malignancy. A wide variety of cancers were represented in the total group, including breast, gastric, ovarian, lung, and a malignant hepatoma. The only cases in which fetal, as opposed to placental, involvement occurred were those of malignant melanoma, leukemia, and lymphoma. The most common neoplasm with fetal involvement was malignant melanoma (6 of 11). There were two newborns with leukemia and lymphoma. All of these children died of metastatic disease.

Rothman et al. also reviewed the evidence concerning the usefulness of placental examination as a predictor of fetal involvement. Unfortunately, not all of the placentas were examined in detail, making generalizations difficult. In this series intervillous involvement, without invasion of the villi, was found in 15 of the 26 placentas examined. Despite the lack of villus invasion, two placentas were found to contain maternal malignant cells in capillaries, and in one of these cases the infant died of disseminated malignant melanoma. A further six placentas were found to have villus invasion but in only one case was the child affected, again in a mother with disseminated malignant melanoma. Thus, on the basis of these data, the predictive value of the presence or absence of villus invasion for determining fetal involvement is limited. The most important predictor appeared to be the type of malignancy and its stage.

It is interesting that the transmission of neoplastic disease from the mother to the offspring has not been reported more frequently, particularly in acute leukemia. Maternal transmission of blood cells, including leukocytes, has been well demonstrated. Rothman and his colleagues speculated that "the rare cases of fetal dissemination of malignant disease could be isolated examples of acquired antigen tolerance in which the fetuses were exposed to maternal tumor antigen prior to immunologic competence and as a result did not recognize the maternal tumor cells as a foreign antigen to be rejected" [1]. This indeed seems to be the most likely explanation but does not account for the large number of cases in which leukemia has been diagnosed during early pregnancy without transmission to the fetus.

In addition to direct involvement of the fetus by maternal neoplasia, the concomitant development of cancer in pregnancy may lead to a high incidence of fetal wastage and growth retardation [4–6]. This is obviously most prevalent in malignancies that are widespread. When a cancer is localized, such as breast cancer confined to the breast, there is often little or no effect on the fetus. On the other hand, when the neoplasm is disseminated, such as acute leukemia or widespread malignant melanoma, spontaneous abortions and preterm birth are common [4].

GENERAL PRINCIPLES OF CANCER TREATMENT
Chemotherapy
One of the most frequently asked questions, and one of the most difficult to answer, is "What are the effects of chemotherapy and radiation therapy on the development of the fetus?" Some answers are currently available [7]. The majority of chemotherapeutic agents act on dividing cells. Since the fetus contains a high proportion of dividing cells, one would anticipate significant effects of such drugs on the developing embryo and the potential for long-term side effects in later life. What is also clear, however, is that the DNA repair mechanisms in developing embryos are extremely competent and may rapidly repair chromosomal injuries that have occurred. A large number of case reports have appeared in the literature in which pregnant patients have been given chemotherapy during all stages of pregnancy [4–6,8–16]. The most extensive review of the subject is by Nicholson, who collected reports of 185 cases of pregnant women treated with chemotherapy [15]. Of 85 women who received cancer drugs in the first trimester, 15 had fetal abnormalities. The most commonly implicated drugs were the folic acid antagonists (10 patients). Alkylating agents (busulfan, cyclophosphamide, chlorambucil) were implicated in four others, and one patient had received 6-mercaptopurine. No fetal abnormalities were reported in 75 pregnant women who received cancer chemotherapy during the second or third trimester. From this and other studies it is quite clear that the administration of certain cancer chemotherapeutic agents, particularly the folic acid antagonists such as methotrexate, the alkylating agents, and cytosine arabinoside, may result in significant fetal abnormalities when given during the first trimester [7,16,17] (Table 23-1). In addition to the Nicholson study, there are many case reports of pregnant women receiving multidrug chemotherapy for a wide variety of neoplasms during the second and third trimesters of pregnancy without fetal abnormalities. It is our feeling, based on the available data, that the risk of fetal abnormalities resulting from chemotherapy administered during the first 20 weeks of pregnancy is unacceptable. We recommend therapeutic abortion for all patients who require the administration of any chemotherapeutic agent during this time. For most

*Table 23-1. Cancer chemotherapy
drugs associated with fetal anomalies*

Drugs	Trimester	Abnormalities
Folic acid antagonists Methotrexate Aminopterin	First	Hydrocephalus, cleft palate, skeletal mal- formations
Alkylating agents Cyclophosphamide Busulfan Chlorambucil	First	Skeletal malfor- mations, spon- taneous abor- tion
Antimetabolites 6-Mercaptopurine Cytosine arabinoside	First	Skeletal malfor- mations, spon- taneous abor- tion
Procarbazine	First	Atrial septal defect

patients in the second twenty weeks of pregnancy the dangers do not seem excessively great, and they can probably be treated without fear of significant fetal anomalies.

It must be remembered, however, that the long-term effects of cancer chemotherapy on offspring exposed in utero have not been determined. Absolutely no assurance can as yet be given that the birth of a child exposed in utero to chemotherapy will have continued normal growth and development [18]. In recent years there have been numerous reports of the development of second neoplasms, particularly acute leukemia, after the administration of cancer chemotherapy particularly when combined with radiation therapy [19]. These second neoplasms can appear years after the initial cancer treatment. Thus, it is important that children born under this circumstance be examined at regular intervals throughout their lives. The total incidence of this problem has yet to be determined.

Besides the potential effect of cancer treatment on fetal development, the effects of such treatment on the hematopoietic, immune, and other systems of both mother and fetus must be considered. The major complication of most cancer chemotherapy is hematopoietic cell suppression, with resultant anemia, leukopenia, and thrombocytopenia. Moreover, each individual chemotherapeutic agent may have other unique side effects, which must be familiar to the chemotherapist and obstetrician. No simple guidelines can be given for dealing with these side effects, but they must be searched for throughout the course of treatment. Anemia in the mother will require blood transfusion to prevent

fetal underdevelopment, and prophylactic platelet transfusions may be necessary to prevent bleeding. The white blood cell count must also be monitored continually during the course of therapy. Fever accompanying leukopenia should be presumed to be the result of a bacterial infection. When this occurs, appropriate cultures must be obtained and the patient put on broad-spectrum antibiotics without awaiting culture results. Many patients receiving chemotherapy will require continuous hospitalization throughout the course of their treatment to prevent or combat the side effects of chemotherapy. Further, at the time of delivery, the newborn infant should be immediately evaluated with a complete blood count (CBC) for effects of the chemotherapeutic agents on the hematopoietic system. Several cases of blood cell suppression in infants born in this situation have been noted [20].

Radiation Therapy

Like chemotherapy, radiation of any kind has its major effect on rapidly dividing cells and has potentially deleterious effects on the developing fetus [7]. Ample laboratory and clinical data support the fear of any form of radiation therapy during pregnancy, and it should be avoided if at all possible. Radiation of mouse embryos in therapeutic dosages during the early stages of development results in a broad spectrum of congenital anomalies, particularly of the nervous system. Occasionally radiation to localized areas (e.g., brain metastases) may be necessary and indicated to save the life of the mother. This can usually be accomplished with appropriate fetal shielding. A complete discussion of the effects of radiation during pregnancy is presented in Chapter 8.

Transfusion of Blood
and Blood Products

Many of the neoplastic diseases and the treatments discussed here will necessitate the use of multiple red cell, platelet, and perhaps white blood cell transfusions, imparting the risk of isoimmunization. Every effort should be made to ensure donor compatibility for all transfused blood products. Single donors, particularly for platelets, should be used whenever possible. Modern blood banking techniques and the use of plateletpheresis make this procedure both possible and desirable.

White blood cell (WBC) transfusions have been used with increasing frequency in recent years to treat infected leukopenic patients who have not responded to antibiotic therapy. The efficacy of white blood cell transfusions in this setting is debatable. Their administration has been associated with a high incidence of pulmonary infiltrates and interstitial pneumonitis [21]. Some authors feel that the risks of WBC transfusions outweigh the benefit. We do not recommend their use in pregnant women except when a life-threatening infection has clearly not responded to all other treatment. In the unusual instance in which WBC transfusion is indicated, the best donor would be an identical twin, a sibling, or a parent, in that order.

SPECIFIC NEOPLASTIC DISEASES
Breast Cancer and Pregnancy

Several reviews of this subject are available [22–25]. Breast cancer is the most common cancer in females between the ages of 25 and 74, and the most common cancer to complicate pregnancy. Studies by White have shown that 1 out of every 35 women presenting with breast cancer is pregnant at the time of diagnosis [26]. If one considers only women in the reproductive years, however, the incidence is considerably higher; that is, one in three women presenting with breast cancer is pregnant at the time of diagnosis. Conversely, breast cancer will develop in only 1 in 10,000 pregnant women.

The effect of pregnancy on the development and progression of breast cancer is unclear at the present time. Probably, however, the hormonal changes that occur during pregnancy have significant effects on certain breast cancers. From a wide variety of clinical and laboratory evidence, it is clear that some mammary carcinoma cells retain responsiveness to estrogen and progesterone, both of which increase dramatically during pregnancy. Data regarding the presence or absence of estrogen-binding receptors in breast cancers arising during pregnancy are not yet available. What is clear is that the overall prognosis for women in whom breast cancer develops during pregnancy is poorer than for nonpregnant women. Part of the explanation for this observation is that breast cancer in young women, pregnant or not, usually has a worse prognosis [22]. Potential exacerbating factors include increased vascular and lymphatic permeability, changes in immune status during pregnancy, and delay in diagnosis. It does not appear that breast cancers arising in pregnancy are more malignant or aggressive on the basis of different histologic types. They are similar to those arising in nonpregnant females. The majority are infiltrating ductal carcinomas.

Perhaps one of the most important reasons for the poor prognosis of breast cancer in pregnant women is delayed diagnosis. Applewhite et al. esti-

mated that in pregnant or lactating women there was an 11-month delay before the seeking of medical attention for a breast lump compared to four months in other women [27]. The enlargement of the breast during pregnancy and lactation makes diagnosis more difficult. It is our strong feeling that any lump in the breast must be evaluated until a satisfactory diagnosis is made. Early diagnosis and removal of mammary carcinoma remains the most important factor in cure. If there is any doubt about whether a lump is present, mammography should be done, with appropriate fetal shielding. Any lump present for three weeks should be biopsied.

Once the diagnosis of breast cancer is established, treatment should be initiated without delay. For those patients with stage I disease (primary less than 2 cm in diameter) and clinically negative nodes, a simple mastectomy should be done with an axillary node biopsy. If the nodes are negative, no further therapy is indicated until after delivery, when local radiation should be considered. For patients with stage II disease, or those in whom axillary nodes are positive for metastatic disease, treatment becomes more complex. The initial treatment, carried out promptly, should be a modified radical mastectomy. Difficulty arises because of the increasing evidence of the benefit of adjuvant chemotherapy in premenopausal women after surgical removal of all evidence of disease [28]. Such therapy decreases recurrence rates and appears to confer a significant survival advantage. The most commonly employed regimen includes a combination of cyclophosphamide, methotrexate, and 5-fluorouracil (5-FU). Two of these drugs, methotrexate and 5-FU, have been associated with significant fetal abnormalities when given during the first trimester of pregnancy [7,16,29]. For this reason, we advise therapeutic abortion for women requiring treatment in the first 20 weeks of pregnancy. In the latter half of pregnancy, chemotherapy with these drugs may be given as in the nonpregnant patient. Radiation therapy to prevent local recurrence is not indicated for women with stage II disease. Such treatment does not result in any survival advantage and can be given when, and if, local recurrence arises. For patients presenting with advanced or metastatic disease at diagnosis, tissue must be obtained from either the primary site or metastatic deposits to determine estrogen- and progesterone-binding status. For patients who have positive estrogen- or progesterone-binding tumors, endocrine manipulation alone should be undertaken until term. For patients whose estrogen-binding status is unknown or negative, a regimen including Adriamycin should be instituted.

An exception to this would be the patient who is near term and can be considered for early delivery and postpartum chemotherapy.

The overall prognosis of patients presenting with breast cancer during pregnancy is poor. In one series 75% of such patients had positive axillary nodes at the time of diagnosis [24]. More recent evidence has suggested that with earlier diagnosis and treatment the outcome may not be as poor as initially reported. The overall five-year survival reported by Peters was 30% [30]. When she compared pregnant with nonpregnant patients matched for age and tumor size, the outcome was the same, showing the need for early diagnosis of any breast lump discovered during pregnancy.

A difficult question is whether the patient in whom breast cancer develops during pregnancy should be allowed to become pregnant again [31]. An important factor in counseling such a patient is the interval after the initial cancer and the presence or absence of axillary metastases. Most breast cancers recur within the first two years after diagnosis. Patients with negative axillary nodes at the time of diagnosis should be cautioned not to become pregnant for three years after the initial diagnosis. For patients with positive axillary nodes, this time should be extended to five years. Such patients are at risk not only for the development of recurrence of their initial cancer but also for the development of a second cancer in the remaining breast. For patients who choose to become pregnant again, a mammogram of the remaining breast, and careful physical examination, should be obtained prior to pregnancy.

Hodgkin's Disease

Hodgkin's disease is largely an illness of young adults and affects women during their reproductive years. The association between pregnancy and Hodgkin's disease is, however, uncommon, with less than 150 cases reported in the literature. The subject has been reviewed by Jacobs et al. [32] and Thomas and Peckham [33]. Hodgkin's disease in young women most often presents as cervical or supraclavicular lymphadenopathy discovered by physical examination or as mediastinal lymph node enlargement on a routine chest roentgenogram. Diagnosis is established by biopsy. When Hodgkin's disease is discovered in a pregnant woman, there is no evidence to suggest that therapeutic abortion is beneficial in preventing progression of the disease.

Once the diagnosis of Hodgkin's disease is established, limited staging should be undertaken. In stage I, the disease is confined to a single lymph node region. In stage II, two or more lymphatic areas on the same side of the diaphragm are involved. In stage III, there is involvement of lymphatic tissue on both sides of the diaphragm. In stage IV, it has spread beyond lymphatic tissue to other organs. The spleen and Waldeyer's ring are considered part of the lymphatic system. Further, patients are subclassified depending on the absence (A) or presence (B) of symptoms (fever, night sweats, or weight loss).

Recommendations for staging include a detailed physical examination, roentgenogram of the chest, liver function tests, and bone marrow aspiration and biopsy. Radionuclide scans are generally not recommended in pregnant patients. The treatment will be based on the stage of the disease and stage of gestation. An approach to the management of Hodgkin's disease during pregnancy is outlined in Figure 23-1. This approach is based on the detailed recommendation of Jacobs et al. [32].

Patients prior to 20 weeks' gestation should be encouraged to have a therapeutic abortion. Jacobs suggests that the only exception to this rule might be the woman with stage IA, nonbulky disease in the neck or axilla, who can be given a limited dose of radiation therapy. During the last half of the pregnancy, if the patient has clinical stage IA or IIA supradiaphragmatic disease, Jacobs recommends postponing treatment until post partum. Delivery should be as soon as possible after 33 weeks. In patients with the same stages who are symptomatic or in whom there is rapidly progressive disease, radiation therapy with appropriate shielding should be undertaken. For patients with more advanced disease (stages IIIA, IIIB, IVA, and IVB) Jacobs recommends chemotherapy with a single drug, vinblastine, until delivery can be accomplished. Chemotherapy with Mustargen, Oncovin, prednisone and procarbazine hydrochloride (MOPP) has been given in a few cases without adverse effects [9,34]; however, the individual drugs in this combination have been associated with fetal anomalies while vinblastine has not. More intensive therapy can be given post partum. According to the findings of Jacobs and her colleagues, and other reports in the literature, the long-term prognosis for patients who acquire Hodgkin's disease during pregnancy is not significantly different from that of nonpregnant patients with comparable stage disease. The majority of such patients will be cured and lead long, useful lives.

The Non-Hodgkin's Lymphomas

The non-Hodgkin's lymphomas (NHL) are a heterogeneous group of disorders with variable clinical manifestations and prognoses, as well as a bewildering array of names. They have in common only

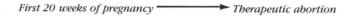

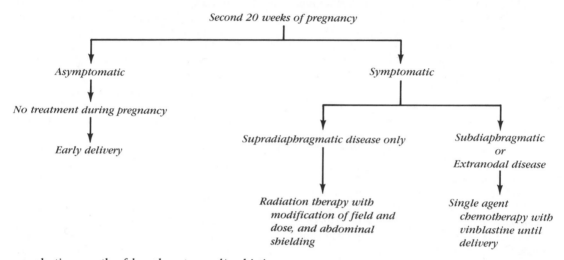

Fig. 23-1. Recommended management of the pregnant patient with Hodgkin's disease. (Modified from Jacobs et al. [32].)

neoplastic growth of lymphocytes and/or histiocytes. Unlike Hodgkin's disease, most NHLs are widespread at diagnosis, and although most respond well to initial treatment, cure is unlikely. Most NHLs occur in older persons and are uncommon in pregnancy. Falkson et al. reviewed the world's literature before 1980 and found only 13 cases plus one of their own [35]. Recommendations for staging and treatment of a pregnant woman with NHL will depend considerably on the histologic type of disease; thus, expert guidance in subclassifying the type of lymphoma is absolutely essential. For the least aggressive forms of NHL (e.g., nodular, lymphocytic lymphoma), previous studies in nonpregnant patients have shown no benefit of early treatment in prolonging survival. Patients may not require any treatment until after delivery. It is of interest, however, that most of the cases reported in pregnancy have been the more aggressive forms. Of the 14 cases reviewed by Falkson et al., 11 had histiocytic lymphoma, and one each had Burkitt's lymphoma, mixed histiocytic-lymphocytic lymphoma, and diffuse convoluted lymphoblastic lymphoma. All of these portend a poor prognosis, although recent years have seen increasing long-term survival for patients with histiocytic lymphomas.

Unlike Hodgkin's disease, NHL will usually show multiple areas of involvement at the time of diagnosis. Thus the extensive staging done in Hodgkin's disease is not so essential for patients with NHL. Since these diseases are widespread, the treatment is primarily chemotherapy. Patients found to have an aggressive type of NHL (e.g., histiocytic lymphoma) during the first 20 weeks

should be advised to have therapeutic abortion. Most drug protocols for the treatment of NHL impart a high risk of teratogenesis when used during organogenesis.

Three final words of caution are in order. First, the placenta and infant must be carefully evaluated for evidence of lymphoma, since involvement of each has been reported [1–3]. Second, back pain in a patient with lymphoma is always a cause for alarm for it is frequently the earliest sign of spinal cord or nerve root involvement [36]. Persistent back pain in such a patient must be carefully and continually evaluated. Since back pain is such a common complaint during pregnancy, myelography may be necessary to confirm neurologic involvement. Finally, patients with NHL should be urged not to become pregnant again. There is no evidence that the diseases are adversely affected by pregnancy, but the long-term prognosis for most patients is poor; despite treatment, most will ultimately relapse and succumb to their disease.

Malignant Melanoma
The incidence of this neoplasm has risen dramatically in the United States in the past 20 years. Malignant melanomas most frequently develop in preexisting moles. In pregnant women, melanomas are most often found in truncal areas, including the shoulders and back. Any change in a mole occurring during pregnancy should be a sig-

nal for alarm to the obstetrician and requires immediate biopsy.

The effects of hormonal changes associated with pregnancy on the development of melanoma have been studied by several investigators [37,38]. Perhaps most intriguing is the possible relationship between melanocyte-stimulating hormone (MSH) and the development of malignant melanoma. In individuals who are able to acquire a suntan, exposure to ultraviolet radiation leads to darkening of the skin, with subsequent suppression of MSH. In contrast, individuals who are unable to develop melanotic changes in the skin have unopposed and constant stimulation of MSH, which continuously acts on the few melanin-producing cells in the body: those present in preexisting moles. It has been suggested that this unopposed and continuous stimulation of MSH may be involved in the development of melanoma. If this hypothesis is valid, pregnancy with the attendant rise in MSH would predictably have a potentiating effect on the development and growth of a malignant melanoma.

Fair-skinned women who are at high risk for the development of malignant melanoma should be observed carefully by their physicians throughout pregnancy and cautioned to limit ultraviolet exposure. Patients should be advised to note any change in preexisting moles and to call it to the attention of a physician. When the diagnosis of melanoma is made, therapy should be instituted without delay. This includes a wide local excision and perhaps regional lymph node dissection.

The prognosis for patients in whom malignant melanoma develops during pregnancy has been reported to be worse than for nonpregnant women [39,40]. Data from the Connecticut Tumor Registry revealed 12 patients with melanomas that developed during pregnancy [40]. These patients were compared with 175 nonpregnant controls. Five-year survival for pregnant women was 55% compared to 83% for controls. The investigators attributed this difference to the fact that melanomas occurring in pregnancy tended to appear most often on the trunk, a prognostically poor site, and at a more advanced stage of disease than in nonpregnant women. When they compared pregnant patients to nonpregnant controls matched by age, anatomic site of primary lesion, and stage at diagnosis, the three- and five-year survivals were not significantly different. Somewhat conflicting data have been reported by Shaw et al. from the Sydney Hospital in Australia [41]. In their study, pregnant women were actually seen at an earlier stage of the disease than nonpregnant controls and had a better five-year survival rate than nonpregnant controls. This may be due to the fact that melanoma is relatively common in Australia and has received considerable attention. The effect of widespread knowledge about the development of the disease and earlier diagnosis probably has a favorable effect on outcome.

Houghton et al. concluded their recent article with the recommendation that women who acquired malignant melanoma during pregnancy not be allowed to become pregnant again for at least several years after the diagnosis of their primary melanoma [40]. In addition, these authors suggest that such patients not receive oral contraceptives because of the potential effect of estrogens on the development of melanoma. We agree with these recommendations.

Treatment of advanced or metastatic melanoma presents a considerably more difficult problem and fortunately a rare one. The benefit of chemotherapy in metastatic melanoma is marginal at best, and never curative. The most effective single drug is imidazole carboxamide (DTIC), with reported response rates of 20 to 30% in nonpregnant patients. More recent multidrug combinations produce similar results. We advise therapeutic abortion for patients in the first 20 weeks of pregnancy. For patients in the last half of pregnancy we suggest postponement of chemotherapy and early delivery unless life-threatening complications arise. In melanoma these most frequently occur because of brain metastases, which can be treated by local radiation rather than chemotherapy. Other complications must be dealt with individually, but it should be remembered that the patients have an extremely poor prognosis with or without treatment. Aggressive therapy is not indicated in the hope of curing the mother. Finally, in women with melanoma the placenta and newborn should be examined carefully for the presence of metastatic disease. Several cases of melanoma in the newborn have been reported [1,3].

Acute Leukemia

More than 300 cases of acute leukemia (myeloid and lymphoblastic) have been reported during pregnancy [4–6,10,42–46]. This combination represents a special problem, for despite many recent advances in the treatment of the adult acute leukemias they remain, for the most part, rapidly fatal illnesses with median survivals of one year or less. To quote Lilleyman et al., "Unless survival times improve dramatically, children born in this situation will soon be motherless and it could be argued that termination of pregnancy on humanitarian and social grounds alone is justifiable if requested by the parents in full knowledge of their situation" [4].

Lilleyman and colleagues reviewed the literature on this subject up to 1977 and discussed in detail 32 cases of acute leukemia complicating pregnancy [4]. They concluded that there is a slightly less than 50% chance of delivering a healthy live baby in this situation. Further, of these 32 cases, 26 of the mothers were dead within seven months following delivery, 12 within two weeks. The fate of four was unknown, and of the total group only two were alive at the time of his report. More recent reports have been more encouraging, but the overall outlook must remain extremely guarded.

Fortunately, the acute leukemias are rare illnesses. Together with the lymphomas, however, they are the major cause of cancer-related deaths in women between the ages of 15 and 35. Acute lymphoblastic leukemia (ALL) is largely a disease of children and in childhood has a relatively good prognosis following treatment. In adults, however, the prognosis is poor. Most patients succumb to the disease within two years. The most common leukemia in young adults is acute myeloid or acute nonlymphocytic leukemia (ANLL). There are many subvarieties that have little prognostic or therapeutic significance. Most nonpregnant patients (approximately 70%) can achieve a remission with present-day chemotherapy, but more than 90% will relapse and die of leukemia within two years.

The diagnosis of acute leukemia is usually not difficult. The major clinical manifestations result from a lack of normal blood formation, resulting in anemia, thrombocytopenia, and leukopenia. Thus, the patient presents with fatigue, bleeding, purpura and petechiae, fever, and infection. Diagnosis is confirmed by bone marrow aspiration and biopsy. Unlike many of the other diseases discussed in this chapter, acute leukemia is rapidly fatal if left untreated—within a few weeks at most and frequently days. Thus, a therapeutic plan must be decided upon quickly if the life of the mother is to be spared. Initial treatment, once the diagnosis is established, should be aimed at life-threatening complications from the hematopoietic dysfunction. Red blood cells should be given to correct the anemia. If the platelet count is less than 10,000/mm^3 or the patient has any evidence of bleeding, platelet transfusions should be given on a daily or every-other-day basis. Any temperature elevation above 38°C should be considered a sign of infection and broad-spectrum antibiotics started immediately after taking blood and other appropriate cultures, but without waiting for the culture results. Serum uric acid level should be measured and allopurinol given by mouth to correct hyperuricemia. Perirectal abscess is a major complication in acute leukemia, and all rectal insertions, probes, and thermometers should be avoided.

If the mother is in the first 20 weeks of pregnancy, therapeutic abortion immediately upon diagnosis is strongly advised. The current multidrug chemotherapy regimens used to treat acute leukemia undoubtedly have major effects on the developing fetus, and the chance for spontaneous abortion or fetal abnormalities is high [4,5,7,17]. In addition, chemotherapy for acute leukemia initially results in further suppression of all peripheral blood cell counts, compounding the complications of bleeding and infection noted previously.

For patients in the second twenty weeks of pregnancy, the risk of fetal abnormalities resulting from administration of chemotherapy does not appear to be high [5–7,42,43,45,46]. No overall estimate can be given, but there are many instances of healthy children born to mothers given multidrug chemotherapy after the twentieth week of gestation. The greatest risk appears to be fetal death. Of the 32 cases reported by Lilleyman et al., eight had spontaneous abortions or stillbirths. Another six patients had premature live infants, one of whom died within 12 hours.

A number of effective chemotherapy regimens for ANLL are currently in use. Most employ a combination of cytosine arabinoside, 6-thioguanine, and daunorubicin or adriamycin. Once the decision to treat has been made, chemotherapy should be started promptly with full dosages similar to those employed in nonpregnant patients. Treatment will probably entail continuous hospitalization until delivery, with scrupulous attention to the recognition and management of the numerous complications that may arise.

Most chemotherapy drugs cross the placenta. Immediately following delivery the hematologic status of the neonate should be determined, particularly if the interval between the last administration of drugs and delivery was within three weeks. The newborn should also be checked for the presence of leukemia. Maternal-fetal transmission of leukemia has been reported, but this appears to be a rare complication.

Chronic Lymphoid Leukemia

Chronic lymphoid leukemia (CLL) is largely a disease of the elderly although a few cases associated with pregnancy have been reported [43]. Early treatment is usually unnecessary in CLL, and therapy should be withheld, in most instances, until after delivery. Indications for treatment include severe systemic symptoms (fever, weight loss), the development of autoimmune hemolytic anemia or thrombocytopenia, recurrent infections, and impingement by lymphatic tissue on vital organs. An elevated white blood cell count, even above 100,000, or simple lymphadenopathy is not by itself an indication for treatment. If therapy is necessary, it should be started with chlorambucil and prednisone, but only in the second 20 weeks of pregnancy. Patients seen before 20 weeks who require treatment should be advised to have a therapeutic abortion for reasons cited earlier. It is important to note that most patients with CLL have associated hypogammaglobulinemia and are particularly prone to the development of various kinds of infections. There is no evidence that administration of gamma globulin is beneficial in preventing infections, and its use cannot be routinely recommended. It has not been determined, however, whether maternal hypogammaglobulinemia leads to any degree of depressed immunity in the neonate. Neonatal gamma globulin levels should be measured at birth and infection in both the infant and mother searched for by appropriate means.

Chronic Myeloid Leukemia

Chronic myeloid leukemia (CML) occurs in women with a median age of 35, therefore falling well into the childbearing years. It accounts for approximately 50% of all leukemias complicating pregnancy [43]. CML differs from acute leukemia in that early and aggressive treatment with chemotherapy does not influence survival or outcome; most patients live approximately four years with minimal therapy. The disease terminates by the development of acute leukemia or so-called blast crisis, for which there is no effective treatment. The drug most commonly used to treat CML is the aklylating agent busulfan [7]. Severe congenital defects have been reported in viable infants of mothers treated with busulfan. The risk of teratogenesis combined with the evidence that delay in treatment of CML does not reduce or alter survival leads us to recommend withholding chemotherapy until after delivery. Exceptions to this advice are patients with extremely high WBC count (greater than 250,000), who are in danger of vascular "sludging" and cerebral problems, and those with early evidence of metamorphosis to acute leukemia (blast crisis). The former should be treated only with periodic leukopheresis until the WBC count is maintained below 100,000. Those developing blast crisis should be treated in a manner similar to that for acute leukemia.

GYNECOLOGIC MALIGNANCIES
Vulvar Cancer

Invasive cancer of the vulva occurring during pregnancy is an extremely rare event with less than 50 cases reported. The majority of these are epidermoid carcinomas, and the patients range in age from 25 to 35. Therapy during the first trimester does not differ from therapy in the nonpregnant patient, a radical vulvectomy and bilateral superficial and deep groin node dissection being the common mode of treatment. It is suggested, however, that this therapy be done preferably after the fourteenth week of pregnancy [47]. Barber states that during the second trimester the therapy will need to be tailored to the size of the uterus; it may be possible to do only the radical vulvectomy, waiting until the postpartum period to do the groin dissection [48]. During the third trimester, it may be best either to defer surgery if the lesion is small [48], or to perform a wide local excision if the lesion is larger [47]. In both cases definitive therapy is carried out post partum. In all pregnancies associated with a vulvar malignancy vaginal delivery is indicated unless there is postsurgical scarring, obstetric contraindication, or a lesion that might interfere with delivery [47].

Vaginal Cancer

Vaginal cancer occurring during pregnancy is also uncommon, with few cases reported in the literature. It is recommended by DiSaia and Creasman that early lesions involving the upper half of the vagina (with or without cervical involvement) discovered during the first trimester or early second trimester be treated by radical hysterectomy, upper vaginectomy, and bilateral pelvic lymphadenectomy, followed by postoperative chemotherapy [47]. In the late second and third trimesters it is possible to successfully reach term with a small lesion. However, for an extensive lesion evacuation of the uterus by hysterotomy or cesarean delivery followed by standard therapy certainly should be considered.

Jones et al. reported a case of DES-related clear cell carcinoma diagnosed in a woman 16 weeks pregnant; malignant cells had been noted by Pap smear at nine weeks [49]. The woman refused therapy at that time. She was observed clinically with frequent pelvic examinations until cesarean delivery was performed at 36 weeks. Immediately following cesarean delivery, the patient underwent a radical hysterectomy, bilateral pelvic lymphadenectomy, and total vaginectomy. She and her child are alive and well without evidence of disease at 72 months.

Cervical Cancer

Carcinoma of the cervix is the fourth most common malignancy in women. The incidence is approximately 20,000 cases of invasive cancer per year and accounts for two-thirds of all cancers of the female genital tract. The average age of patients with invasive cancer at diagnosis is 45 years. Most patients who are pregnant at the time of diagnosis have carcinoma in situ (CIS) rather than invasive disease; indeed, the peak incidence of carcinoma in situ of the cervix nearly coincides with the most active childbearing years. This form of cervical cancer is as common in pregnant females as in nonpregnant females [50].

Invasive cervical cancer is relatively rare during pregnancy. Graham et al. determined a worldwide prevalence for invasive cervical cancer of 0.04% in 504,000 pregnancies [51]. The percentage of patients with invasive cancer who were pregnant at the time of diagnosis varied between 1 and 5% [51]. In a series reported by Creasman et al. the mean age was 33, and 60% of the patients were diagnosed as stage I or II [52]. Symptoms tended to be the same as those found in the nonpregnant woman, vaginal bleeding being the most common. However, 30% of the patients had no symptoms at the time of diagnosis [52].

The diagnosis of cervical cancer in the pregnant female is made in exactly the same way as it is made in the nonpregnant woman. When the Pap smear has been reported to be dysplastic or a lesion can be seen, the diagnosis should be confirmed by cervical biopsy. If possible, colposcopy-directed cervical biopsies should be done, followed by staging to determine the extent of the disease. For details of the diagnosis, staging, and treatment of cervical cancer complicating pregnancy, see the excellent article by Green [50].

The treatment of CIS of the cervix in pregnancy is well described by Fowler et al. from the Dysplasia Clinic at North Carolina Memorial Hospital [53]. In general, if there was no evidence of invasion and the extent of the lesion could be clearly seen, the patients were followed until term and allowed to deliver vaginally. Treatment was undertaken post partum. In the series by Fowler et al. 84 of the original 109 patients have been followed for 2 to 114 months post partum, none has had recurrent disease, but two have had persistent disease. Treatment consisted of conization, cryosurgery, hysterectomy, electrocautery, biopsy only, or no further therapy [47,50,53].

Cone biopsy has been a topic of much discussion; the issues of bleeding and premature delivery are the prime concern. Green feels that conization after the twelfth week and before the third trimester is the treatment of choice for CIS of the cervix [50]. He reported five cases of CIS during pregnancy, all of whom are alive, well, and free of disease 7 to 13 years after diagnosis. DiSaia and Creasman [47] state that cone biopsy should be used only when a microinvasive lesion is found and frank invasion must be ruled out, and Fowler et al. used the cone biopsy only when there was a marked discrepancy between cytology, colposcopic findings, and biopsy results. None of the 13 patients with cone biopsy in the latter series required blood transfusion although one patient did deliver prematurely [53].

For patients with clinically invasive cancer, much controversy exists over the appropriate form of therapy—surgery or radiation [47,48,50, 55–57]. Green favors radical surgery and suggests that patients in their first 20 weeks of pregnancy have a radical hysterectomy plus pelvic lymphadenectomy with the fetus in utero [50]. For patients in the second half of pregnancy, the radical hysterectomy and pelvic lymphadenectomy should be preceded by a hysterotomy or, when near term, a cesarean delivery. Many other authorities argue for radiation therapy and suggest that in the first 20 weeks abortion not be induced but allowed to come about as the result of external radiation therapy [54,56,57]. For those in the last 20 weeks of pregnancy, radiation should be preceded by hysterotomy (or if near term, a cesarean delivery). Following external radiation, internal radiation with colpostats and tandem is completed. In early stages, it appears that radiation therapy and surgery have equal survival rates; however, many physicians argue for radical surgery because of the possible late effects of radiation therapy [48].

Controversy exists over the issue of vaginal delivery versus cesarean delivery, which has been discussed by many authors [47,57]. Some authors suggest that patients who deliver vaginally have a better survival rate than those having cesarean delivery, but major concern has been raised because of the possibility of bleeding, infection, or dissemination of the cancer from vaginal delivery [47,57].

Of prime importance in cervical carcinoma associated with pregnancy is early diagnosis and prompt treatment. Green and others have noted that in patients diagnosed early and adequately treated, stage-for-stage survival is similar to that obtained in the nonpregnant female [47,48,50].

Endometrial Cancer

Endometrial cancer occurring during pregnancy

has been reported only rarely. Sandstrom et al. [58] studied the seventh case of endometrial adenocarcinoma associated with pregnancy and presented follow-up data on four of six cases reported by Karlen et al. in 1972 [59]. The patients ranged in age from 21 to 43 years, and the majority were noted to have only a small focus of well-differentiated tumor. Symptoms prior to diagnosis, most of short duration, were dysmenorrhea, irregular menses, and hypermenorrhea. In general, therapy involved an immediate total abdominal hysterectomy (TAH) with or without bilateral salpingo-oophorectomy (BSO). Only one of the seven patients expired from her disease following TAH and BSO and radiation therapy. It is of interest that this patient had the only reported instance of deep myometrial invasion [58].

Fallopian Tube Cancer

The possibility that fallopian tube carcinoma will occur during pregnancy is remote. Most cases reported are incidental findings at laparotomy or tubal ligation. The standard treatment is TAH and BSO for in situ lesions with the addition of postoperative radiation therapy or chemotherapy for invasive cancer [60].

Schinfeld and Winston reported a case of primary tubal cancer found incidentally at cesarean delivery for a term breech pregnancy [61]. The patient was treated with TAH-BSO, partial omentectomy, and postoperative chemotherapy. At 18 months after the original surgery she was noted to have a solitary nodule of carcinoma in her pelvis. This was excised along with the rest of the omentum, and combined treatment with chemotherapy and radiation therapy was instituted postoperatively. Chemotherapy was discontinued 18 months later, and at present the patient still has no evidence of disease.

Ovarian Cancer

Ovarian cancer is the third most common gynecologic malignancy but accounts for the largest number of deaths. The incidence of this disease declined between 1947 and 1967 but in recent years has risen to approximately 17 cases per 100,000. The peak age of patients with ovarian cancer is somewhat older than the childbearing years; 60% of ovarian tumors develop in women between the ages of 40 and 60 years.

A large number of ovarian growths occur during pregnancy. While it is estimated by Eastman and Hellman that they occur in approximately 1 out of every 81 pregnancies, only 2 to 5% of them will be malignant [62]. In general, the patient is noted to have an adnexal mass at the time of her first ante-partum visit, although in many cases the diagnosis will not be made until delivery when an exploratory laparotomy must be done because of an obstructed birth canal [48]. From the time the mass is noted, accurate diagnosis, staging, and treatment are of prime importance.

Barber suggests that if the tumor is of uniform consistency, mobile, unilateral, encapsulated, and less than 10 cm in size the patient can be closely followed until the second trimester, when laparotomy is less likely to cause abortion [48]. Surgical intervention should be undertaken for any complication such as torsion, which occurs in 10 to 15% of all ovarian tumors found in pregnancy. If the mass is hard, knobby, bilateral, greater than 10 cm or if ascites is present, surgical intervention should be carried out immediately regardless of trimester.

If malignancy is diagnosed at laparotomy, the surgeon's first obligation is to accurately stage the disease. Many tumors are found to be localized, but one-third to one-half will be diagnosed as stage III or IV [48]. Barber suggests that in an early (IA) lesion of low-grade malignancy unilateral oophorectomy be done. The other ovary should be split and subjected to biopsy. Omental and nodal biopsies, and peritoneal washings should be obtained; if there is no evidence of spread, the pregnancy can be allowed to continue. Following delivery, appropriate therapy, including a TAH and removal of the remaining ovary, should be completed. If the tumor is not stage IA or is not histologically of low-grade malignancy, immediate TAH, BSO, omentectomy, and nodal biopsy should be done. The addition of postoperative radiation therapy or chemotherapy or both will be dependent on the stage of disease and the protocols of the institution; however, in general, multidrug chemotherapy is used at most institutions for stage III and stage IV ovarian malignancies.

Pregnancy does not alter the outcome of the ovarian malignancy. Stage for stage, pregnant and nonpregnant patients have the same survival rate [48].

Miscellaneous Neoplasms

A large number of other neoplasms have been reported to occur rarely in association with pregnancy. These include carcinoma of the bowel [63], pituitary tumors [64], neuroblastoma [65], gastric carcinoma [66], sarcomas [67,68], parathyroid carcinoma [69], choriocarcinoma [70–72], endodermal sinus tumors [73–75], carcinoma of the lung [76], and oat cell carcinoma of the uterine cervix [77]. Diagnosis, management, and outcome are discussed in the articles listed.

REFERENCES

1. Rothman LA, Cohen CJ, Astarloa J. Placental and fetal involvement by maternal malignancy: a report of rectal carcinoma and review of the literature. Am J Obstet Gynecol. 1973; 116:1023–4.

2. Cramblett HG, Friedman JL, Najjar S. Leukemia in an infant born of a mother with leukemia. N Engl J Med. 1958; 259:727–9.

3. Potter JF, Schoeneman M. Metastasis of maternal cancer to the placenta and fetus. Cancer. 1970; 25:380–8.

4. Lilleyman JS, Hill AS, Anderton KJ. Consequences of acute myelogenous leukemia in early pregnancy. Cancer. 1977; 40:1300–3.

5. Pizzuto J, Aviles A, Noriega L, Niz J, Morales M, Romero F. Treatment of acute leukemia during pregnancy: presentation of nine cases. Cancer Treat Rep. 1980; 64:679–83.

6. Dara P, Satler LM, Armentrout SA. Successful pregnancy during chemotherapy for acute leukemia. Cancer. 1981; 47:845–6.

7. Sweet DL, Kinzie J. Consequences of radiotherapy and antineoplastic therapy for the fetus. J Reprod Med. 1976; 17:241–6.

8. Blatt J, Mulvihill JJ, Ziegler JL, Young RC, Poplack DG. Pregnancy outcome following cancer chemotherapy. Am J Med. 1980; 69:828–32.

9. Daly H, McCann SR, Hanratty TD, Temperley IJ. Successful pregnancy during combination chemotherapy for Hodgkin's disease. Acta Haematol (Basel). 1980; 64:154–6.

10. Alegre A, Chunchurreta R, Rodriguez-Alarcon J, Cruz E, Prada M. Successful pregnancy in acute promyelocytic leukemia. Cancer. 1982; 49:152–3.

11. Durodola JI. Administration of cyclophosphamide during late pregnancy and early lactation: a case report. J Natl Med Assoc. 1979; 71:165–6.

12. Hardin JS. Cyclophosphamide treatment of lymphoma during third trimester of pregnancy. Obstet Gynecol. 1971; 39:850–1.

13. Boros SJ, Reynolds JW. Intrauterine growth retardation following third-trimester exposure to busulfan. Am J Obstet Gynecol. 1977; 129:111–2.

14. Doney KC, Kraemer KG, Shepard TH. Combination chemotherapy for acute myelocytic leukemia during pregnancy: three case reports. Cancer Treat Rep. 1979; 63:369–71.

15. Nicholson HO. Cytotoxic drugs in pregnancy. J Obstet Gynaecol Br Comm. 1968; 75:307–12.

16. Kaempfer SH. The effects of cancer chemotherapy on reproduction: a review of the literature. Oncol Nurs Forum. 1981; 8:11–8.

17. Schafer AI. Teratogenic effects of antileukemic chemotherapy. Arch Intern Med. 1981; 141:514–5.

18. Ask-Upmark E. Another follow-up study of children born of mothers with leukemia. Acta Med Scand. 1964; 175:391–4.

19. DeVita VT, Hellman S, Rosenberg SA. Cancer. Principles and practice of oncology. Philadelphia: Lippincott, 1982.

20. Okun DB, Groncy PK, Seiger L, Tanaka KR. Acute leukemia in pregnancy: transient neonatal myelosuppression after combination chemotherapy in the mother. Med Pediatr Oncol. 1979; 7:315–9.

21. Winston DJ, Ho WG, Gale RP. Prophylactic granulocyte transfusions during chemotherapy of acute nonlymphocytic leukemia. Ann Intern Med. 1981; 94:616–22.

22. Donegan WL. Mammary carcinoma and pregnancy. In: Donegan WL, Spratt JS, eds. Cancer of the breast. 2nd ed. Philadelphia: Saunders, 1979:448–63.

23. Anderson JM. Mammary cancers and pregnancy. Br Med J. 1979; 1:1124–7.

24. Ribeiro GG, Palmer MK. Breast carcinoma associated with pregnancy: a clinician's dilemma. Br Med J. 1977; 2:1524–7.

25. Zinns JS. The association of pregnancy and breast cancer. J Reprod Med. 1979; 22:297–301.

26. White TT. Prognosis of breast cancer for pregnant and nursing women: analysis of 1413 cases. Surg Gynecol Obstet. 1955; 100:661–6.

27. Applewhite RR, Smith LR, DiVincenti F. Carcinoma of the breast associated with pregnancy and lactation. Am Surg. 1973; 39:101–4.

28. Bonadonna G, Valagussa P. Dose-response effect of adjuvant chemotherapy in breast cancer. N Engl J Med. 1981; 304:10–5.

29. Stephens JD, Golbus MS, Miller TR, Wilber RR, Epstein CJ. Multiple congenital anomalies in a fetus exposed to 5-fluorouracil during the first trimester. Am J Obstet Gynecol. 1980; 137:747–9.

30. Peters MV. The effect of pregnancy in breast cancer. In: Forrest APM, Kunkler PB, eds. Prognostic factors in breast cancer. Edinburgh: Livingstone, 1968:65–89.

31. Harvey JC, Rosen PP, Ashikari R, Robbins GF, Kinne DW. The effect of pregnancy on the prognosis of carcinoma of the breast following radical mastectomy. Surg Gynecol Obstet. 1981; 153:723–5.

32. Jacobs C, Donaldson SS, Rosenberg SA, Kaplan HS. Management of the pregnant patient with Hodgkin's disease. Ann Intern Med. 1981; 95:669–75.

33. Thomas PR, Peckham MJ. The investigation and management of Hodgkin's disease in the pregnant patient. Cancer. 1976; 38:1443–51.

34. Jones RT, Weinerman BH. MOPP (nitrogen mustard, vincristine, procarbazine, and prednisone) given during pregnancy. Obstet Gynecol. 1979; 54:477–8.

35. Falkson HC, Simson IW, Falkson G. Non-Hodgkin's lymphoma in pregnancy. Cancer. 1980; 45:1679–82.

36. Rodichok LD, Harper GR, Ruckdeschel JC, Price A, Roberson G, Barron KD, Horton J. Early diagnosis of spinal epidural metastases. Am J Med. 1981; 70:1181–8.

37. Shaw HM, Milton GW, Farago G, McCarthy WH. Endocrine influences on survival from malignant melanoma. Cancer. 1978; 42:669–77.

38. Mirimanoff RO, Wagenknecht L, Hunziker N. Long-term complete remission of malignant melanoma with tamoxifen. Lancet. 1981; 1:1368–9. letter.

39. Shiu MH, Schottenfeld D, Maclean B, Fortner JG. Adverse effect of pregnancy on melanoma: a reappraisal. Cancer. 1976; 37:181–7.

40. Houghton AN, Flannery J, Viola MV. Malignant melanoma of the skin occurring during pregnancy. Cancer. 1981; 48:407–10.

41. Shaw HM, Milton GW, Garago G, McCarthy WH. Endocrine influences on survival from malignant melanoma. Cancer. 1978; 42:669–77.

42. Raich PC, Curet LB. Treatment of acute leukemia during pregnancy. Cancer. 1975; 36:861–2.

43. O'Dell RF. Leukemia and lymphoma complicating pregnancy. Clin Obstet Gynecol. 1979; 22:859–70.

44. O'Donnell R, Costigan C, O'Connell LG. Two cases of acute leukaemia in pregnancy. Acta Haematol (Basel). 1979; 61:298–300.

45. Hamer JW, Beard ME, Duff GB. Pregnancy complicated by acute myeloid leukaemia. NZ Med J. 1979; 89:212–3.

46. Monoharan A, Leyden MJ. Acute non-lymphocytic leukaemia in the third trimester of pregnancy. Aust NZ J Med. 1979; 9:71–4.

47. DiSaia PJ, Creasman WT. Clinical gynecologic oncology. St. Louis: Mosby, 1981:376–400.

48. Barber HRK. Manual of gynecologic oncology. Philadelphia: Lippincott, 1980.

49. Jones WB, Woodruff JM, Erlandson RA, Lewis JL. DES-related clear cell adenocarcinoma of the vagina in pregnancy. Obstet Gynecol. 1981; 57:76S–80S.

50. Green TH. Surgical management of carcinoma of the cervix in pregnancy. Prog Gynecol. 1975; 6:607–26.

51. Graham JB, Sotto LS Jr, Paloucek FP. Carcinoma of the cervix. Philadelphia: Saunders, 1962.

52. Creasman WT, Rutledge FN, Fletcher GH. Carcinoma of the cervix associated with pregnancy. Obstet Gynecol. 1970; 36:495–501.

53. Fowler WC, Walton LA, Edelman DA. Cervical intraepithelial neoplasia during pregnancy. South Med J. 1980; 73:1180–5.

54. Bosch A, Marcial VA. Carcinoma of the uterine cervix associated with pregnancy. Am J Roentgenol. 1966; 96:92–9.

55. Funnell JD, Puchett TG, Strebel GF, Kelso JW. Carcinoma of the cervix complicating pregnancy. South Med J. 1980; 73:1308–10.

56. Lee RB, Neglia W, Park RC. Cervical carcinoma in pregnancy. Obstet Gynecol. 1981; 58:584–9.

57. Waldrop GM, Palmer JP. Carcinoma of the cervix associated with pregnancy. Am J Obstet Gynecol. 1963; 86:201–12.

58. Sandstrom RE, Welch WR, Green TH. Adenocarcinoma of the endometrium in pregnancy. Obstet Gynecol. 1979; 53:73S–76S.

59. Karlen JR, Sternberg LB, Abbott JN. Carcinoma of the endometrium co-existing with pregnancy. Obstet Gynecol. 1972; 40:334–9.

60. Saffos RO, Rhatigan RM, Scully RE. Metaplastic papillary tumor of the fallopian tube—a distinctive lesion of pregnancy. Am J Clin Pathol. 1980; 74:232–6.

61. Schinfeld JS, Winston HG. Primary tubal carcinoma in pregnancy. Am J Obstet Gynecol. 1980; 137:512–4.

62. Eastman NJ, Hellman LM. Ovarian tumors in pregnancy. In: Eastman NJ, Hellman LM, eds. Williams obstetrics. 13th ed. New York: Appleton-Century-Crofts, 1966.

63. Barber HR, Brunschwig A. Carcinoma of the bowel. Am J Obstet Gynecol. 1968; 100:926–33.

64. Bloch B. Pituitary tumours in pregnancy. A case report. S Afr Med J. 1979; 55:57–9.

65. Besana C, Ciboddo G, Gromo G, Salmaggi C. Neuroblastoma in pregnancy. Lancet. 1981; 2:534. letter.

66. Sims EH, Schlater TL, Sims M, Lou MA. Obstructing gastric carcinoma complicating pregnancy. J Natl Med Assoc. 1980; 72:21–3.

67. Ginsburg DS, Hernandez E, Johnson JW. Sarcoma complicating von Recklinghausen disease in pregnancy. Obstet Gynecol. 1981; 58:385–7.

68. Johnston GA, Simon MA, Azizi F. Giant cell tumors of bone in pregnancy: report of two cases. J Reprod Med. 1980; 24:43–5.

69. Hess HM, Dickson J, Fox HE. Hyperfunctioning parathyroid carcinoma presenting as acute pancreatitis in pregnancy. J Reprod Med. 1980; 25:83–7.

70. Cunanan RG Jr, Lippes J, Tancinco PA. Choriocarcinoma of the ovary with coexisting normal pregnancy. Obstet Gynecol. 1980; 55:669–72.

71. Rolon PA, Hochsztajn de Lopez BH. Malignant trophoblastic disease in Paraguay. J Reprod Med. 1979; 23:94–6.

72. McCue SA, Greene JB. Metastatic cerebral choriocarcinoma during pregnancy. Minn Med. 1980; 63:164–6.

73. Weed JC, Roh RA, Mendenhall HW. Recurrent endodermal sinus tumor during pregnancy. Obstet Gynecol. 1979; 54:653–5.

74. Krishnamurthy SC, Sampat MB. Endodermal sinus (yolk sac) tumor of the vulva in a pregnant female. Gynecol Oncol. 1981; 11:379–82.

75. Petrucha RA, Ruffolo E, Messina AM, Bouis PJ, Praphat H. Endodermal sinus tumor: report of a case associated with pregnancy. Obstet Gynecol. 1980; 55:90S–93S.

76. Read EJ, Platzer PB. Placental metastasis from maternal carcinoma of the lung. Obstet Gynecol. 1980; 58:387–91.

77. Jacobs AJ, Marchevsky A, Gordon RE, Deppe G, Cohen CJ. Oat cell carcinoma of the uterine cervix in a pregnant woman treated with cis-diamminedichloroplatinum. Gynecol Oncol. 1980; 9:405–10.

24. INFECTIOUS DISEASES

James A. McGregor, Robert E. Wall, and F. Marc LaForce

Immunologic and anatomic changes during pregnancy alter the pregnant patient's response to infection [1–5]. These changes can result in increased susceptibility to infection or increased severity of certain infections. The effects of maternal infection on the fetus are dependent on multiple factors, including the type of the organism, the inoculum, preexisting host immunity, and host defenses. These factors, among others, help to determine whether the infectious agent can infect and traverse the placenta. Also, fetuses vary from their mothers and one from another in their ability to avoid or overcome infection. Overwhelming infections usually result in abortion or fetal death. Less frequently, infection can result in structural or developmental abnormalities.

The discussion of infectious diseases complicating pregnancy is grouped according to the infectious agent or the mode of transmission. Clinical and laboratory diagnosis of specific diseases and their management are presented.

IMMUNIZATION

The single most effective means of disease prevention is active vaccination. Preferably, vaccination status should be reviewed prior to conception.

Active Immunization

Active immunization may be defined as the induction of specific immunity by stimulation of antibody production within the recipient. Active immunity may be induced in several ways. *Toxoids* are preparations of bacterial exotoxin that have been altered in order to retain their antigenicity without significant toxicity. Tetanus-diphtheria toxoid is an example. Antigenic killed whole bacteria or viruses (*killed vaccine*), or portions of them, can be used to induce prolonged immunity. Heat or chemicals can be used to treat these organisms prior to inoculation of a host. Typhoid, meningococcus, and rabies vaccines are examples.

Vaccines that protect against viral infections have been developed by repeated passage of the wild virus through animal or human tissue culture so as to retain virus antigenicity while eliminating virulence (*attenuated live vaccine*). Rubella, mumps, measles, and yellow fever vaccines are examples. The Centers for Disease Control (CDC) in Atlanta maintains a registry of women who received live virus vaccines three months prior to or following conception. Physicians are urged to report such cases immediately.

A decision to vaccinate during pregnancy should be based on the woman's relative risk of exposure to the disease, susceptibility to the disease, gestational age, and the relative risk of the vaccine being considered. Some general principles do apply. Killed vaccines are probably safe. Live virus vaccines are best withheld during pregnancy unless absolutely indicated. When live virus vaccines are necessary, their use should be postponed until after the first trimester [6].

Passive Immunization

Passive immunization involves the administration of preformed antibody, either human or animal, to prevent illness. Specific examples include immune serum globulin (IG), which confers nonspecific passive immunity, and specific hyperimmune globulin, which confers immunity against infections such as varicella-zoster or rabies.

Passive immunization with hyperimmune globulin may be used in pregnancy for postexposure protection (hepatitis, rabies, tetanus). Varicella-zoster immune globulin (VZIG) is used for newborns whose mothers contracted varicella in the period ranging from four days before to two days following delivery, since passive transport of maternal antibody to the fetus will be incomplete or nonexistent then. It is not indicated for pregnant women exposed to the disease at other times during gestation.

In May 1982, the American College of Obstetricians and Gynecologists issued a comprehensive technical bulletin with updated recommendations for immunization during pregnancy [6]. Table 24-1 is a reproduction of those recommendations.

Table 24-1. Immunization during pregnancy

Immunizing agent	Risk from disease to pregnant female	Risk from disease to fetus or neonate	Type of immunizing agent	Risk from immunizing agent to fetus	Indications for immunization during pregnancy	Dose schedule	Comments
Live Virus Vaccines							
Measles	Significant morbidity, low mortality; not altered by pregnancy	Significant increase in abortion rate; may cause malformations	Live attenuated virus vaccine	None confirmed	Contraindicated (See Immune Globulins)	Single dose	Vaccination of susceptible women should be part of postpartum care
Mumps	Low morbidity and mortality; not altered by pregnancy	Probable increased rate of abortion in 1st trimester. Questionable association of fibroelastosis in neonates	Live attenuated virus vaccine	None confirmed	Contraindicated	Single dose	
Polio-myelitis	No increased incidence in pregnancy, but may be more severe if it does occur	Anoxic fetal damage reported; 50% mortality in neonatal disease	Live attenuated virus (OPV) and inactivated virus (IPV) vaccine*	None confirmed	Not routinely recommended for adults in US, except persons at increased risk of exposure	*Primary:* 3 doses of IPV at 4–8 wk intervals and a 4th dose 6–12 mo after the 3rd dose; 2 doses of OPV with a 6–8 wk interval and a 3rd dose at least 6 wk later, customarily 8–12 mo later *Booster:* Every 5 yr until 18 yr of age for IPV	Vaccine indicated for susceptible pregnant women traveling in endemic areas or in other high-risk situations
Rubella	Low morbidity and mortality; not altered by pregnancy	High rate of abortion and congenital rubella syndrome	Live attenuated virus vaccine	None confirmed	Contraindicated	Single dose	Teratogenicity of vaccine is theoretical, not confirmed to date. Vaccination of susceptible women should be part of postpartum care

Vaccine	Effect of disease on pregnancy	Effect on fetus	Type of vaccine	Risk to fetus from vaccine	Indications during pregnancy	Dose	Comments
Yellow fever	Significant morbidity and mortality; not altered by pregnancy	Unknown	Live attenuated virus vaccine	Unknown	Contraindicated except if exposure unavoidable	Single dose	Postponement of travel preferable to vaccination, if possible
Inactivated Virus Vaccines							
Influenza	Possible increase in morbidity and mortality during epidemic of new antigenic strain	Possible increased abortion rate; no malformations confirmed	Inactivated type A and type B virus vaccines	None confirmed	Usually recommended only for patients with serious underlying diseases; public health authorities to be consulted for current recommendation	Consult with public health authorities since recommendations change each year	Criteria for vaccination of pregnant women same as for all adults
Rabies	Near 100% fatality; not altered by pregnancy	Determined by maternal disease	Killed virus vaccine	Unknown	Indications for prophylaxis not altered by pregnancy; each case considered individually	Public health authorities to be consulted for indications and dosage	
Inactivated Bacterial Vaccines							
Cholera	Significant morbidity and mortality; more severe during 3rd trimester	Increased risk of fetal death during 3rd trimester maternal illness	Killed bacterial vaccine	Unknown	Only to meet international travel requirements	2 injections, 4–8 wk apart	Vaccine of low efficacy
Meningococcus	No increased risk during pregnancy; no increase in severity of disease	Unknown	Killed bacterial vaccine	No data available on use during pregnancy	Indications not altered by pregnancy; vaccination recommended only in unusual outbreak situations	Public health authorities to be consulted	
Plague	Significant morbidity and mortality; not altered by pregnancy	Determined by maternal disease	Killed bacterial vaccine	None reported	Very selective vaccination of exposed persons	Public health authorities to be consulted for indications and dosage	

Table 24-1. Immunization during pregnancy (continued)

Immunizing agent	Risk from disease to pregnant female	Risk from disease to fetus or neonate	Type of immunizing agent	Risk from immunizing agent to fetus	Indications for immunization during pregnancy	Dose schedule	Comments
Pneumo- coccus	No increased risk during pregnancy; no increase in severity of disease	Unknown	Polyvalent polysaccha- ride vaccine	No data avail- able on use during preg- nancy	Indications not al- tered by preg- nancy; vaccine used only for high-risk indi- viduals	In adults 1 dose only	
Typhoid	Significant morbid- ity and mortality; not altered by pregnancy	Unknown	Killed bacterial vaccine	None confirmed	Not recommended routinely ex- cept for close, continued expo- sure or travel to endemic areas	*Primary:* 2 injec- tions, 4 wk apart *Booster:* single dose	
Toxoids							
Tetanus- diph- theria	Severe morbidity; tetanus mortality 60%; diphtheria mortality 10%; unaltered by pregnancy	Neonatal tetanus mortality 60%	Combined tet- anus-diph- theria tox- oids pre- ferred: adult tetanus-diph- theria formu- lation	None confirmed	Lack of primary series, or no booster within past 10 yr	*Primary:* 2 doses at 1- to 2-mo in- terval with a 3rd dose 6–12 mo after the second *Booster:* single dose every 10 yr after comple- tion of the pri- mary series	Updating of immune status should be part of antepartum care
Immune Globulins: Hyperimmune							
Hepatitis B	Possible increased severity during 3rd trimester	Possible increase in abortion rate and prematurity. Neonatal hepa- titis can occur if mother is a chronic carrier or is acutely infected	Hepatitis B im- mune globu- lin (HBIG)	None reported	Postexposure prophylaxis	.06 mL/kg immedi- ately and 1 mo later of HBIG	Infants born to HBsAg- positive mothers should receive 0.5 mL of HBIG as soon after birth as possible and the same dose repeated 3 and 6 mo later
Rabies	Near 100% fatality; not altered by pregnancy	Determined by maternal disease	Rabies immune globulin (RIG)	None reported	Postexposure prophylaxis	20 IU/kg in one dose of RIG	Used in conjunction with rabies killed virus vaccine

Disease	Maternal effects	Fetal/neonatal effects	Immune globulin	Adverse effects	Indication	Dose	Comments
Tetanus	Severe morbidity; mortality 60%	Neonatal tetanus mortality 60%	Tetanus immune globulin (TIG)	None reported	Postexposure prophylaxis	250 units in one dose of TIG	Used in conjunction with tetanus toxoid
Varicella	Possible increase in severe varicella pneumonia	Can cause congenital varicella with increased mortality in neonatal period; very rarely causes congenital defects	Varicella-zoster immune globulin (VZIG)	None reported	Not routinely indicated in healthy pregnant women exposed to varicella	1 vial/kg in one dose of VZIG, up to 5 vials	Only indicated for newborns of mothers who developed varicella within 4 days prior to delivery or 2 days following delivery. Approximately 90–95% of adults are immune to varicella

Immune Globulins: Pooled

Disease	Maternal effects	Fetal/neonatal effects	Immune globulin	Adverse effects	Indication	Dose	Comments
Hepatitis A	Possible increased severity during 3rd trimester	Probable increase in abortion rate and prematurity. Possible transmission to neonate at delivery if mother is incubating the virus or is acutely ill at that time	Pooled immune globulin (IG)	None reported	Postexposure prophylaxis	.02 mL/kg in one dose of IG	IG should be given as soon as possible and within 2 wk of exposure. Infants born to mothers who are incubating the virus or are acutely ill at delivery should receive one dose of 0.5 mL as soon as possible after birth
Measles	Significant morbidity, low mortality; not altered by pregnancy	Significant increase in abortion rate; may cause malformations	Pooled immune globulin (IG)	None reported	Postexposure prophylaxis	.25 mL/kg in one dose of IG, up to 15 mL	Unclear if it prevents abortion. Must be given within 6 days of exposure

*Inactivated polio vaccine (IPV) recommended for unimmunized adults at increased risk.

Source: Committee on Technical Bulletins of the American College of Obstetricians and Gynecologists [6]. Reprinted with permission of American College of Obstetricians and Gynecologists.

ANTIBIOTICS

The aim of antibiotic therapy is augmentation of host defense mechanisms by establishing effective and safe concentrations of appropriate antimicrobial agents in the blood and infected tissues. Guidelines for bacteriologically appropriate, cost-effective use of antimicrobials are available for the general population, but rarely address use in pregnant, puerperal, or lactating women [7–17]. This section includes basic information regarding the pharmacokinetics of antibiotics in pregnancy as well as some practical recommendations for their use.

Altered maternal physiology profoundly affects antimicrobial pharmacokinetics (Table 24-2). Many of these changes, such as increase in blood volume, development of the "fetoplacental unit," increased cardiac output, and increased glomerular filtration rate, occur shortly after conception. Expansion of the blood volume reduces the effective circulating drug concentration. Increased glomerular filtration and renal excretion hasten the clearance of many agents, especially the aminoglycosides, making dosage calculations difficult. Increased gastric emptying time may diminish the absorption and bioavailability of orally administered agents [18].

Decreased levels of serum proteins in pregnancy may profoundly affect concentrations of "active" antibiotic in the tissues, as well as the amount of drug that crosses the placenta. The more avidly and completely bound an antibiotic is to plasma proteins, the less will be available as free drug to traverse the placenta. Antimicrobials with avid protein binding, such as cefazolin or dicloxacillin, are less likely to cross the placenta in significant amounts than antibiotics with low protein binding, such as methicillin [19]. Measurement of maternal serum antibiotic levels is desirable in patients with severe infections or in patients who require prolonged therapy.

Antibiotics are chemicals that are not part of a pregnant woman's normal internal milieu. It is likely that all substances administered to pregnant or lactating women cross the placenta or enter breast milk to some degree. Since drug interactions with embryonic and fetal tissues have been incompletely studied and in fact may change along with intrauterine growth and differentiation, it is best to consider even the most innocuous antimicrobial agent as potentially toxic. It is possible that many untoward embryonic or fetal reactions are not presently recognized or may be expressed as subtle alterations in central nervous system–mediated behavior. Some common antibiotics and their special considerations during pregnancy are listed in Table 24-3. Selected antibiotics are discussed in greater detail below.

Tetracyclines

Tetracyclines act by binding to the bacterial 30s ribosome thereby interfering with bacterial protein synthesis. The teratogenic potential of tetracyclines in humans is poorly documented, although several reports suggest that there may be some risk to their use in the first trimester [20–22]. Tetracyclines are known to be efficient chelators of various heavy metals, most prominently calcium. They can produce irreversible discoloration and weakening of deciduous teeth in the fetus if used during pregnancy, and in permanent teeth if given to an infant or child during the first eight years of life. These effects appear to be dose-related and occur with greatest frequency when the total tetracycline dosage exceeds 3 g, when the drug is administered for more than ten days or when treatment is begun after the 25th week of gestation. Tetracyclines are also known to deposit in the calcifying skeleton after the 12th week of gestation, where they inhibit bony elongation and calcium uptake into the bone matrix [23,24].

Pregnant women may also experience untoward reactions to tetracyclines. Hepatic failure, and perhaps pancreatitis, has been reported in pregnant women treated near term with large doses of intravenous tetracycline for pyelonephritis [25, 26]. Tetracyclines should be excluded from use in pregnant women and in children up to the age of

Table 24-2. Effect of altered maternal physiology on antimicrobial pharmacokinetics

Physiologic alteration	Pharmacokinetic effect
Expanded blood volume	Expanded volume of distribution; lower maternal blood levels
Increased glomerular filtration rate	More rapid renal drug clearance
Altered gastric emptying (increased or decreased)	Altered drug absorption (increased or decreased)
Decreased albumin and total protein	Increased maternal blood levels of "free" drug; altered placental transport
Decreased feto-maternal barriers with advancing gestation	Increased placental transport
Immature fetal liver function	Increased fetal blood levels

Table 24-3. Antibiotic use during pregnancy

Antibiotic	Uses	Special considerations during pregnancy
Penicillin G	Susceptible gram-positive infections	Safe in non-allergic patients; dosage requirements increased during pregnancy
Ampicillin	Effective in UTI secondary to susceptible enteric pathogens	Dosage requirements increased during pregnancy; can lower urinary estriols; unconjugated serum estriol unaffected
Amoxicillin	Same spectrum as ampicillin; provides higher tissue concentration than ampicillin	Same as ampicillin
Oxacillin	Effective against penicillinase-producing organisms	Dosage requirements increased during pregnancy
Cephalosporins	Effective against many gram-negative and gram-positive organisms	Dosage requirements increased during pregnancy; some cross-sensitivity in penicillin-allergic patients; may affect urinary estriols; no effect on unconjugated serum estriol
Erythromycin	Most useful against gram-positive cocci in penicillin-allergic patients	Generally safe; placental transfer is erratic, but the fetal liver concentrates the drug
Tetracycline	Contraindicated during pregnancy and lactation	Abnormal fetal teeth and bone development; increased risk of maternal liver and pancreatic disease
Chloramphenicol	Avoid during pregnancy and lactation	May cause "gray baby syndrome"
Clindamycin	Effective against serious anaerobic infections; including those caused by resistant *Bacteroides*	Fetal effects are unknown; may rarely cause pseudomembranous colitis in the mother
Vancomycin	Effective against penicillinase-producing organisms; bacterial endocarditis prophylaxis at delivery in penicillin-allergic patients	Potential fetal ototoxicity; should be reserved for life-threatening infections in patients allergic to penicillin
Metronidazole	Contraindicated in first trimester	Mutagenic and carcinogenic in animals; may be necessary to use for symptomatic parasitic infections during second and third trimesters
Nitrofurantoin	Effective principally against organisms responsible for UTI, including enterococcus	Generally safe, but has been rarely associated with hemolytic anemia in the newborn; few systemic effects
Sulfanomides	Effective in most uncomplicated UTIs	Competes with bilirubin for albumin binding; should not be used in last trimester to avoid neonatal kernicterus
Trimethoprim	Effective in most lower UTIs	Folic acid antagonist; should be avoided during pregnancy unless no alternative available
Aminoglycosides amikacin gentamicin kanamycin streptomycin tobramycin	Effective in serious gram-negative infections	Possible fetal and maternal ototoxicity and renal toxicity; maternal serum levels should be monitored closely

UTI = urinary tract infection

eight unless no other antimicrobial agent can be effectively substituted.

Sulfonamides and Trimethoprim

Sulfonamides are bacteriostatic and act by inhibiting the intracellular synthesis of folic acid by bacteria. They can be particularly useful for treating lower urinary tract infections during the first two trimesters. Trimethoprim blocks the production of folic acid by binding to and inhibiting the enzyme dihydrofolate reductase.

The highly useful fixed combination of trimethoprim and sulfamethoxazole (TMP/SMZ) is commonly used to treat nonpregnant patients with urinary tract infection, sinusitis, pneumocystis, or shigellosis. It may also be useful against toxoplasmosis. Maternal treatment with trimethoprim should be avoided throughout pregnancy because of the possibility of a synergistic antifolate effect on rapidly dividing cells. During the third trimester, sulfa-containing preparations have been avoided because of the possible displacement of free bilirubin from albumin binding sites, predisposing the newborn to kernicterus. The clinical practice of avoiding TMP/SMZ and other sulfa preparations near term stems from studies on more avid albumin-binding sulfa preparations used during the late 1950s and early 1960s. More recently, Springer and colleagues investigated the pharmacokinetic effects of direct TMP/SMZ neonatal therapy during a nursery outbreak of a resistant strain of *Klebsiella pneumoniae* that was sensitive only to this combination [27]. They noted no adverse effects and found the bilirubin-binding capacity of albumin was unchanged at the therapeutic concentrations achieved in 12 neonates. These preliminary observations suggest that both neonatal and maternal therapy with TMP/SMZ may be safe in the latter part of pregnancy in women with normally functioning kidneys, as well as in the newborn period when dosages are calculated on the basis of measured blood levels. The passage of TMP/SMZ across the placenta and blood-brain barrier also allows for the possibility of fetal therapy for intrauterine infections with such organisms as *Toxoplasma gondii*. In utero, free bilirubin traverses the placenta so that displaced bilirubin is less of a threat to the fetus. However, until these studies can be corroborated, alternatives to sulfa-containing preparations should be considered first when needed near term.

All sulfa preparations should be avoided in both women and their offspring who have glucose-6-phosphate dehydrogenase deficiency because of the possibility of massive red cell hemolysis. During lactation sulfa may pass through breast milk in recoverable amounts and be absorbed by the infant.

Penicillins

The penicillins are probably the most widely used antimicrobials during pregnancy. As a group, they have a wide margin of safety for both the pregnant woman and the fetus. No teratogenic effects were demonstrated with first-trimester administration of penicillin derivatives in over 3,500 gravidas in the Collaborative Perinatal Project [10].

Serum levels of penicillins are lower and renal clearance is higher throughout pregnancy. Penicillins are bound to plasma proteins to varying degrees; the free drug appears to be the active form. Maternal administration of penicillins with high protein binding, including nafcillin, oxacillin, cloxacillin, and dicloxacillin, result in lower amniotic fluid levels and lower fetal tissue levels than penicillins that are poorly protein bound, such as ampicillin and methicillin.

Erythromycin

Erythromycin is generally safe for use during pregnancy (except for the estolate form, which has been associated with hepatotoxicity) and offers an alternative for the treatment of gonorrhea and syphilis in penicillin-allergic patients. Since erythromycin does not reliably achieve significant fetal serum levels, it is recommended that penicillin be administered to every newborn whose mother received erythromycin for the treatment of syphilis during pregnancy [28].

Cephalosporins

Cephalosporins have been used extensively during pregnancy and have been demonstrated to have a wide margin of safety. Maternal levels of cephalosporins are considerably lower than levels measured in nonpregnant patients. Transplacental transfer of cephalothin is rapid, and bactericidal concentrations are attainable in fetal tissues and amniotic fluid [29].

Metronidazole

Even though metronidazole and its metabolites traverse the placenta readily and interfere with DNA synthesis, no excess malformations have been noted with second- or third-trimester treatment of several hundred women [32]. Experience with metronidazole use in the first trimester of human pregnancy remains unreported. Nevertheless, the increased incidence of various tumors in rodents and increased mutation rates in various bacteria should give considerable pause to the use of metronidazole in pregnancy, especially during organogenesis [30,31]. The duration of elevated maternal, and presumably fetal, metronidazole blood levels may be shortened by use of a single 2-g dose of metronidazole for the treatment of severe symptomatic trichomoniasis.

Chloramphenicol

A general proscription of chloramphenicol usage in pregnancy and lactation rests on the observations of transient bone marrow suppression and the "gray baby syndrome," as well as the unpredictable, but rare, complication of aplastic anemia. Avoidance of chloramphenicol usage during pregnancy is not difficult since less toxic drugs may be used in place of this agent. However, when chloramphenicol is the best choice on the basis of microbiologic sensitivities, the risk of its use may be reduced by careful monitoring of serum drug levels [33].

Aminoglycosides

Aminoglycosides should be used during gestation for initial therapy of severe maternal infections, and for treatment when less toxic agents cannot be substituted. These drugs readily cross the placenta and are potentially ototoxic. Because of unpredictable serum levels and increased renal clearance during pregnancy, aminoglycoside levels should be obtained when these agents are used to treat infections in pregnant women. Because of negligible absorption from the gastrointestinal tract, they appear to be safe for use during lactation [16,34].

ISOLATION PROCEDURES

Maternal and fetal isolation procedures vary at different institutions. Procedures are often governed by hospital infectious disease committees. Some guidelines for isolation have been listed in Table 24-5 [35].

SEXUALLY TRANSMITTED DISEASES
Gonorrhea

Maternal genital tract infections with *Neisseria gonorrhoeae* occur in 1 to 7% of pregnant women in prenatal clinics [36–37]. Gonorrhea places the pregnant woman and her fetus at considerable risk. Preterm rupture of membranes, preterm labor, chorioamnionitis, intrauterine growth retardation, ophthalmia neonatorum, disseminated gonococcal infection, and sepsis of mother or newborn can result [38,39]. Routine endocervical culture for gonorrhea is essential during pregnancy since the majority of infections are asymptomatic. Purulent endocervicitis, Bartholin's duct abscess, or fulminant postpartum endometritis are frequently caused by *Neisseria gonorrhoeae*. Because of the increasing incidence of penicillinase-producing *Neisseria gonorrhoeae* (PPNG) in the United States, all culture isolates must be tested for penicillinase production [40,41].

Dosage schedules for treatment of *Neisseria gonorrhoeae* during pregnancy are presented in Table 24-4 [42]. Single-dose oral amoxicillin, oral ampicillin, or intramuscular procaine penicillin G, each given concurrently with probenecid 1.0 g, is effective treatment for most cases of maternal genital infection. The presence of PPNG, a history of penicillin allergy, or a positive repeat culture warrants treatment with spectinomycin 2.0 g intra-

muscularly. Treatment of all sexual contacts is necessary, and follow-up culture is mandatory within 4 to 7 days. Reculture in the third trimester is also recommended. Because of the high frequency of concurrent infection with other venereal diseases, appropriate laboratory evaluation should be obtained where possible. Recommended treatment for gonorrhea does not necessarily eradicate other concurrent venereal disease.

Recommended isolation procedures for mothers with gonorrhea and their infants are presented in Table 24-5.

Syphilis

The incidence of syphilis in the United States has shown a small but steady increase since 1977 [43]. Although the majority of the increase is attributed to the rising frequency of this disease in male homosexuals, the incidence in women has also risen. At a large urban county hospital in Los Angeles, the rate of syphilis among antenatal patients increased by 50% between 1971 and 1981 [44].

After passage through the mucosa, *Treponema pallidum* produces an initial spirochetemia followed by the development of a painless chancre at the initial inoculation site, often within several weeks. Local lymphadenopathy usually accompanies the initial lesion. Following healing of the chancre, the secondary stage ensues, with the development of lymphadenopathy, fever, and the classic macular, nonpruritic rash, which commonly involves the palms and soles. Lesions of both the primary and secondary stages are highly contagious.

Transmission of spirochetes across the placenta may occur during any trimester [45]. The complications of untreated intrauterine fetal infections include preterm labor, stillbirth, intrauterine growth retardation, hepatosplenomegaly, abnormal skeletal development, and dermatitis.

The diagnosis of early syphilis during pregnancy is often difficult because of the evanescent, asymptomatic nature of the primary chancre and the nonspecific nature of the rash, fever, and lymphadenopathy in the secondary phase. Dark-field microscopy of lesions by an experienced examiner is considered the most reliable and direct means of establishing the diagnosis.

Serologic diagnosis and confirmation of syphilis during pregnancy is performed initially using nontreponemal tests such as the Venereal Disease Research Laboratory (VDRL) test, rapid plasma reagin (RPR) test, or automated reagin test (ART). Although these tests are inexpensive and easily

Table 24-4. Treatment of sexually transmitted diseases during pregnancy

Disease	Treatment
Gonorrhea	
Local maternal infection	
Uncomplicated	Amoxicillin 3.0 g P.O. and probenecid 1.0 g P.O., immediately
	or
	Ampicillin 3.5 g P.O. and probenecid 1.0 g P.O., immediately
	or
	Procaine penicillin G 2.4 million units IM in *each* buttock and probenecid 1.0 g P.O., immediately
Penicillin allergy	Spectinomycin 2.0 g IM
PPNG or treatment failure	Spectinomycin 2.0 g IM
	or
	Cefotaxime 1.0 g IM, only
	or
	Cefoxitin 2.0 g IM and probenecid 1.0 g P.O., immediately
Disseminated maternal infection	Amoxicillin 3.0 g P.O. and probenecid 1.0 g P.O., immediately *plus* Amoxicillin 500 mg P.O. q.i.d. for 7 days
	or
	Ampicillin 3.5 g P.O. and probenecid 1.0 g P.O., immediately *plus* Ampicillin 500 mg P.O. q.i.d. for 7 days
	or
	Aqueous crystalline penicillin G 10 million units IV daily until improved, followed by amoxicillin 500 mg P.O. q.i.d. for 7 days *or* ampicillin 500 mg P.O. q.i.d. for 7 days
PPNG	Cefoxitin 1.0 g q6h for 7 days
	or
	Cefotaxime 500 mg IV q6h for 7 days
Penicillin allergy	Erythromycin 500 mg P.O. q.i.d. for 7 days
Syphilis	
Maternal infection	
Primary, secondary, latent syphilis of less than 1 yr duration	Benzathine penicillin G 2.4 million units IM; or, for penicillin-allergic patients, erythromycin 500 mg P.O. q.i.d. for 15 days (treat newborn with penicillin)
Syphilis of more than 1 yr duration or syphilis of unknown duration	Benzathine penicillin G 2.4 million units IM once a wk for 3 wk; or for penicillin-allergic patients, erythromycin 500 mg P.O. q.i.d. for 30 days (treat newborn with penicillin)
Neurosyphilis	Aqueous penicillin G 6.0–9.0 million units over 3–4 wk; expert consultation
Chlamydia	
Maternal infection	Erythromycin 500 mg P.O. q.i.d. for 7–10 days; treat partner
Neonatal prophylaxis	Erythromycin ophthalmic ointment 0.5% applied bilaterally at delivery
Mycoplasma	
Maternal infection	Erythromycin 500 mg P.O. q.i.d. for 7–10 days; treat partner
Herpes simplex	Acyclovir has not been tested in pregnant or lactating women
Condyloma acuminata (symptomatic only)	CO_2 laser therapy, cryotherapy, surgical removal. Podophyllin is contraindicated during pregnancy
Nonspecific vaginitis (symptomatic only)	Ampicillin 500 mg P.O. q.i.d. for 7 days for patient and partner, or for penicillin-allergic patients, sulfa cream intravaginally b.i.d.
Trichomonas (symptomatic only)	Metronidazole 2 g P.O. immediately for patient and partner; metronidazole is contraindicated in the 1st trimester of pregnancy
	or
	Clotrimazole 100 mg intravaginally for 7 days; safety of clotrimazole in the 1st trimester has not been established

PPNG = penicillinase-producing *Neisseria gonorrhoeae.*
Source: *Morbidity and Mortality Weekly Report* [42].

*Table 24-5. Recommended isolation procedures for selected infections**

Maternal infection	Maternal isolation	Infant isolation	Mother/infant interaction
Campylobacter	Enteric precautions until 2 negative stool cultures	Enteric precautions	Gown and gloves, careful handwashing
Chicken pox	Strict isolation, preferably in area remote from immunocompromised patients or susceptible staff until 7 days after onset of rash or all lesions crusted	None for the first 7 days following exposure; strict isolation for subsequent 2 wks; if mother contracted varicella less than 5 days before delivery or within 48 hrs after delivery administer VZIG to newborn promptly	None, until newborn receives VZIG or mother out of isolation
Chlamydia	None	Caretakers wear gloves for initial bath	Careful handwashing; mother must wear clean cover gown and have lower part of body covered; breast-feeding may be permitted
Endometritis	Segregation (patients may room together, but not with noninfected patients)	None	Mother must wear clean cover gown; careful handwashing do not place baby on mother's bed or expose directly to lochia
Gonorrhea	Avoid contact until initiation of therapy	Isolation with mother	Careful handwashing; avoid contact with secretions or fomites
Hepatitis	Blood and enteric precautions	Blood and enteric precautions; isolation with mother	Careful handwashing; avoidance of newborn contact with blood, blood products or lochia; gown and gloves when handling infant
Herpes, genital (active herpetic lesions at birth)	Wound and skin isolation for infected area only; private room, if possible	Caretakers wear gloves for initial bath; gown, gloves; rooming in or isolation	Cesarean delivery; careful handwashing
Herpes, oral	None	None	Careful handwashing; mother must wear mask; avoid contact with oral secretions until lesion has healed
Mastitis	No isolation; careful handwashing; individual breast pump	None	No restrictions; encourage breast feeding
Measles	Respiratory isolation until 4 days after onset of rash; exposure with history of measles—no isolation; exposure with no history of measles—no isolation for first 7 days, respiratory isolation for next 7 days	None for first 5 days after exposure; respiratory isolation for next 7 days; measles hyperimmune globulin	Mask until 4 days after onset of rash; careful handwashing; cover gown; avoid contact with lesions and fomites
Mononucleosis (Epstein-Barr Virus)	Respiratory isolation for duration of illness	None	Careful handwashing; avoid direct contact with oral secretions
Mumps	No isolation for first 7 days after exposure; respiratory isolation for next 2 wk or until 9 days after onset of swelling	None for first 7 days after exposure; respiratory isolation for next 2 wk or until 9 days after onset of swelling	Mother should wear mask until 1 wk after onset of swelling; careful handwashing
Mycoplasma	None	None	Careful handwashing

331

Table 24-5. (Continued)

Maternal infection	Mother isolation	Infant isolation	Mother/infant interaction
Pneumonia, bacterial (other than Staphylococcus aureus or group A Streptococcus)	None	None	Careful handwashing; mother should wear mask
Rubella	Respiratory isolation	Isolation with mother	Mask until 3–4 days after rash; careful handwashing
Streptococcus, group B (colonization)	None	None	Careful handwashing
Syphilis	Blood and wound precautions	Isolation with mother	Careful handwashing; avoid contact with lesions
Tuberculosis	Respiratory isolation	Isolation with mother until two maternal sputums negative	Careful handwashing; neonatal chemoprophylaxis

*The purpose of isolation procedures and precautions in handling patients and/or their products is to prevent the transmission of disease. These procedures may be explained as follows. Respiratory isolation: reduce risk of transmission of organisms by droplets dispersed into the environment by the upper respiratory tract or lungs; enteric precautions: avoid contact with feces or objects contaminated with feces; wound precautions: avoid contact with contaminated wounds or secretions from contaminated wounds; blood precautions: avoid contact with blood or objects contaminated with blood.

performed, their lack of specificity requires confirmation of a positive screening test with the fluorescent treponemal antibody absorption test (FTA-ABS) or the more practical and economical microhemagglutination assay for *Treponema pallidum* antibody (MHA-TP) [46,47].

All pregnant women should be screened with a nontreponemal test for syphilis. In patients at high risk of contracting the disease, serology should be repeated in the third trimester. In patients with recent exposure, nontreponemal serologic tests may remain negative for up to six weeks. During pregnancy, the benefits of treating a woman with a recent known exposure may outweigh the risks of awaiting seroconversion [42].

The current guidelines for treating syphilis during pregnancy are presented in Table 24-4 [42]. For early syphilis, benzathine penicillin G, 2.4 million units IM, is given in a single dose. For patients who have a history of penicillin allergy, erythromycin can be substituted. However, because of the increased risk of congenital syphilis in the offspring of these women, despite erythromycin therapy, investigation of the allergic history and skin-testing to substantiate penicillin allergy is appropriate [28,48]. Since erythromycin does not reliably achieve significant fetal serum levels, it is recommended that penicillin be administered to every newborn whose mother received erythromycin for the treatment of syphilis during pregnancy. Latent syphilis of more than one year's duration or syphilis of unknown duration requires prolonged therapy with repeated injections. Cerebrospinal fluid examination should be performed prior to treatment to rule out neurologic involvement. Central nervous system involvement does not consistently resolve with long-term penicillin therapy.

The onset of chills, fever, hyperventilation, headache, tachycardia, and hypotension within 8 to 12 hours of treatment (Jarisch-Herxheimer reaction) is a common complication of syphilis therapy [49]. Patients should be informed of this possible reaction. Since temperatures may become very high, pregnant women and all ill newborns should be pretreated with an antipyretic agent.

Follow-up of patients treated for syphilis during pregnancy consists of monthly nontreponemal serologic examinations. Persistence or recurrence of clinical signs or symptoms requires retreatment. A four-fold increase in the titer of follow-up serology also mandates retreatment. Nontreponemal serologic tests can be expected to become negative within 12 to 24 months of adequate therapy. In a few instances of long-term disease, these tests may remain positive in low titers despite adequate treatment. Treponemal serologic tests, however, will rarely revert to negative despite eradication of syphilis, and are thus of no benefit in following response to therapy. After therapy for neurosyphilis, serologic testing, including examination of the cerebrospinal fluid, must be obtained twice yearly for a minimum of three years.

Chlamydia

Chlamydia trachomatis is a highly successful parasite of man that has assumed increasing importance as a possible etiologic agent in maternal and neonatal disease. It is an obligate intracellular bacterialike organism that has been implicated as a frequent cause of acute and chronic salpingitis, endometritis, cervicitis, and urethritis [50–53].

Prospective studies suggest that up to 18% of pregnant women carry *Chlamydia* in the lower genital tract. The highest carriage rates should be expected in women with other venereal diseases, in those with multiple sex partners, and in women of lower socioeconomic status [54,55]. Although commonly asymptomatic, a mucopurulent endocervical discharge with associated general signs of cervicitis may be present.

Identification of chlamydial infection must be performed by isolation of the organism in tissue culture. Availability of *Chlamydia* culture is not universal and specific arrangements for sampling and transport must be made with each laboratory. Vigorous "scraping" or biopsy of infected tissues must be obtained to insure successful culture of this fastidious intracellular organism.

The effects of maternal chlamydial infection on the outcome of pregnancy are presently unknown. Frommell et al. found no association between maternal infection with *C. trachomatis* and preterm delivery, low birth weight, and postpartum complications [56]. However, Martin et al. found a statistically significant increase in preterm delivery, stillbirth, and neonatal death in mothers who carried *Chlamydia* in their lower genital tract during pregnancy [57]. Wager et al. noted a four-fold increase in intrapartum fever and delayed postpartum endometritis in women who were culture-positive for *C. trachomatis* during gestation [58]. Although the results of these more recent studies are disturbing, controlled, prospective confirmation in a large series of patients is needed.

Vertical transmission of *Chlamydia* from mother to infant during birth is well documented. Ophthalmia neonatorum secondary to *C. trachomatis* appears to occur in 20 to 50% of infants born to mothers carrying *Chlamydia* in the lower genital tract [58,59]. Erythromycin ophthalmic ointment 0.5% soon after delivery has been shown to adequately protect against chlamydial conjunctivitis in addition to providing the necessary prevention against neonatal gonococcal ophthal-

mia [42,60]. Beem and Saxon described the development of a distinctive pneumonia syndrome within three months of delivery in 10 to 20% of children born to mothers with genital *C. trachomatis* [61].

Treatment of pregnant women with documented chlamydial infection during pregnancy is accomplished with erythromycin (see Table 24-4) [42]. Sulfonamides offer a reasonable, though unproven, alternative during pregnancy in erythromycin-allergic patients [62].

The Centers for Disease Control guidelines also recommend empiric treatment for pregnant women whose sexual partners have nongonococcal urethritis [42].

Recommended isolation procedures for women with chlamydial infections and their infants are presented in Table 24-5.

Mycoplasma

Mycoplasma are the smallest organisms capable of independent existence and replication. *Mycoplasma hominis* and *Ureaplasma urealyticum* appear to play a role in genital tract disease in humans. *Mycoplasma* can be commonly cultured from the vagina of an asymptomatic pregnant woman [63]. Higher rates of colonization are found in women with multiple sexual partners and in those from low socioeconomic groups [63].

The effect of genital *Mycoplasma* colonization on the outcome of pregnancy is unclear. Braun et al. found a statistically significant decrease in birth weight in infants of women colonized with *U. urealyticum* during gestation [64]. Colonization with *M. hominis* appeared to have no effect on birth weight. Others have failed to confirm such an association [65]. Investigators have also demonstrated an association between chorioamnionitis and isolation of *U. urealyticum* [66]. Puerperal fever appears to be caused by *M. hominis* in some instances. The true incidence of postpartum endometritis secondary to *Mycoplasma* must still be delineated.

Although serious *M. hominis* infections have been reported in newborns, the exact consequences of mycoplasma infections in newborns remain undefined [67]. Despite the high prevalence of neonatal mycoplasma colonization, the infrequency of clinical infection suggests that this organism is a pathogen of very low virulence.

Isolation of *Mycoplasma* requires inoculation of a special media that is provided by a limited number of clinical laboratories. Specific serologic titers may be helpful in making the diagnosis, although cross-reactivity is common. Because of the poorly defined role of *Mycoplasma* in perinatal disease, routine screening or treatment of the asymptomatic patient is not recommended.

Generally, *Mycoplasma* is sensitive to tetracyclines and erythromycin. Treatment with erythromycin for documented infections during pregnancy is described in Table 24-4.

Genital Herpes

Genital infection with herpes simplex virus (HSV) has reached epidemic proportions in the United States [68]. The devastating morbidity and mortality as a result of disseminated neonatal infection with HSV acquired at delivery has prompted considerable attention from both physicians and the public.

Primary genital herpes infection in women usually presents as multiple, painful, ulcerating blisters on the vulva, perineum, or buttocks. Either type I or type II virus may be responsible, although herpes type II is present in the majority of cases [69]. Local lymphadenopathy and systemic signs of viremia are common in the primary infection. After two to four weeks, the genital lesions resolve and the virus retreats indefinitely to the dorsal ganglia of the nerve roots involved with the initial outbreak. Up to 85 percent of patients experience clinical recurrence of varying frequency and intensity [70]. In up to 10% of asymptomatic women with a history of genital herpes, HSV can be isolated from the cervix [71].

Diagnosis of HSV infection is made by virus isolation and identification in tissue culture. Although use of cytology to make the diagnosis has been proposed, the high incidence of false negative results, as well as occasional false positive smears, renders this technique unreliable [69]. Serology is of limited value because of the high prevalence of HSV antibodies in the general population. Development of an enzyme-linked immunosorbant assay (ELISA) will likely provide rapid diagnosis in the future if present technical problems can be overcome [69].

HSV can be isolated from the cervix of approximately 1% of all asymptomatic pregnant patients [72,73]. In pregnant patients with a history of genital herpes, or in those whose partners have a history of genital herpes, up to 14% of patients will shed HSV from the cervix or vulva asymptomatically [74,75].

The effect of clinically evident genital herpes infection on the developing fetus is not clear. Primary infection early during pregnancy is associated with an increased risk of spontaneous abortion. Teratogenicity, if it occurs at all, appears to be exceedingly rare [69,73]. Primary infection

after 20 weeks gestation has been correlated with an increased risk of preterm birth. It is unlikely that recurrent herpes increases the risk of abortion or preterm birth, although some authors have reported increased perinatal wastage with secondary HSV infections [73,76]. The safety and possible benefits of the antiviral agent acyclovir, either topically or parenterally, for treatment of primary or recurrent disease during human pregnancy remains unstudied. Early reports of the use of the laser to treat genital lesions during pregnancy appear promising [77].

Vertical transmission of HSV to the newborn at the time of delivery represents the greatest risk to the newborn. Fortunately, the incidence of neonatal infection approximates only one in 7500 deliveries [69]. Fifty to seventy percent of the mothers of newborns with HSV infection are asymptomatic at the time of delivery [74,76]. Fifty percent of affected neonates are delivered preterm. Disseminated neonatal disease is most often noted within the first ten days of life, although the onset of clinical infection can be delayed for up to four weeks [69,76]. Cesarean birth appears to minimize, though not eliminate, the risk of acquiring herpes from mothers with primary or recurrent HSV genital infection at delivery [78].

The mortality rate of untreated disseminated neonatal HSV infections exceeds 50%. Of those who survive, neurologic or ophthalmic damage is frequent [74,79]. Early treatment with adenine arabinoside has been shown to decrease mortality and morbidity rates [79].

Optimal management of pregnant patients with a history of genital herpes infection will prevent vertical transmission to the neonate at delivery while minimizing the need for cesarean delivery. Such optimal management has yet to be defined; however, several approaches have been suggested [74,80,81]. All protocols presume the availability of accurate viral cultures. The clinician must locate such facilities and prearrange appropriate sampling, transport, and reporting through direct communication with the virology laboratory. With optimal viral techniques the rate of false negative cultures should be less than 10% [75]. Because of the relative ease and rapidity of HSV culture, results of sampling should be available in two to six days [69,80].

Pregnant women with a history suggestive of genital HSV infection or those with a sexual partner with a history suggestive of genital HSV infection should be managed as outlined below. Adherence to such recommendations should minimize risks of neonatal infection while allowing vaginal delivery in the majority of patients.

1. Educate the patient and her family regarding the potential risks of neonatal herpes infection.
2. Explain the plan of management and the need to maintain close communication and maximal compliance.
3. Explain the venereal nature of HSV infection and the need for sexual abstinence when active lesions are present; explain the risk of transmission of HSV from oral lesions during orogenital intercourse.
4. If suspicious lesions appear during pregnancy, culture the patient or her sexual partner at least once if HSV has not been documented previously by culture.
5. Even for asymptomatic patients, begin weekly cervical and vulvar cultures at 36 weeks. Separate swabs should be used to prevent inadvertent inoculation of an uninvolved site. To minimize cost, both swabs may be used to inoculate the same medium.
6. In patients at high risk for preterm delivery, begin weekly cultures earlier in gestation, (e.g., at 32 weeks).
7. For patients at 36 weeks or later, stress the importance of notifying the physician immediately if symptoms suggestive of HSV infection are noted, or if membranes rupture.
8. At the time labor begins, deliver the fetus vaginally if cultures have remained negative and a thorough examination of the vulva, cervix, and vagina is negative.
9. In patients who have had frequent recurrences during gestation, consider induction of labor near term if fetal maturity is assured and if the two latest cultures have been negative for HSV. (Two negative cultures will minimize the chance of false negative results).
10. If HSV is isolated near term, repeat genital cultures two to three times weekly until two consecutive cultures remain negative for more than 72 hours. Data suggest that only a minority of patients will shed virus for more than five days after recurrent infection begins [70, 82].
11. Following a positive culture near term, cesarean delivery should be performed if labor begins before two negative cultures can be documented.
12. If membranes rupture following a positive culture and before subsequent negative cultures can be documented, cesarean delivery should be performed as soon as possible, *regardless of the duration of ruptured membranes* [69,70,75].
13. If suspicious genital lesions *or symptoms* exist at the onset of labor or at the time of rupture of membranes, cesarean delivery should be performed regardless of previous culture results and *regardless of duration of ruptured membranes.*

Following delivery, mothers with active herpetic infection (genital or nongenital) must avoid all contact between the herpetic lesions and the infant (see Table 24-5). Careful handwashing is recommended. Infants should either remain with their mothers or be isolated from other newborns while in the nursery. Breast feeding is not discouraged [69,75].

Condyloma Acuminata
(Venereal Warts)

Condyloma acuminata are common genital lesions caused by sexually transmitted human papilloma virus. Like most other veneral diseases, the incidence is increasing [84].

Diagnosis is most often made by recognition of typical multiple papillomatous lesions on the vulva, urethra, vagina, cervix, perineum, or rectum. Single lesions, those exhibiting necrosis or bleeding, and those that do not respond to the usual treatment should be biopsied [85].

During pregnancy, condylomas may grow rapidly, although spontaneous regression following delivery is not uncommon [86]. Complications of labor and delivery secondary to large condylomas have been reported [86]. Vertical transmission to the infant has also been reported, although the exact incidence is not known [87,88].

Treatment with podophyllin, a commonly used caustic agent, is contraindicated during pregnancy [84]. A variety of other treatment modalities have also been used, including surgical excision and cryotherapy. Most recently, successful treatment of symptomatic or enlarging vulvar condylomas during pregnancy has been accomplished with the carbon dioxide laser [89,90].

Trichomoniasis

Genital infection with the motile protozoan *Trichomonas vaginalis* is a venereally transmitted disease that may occur in 20% of pregnancies. The organism is best identified on wet smear in symptomatic cases, although identification on routine Pap smear or urinalysis is not uncommon. Vaginal pain, a malodorous discharge, or vulvar itching are the most common symptoms.

Asymptomatic vaginal infestation with trichomonads does not appear to affect the outcome of pregnancy. Treatment of asymptomatic infection during pregnancy is not recommended. The most effective agent for treatment of symptomatic infestation during the second and third trimesters is metronidazole; its use in the first trimester is contraindicated because it has been found to be mutagenic and carcinogenic in animals [30,31]. Clotrimazole is a vaginal antifungal agent that also appears to have limited effectiveness against trichomonads. Its use in the first trimester of pregnancy is not recommended but may be necessary to control severe symptoms. Chronic use of iodide-containing preparations during pregnancy is not suggested because of the reported risk of fetal goiter [83].

Nonspecific Vaginitis

Vaginal infection not attributable to uterine infection, *Candida albicans*, or *Trichomonas vaginalis* has been termed nonspecific vaginitis (NSV). Despite Gardner and Duke's classic association of *Haemophilus vaginalis* (now termed *Gardnerella vaginalis*) with NSV [91], its etiology remains controversial. Current opinion favors an etiologic role for certain anaerobic vaginal bacteria in concert with *G. vaginalis* in NSV [92–95]. Venereal transmission is the most likely mode of infection.

Vaginal colonization with *G. vaginalis* occurs in up to 40% of asymptomatic women [94]. Patients with symptomatic NSV complain of a malodorous discharge often accompanied by itching and burning. The diagnosis of NSV depends not on culture but on the observation of short motile rods and vaginal epithelial cells covered by bacteria called "clue cells" [95]. The "fishy" odor sometimes noted upon application of 10% potassium hydroxide to the discharge may be helpful in making the diagnosis [92].

The therapy of symptomatic NSV during pregnancy is controversial. Although metronidazole has been shown to be the agent of choice, its use in pregnant women is not recommended. Likewise, tetracyclines are contraindicated during pregnancy. Ampicillin, 500 mg orally four times daily for seven days, is the treatment of choice during pregnancy. Antibiotic treatment of the sexual partner is also recommended since NSV appears to be transmitted venereally. In patients who are penicillin-allergic, local application of a sulfa cream twice daily may give partial relief [92,96]. Long-term systemic antibiotic therapy, however, may contribute to the subsequent development of vaginal candidiasis.

As yet, no deleterious effects on infants born to untreated mothers have been published.

GROUP B STREPTOCOCCUS

Over the last two decades, group B streptococcus has emerged as a major cause of neonatal sepsis, morbidity, and death [97]. The estimated incidence of disease caused by this organism is between one and five cases per 1000 live births [98].

Two distinct clinical entities, early- and late-onset disease, have been described. Early-onset disease presents during the first five days of life, often within hours of delivery. Pneumonia and generalized sepsis dominate the clinical picture, with a minority of infants exhibiting meningitis. The presentation may at first be difficult to differentiate from hyaline membrane disease [99]. Preterm and growth-retarded infants are more frequently affected. Vertical transmission of the infecting organism from mother to baby appears to be the most likely mode of transmission. Genital colonization rates during pregnancy approach 35% in some studies [100]. Although most infants are colonized during vaginal delivery, very few show clinical signs of infection [98]. Neonatal mortality rate in early-onset disease is 50%, despite aggressive therapy [98].

Attempts to eliminate genital colonization during pregnancy have been disappointing [101]. Culture and treatment late in gestation have been suggested by some [102]. In a large controlled study, Siegel et al. administered parenteral penicillin to infants at the time of birth [103]. Treated neonates showed lower colonization and clinical infection rates. A more recent study was unable to show benefit from penicillin treatment to low birth weight infants [104].

Late-onset disease occurs after seven days and before three months of age, usually manifests itself as meningitis, and has a mortality rate of 25% [98]. The mode of transmission appears to be nosocomial or community-acquired; colonization at the time of delivery does not appear to be involved.

Treatment of either early- or late-onset disease in neonates requires high parenteral dosages of penicillin G and supportive measures. Multivalent vaccination of all antibody-deficient pregnant women has been proposed and theoretically should be efficacious [98]. Investigation into development of such a vaccine is underway.

Recommended isolation procedures in group B streptococcal infections are presented in Table 24-5.

CHORIOAMNIONITIS

Chorioamnionitis is an inflammation of the placental membranes classically associated with prolonged rupture of the amnion. Although histologic evidence of inflammation is a common finding in normal pregnancies, approximately 1% of all pregnancies appear to be complicated by clinically evident chorioamnionitis [105,106]. With prolonged rupture of membranes, the risk appears to approach 25% [106]. Uterine tenderness, maternal fever, fetal tachycardia, foul vaginal discharge, and elevation in maternal white blood cell count dominate the clinical picture. Despite the improved prognosis for both mother and fetus, this serious complication continues to be a major source of morbidity and mortality for both and must be managed aggressively [107].

The incomplete mechanical barriers to intrauterine infection include the mucous "plug" of the endocervix and the intact amnion. Even in the absence of such barriers, intrauterine sepsis does not develop in the majority of cases, presumably due to the bacteriostatic properties of amniotic fluid [108,109]. Chorioamnionitis has been documented in the presence of intact placental membranes [110]. Infection through hematogenous spread is well known. The organisms involved most often are those found normally in the vagina and cervix. Other organisms, including *Listeria monocytogenes, Neisseria gonorrhoeae,* or group A beta-hemolytic Streptococcus, may be identified.

Increasing evidence points to a major role for subclinical chorioamnionitis in preterm labor and in preterm rupture of membranes [111,112]. Bejar et al. have demonstrated marked phospholipase A_2 activity in bacteria responsible for chorioamnionitis [113]. They theorize that increased production of prostaglandins associated with chorioamnionitis may explain resultant preterm labor or preterm rupture of membranes. Amniotic fluid analysis to rule out chorioamnionitis has been recommended by some in an effort to detect subclinical infection and optimize management of both of these common and difficult obstetric complications [111,112]. However, bacteriologic evaluation of amniotic fluid obtained by amniocentesis can be difficult. The presence of white cells is not always indicative of infection. Nevertheless, observation of organisms on Gram stain of uncentrifuged fluid or culture of fluid growing at least 10^2 organisms/mL indicates chorioamnionitis [114]. In the future, identification of organic acid metabolites of bacteria in amniotic fluid by gas-liquid chromatography may prove valuable in the diagnosis of chorioamnionitis [115].

Chorioamnionitis requires maternal antibiotic therapy and prompt delivery. If there are no signs of imminent fetal or maternal jeopardy, vaginal delivery is preferred in order to minimize subsequent maternal morbidity. Parenteral antibiotics, usually ampicillin and an aminoglycoside, should be initiated. In severely ill patients, or in patients undergoing cesarean delivery, clindamycin should be added to the antibiotic regimen to eradicate resistant anaerobic organisms.

PUERPERAL MASTITIS

Sporadic puerperal mastitis is a cellulitis of the interlobular connective tissue of the breast that usually occurs within several weeks of the initiation of lactation [116]. It is characterized by localized pain and redness, chills, and significant fever. Cracked or fissured nipples allow the entrance of pathogenic organisms, usually *Staphylococcus* or *Streptococcus*, although gram-negative enteric bacteria are occasionally isolated [117]. Early initiation of systemic antibiotics effective against penicillinase-producing organisms is essential in preventing abscess formation. Dicloxacillin (or equivalent) is most often recommended, although cephalosporins are also effective, particularly if the responsible organism is a gram-negative enteric. In penicillin-allergic patients, erythromycin is an appropriate alternative. To facilitate drainage and decrease abscess formation, breast feeding should be continued, although emptying of the affected breast must sometimes be accomplished with breast pumping.

Epidemic puerperal mastitis is an uncommon nosocomial infection usually developing within several days of delivery and associated with a highly virulent strain of *Staphylococcus aureus*. Since infants are also affected, prompt treatment of both mother and baby with a penicillinase-resistant penicillin is mandatory. The source of the epidemic must be identified immediately to control the outbreak [118].

Superficial mastitis due to *Candida albicans* is not uncommon. Topical antifungal agents containing nystatin, clotrimazole, or miconazole must be applied to both the mother's nipples, as well as to the infant's oropharynx, which is often infected concurrently.

URINARY TRACT INFECTIONS
Epidemiology and Pathogenesis

Urinary tract infections are among the most common infections associated with pregnancy; likewise, they represent the most frequently observed renal complication of pregnancy. Three types of urinary tract infections are seen: asymptomatic bacteriuria, acute cystitis, and pyelonephritis. Approximately 5 to 10% of pregnant women have significant bacteriuria ($>10^5$ colonies of bacteria per milliliter of urine). The responsible organism in more than 85% of these infections is *Escherichia coli*. The incidence of bacteriuria is higher in the presence of any of the following factors: history of childhood urinary tract infections, advanced maternal age, multiparity, low socioeconomic status, underlying chronic disease (e.g., diabetes mellitus or sickle cell disorders), nonglomerular renal disease (e.g., obstructive uropathy, analgesic nephropathy, and reflux nephropathy), and hypertension [119]. Pregnancy itself can create a predisposition to bacteriuria by causing alteration, including dilatation of the ureters and collecting system, glycosuria, aminoaciduria, and dehydration in patients with persistent vomiting. In addition to a high incidence of bacteriuria, pregnancy is associated with a high propensity for infection involving the upper urinary tract. As many as 25% of pregnant women with bacteriuria will develop acute pyelonephritis later in pregnancy if they are not treated effectively during the asymptomatic bacteriuric stage. Also, as many as 30% of pregnant women with asymptomatic bacteriuria have roentgenographic evidence of abnormalities of the urinary tract.

Current data suggest that 80 to 90% of all cases of acute pyelonephritis can be prevented by treatment of symptomatic bacteriuria in early gestation [120]. If asymptomatic bacteriuria is not present in early pregnancy the likelihood of acquiring bacteriuria later in pregnancy is less than 2%. Similarly, only 2 to 3% of patients treated during early pregnancy for bacteriuria will develop pyelonephritis in later pregnancy. Several studies have shown that women who suffer pyelonephritis during pregnancy have twice the preterm delivery rate of either nonbacteriurics or asymptomatic bacteriuric controls [120]. Since pregnancy sets the stage for renal parenchymal infection in patients with bacteriuria, it is essential that the first prenatal examination include a screening test for bacteriuria with effective treatment and followup of infected patients.

Diagnosis

To facilitate discussion of urinary tract infections, several terms should first be defined. *Significant bacteriuria* means recovery of greater than 10^5 organisms per mL of urine. This is a convenient number with which to distinguish true infection from urethral bacterial contamination. *Asymptomatic bacteriuria* applies to women with greater than 10^5 bacteria per mL on two consecutive urine samples who are completely asymptomatic and who are identified only through routine quantitative urine culture.

By quantitating bacteria in urine it is possible to reliably differentiate urine contamination from true urinary tract infection. The most commonly used method to quantitate bacteria is urine culture, which can be performed in all microbiology laboratories. If there are more than 10^5 bacteria per mL in a clean-catch urine specimen from an asymptomatic woman, there is an 80% probability that this finding represents true bacteriuria. If the original finding is confirmed by a second culture, the probability is increased to 95%. Another simple, reliable, and inexpensive office technique is the dip slide culture.

Microscopic examination of a centrifuged, midstream urine specimen can be performed to investigate the presence of pyuria. The majority of patients with symptomatic infection and significant bacteriuria will demonstrate significant pyuria (>5 white cells per high-powered field), although approximately 20% of patients who have urine samples with insignificant bacteriuria may also demonstrate pyuria.

Another useful test for a presumptive diagnosis of urinary tract infection is microscopic examination for bacteria. A drop of urine that has not been spun in the centrifuge is placed on a slide, allowed to dry, and then stained. The slide is then scanned using the oil immersion lens. The presence of any bacteria suggests that greater than 10^5 bacteria per mL of urine will be demonstrated by quantitative methods.

Localization of the site of urinary tract infection can be important for determining appropriate dosage and duration of antibiotic therapy. One of the most promising noninvasive tests for distinguishing upper from lower urinary tract infections is the antibody-coated bacteria assay [202,203]. Unfortunately, this test requires further standardization and wider availability to be clinically useful.

Clinical Manifestations

Lower urinary tract infections are characterized primarily by dysuria and urinary frequency with normal body temperature. Bacterial cystitis and the *anterior urethral syndrome* present as lower urinary tract infections and are indistinguishable clinically. The anterior urethral syndrome is characterized by pyuria in patients whose urine cultures are negative for bacterial growth. These patients often have symptoms typical of lower urinary tract infection. *Chlamydia trachomatis, Staphylococcus saprophyticus*, or *E. coli* may be recovered in a high percentage of these cases [121].

Systemic symptoms such as fever and chills are common in patients with acute pyelonephritis (upper urinary tract infection). The presentation of acute pyelonephritis is essentially unaltered by pregnancy.

Treatment
Because of the certainty of decreasing the incidence of symptomatic pyelonephritis, it is necessary that pregnant bacteriuric patients be identified and treated. Urine cultures should be obtained in all women during early prenatal visits. There is no evidence to support the superiority of bactericidal over bacteriostatic antibiotics in urinary tract infection. These infections respond promptly to virtually all antimicrobials. Cost and safety to the fetus are thus the two most important criteria in choosing an antimicrobial agent.

Recently, the length of treatment of asymptomatic bacteriuria has come under close scrutiny [122]. It is now clear that the majority of uncomplicated urinary tract infections in nonpregnant patients can be treated with a single dose of ampicillin or amoxicillin. Harris et al. treated 86 pregnant patients who had confirmed asymptomatic bacteriuria with a single-dose, single-antimicrobial regimen [123]. Overall, the immediate rate of failure for the single-dose regimen was 31%, with a subsequent recurrence rate of 3.5%.

Because large studies of single dose therapy have not been done in pregnant women with symptomatic urinary tract infections, it would seem prudent that therapy be given for five to seven days. Urine culture should be repeated 48 hours after the completion of therapy. If the urine culture is positive, repeat sensitivity studies should be performed and therapy chosen according to the results. Reinfection (presence of bacteria of a different strain and/or a different pattern of antibiotic sensitivity than the original bacteria) usually occurs within a few weeks of the initial infection and should be treated. True relapse with the same bacterium is often indicative of a chronic renal parenchymal infection. Patients with relapses should be treated with prolonged antibiotic therapy (14 to 21 days) and followed up with monthly cultures. Some patients who have demonstrated relapse may require suppressive antibiotic therapy throughout the remainder of pregnancy. Patients with relapse should also be considered for postpartum urologic evaluation.

Patients with symptomatic pyelonephritis should be hospitalized. After blood and urine cultures are obtained, parenteral antibiotics, such as ampicillin or amoxicillin, should be given. An aminoglycoside should be added if the patient appears toxic. Patients usually respond promptly and are afebrile within 48 hours. Since 25% of these patients may become reinfected during the same

pregnancy [124], repeat urine cultures should be obtained at intervals throughout pregnancy. Many authors favor continuous antibiotic therapy for the remainder of pregnancy; however, the usefulness of prolonged therapy remains to be established.

PNEUMONIA
In the preantibiotic era, pneumonia during pregnancy caused extensive maternal and perinatal mortality [125–128]. Today, pneumonia, especially pneumococcal lobar pneumonia, has become an uncommon cause of maternal death. Nevertheless, as women with a great variety of chronic systemic illnesses or immunocompromised states have become pregnant, pneumonias caused by previously uncommon organisms are recognized more frequently.

Normal pulmonary defense mechanisms keep lung tissue essentially sterile. The occurrence of pneumonia suggests either an alteration in host defenses, exposure to a virulent microorganism, or challenge by a large inoculum of less virulent microorganisms. Maternal mortality from pneumonia is most likely to occur after 25 weeks gestation, which is the period of maximal, pregnancy-induced alterations in the respiratory system [129]. These alterations include diaphragmatic elevation of approximately 4 cm and moderate pulmonary vascular engorgement with a consequent decrease in average residual volume. This is associated with a significantly decreased functional residual capacity that causes diminished functional respiratory reserve [130]. A physiologic predisposition to airway closure during pregnancy may lead to air trapping and decreased ventilation with shunting of lung perfusion. These changes may worsen existing hypoxia in pregnant women with acute lung disease.

Despite the fetus' compensatory mechanisms for dealing with its relatively hypoxic environment, maternal respiratory embarrassment may lead to heightened fetal hypoxia and acidosis and possible death in utero. The fetus is also at risk from hyperthermia, which commonly accompanies maternal pneumonitis [131,132].

Clinical Manifestations
Other than accentuating tachycardia and tachypnea, pregnancy does not alter the physical findings in pneumonia. Examination of the chest may show "splinting," with an inspiratory lag on the side of the consolidation. Fine rales may be the only auscultatory finding in early bacterial pneumonia. Auscultatory findings of consolidation such as egophony, bronchial breath sounds, and dull-

ness on percussion strongly suggest bacterial pneumonitis. Frank cyanosis, use of accessory muscles of respiration, nasal flaring, and sternal retractions imply severe lung involvement.

In the presence of findings compatible with pneumonia, a roentgenogram of the chest with abdominal shielding can provide confirmation of the diagnosis with minimal risk to the fetus (see Chap. 8).

"Atypical pneumonia," commonly caused by *Mycoplasma pneumoniae*, may occur during pregnancy. Oxorn's series on pneumonia in pregnant women treated at the Royal Victoria Hospital, London, in both the pre- and postantibiotic eras identified 24% as having atypical pneumonia [127]. The symptom complex for the disease commonly includes fever, malaise, coryza, headache, cough, and often a rash or diarrhea. Adenoviruses, parainfluenza viruses, Epstein-Barr viruses, respiratory syncytial virus, and presumably *Legionella pneumophila* may cause similar respiratory syndromes. "Atypical pneumonia" is marked by scant auscultatory findings and, commonly, substantial radiographic changes.

Influenza-virus pneumonia is characterized by a short antecedent history of myalgia, malaise, and chills, followed by fever, headache, nasal congestion, and mild sore throat. Physical exam often reveals diffuse, bilateral, crepitant rales. Roentgenographic findings are characterized by diffuse, bilateral, fluffy infiltrates originating at the hilum and radiating to the periphery.

Pneumococcal pneumonia is characterized by productive cough, fever, and rigors. Roentgenographic findings usually include lobar consolidation. Gram-stained sputum may show sheets of white cells and encapsulated, lancet-shaped, gram-positive diplococci.

Varicella-zoster (chickenpox) pneumonia is characterized by a dry, nonproductive cough that begins two to five days after the appearance of the typical cutaneous lesions. Physical findings are often minimal despite extensive roentgenographic evidence of parenchymal involvement. Typical roentgenographic findings include diffuse, bilateral, nodular infiltrates.

Pneumonitis may also be due to parasitic infestations in patients from Southeast Asia or other areas of the world where these diseases are endemic. Tuberculosis, sarcoidosis, brucellosis, and psittacosis must also be considered.

Sputum culture and Gram stain should be done early in the course of the disease. Blood cultures are important since they may yield definitive microbiologic data. Transtracheal aspiration is not recommended unless the patient is immunocompromised and a variety of organisms are possible etiologic agents. Examination of pleural fluid in pregnant women with pneumonia is strongly recommended since this material may yield reliable bacteriologic data.

Treatment

Little modification needs to be made for antibiotic treatment of pneumonia in pregnant women except for the substitution of erythromycin for tetracycline when *Mycoplasma* or *Chlamydia* is suspected. Initial therapy tends to be empiric. Generally, penicillin, ampicillin, or erythromycin are used in community-acquired pneumonias, which are frequently due to pneumococcus or mycoplasmas. Supportive therapy is important in all cases of pneumonia regardless of the etiologic agent. Such supportive therapy should include the following:

1. Supplemental oxygen with follow-up determination of arterial PO_2
2. Adequate restoration of fluid and electrolyte balance
3. Use of physical measures such as postural drainage and back clapping to assist in clearance of secretions
4. Use of bronchodilating drugs when bronchospasm is present
5. Correction of anemia if present in order to increase oxygen-carrying capacity
6. Careful attention to skin color
7. Frequent assessment of fetal well-being. Deterioration of the fetus can be remarkably rapid

Recommended isolation procedures for women with pneumonia and their infants are presented in Table 24-5.

VIRAL INFECTIONS
Cytomegalovirus
Cytomegalovirus (CMV), is a member of the herpesvirus group, and is a common, usually asymptomatic illness. CMV has been isolated from saliva, breast milk, cervical mucus, and semen and can be transmitted venereally.

Epidemiologic studies in pregnant women have shown that the rate of cervical cytomegalovirus infection during pregnancy increases with gestational age. Approximately 1 to 2% of urban North American women have positive cervical cultures during their first trimester. This figures rises to 7% and 14% in the second and third trimester, respectively [133].

Congenital Infection
The incidence of congenital CMV infections in the

United States ranges from 0.5 to 2% of all live births, but only 5 to 10% of these infected infants manifest a symptomatic infection at birth [134]. The majority of these have major developmental defects or central nervous system sequelae, while 5 to 17% of those with silent congenital infection develop varying degrees of complications during their preschool years [135].

Intrauterine infection due to secondary or reactivated infection may rarely occur in immune mothers. There have been reports of congenital cytomegalovirus disease in consecutive pregnancies. These cases would suggest that immunity is not complete, although it still appears to be important in reducing the extent and severity of infection.

Symptomatic congenital cytomegalovirus disease is characterized by jaundice and multiple organ involvement. Microcephaly, motor disability, cerebral calcifications, chorioretinitis, and hepatosplenomegaly are also seen. Respiratory distress and seizures develop soon after birth and most infants with the fulminant form of disease die. In survivors, neurologic sequelae may become apparent later [134].

Newborns may acquire CMV from sources other than their mothers, including blood products. Acquisition of CMV by the newborn shortly after birth or while passing through the birth canal does not usually cause severe disease. Therefore, vaginal delivery of CMV-infected mothers is preferred.

Asymptomatic infections

Hanshaw identified 53 children with IgM antibodies to CMV in cord blood [135]. He evaluated 44 of these children at 3½ to 7 years of age. The mean I.Q. of 103 was significantly lower than matched controls. The predicted school failure based on I.Q., behavioral, neurologic, and auditory data was two and one half times greater than that in controls matched by socioeconomic status. These data suggest that asymptomatic CMV infection may have important sequelae.

Breast feeding

CMV can be cultured, at least transiently, from breast milk, in up to 27% of seropositive postpartum mothers and from 18% of all mothers. In a study of 17 infants born to women excreting detectable CMV in colostrum or milk, nine (52%) acquired CMV between three weeks and nine months of age. None of these infants developed detectable morbidity after a mean follow-up time of two years [136]. Donations of milk to a milk bank by known CMV-seropositive mothers are inadvisable.

Varicella-Zoster

Chickenpox, caused by the varicella-zoster virus, is uncommon during pregnancy, but can result in serious maternal infection, particularly pneumonia. Infection in early pregnancy has been implicated in the development of congenital abnormalities. Reported congenital defects include skin scarring, hypoplastic limbs, eye abnormalities, microcephaly, and severe motor and growth retardation [137]. Infection in late gestation can result in transplacental passage of virus to the fetus. However, neonatal chickenpox is not inevitable following maternal disease in late gestation. From data reported to the Centers for Disease Control, Meyers found that only 11 of 46 infants born to mothers who had the onset of chickenpox within 17 days before delivery developed neonatal chickenpox within the first ten days of life [138].

Nonimmune pregnant women should not be exposed to persons with active varicella-zoster infection. If close exposure does occur, zoster immune globulin may be administered. Passive immunization with zoster immune serum globulin (ZIG) or zoster immune plasma (ZIP) may ameliorate maternal disease, but because of the delay in placental antibody transport, it is unlikely that it will completely protect the newborn against infection. Administration of ZIG to newborns whose mothers developed chickenpox in the period between five days before and two days after delivery may lessen any ensuing neonatal illness. Currently, varicella-zoster immune globulin (VZIG) is available at some centers for passive immunization. Mothers with infectious chickenpox at birth should be kept in isolation and be attended to by staff known to have had prior varicella-zoster infection (see Table 24-5). The unprotected newborn should be isolated from its infectious mother until passive immunoprophylaxis has been administered. Rooming-in, prompt discharge, and follow-up are recommended.

Rubella

Until the 1940s rubella was considered a mild disease with epidemic potential, but of no great public health importance. Then, in 1942, an association between maternal rubella and congenital defects was recognized [139]. This observation helped to identify rubella as an important and preventable cause of congenital malformation.

Rubella virus is spread by respiratory secretions. Some infected individuals are asymptomatic. Therefore, tracking the source of infection in a partially immunized population is difficult. Children with congenital rubella shed large quantities of virus for many months and can be an important source of infection. Recipients of rubella vaccine do not transmit the virus to others.

The incidence of rubella is highest in the spring. Although it is more common in school-age children, it is being seen with increasing frequency in older age groups. In unvaccinated populations rubella epidemics occur every six to nine years; major epidemics have occurred every 30 years.

The incubation period for rubella is 12 to 24 days (average is 18 days). Children and young adults have malaise, fever, and anorexia early in the clinical course of the disease. The posterior auricular, posterior cervical, and suboccipital lymph nodes are commonly involved. A maculopapular, nonconfluent rash begins on the face and spreads to the trunk. The rash usually lasts three to five days. Fever, if present, rarely persists beyond the first day of the rash.

The most common complications of rubella in adult women are arthritis and arthralgia which may affect up to one-third of these patients [139]. Joint symptoms are not usually seen in children or adult men.

Congenital Rubella

Rubella can be a devastating disease in early gestation and may lead to preterm delivery, congenital defects, or fetal or neonatal death. Rubella vaccine has, however, virtually eliminated the risk of epidemic.

The effects of rubella virus on a fetus vary with the stage of gestation. Generally, the earlier in gestation the infection occurs, the more severe the illness. In the first two months of gestation, the fetus has approximately a 50% chance of being affected, whereas rubella infection during the fourth month of gestation carries a 10% risk of a single congenital defect. Mann et al. have developed algorithms for assessing risks of rubella infection during pregnancy [140].

Congenital rubella may cause low birth weight and congenital defects, including myopia, deafness, cataracts, glaucoma, congenital heart disease, and mental retardation. Some children whose mothers had rubella during pregnancy and who seemed normal at birth have been found to have abnormalities such as deafness on reaching school age.

Rubella Vaccine

An excellent live attenuated rubella vaccine is available. The major immunization strategy in the United States has been to vaccinate prepubertal children in order to reduce the number of susceptible pregnant women. Recently, proposals to vaccinate susceptible adolescent females have been advanced [141]. Rubella vaccine may cause viremia, adenopathy, arthritis, and arthralgia. All of these complications are more common in adults than in children (see Immunization).

Rubella virus has been isolated from fetal tissue at abortion following inadvertent vaccination of pregnant women. No infant with congenital rubella syndrome has been born to a woman given rubella vaccine during pregnancy [142]. However, since a theoretical risk remains, women inadvertently vaccinated during the first or second trimester should be counseled with current information regarding risk of congenital anomalies. Women should not become pregnant for at least three months following rubella vaccination. Premarital screening of blood for antibody to rubella virus should be performed and vaccination offered to those found to be seronegative. Vaccinated women should be counseled to use contraception for at least three months. Seronegative women may be vaccinated in the immediate postpartum period since few will become pregnant again within three months. Vaccination is not a contraindication to breast feeding.

Measles

Measles in pregnancy has been implicated in congenital malformation, but no causal relationship has been established. There is an apparent increase in abortion, preterm birth, and perinatal death. The infant may acquire the disease in utero and be born with the characteristic morbilliform rash or develop the rash in the first few days of life.

The measles vaccine has significantly reduced the occurrence of the disease during pregnancy. Women who have never received the vaccine or had the disease should be offered immunity before becoming pregnant. Susceptible pregnant women who have been exposed to the disease should receive immune serum globulin promptly (see Immunization) [143]. Recommended isolation procedures for women with measles and their infants are presented in Table 24-5.

Mumps

Mumps is a highly contagious infection caused by a paramyxovirus. It is spread by respiratory droplets, and is most common in the winter and spring. After an 18-day incubation period, unilateral or bilateral parotitis develops, accompanied by myalgia, fever, anorexia, and, occasionally, earaches.

A diagnosis of mumps is usually established by clinical characteristics and can be confirmed by detecting a rise in complement-fixing mumps antibodies.

The clinical course and severity of mumps do

not appear to be affected by pregnancy; however, Siegel and Fuerst demonstrated an increase in early fetal deaths [144]. Although congenital malformations such as endocardial fibrosis can be induced in experimental animals by mumps virus, no convincing association has been made in humans. Mumps infection in neonates can cause considerable morbidity. Isolation of the mother and infant from other mothers and infants is recommended [145] (see Table 24-5). (see Immunization for information on vaccines.)

Influenza

Influenza may constitute a special hazard to pregnant women. The 1918–1919 and 1957–1958 influenza epidemics were associated with increased maternal mortality.

Signs and symptoms of influenza consist of a short antecedent illness characterized by malaise, myalgia, and chills, followed by the onset of fever, pain on ocular movements, and a mild sore throat. Two to three days later, cough, substernal soreness, and chest pain may develop. Most patients with clinical influenza will improve by the fifth or sixth day of illness and recover completely.

The association between congenital abnormalities and influenza infection during pregnancy is uncertain, although most of the data suggest that there is no association.

Studies have shown that killed influenza virus vaccines can be safely administered during pregnancy [146,147]. In the absence of an epidemic, physicians should evaluate the need for influenza immunization in pregnant patients on the same basis used for other individuals. Vaccination is mandatory for pregnant women with high risk medical conditions such as heart or lung disease. When epidemic influenza is anticipated, routine immunization of pregnant women using killed vaccine is recommended (see Immunization).

Hepatitis B Virus

For a complete discussion of hepatitis B virus, see Chapter 15.

Enteroviruses

All of the enteroviruses (Coxsackie viruses A and B, echoviruses, poliovirus) have been implicated in serious neonatal disease.

Coxsackie virus

Neonatal Coxsackie A infection, particularly types A4, A5, A8, and A9, have been implicated in febrile illnesses, bronchopneumonia, and sudden infant death [148]. Coxsackie A9 virus infection has also been associated with an increased incidence of

congenital gastrointestinal malformations [149].

Maternal Coxsackie B infections, especially types B2, B3, and B4, can result in fatal neonatal infection with myocarditis being the usual cause of death. Meningoencephalitis and, less frequently, hepatitis and pancreatitis can occur. Coxsackie B viruses (types B1–B5) were associated with an increased incidence of congenital heart disease, particularly when maternal infection was with two or more Coxsackie viruses [149].

Echoviruses

Echoviruses were previously believed to be an uncommon cause of neonatal infection. Increasing numbers of reports of sporadic cases or limited epidemics among nursery populations have required a reassessment of the pathogenicity of these organisms [150–153]. Types 6, 9, 11, 14, 19, and 22 have been implicated in neonatal disease.

Maternal illness is usually manifested by fever, pleuritic pain, and abdominal pain and distention. Most neonatal infections have occurred in newborns of mothers who have acquired their infection within five days of parturition. Although passive transfer of specific IgG immunoglobulin may not prevent colonization of the neonate, it may prevent serious systemic disease. Maternal and cord immunoglobulin levels are closely correlated [149].

The clinical manifestations of neonatal echovirus infection include hepatic necrosis and failure, disseminated intravascular coagulopathy, and parenchymal hemorrhage, particularly of the renal medulla and the adrenal glands [152,153].

Poliovirus

Maternal poliovirus infection has been associated with an increased incidence of abortion or fetal death. There is no evidence that poliovirus infection or the inactivated virus vaccines are teratogenic (see Immunization).

TUBERCULOSIS

Few concepts in infectious disease have changed as much as those relating to the effect of pregnancy on tuberculosis. For centuries, pregnancy was felt to be beneficial for the woman with tuberculosis. Then, during the early decades of this century, the opposite opinion was vigorously proposed. However, several clinical studies completed prior to the widespread use of antituberculous agents have now firmly established the principle that pregnancy has little or no effect on the course of tuberculosis. With the development of excellent chemotherapeutics against the tubercle bacillus, the outlook for the control and cure of tuberculosis in the pregnant woman has improved considerably [154].

Diagnosis and Treatment

Since pulmonary tuberculosis is a relatively rare disease in this country, it is no longer recommended that all women receive a routine chest roentgenogram as part of prenatal care. A study performed at the Mayo Clinic demonstrated that all of the conditions detected by routine chest roentgenogram could have been revealed by careful history or physical examination [155].

Tuberculin skin testing remains useful as a screen for tuberculosis; however, it must be kept in mind that 20% of patients with reactivation tuberculosis have a negative skin test. Certain populations, including recent Asian immigrants, migrant workers, American Indians, or women from urban low socioeconomic groups, have a much greater risk of having either quiescent or active tuberculosis than the population as a whole. Certainly, for these individuals at high risk for tuberculosis, tuberculin skin testing is appropriate. The Mantoux test is much more reliable for this purpose than the tine test and should be the only test employed [156]. Patients with a reactive tuberculin skin test who were previously known to be negative or patients whose prior response to testing is unknown should receive a chest roentgenogram. Patients with strong clinical evidence of tuberculosis should have a chest roentgenogram performed even if the skin test is negative. If indicated, a roentgenogram can be performed during any trimester with appropriate abdominal shielding. The definitive diagnosis of active tuberculosis is dependent upon growth of *Mycobacterium tuberculosis* on culture.

A variety of conflicting data have been published regarding the interaction of pregnancy and tuberculosis. Currently, most investigators feel that pregnancy itself is not a factor predisposing to the development of tuberculosis [157]. Several studies have shown that, when standard chemotherapy is administered, pregnancy does not have a deleterious effect on the course of tuberculosis [158,159].

Reports have also varied concerning the specific effect of tuberculosis on the course of pregnancy and on the newborn. In a Norwegian study conducted by Bjerkedal and associates, women with active tuberculosis or a previous history of tuberculosis were found to have an excessive rate of pregnancy complications, miscarriage, and difficult labor [160]. Good et al. studied a group of women with tuberculosis during pregnancy by comparing the outcomes of patients with drug-resistant disease and drug-susceptible disease [154]. Six of the 16 offspring of the drug-resistant group suffered fetal or neonatal complications, while these complications occurred in two of 11 offspring of the drug-susceptible group. In one large series, 600 out of 616 pregnancies in patients with tuberculosis resulted in the birth of normal live infants [161].

Positive Tuberculin Test with Negative Chest Roentgenogram

Patients with positive tuberculin tests and negative chest roentgenograms represent either a recent tuberculin conversion or well-contained tuberculosis. These women should be carefully questioned about exposure to individuals with possible active tuberculosis. If they have not been skin tested in the past it is prudent to assume that a recent tuberculin conversion has occurred. Epidemiologic investigation of their immediate family should be promptly carried out in an attempt to establish if an active case of tuberculosis is present. This is particularly important because patients with active tuberculosis present a significant health hazard to the newborn. These women should be treated with isoniazid 300 mg and pyridoxine 50 to 100 mg daily for one year. Treatment can usually be deferred until postpartum. Tuberculosis chemoprophylaxis is not a contraindication to breast feeding.

Positive Tuberculin Test with Roentgenographic Evidence of Tuberculosis

The most important information in this circumstance is the determination of the bacteriologic activity of the disease. Sputum stains and cultures are vital. Patients with active tuberculosis are best hospitalized for initial evaluation. For patients with minimally active disease, therapy with isoniazid and ethambutol should be begun immediately. Each of these drugs has been shown to be safe for use during pregnancy [162]. If sputum smears are negative, these patients have a low rate of infectivity and can be followed on an outpatient basis for the remainder of their pregnancy. All pregnant women with advanced pulmonary tuberculosis should be begun on isoniazid, ethambutol, and rifampin after sputum smears and cultures are obtained. A list of antituberculosis drugs and their potential adverse effects is presented in Table 24-6. Rifampin has been shown to be teratogenic in laboratory animals and should be avoided during embryogenesis, if possible. It has also been reported that the efficacy of oral contraceptives may be af-

Table 24-6. Antituberculosis drugs: dosage and adverse effects

Drugs	Usual adult dosages and route of administration	Adverse effect of drug in host	Teratogenic effects
Isoniazid	300 mg/day PO	Gastrointestinal disturbances, peripheral neuropathy, hepatitis	Not teratogenic but may be embryocidal in rabbits and rats
Para-aminosalicylic acid (PAS)	10–12 g/day PO	Nausea, vomiting, diarrhea; rarely myxedema	Unknown
Ethambutol	25 mg/kg for 1 mo, then 10–15 mg/kg/day PO	Decreased visual acuity (optic neuritis)	Rats—decreased fertility; mice—cleft palate and exencephaly; rabbits—monophthalmia
Rifampin	600 mg/day PO	Gastrointestinal disturbances, headache; rarely hepatitis	Rodents—spina bifida and cleft palates. Avoid use during embryogenesis
Streptomycin	0.75–1 g daily for 14 to 21 days, then 1 g 3 times/wk IM	Ototoxicity (vestibular and cochlear), headache, pain at site of injection; rarely nephrotoxicity	Unknown
Capreomycin	0.75–1 g/day for 60 to 120 days, then 1 g 3 times/wk IM	Nephrotoxicity and ototoxicity	"Wavy ribs" in litter of female rats
Viomycin	1–2 g/day for 2 to 4 wk, then 1–2 g 2 to 3 times/wk IM	Nephrotoxicity, ototoxicity	Unknown
Ethionamide	0.5–1 g/day in divided doses PO	Gastrointestinal disturbances, hepatitis, optic and peripheral neuritis	Teratogenic effects in rabbits and rats
Pyrazinamide	20–35 mg/kg/day PO	Hepatic toxicity, hyperuricemia	Unknown
Cycloserine	250 mg twice a day	Central nervous system psychoses, drowsiness, headache, convulsions	Unknown

Source: Good [154]. Reprinted with permission.

fected in some patients being treated for tuberculosis with rifampin. In such cases alternative contraceptive measures should be employed [163].

Neonatal Care
Death rates for tuberculosis are highest in newborns. Because of this, it is imperative that both the obstetrician and the pediatrician understand that the child whose mother has active tuberculosis must be protected from exposure and infection. The child born to a mother with suspected active tuberculosis should be separated from the mother at birth. Generally, an adult is considered noninfectious after three weeks of therapy with at least two bactericidal agents. Continued follow-up for these children is crucial.

At birth, a tuberculin test must be done. If the tuberculin test is positive, the infant is treated for congenital tuberculosis. If the tuberculin test is negative, several alternatives are available: The child may receive prophylactic isoniazid for one year, or may be followed with serial chest roentgenograms and tuberculin tests every three months for one year, or the child can be vaccinated with Bacillus Calmette-Guérin (BCG). If a child is born to a family where therapeutic and preventive measures cannot be guaranteed or if epidemiologic investigation of that family cannot be completed, it would seem more prudent to vaccinate the newborn with BCG.

FUNGAL INFECTIONS
Coccidioidomycosis
Coccidioidomycosis is a common fungal infection in the San Joaquin valley of California and northern Mexico. Fortunately, the vast majority of infec-

tions are controlled by host immunologic defenses. Women who acquire the infection during pregnancy are at increased risk of serious infectious complications, including dissemination [164].

The pathophysiology of infection due to *Coccidioides immitis* is similar to tuberculosis. The organism is found in soil and produces spores that are infectious once inhaled. Spores multiply within lung tissue and set up an inflammatory response. Over a period of time, cellular defense mechanisms become activated, usually bringing the disease under control.

More than one-half of individuals infected are asymptomatic or suffer a mild viral-like respiratory tract infection that is sometimes called "valley fever." These persons can be identified by the conversion of their coccidioidin skin test.

About 40% of primary infections will be associated with systemic findings. Usually, about two weeks following exposure the individual develops malaise, fever, night sweats, increased sputum production, and chills. Erythema nodosum may also occur. Roentgenographic findings are quite variable and may include hilar adenopathy, pleural effusions, and infiltrates. In greater than 90% of patients, the findings resolve spontaneously. Some patients develop chronic pulmonary coccidioidomycosis infections characterized by chronic cavitary disease, and a few patients will develop disseminated disease. Any organ system may be involved, with the most serious complication being coccidioidal meningitis. Extensive reviews have summarized the various syndromes associated with dissemination [164]. Previously resolved coccidioidomycosis is not a problem to a woman who becomes pregnant. On the other hand, acquiring coccidioidomycosis during pregnancy or becoming pregnant during active infection can be dangerous.

Dissemination is 40 to 100 times more common in pregnant than nonpregnant patients, and the risk of dissemination increases the later in gestation the disease is acquired. In one study of 65 patients with coincidental pregnancy and coccidioidomycosis, 37 developed disseminated disease and 29 of these patients died [165]. Thus, in patients with recent travel to endemic areas who develop acute pulmonary symptoms, primary coccidioidomycosis should be considered. Serum should be obtained for a coccidioidomycosis complement fixation text. An elevated titer is suggestive, though not diagnostic, of acute infection.

Treatment

Amphotericin B is the drug of choice for coccidioidomycosis [166]. All pregnant women with active disease must be treated. Therapy is begun with a small test dose of 1 mg given intravenously in 20 mL of 5% dextrose in water. If there is no reaction or only mild reactions the dose is gradually increased from 0.2 mg/kg/day to 1 mg/kg/day. Infusions are given in 500 mL of 5% dextrose in water over a four-hour period. Biweekly determinations of creatinine, hematocrit, and potassium are necessary. Azotemia normally accompanies amphotericin B therapy, and a therapeutic course of the drug is usually followed by a permanent reduction in glomerular filtration rate. The reduction is related to the total dosage. During a course of therapy, creatinine levels may rise up to 2 to 3 mg/dL. Hematocrit values may fall and hypokalemia requiring potassium supplementation may develop. Although such alterations may be alarming, the use of amphotericin B during pregnancy does not appear to cause specific detrimental effects to the fetus [167,168].

Other opportunistic mycotic infections have been reported during pregnancy, including aspergillosis, blastomycosis, mucormycosis, and histoplasmosis [169]. However, coccidioidomycosis has been shown to be the only mycosis associated with pregnancies not altered by immunosuppression.

Candidiasis

Vulvovaginitis secondary to *Candida albicans* may affect as many as 30% of pregnancies [170]. Fortunately, most candidal infections are asymptomatic during pregnancy and do not require treatment.

Itching, burning, soreness, dyspareunia, and dysuria represent the most common symptomatology. Only rarely does candidal vaginitis alone cause a foul-smelling discharge.

Diagnosis must be accomplished using laboratory methods. The classic appearance of a white curdlike discharge may not be evident. In most instances, microscopic examination of vulvar or vaginal secretions in 10% potassium hydroxide solution should reveal hyphae. Because of high vaginal colonization rates, interpretation of cultures may be difficult [171]. Frequently, *Candida* organisms may be observed on routine Pap smear or urinalysis.

Treatment of symptomatic candidal infections during pregnancy should be initiated locally with miconazole or clotrimazole. These preparations appear to be more effective than nystatin. Although no adverse effects on mother or fetus have been demonstrated, any of these preparations should be used cautiously in the first trimester.

Table 24-7. Treatment of intestinal infestations

Infestation	Drug	Dosage	Comment
Hookworm	Pyrantel pamoate *or*	11 mg/kg single dose (maximum of 1 g)	Treatment of asymptomatic infestations should be postponed until after delivery
	Mebendazole	100 mg b.i.d. for 3 days	Avoid during organogenesis
Roundworm	Piperazine *or*	4 g single dose	Treatment during pregnancy reserved for heavy or symptomatic infestations
	Mebendazole	100 mg b.i.d. for 3 days	Avoid during organogenesis
Pinworm	Pyrantel pamoate *or*	11 mg/kg single dose; repeat in 3 wk	Also treat all family members
	Mebendazole	100 mg b.i.d. for 3 days	Avoid during organogenesis
Whipworm	Pyrantel pamoate *or*	11 mg/kg single dose; repeat in 3 wk	Also treat all family members
	Mebendazole	100 mg b.i.d. for 3 days	Avoid during organogenesis
Tapeworms	Niclosamide	2 g single dose 1 hr before breakfast	Treatment of mild infestations should be delayed until after delivery; treatment should be followed by mild purgation
Strongyloides	Thiabendazole	25 mg/kg b.i.d. for 2 days	Infestation may cause anemia and malabsorption and should be treated during pregnancy

PARASITIC INFESTATIONS

Parasitic diseases are among the most common and destructive, yet neglected, diseases of our species. Pregnant women and their progeny, both those who live in or travel to endemic areas, are among the most vulnerable to these diseases. Morbidity may vary from mild pruritus due to lice or mite infestations to abortion and maternal mortality from malaria. On the other hand, it must be remembered that the mere presence of parasites does not always require treatment when infestations are mild.

Much attention has recently been focused on "geographic medicine" because of increasing numbers of refugees and immigrants resettling in this country from Southeast Asia, Central and South America, Africa, and the Caribbean [172, 173,174]. The prevalence of treponematosis (10%), tuberculosis (55% positive PPD), and hepatitis B antigenemia (14%) in many of these immigrants may indeed pose significant public health threats [175].

Since complete descriptions of each parasitic disease are available elsewhere, this discussion will be limited to the implications of some of these disorders during pregnancy. Recent or updated information sources on individual diseases and therapy should be consulted for specific problems since treatment recommendations may change rapidly [176,177,178]. The treatment of several types of intestinal infestations is outlined in Table 24-7.

Hookworm

Hookworm (*Ancylostoma duodenale* or *Necator americanus*) disease in pregnancy may be an important cause of anemia and protein loss, especially in malnourished women. In Venezuela, a study of 1600 gravidas showed 73.8% had intestinal parasites [179]. Of these women, 22% had hookworms alone or in combination with other helminths. An Indian study found 35% of anemic women parasitized by hookworms [180]. Cardiac failure from anemia induced by hookworm infestation is one of the most common causes of maternal death in West Africa [181]. Each worm extracts roughly 0.05 mL of blood per day, so women with heavy infestations may lose up to 150 mL of blood daily.

Loss of serum proteins, including albumin, occurs with blood loss and may be a cause of hypoalbuminemia with edema or worsened maternal malnutrition. Malnutrition and anemia in pregnancy correlate with poor reproductive outcome and increased risk of postpartum maternal death. Nevertheless, only a minority of hookworm infestations cause significant nutritional loss. Because of inadequate knowledge about effective antihelminthic agents in pregnancy, it is suggested that treatment of asymptomatic infestations may be postponed until after delivery. In cases where treatment is indicated, pyrantel pamoate and mebendazole are both useful against hookworms, as well as against roundworms, pinworms, and whipworms. Both drugs are minimally absorbed across the intestinal wall. Mebendazole has the disadvantage of having been shown to be teratogenic in rats, which should preclude its use at least during organogenesis. Any anemia secondary to hookworms should be treated with iron and folic acid supplements. Since all of these antihelminthic agents are minimally absorbed by the gastrointestinal tract, breast-feeding is not contraindicated.

Roundworm

Roundworms (*Ascaris lumbricoides*) infestations occur commonly and remain unnoticed unless a worm migrates to an anatomically important site, such as the appendix, biliary tree, or lung. Occasionally they are identified in the stool. Treatment considerations are similar to hookworms, with therapy during pregnancy reserved for heavy or symptomatic infestations. Mebendazole and piperazine are both effective drugs for the treatment of roundworm.

Pinworm and Whipworm

Although rarely symptomatic during pregnancy, treatment of pinworms (*Enterobius vermicularis*) and whipworms (*Trichuris trichiura*) may be demanded by the patient on strongly expressed emotional or aesthetic grounds. Pinworms may be treated with pyrantel pamoate or mebendazole, avoiding the first trimester if possible. All family members should be similarly treated. Rarely, in prolonged infestations, pinworms can spread to the upper genital tract and pelvic peritoneum, where resultant granulomatous peritonitis, salpingitis, and endometritis can cause infertility [182]. If this condition is diagnosed at laparotomy, strong consideration should be given to medical therapy with high doses of oral mebendazole prior to surgery [183].

Tapeworms

Intestinal tapeworms (*Taenia saginata, Taenia solium, Diphyllobothrium latum*) are acquired by ingestion of viable cysticerci in undercooked food. Niclosamide is effective against all tapeworms but has not been studied in pregnancy or lactation. Therapy can generally be delayed until after delivery. When *T. solium* is noted, a single 2 g dose of niclosamide should be followed in two hours by mild purgation to prevent cysticercosis. In all tapeworm infestations, the stool should be reexamined in two months and treatment repeated if eggs are still present [184].

Malaria

Malaria presents an immense health problem for pregnant women who live in endemic regions of the world as well as for pregnant travelers. Alteration of host resistance factors during pregnancy appears to predispose to infection and increased blood density of all four types of malaria [185,186]. Normally immune mothers living in an endemic area, may suffer a relative loss of immunity, with subsequent relapse even if many years have elapsed since the initial attack [187].

Infection with *Plasmodium falciparum* is the most serious and life-threatening. This fact is further complicated by the emergence of strains of *P. falciparum* resistant not only to chloroquine but also to sulfonamide and pyrimethamine. Additionally, acute renal failure associated with *P. falciparum* may occur from massive hemoglobinuria ("Black water fever"). Cerebral involvement may also occur leading to delirium and seizures, occasionally mistaken for eclampsia.

Malarial infection of the placenta occurs in 25 to 80% of infected women [186,188]. Marked placental infection and congenital disease may occur even in women without detectable blood parasitemia [189]. Damage to the placenta can be highly variable and may be responsible for some perinatal complications, including preterm delivery and growth-retarded newborns [186,188]. Reproductive wastage from abortion has also been frequently reported [186].

Transplacental passage of malaria occurs frequently but in small inoculums [188]. It is rare to find malaria in the newborn's peripheral blood even if it is noted in the cord blood [185]. Transplacental passive malaria immunization by maternal antimalarial antibody likely protects the newborn from congenital malaria. Active fetal immunization by malarial antigen, which crosses the placenta, also occurs. Overall, clinically apparent congenital malaria occurs rarely, probably in the range of 1 in 1,000 infants of infected mothers [186].

Congenital malaria may be difficult to diagnose in the absence of a positive maternal history. Microscopic examination of the placenta may aid greatly in the diagnosis. As with most newborn septicemias, the presenting signs and symptoms are subtle and varied. Classic malarial paroxysms of chills and sweats are absent in the newborn. Poor feeding, lethargy, vomiting, diarrhea, hepatosplenomegaly, and fever may be present [189].

None of the antimalarial drugs is completely safe during pregnancy. Pyrimethamine and proquanil are folic acid antagonists and should be avoided during organogenesis, although confirmation of the teratogenic effects of these drugs in the dosages used to treat malaria is lacking. Both quinine and chloroquine are suspected of being ototoxic to the fetus. Sulfonamides, dapsone, and primaquine produce hemolysis in patients with glucose-6-phosphate dehydrogenase (G6PD) deficiency and may produce hemolysis in neonates even without G6PD deficiency. Additionally, sulfonamides have the theoretic potential of causing kernicterus in neonates when used near term.

Clearly the best prophylaxis against malaria for pregnant women is avoidance of travel to known endemic areas, especially regions of the world known to have drug-resistant *P. falciparum*. Currently these areas include the interiors of Brazil, Colombia, Ecuador, Guyana, Panama, Surinam, Venezuela, Bangladesh, India, Indonesia, and all of Burma, Cambodia, Viet Nam, and certain Philippine islands [190]. For pregnant women who must travel to endemic areas (other than areas with drug-resistant *P. falciparum*), weekly chemoprophylaxis must be assiduously observed. Adequate protection is usually achieved with chloroquine phosphate, 500 mg orally once each week, beginning one week prior to departure and continued for eight weeks after leaving the endemic region. Prophylaxis should not be withheld, regardless of the stage of gestation, since fetal and neonatal hazard from the drug is probably less than the risk from acute malaria.

Treatment of acute malaria is accomplished with chloroquine phosphate, 1 g given initially, followed six hours later by 500 mg, and then 50 mg given once a day for two days. Initial chloroquine therapy should be followed by a 14-day course of primaquine phosphate. An acute attack of falciparum malaria constitutes a medical emergency. A single case report of chloroquine-resistant malaria has been successfully treated during pregnancy with pyrimethamine and sulfonamide [193].

Schistosomiasis
Roughly 200 million of the world's population suffers from schistosomiasis (*Schistosoma mansoni, Schistosoma haematobium, Schistosoma japonicum*). While pregnancy does not alter schistosomiasis, the disease may prevent pregnancy. Longstanding schistosomiasis can cause fibrosis and granulomatous scarring of both the upper and lower genital tracts, making conception unlikely and occasionally interfering with vaginal delivery. Niridazole is effective against schistosomiasis, although little is known about its use during pregnancy or lactation. Treatment for schistosomiasis and various flukes should optimally be delayed until after delivery [184].

Amebiasis
Amebiasis is endemic in much of the world. Lawson and Steward reported increased invasiveness of latent amebiasis during pregnancy [191]. For invasive amebiasis and amebic abscesses, metronidazole appears to be the drug of choice, and diloxanid may be added to help eradicate intestinal amebas. Use of metronidazole during pregnancy should be restricted to proven infestations and then only after the completion of organogenesis.

Giardiasis
Symptomatic infestation with *Giardia lamblia* may lead to acute weight loss and gastrointestinal malabsorption. Atabrine hydrochloride reacts so avidly with DNA that it is used as a stain in chromosomal analysis and should thus be avoided in pregnancy. Metronidazole, 250 mg three times daily for five days, is the treatment of choice for giardiasis during pregnancy (after the first trimester) and lactation [192]. If giardiasis is asymptomatic, treatment may be deferred until following delivery.

Toxoplasmosis
Toxoplasma gondii, an obligate intracellular parasite, is distributed worldwide and can infect virtually all mammalian species. The disease is commonly acquired from the ingestion of incompletely cooked meat or oocysts from cat feces [194–196]. Acquired toxoplasmosis is asymptomatic up to 90% of the time and occurs primarily in children and young adults. In two prospective studies in the United States and a larger similar study in Norway, the observed incidence of congenital toxoplasmosis was approximately 1 per 1000 live births [197,198,199]. These studies suggest that 45% of women who acquire primary toxoplasmosis during pregnancy and who are not treated will give birth to congenitally infected infants. Of congenitally infected infants born alive, 8% will become severely mentally retarded [200]. In the most rigorously followed group of children with congenital toxoplasmosis, 11 of 13 (85%) developed a major neurologic deficit such as unilateral blindness or mental retardation. Each of six children who had sequential I.Q. testing showed a decrease in test scores despite specific antitoxoplasma therapy [200].

Before maternal or fetal intervention can be contemplated, a diagnosis of primary toxoplasmosis must be made with some assurance. Only about 10% of pregnant women with toxoplasmosis develop clinical illness. There are no pathognomonic signs and the most common presentation is one of "seronegative mononucleosis" with fever, malaise, lymphadenopathy, and, occasionally, evidence of hepatitis. Even if there are clinical signs of disease, the diagnosis must be made serologically. Since 90% of primary cases are asymptomatic, serologic methods for diagnosis or screening assume great importance.

The Sabin-Feldman dye test remains the single most reliable test; however, it is not commonly available to the practitioner. The conventional indirect fluorescent antibody (IFA) test is more frequently employed. IFA testing can provide reliable results if performed with careful standardization. The diagnosis of acute acquired toxoplasmosis can be established by showing rising serologic titers in maternal serum. A single high serologic titer (even as high as 1 : 4000) does not establish the diagnosis since high titers may persist for several years following an acute infection.

Since the initial antibody response to toxoplasmosis infection is mostly IgM, performance of an IgM-IFA can be helpful in confirming an acute infection. The absence of IgM antibody is strong evidence against acute toxoplasmosis in an immunologically competent patient. A rising IgM antibody titer or a single titer of 1 : 512 or more strongly suggests recent infection. Before proceeding with therapy, consultation on interpretation of serologic results is advisable. It is mandatory that any serologic screening procedures be done only with laboratory techniques that have been proved reliable. Such tests are available through the Centers for Disease Control in Atlanta. Unstandardized testing with erratic results only adds confusion to the problem.

In the face of such diagnostic and therapeutic difficulties, it is apparent that prevention of primary toxoplasmosis during pregnancy is highly desirable. Wilson and Remington suggest that pregnant women take the following hygienic measures [200]:

1. Adequately cook or cure all meat.
2. Wash hands after touching raw meat and avoid touching eyes or mucous membranes while preparing meat.
3. Wash all kitchen surfaces that come in contact with uncooked meat.
4. Avoid contact with cat feces in litter boxes and avoid gardening in soil contaminated with cat droppings.
5. Have husband or another nonpregnant individual disinfect and empty cat litter box at least every other day.

Firm guidelines regarding treatment of acute toxoplasmosis during pregnancy with either pyrimethamine and sulfa or with the less toxic spiramycin have not been established. The use of these drugs may reduce the incidence of congenital infection and abortion. Acute infection with toxoplasmosis does not represent a clear indication for therapeutic abortion since the risk of serious congenital disease is small. Acute infection can be effectively treated with pyrimethamine, 25 mg/day, along with the fixed combination trimethoprim/sulfamethoxazole for at least three to four weeks.

Lice and Scabies Infestations

Infestations with various insects, including lice (*Pediculus humanus* and *Phthirius pubis*) or mites (*Sarcoptes scabiei*) may be as alarming as they are common. An estimated six million cases of head lice occurred in this country in 1976, and infestation with lice seems to be increasing as the pandemic of scabies abates [201]. Treatment in pregnancy has become somewhat uncertain since concern has been voiced that gamma benzene hexachloride (lindane [Kwell]) may cause damage to the central nervous system in small children, infants, and, inferentially, fetuses. Gamma benzene hexachloride is a highly lipid soluble that accumulates in the central nervous systems of guinea pigs and rats, leading to neurophysiologic abnormalities. Alternative therapies for insect infestation during pregnancy and in small children include piperonyl butoxide (Rid) or 0.03% copper oleate (Cuprex). Ovicidal effects of piperonyl butoxide remain in doubt, so a second application is recommended five to seven days after initial dose to kill hatching progeny. None of these drugs has been adequately tested in humans to establish their safety during pregnancy.

REFERENCES

1. Millar KG, Mills P, Baines MG. A study of the influence of pregnancy on the thymus gland of the mouse. Am J Obstet Gynecol. 1973; 117:913–8.
2. Smith JK, Caspary EA, Field EJ. Lymphocyte reactivity to antigen in pregnancy. Am J Obstet Gynecol. 1972; 113:602–6.
3. Finn R, St. Hill CA, Govan AJ, et al. Immunological responses in pregnancy and survival of fetal homograft. Br Med J. 1972; 3:150–2.
4. Gusdon JP. Maternal immune responses in pregnancy. In: Scott JS, Jones WR, eds. Immunology of human reproduction. London: Academic Press, 1975:103–25.
5. Baines MG, Millar KG, Mills P. Studies of complement levels in normal human pregnancy. Obstet Gynecol. 1974; 43:806–10.
6. Committee on technical bulletins of the American

College of Obstetricians and Gynecologists. Immunization during pregnancy. ACOG Tech Bull. 1982; 64:1–8.

7. Pratt WB. Chemotherapy of infection. New York: Oxford University Press, 1977.

8. Antimicrobial agents, Part 1. Mayo Clin Proc. 1977; 52:601–40.

9. Editorial Board. The choice of antimicrobial drugs. Med Lett Drugs Ther. 1982; 24:21–8.

10. Heinonen OP, Shapiro S, Slone D. Birth defects and drugs in pregnancy. Littleton, Mass.: Publishing Sciences Group, 1977.

11. Ledger WJ. Antibiotics in pregnancy. Clin Obstet Gynecol. 1977; 20:411–21.

12. Landers DV, Green JR, Sweet RL. Antibiotic use during pregnancy and the postpartum period. Clin Obstet Gynecol. 1983; 26: 391–406.

13. Hill RM, Stern L. Drugs in pregnancy: Effects on the fetus and newborn. Drugs. 1979; 17:182–97.

14. Howard FM, Hill JM. Drugs in pregnancy. Obstet Gynecol Surv. 1979; 34:643–53.

15. Weinstein AJ. Treatment of bacterial infections in pregnancy. Drugs. 1979; 17:56–65.

16. Drugs excreted in mother's milk. Patient Care. 1980; 14:87–105.

17. White GJ, White MK. Breastfeeding and drugs in human milk. Vet Hum Toxicol. 1980; 22(Suppl. 1):1–43.

18. Philipson A. Pharmacokinetics of ampicillin during pregnancy. J Infect Dis. 1977; 136:370–6.

19. Depp R, Kind AC, Kirby W, Johnson WL. Transplacental passage of methicillin and dicloxacillin into the fetus and amniotic fluid. Am J Obstet Gynecol. 1970; 107:1054–7.

20. Carter MP, Wilson F. Tetracycline and congenital limb abnormalities. Br Med J. 1962; 2:407–8.

21. Woollam DH, Millen JW. Experimental mammalian teratology and the effect of drugs on the embryo. Proc R Soc Med. 1963; 56:597–600.

22. Corcoran R, Castles JM. Tetracycline for acne vulgaris and possible teratogenesis. Br Med J. 1977; 2:807–8.

23. Rendle-Short TJ. Tetracycline in teeth and bone. Lancet. 1962; 1:1188.

24. Weyman J. The clinical appearances of tetracycline staining of the teeth. Br Dent J. 1965; 118:289–91.

25. Schultz JC, Adamson JS Jr, Workman WW, Norman TD. Fatal liver disease after intravenous administration of tetracycline in high dosage. N Engl J Med. 1963; 269:999–1004.

26. Tetracyclines and the liver in pregnancy. Lancet. 1966; 1:357–8.

27. Springer C, Eyal F, Michel J. Pharmacology of trimethoprim-sulfamethoxazole in newborn infants. J Pediatr. 1982; 100:647–50.

28. Fenton LJ, Light IJ. Congenital syphilis after maternal treatment with erythromycin. Obstet Gynecol. 1976; 47:472–4.

29. MacAulay MA, Charles D. Placental transfer of cephalothin. Am J Obstet Gynecol. 1968; 100:940–6.

30. Rustia M, Shubik P. Induction of lung tumors and malignant lymphomas in mice by metronidazole. J Natl Cancer Inst. 1972; 48:721–9.

31. Legator MS, Connor TH, Stoeckel M. Detection of mutagenic activity of metronidazole and niridazole in body fluids of humans and mice. Science. 1975; 188:1118–9.

32. Adamsons K, Joelsson I. The effects of pharmacologic agents upon the fetus and newborn. Am J Obstet Gynecol. 1966; 96:437–60.

33. Marks M, Laferriere C. Chloramphemicol: Recent developments and clinical indications. Drug Rev. 1982; 1:315–30.

34. Conway N, Birt BD. Streptomycin in pregnancy: Effect on the foetal ear. Br Med J. 1965; 2:260–3.

35. Weinstein RA, Boyer KM, Linn ES. Isolation guidelines for obstetric patients and newborn infants. Am J Obstet Gynecol. 1983; 146:353–60.

36. Spence MR. Gonorrhea in a military prenatal population. Obstet Gynecol. 1975; 42:223–6.

37. Jones DE, Brame RG, Jones CP. Gonorrhea in obstetric patients. J Am Vener Dis Assoc. 1976; 2:30–2.

38. Israel KS, Rissing KB, Brooks GF. Neonatal and childhood gonococcal infections. Clin Obstet Gynecol. 1975; 18:143–51.

39. Handsfield HH, Hodson WA, Holmes KK. Neonatal gonococcal infection. I. Orogastric contamination with *Neisseria gonorrhoeae.* JAMA. 1973; 225:697–701.

40. Centers for Disease Control. Global distribution of penicillinase-producing *Neisseria gonorrhoeae* (PPNG). MMWR 1982; 31:1–3.

41. McCormack WM. Penicillinase-producing *Neisseria gonorrhoeae*—A retrospective. N Engl J Med. 1982; 307:438–9.

42. Centers for Disease Control. Sexually transmitted diseases. Treatment guidelines 1982. MMWR Suppl. 1982; 31:32s–60s.

43. Centers for Disease Control. Syphilis trends in the United States. MMWR. 1981; 30:441–4.

44. Personal communication. Dr. Betty Bernard. 1982.

45. Harter C, Bernirschke K. Fetal syphilis in the first trimester. Am J Obstet Gynecol. 1976; 124:705–11.

46. Shore RN. Hemagglutination tests and related advances in serodiagnosis of syphilis. Arch Dermatol. 1974; 109:854–7.

47. Salo OP, Aho K, Nieminen E, Harmila P. False-positive serological test for syphilis in pregnancy. Acta Derm Venereol. 1969; 49:332–5.

48. Improved tracking of penicillin allergies. [NEWS] JAMA. 1981; 245:2000.

49. Gelfand JA, Elin RJ, Berry FW, Frank MM. Endotoxemia associated with the Jarisch-Herxheimer reaction. N Engl J Med. 1976; 295:211–3.

50. Henry-Suchet J, Catalan F, Loffredo V, et al. Microbiology of specimens obtained by laparoscopy from controls and from patients with pelvic inflammatory disease or infertility with tubal obstruction.

Am J Obstet Gynecol. 1980; 138:1022–5.

51. Stamm WE, Wagner KF, Amsel R, et al. Causes of the acute urethral syndrome in women. N Engl J Med. 1980; 303:409–15.

52. Paavonen J. Chlamydial infections of the female genital tract and neonate. Infectious Disease Letters for Obstetrics-Gynecology. 1982; 4:19–30.

53. Sweet RL. Chlamydial salpingitis and infertility. Fertil Steril. 1982; 38:550–3.

54. Schachter J. Chlamydial infections (second of three parts). N Engl J Med. 1978; 298:490–5.

55. Heggie AD, Lumicao GG, Stuart LA, Gyves MT. *Chlamydia trachomatis* infection in mothers and infants. Am J Dis Child. 1981; 135:507–11.

56. Frommell GT, Rothenberg R, Wang S, McIntosh K. Chlamydial infection of mothers and their infants. J Pediatr 1979; 95:28–32.

57. Martin DH, Koutsky L, Eschenbach DA, et al. Prematurity and perinatal mortality in pregnancies complicated by maternal *Chlamydia trachomatis* infections. JAMA. 1982; 247:1585–8.

58. Wager GP, Martin DH, Koutsky L, et al. Puerperal infectious morbidity: Relationship to route of delivery and to antepartum *Chlamydia trachomatis* infection. Am J Obstet Gynecol. 1980; 138:1028–33.

59. Schachter J. Chlamydial infections (third of three parts). N Engl J Med. 1978; 298:540–9.

60. Hammerschlag MR, Chandler JW, Alexander ER, et al. Erythromycin ointment for ocular prophylaxis of neonatal chlamydial infection. JAMA. 1980; 244:2291–3.

61. Beem MO, Saxon EM. Respiratory-tract colonization and distinctive pneumonia syndrome in infants infected with *Chlamydia trachomatis*. N Engl J Med. 1977; 296:306–10.

62. Blackman HJ, Yoneda C, Dawson CR, Schachter J. Antibiotic susceptibility of *Chlamydia trachomatis*. Antimicrob Agents Chemother. 1977; 12:673–7.

63. Taylor-Robinson D, McCormack WM. The genital mycoplasmas (first of two parts). N Engl J Med. 1980; 302:1003–10.

64. Braun P, Lee YH, Klein JO, et al. Birth weight and genital mycoplasmas in pregnancy. N Engl J Med. 1971; 284:167–71.

65. Taylor-Robinson D, McCormack WM. The genital mycoplasmas (second of two parts). N Engl J Med. 1980; 302:1063–7.

66. Shurin PA, Alpert S, Rosner B, Driscoll SG, Lee YH. Chorioamnionitis and colonization of the newborn infant with genital mycoplasmas. N Engl J Med. 1975; 293:5–8.

67. Cassell GH, Cole BC. Mycoplasmas as agents of human disease. N Engl J Med. 1981; 304:80–9.

68. Centers for Disease Control. Genital herpes infection—United States, 1966–1979. MMWR. 1982; 31:137–9.

69. Grossman JH. Herpes simplex virus (HSV) infections. Clin Obstet Gynecol. 1982; 25:555–61.

70. Corey L, Adams HG, Brown ZA, Holmes KK. Genital herpes simplex virus infections: Clinical manifestations, course and complications. Ann Intern Med. 1983; 98:958–72.

71. Adam E, Kaufman RH, Mirkovic RR, Melnick JL. Persistence of virus shedding in asymptomatic women after recovery from herpes genitalis. Obstet Gynecol. 1979; 54:171–3.

72. Bolognese RJ, Corson SL, Fuccillo DA, Traub R, Moder F, Sever JL. Herpesvirus hominis type II infections in asymptomatic pregnant women. Obstet Gynecol. 1976; 48:507–10.

73. Nahmias AJ, Josey WE, Naib ZM, et al. Perinatal risk associated with maternal genital herpes simplex virus infection. Am J Obstet Gynecol. 1971; 110:825–37.

74. Grossman JH, Wallen WC, Sever JL. Management of genital herpes simplex virus infection during pregnancy. Obstet Gynecol. 1981; 58:1–4.

75. Vontver LA, Hickok DE, Brown Z, Reid L, Corey L. Recurrent genital herpes simplex virus infection in pregnancy: Infant outcome and frequency of asymptomatic recurrences. Am J Obstet Gynecol. 1982; 143:75–84.

76. Whitley RJ, Nahmias AJ, Visintine AM, Fleming CL, Alford CA. The natural history of herpes simplex virus infection of mother and newborn. Pediatrics. 1980; 66:489–94.

77. International Medical News Service. Laser treatment termed extremely effective against viral STD. Obstet Gynecol News. 1982; 17:No. 1.

78. Amstey MS, Monif GR, Nahmias AJ, Josey WE. Cesarean section and genital herpesvirus infection. Obstet Gynecol. 1979; 53:641–2.

79. Whitley RJ, Nahmias AJ, Soong SJ, Galasso GG, Fleming CL, Alford CA. Vidarabine therapy of neonatal herpes simplex virus infection. Pediatrics. 1980; 66:495–501.

80. Boehm FM, Estes W, Wright PF, Growdon JF. Management of genital herpes simplex virus infection occurring during pregnancy.

81. American Academy of Pediatrics. Committee on Fetus and Newborn and Committee on Infectious Diseases. Perinatal herpes simplex virus infections. Pediatrics. 1980; 66:147–9.

82. Guinan ME, MacCalman J, Kern ER, Overall JC, Spruance SL. The course of untreated recurrent genital herpes simplex infection in 27 women. N Engl J Med. 1981; 304:759–63.

83. Vorherr H, Vorherr UF, Mehta P, Ulrich JA, Messer RH. Vaginal absorption of povidone-iodine. JAMA. 1980; 244:2628–9.

84. Powell LC. Condyloma acuminatum: Recent advances in development, carcinogenesis, and treatment. Clin Obstet Gynecol. 1978; 21:1061–79.

85. Kovar WR. Condyloma acuminatum—Diagnosis, precautions, treatment. Nebr Med J. 1979; 64:306–8.

86. Oriel JD. Genital warts. Sex Transm Dis. 1977; 4:153–9.

87. Patel R, Groff DB. Condyloma acuminata in childhood. Pediatrics. 1972; 50:153–4.

88. Cook TA, Cohn AM, Brunschwig JP, Butl JS, Rawls WE. Wart viruses and laryngeal papillomas. Lancet. 1973; 1:782.

89. Malfetano JH, Marin AC, Malfetano JH, Jr. Laser treatment of condylomata acuminata in pregnancy. J Reprod Med. 1981; 26:574–6.

90. Calkins JW, Masterson BJ, Magrina JF, Capen CV. Management of condylomata acuminata with the carbon dioxide laser. Obstet Gynecol. 1982; 59:105–8.

91. Gardner HL, Dukes CD. *Haemophilus vaginalis* vaginitis. A newly defined specific infection previously classified non-specific vaginitis. Am J Obstet Gynecol. 1955; 69:962–76.

92. Vontver LA, Eschenbach DA. The role of *Gardnerella vaginalis* in nonspecific vaginitis. Clin Obstet Gynecol. 1981; 24:539–60.

93. Pheifer TA, Forsyth PS, Durfee MA, Pollock HM, Holmes KK. Nonspecific vaginitis: Role of *Haemophilus vaginalis* and treatment with metronidazole. N Engl J Med. 1978; 298:1429–34.

94. Spiegel CA, Amsel R, Eschenbach D, Schoenknecht F, Holmes KK. Anaerobic bacteria in nonspecific vaginitis. N Engl J Med. 1980; 303:601–7.

95. Kaufman RH. The origin and diagnosis of "nonspecific vaginitis." N Engl J Med. 1980; 303:637–8.

96. Malouf M, Fortier M, Morin G, Dube JL. Treatment of *Hemophilus vaginalis* vaginitis. Obstet Gynecol. 1981; 57:711–4.

97. Eickhoff TC, Klein JO, Daley AK, et al. Neonatal sepsis and other infections due to group B beta-hemolytic streptococci. N Engl J Med. 1964; 271:1221–8.

98. Baker CJ. Group B Streptococcal infections in neonates. Pediatr Rev. 1979; 1:5–15.

99. Ablow RC, Driscoll SG, Effmann EL, et al. A comparison of early-onset group B streptococcal neonatal infection and the respiratory-distress syndrome of the newborn. N Engl J Med. 1976; 294:65–70.

100. Anthony BF, Okada DM, Hobel CJ. Epidemiology of group B Streptococcus: Longitudinal observations during pregnancy. J Infect Dis. 1978; 137:524–30.

101. Hall RT, Barnes W, Kirshnan L, et al. Antibiotic treatment of parturient women colonized with group B streptococci. Am J Obstet Gynecol. 1976; 124:630–4.

102. Merenstein GB, Todd WA, Brown G, Yost CC, Luzier T. Group B beta-hemolytic streptococcus: Randomized controlled treatment study at term. Obstet Gynecol. 1980; 55:315–8.

103. Siegel JD, McCracken GH, Threlkeld N, Milvenan B, Rosenfeld CR. Single-dose penicillin prophylaxis against neonatal group B streptococcal infections. N Engl J Med. 1980; 303:769–75.

104. Pyati SP, Pildes RS, Jacobs NM et al. Penicillin in infants weighing two kilograms or less with early onset group B streptococcal disease. N Engl J Med. 1983; 309:1383–9.

105. Maudsley RF, Brix GA, Hinton NA, Robertson EM, Bryans AM, Haust MD. Placental inflammation and infection. A prospective bacteriologic and histologic study. Am J Obstet Gynecol. 1966; 95:648–59.

106. Gibbs RS, Castillo MS, Rodgers PJ. Management of acute chorioamnionitis. Am J Obstet Gynecol. 1980; 136:709–13.

107. Koh KS, Chan FH, Monfared AH, Ledger WJ, Paul RH. The changing perinatal and maternal outcome in chorioamnionitis. Obstet Gynecol. 1979; 53:730–4.

108. Daikoku NH, Kaltreider DF, Johnson TR, Johnson JW, Simmons MA. Premature rupture of membranes and preterm labor: Neonatal infection and perinatal mortality risks. Obstet Gynecol. 1981; 58:417–25.

109. Larsen B. How does amniotic fluid protect mother and fetus against infection? Contemp Obstet Gynecol. 1980; 15:127–44.

110. Driscoll SG. Significance of acute chorioamnionitis. Clin Obstet Gynecol. 1979; 22:339–49.

111. Bobitt JR, Hayslip CC, Damato JD. Amniotic fluid infection as determined by transabdominal amniocentesis in patients with intact membranes in premature labor. Am J Obstet Gynecol. 1981; 140:947–52.

112. Garite TJ, Freeman RK, Linzey EM, Braly P. The use of amniocentesis in patients with premature rupture of membranes. Obstet Gynecol. 1979; 54:226–30.

113. Bejar R, Curbelo V, Davis C, Gluck L. Premature labor. II. Bacterial sources of phospholipase. Obstet Gynecol. 1981; 57:479–82.

114. Mead PB. Management of the patient with premature rupture of the membranes. Clin Perinatol. 1980; 7:243–55.

115. Gravett MG, Eschenbach DA, Spiegel-Brown CA, Holmes KK. Rapid diagnosis of amniotic fluid infection by gas-liquid chromatography. N Engl J Med. 1982; 306:725–8.

116. Niebyl JR, Spence MR, Parmley TH. Sporadic (non-epidemic) puerperal mastitis. J Reprod Med. 1978; 20:97–100.

117. Marshall BR, Hepper JK, Zirbel CC. Sporadic puerperal mastitis. An infection that need not interrupt lactation. JAMA. 1975; 233:1377–9.

118. Gibberd GF. Sporadic and epidemic puerperal breast infections. A contrast in morbid anatomy and clinical signs. Am J Obstet Gynecol. 1953; 65:1038–41.

119. Norden CW, Kass EH. Bacteriuria of pregnancy—A critical appraisal. Annu Rev Med. 1968; 19:431–70.

120. Kass EH. Horatio at the orifice: The significance of bacteriuria. J Infect Dis. 1978; 138:546–57.

121. Stamm WE, Wagner KF, Amsel R, et al. Causes of the acute urethral syndrome in women. N Engl J Med. 1980; 303:409–15.

122. Kunin CM. Duration of treatment of urinary tract infections. Am J Med. 1981; 71:849–54.

123. Harris RE, Gilstrap LC, Pretty A. Single-dose antimicrobial therapy for asymptomatic bacteriuria during pregnancy. Obstet Gynecol. 1982; 59:546–9.

124. Gilstrap LC, Cunningham FG, Whalley PJ. Acute pyelonephritis in pregnancy: An anterospective study. Obstet Gynecol. 1981; 57:409–13.

125. Ransdell RC. Pneumonia and pregnancy. Am Med. 1905; 9:237–9.

126. Hopwood HG. Pneumonia in pregnancy. Obstet Gynecol. 1965; 25:875–9.

127. Oxorn H. The changing aspects of pneumonia complicating pregnancy. Am J Obstet Gynecol. 1955; 70:1057–63.

128. Primrose T. Maternal mortality: The non-obstetric death. Clin Obstet Gynecol. 1963; 6:893–9.

129. Monif GR. Infectious diseases in obstetrics and gynecology. Hagerstown: Harper & Row, 1974; 357–67.

130. Fishburne JI. Physiology and disease of the respiratory system in pregnancy. J Reprod Med. 1979; 22:177–89.

131. Abrams RM. Energy metabolism. Semin Perinatol. 1979; 3:109–19.

132. Edwards MJ, Wanner RA. Extremes of temperature. In: Wilson JG, Fraser FC, eds. Handbook of Teratology. Vol 1. New York: Plenum, 1977:421–44.

133. Ho M. Cytomegalovirus infections and diseases. DM. 1978; 24(12):1–61.

134. Hanshaw JB. Congenital cytomegalovirus infection: A fifteen year perspective. J Infect Dis. 1971; 123:555–61.

135. Hanshaw JB, Scheiner AP, Moxley AW, Gaev L, Abel V, Scheiner B. School failure and deafness after "silent" congenital cytomegalovirus infection. N Engl J Med. 1976; 295:468–70.

136. Hayes K, Danks DM, Gibas H, Jack I. Cytomegalovirus in human milk. N Engl J Med. 1972; 287:17–8.

137. Herrmann KL. Congenital and perinatal varicella. Clin Obstet Gynecol. 1982; 25:605–9.

138. Meyers JD. Congenital varicella in term infants: Risk reconsidered. J Infect Dis. 1974; 129:215–7.

139. Horstmann DM. Controlling rubella: Problems and perspectives. Ann Intern Med. 1975; 83:412–7.

140. Mann JM, Preblud SR, Hoffman RE, Brandling-Bennett AD, Hinman AR, Herrman KL. Assessing risks of rubella infection during pregnancy. A standardized approach. JAMA. 1981; 245:1647–52.

141. Schoenbaum SC, Biano S, Mack T. Epidemiology of congenital rubella syndrome: The role of maternal parity. JAMA. 1975; 233:151–5.

142. Preblud SR, Stetler HC, Frank JA, Greaves WL, Hinman AR, Herrmann KL. Fetal risk associated with vaccine. JAMA. 1981; 246:1413–7.

143. Yeager AS, Davis JH, Ross LA, Harvey B. Measles immunization: Successes and failures. JAMA. 1977; 237:347–51.

144. Siegel M, Fuerst HT. Low birth weight and maternal virus diseases. JAMA. 1966; 197:680–4.

145. Jones JF, Ray CG, Fulginiti VA. Perinatal mumps infection. J Pediatr. 1980; 96:912–4.

146. Sumaya CV, Gibbs RS. Immunization of pregnant women with influenza A/New Jersey/76 virus vaccine: Reactogenicity and immunogenicity in mother and infant. J Infect Dis. 1979; 140:141–6.

147. Centers for Disease Control. Influenza vaccine 1981–1982: Recommendations of the Public Health Service Immunization Practices Advisory Committee. Ann Intern Med. 1981; 95:461–3.

148. Balduzzi PC, Greendyke RM. Sudden unexpected death in infancy and viral infection. Pediatrics. 1966; 38:201–6.

149. Brown GC, Karunas RS. Relationship of congenital anomalies and maternal infection with selected enteroviruses. Am J Epidemiol. 1972; 95:207–17.

150. Modlin JF, Polk BF, Horton P, Etkind P, Crane E, Spiliotes A. Perinatal echovirus infection: Risk of transmission during a community outbreak. N Engl J Med. 1981; 305:368–71.

151. Modlin JF. Fatal echovirus 11 disease in premature neonates. Pediatrics. 1980; 66:775–80.

152. Rawls WE, Shorter RG, Herrmann EC. Fatal neonatal illness associated with ECHO 9 Coxsackie A-23 virus. Pediatrics. 1964; 33:278–80.

153. Hughes JR, Wilfert CM, Moore M, Benirschke K, Hoyos-Guevara E de. Echovirus 14 infection associated with fatal neonatal hepatic necrosis. Am J Dis Child. 1972; 123:61–7.

154. Good JT, Iseman MD, Davidson PT, Lakshminarayan S, Sahn SA. Tuberculosis in association with pregnancy. Am J Obstet Gynecol. 1981; 140:492–8.

155. Bonebrake CR, Noller KL, Loehnen CP, Muhm JR, Fish CR. Routine chest roentgenography in pregnancy. JAMA. 1978; 240:2747–8.

156. Lunn JA, Johnson AJ. Comparison of the tine and Mantoux tuberculin tests. Br Med J. 1978; 1:1451–3.

157. Schaefer G, Zervoudakis IA, Fuchs FF, David S. Pregnancy and pulmonary tuberculosis. Obstet Gynecol. 1975; 46:706–15.

158. Pridie RB, Stradling P. Management of pulmonary tuberculosis during pregnancy. Br Med J. 1961; 2:78–9.

159. de March AP. Tuberculosis and pregnancy. Chest. 1975; 68:800–4.

160. Bjerkedal T, Bahna SL, Lehmann EH. Course and outcome of pregnancy in women with pulmonary tuberculosis. Scand J Respir Dis. 1975; 56:245–50.

161. Selikoff IJ, Dorfmann HL. Management of tuberculosis. In: Rovinsky JJ, Guttmacher AF, eds. Medical, surgical, and gynecologic complications of pregnancy. 2nd ed. Baltimore: Williams & Wilkins, 1965:111–43.

162. Snider DE, Layde PM, Johnson MW, Lyle MA. Treatment of tuberculosis during pregnancy. Am Rev Respir Dis. 1980; 122:65–79.

163. Skolnick JL, Stoler BS, Katz DB, Anderson WH. Rifampin, oral contraceptives, and pregnancy. JAMA. 1976; 236:1382.

164. Stevens DA. *Coccidioides immitis.* In: Mandell GL, Douglas RG, Bennett JE, eds. Principles and practice of infectious diseases. New York: Wiley, 1979:2053–66.

165. Harris RE. Coccidioidomycosis complicating pregnancy. Obstet Gynecol. 1966; 28:401–5.

166. Treatment of fungal diseases. Am Rev Respir Dis. 1979; 120:1393–7.

167. Ellinoy BR. Amphotericin B usage in pregnancy complicated by cryptococcosis. Am J Obstet Gynecol. 1973; 115:285–6.

168. Silberfarb PM, Sarosi GA, Tosh FE. Cryptococcosis and pregnancy. Am J Obstet Gynecol. 1972; 112:714–20.

169. Purtilo DT. Opportunistic mycotic infections in pregnant women. Am J Obstet Gynecol. 1975; 122:607–10.

170. Fleury FJ. Adult vaginitis. Clin Obstet Gynecol. 1981; 24:407–38.

171. Knox JM. Evaluation and management of diseases of the vulva: Cutaneous inflammations and infections. Clin Obstet Gynecol. 1978; 21:991–1005.

172. Heyneman D. New Americans—New diseases? West J Med. 1981; 135:231–3.

173. Barrett-Connor E. Latent and chronic infections imported from Southeast Asia. JAMA. 1978; 239:1901–6.

174. Wiesenthal AM, Nickels MK, Hashimoto KG, Endo T, Ehrhard HB. Intestinal parasites in Southeast-Asian refugees. JAMA. 1980; 244:2543–4.

175. Catanzaro A, Moser RJ. Health status of refugees from Vietnam, Laos, and Cambodia. JAMA. 1982; 247:1303–8.

176. Schultz MG. Current concepts in parasitology: Parasitic diseases. N Engl J Med. 1977; 297:1259–61.

177. Peters W. Current concepts in parasitology: Malaria. N Engl J Med. 1977; 297:1261–4.

178. Drugs for parasitic infections. Med Lett Drugs Ther. 1982; 24:5–12.

179. Aguero O, Aure M, Sosa M. Parasitosis intestinal y embarazo. Rev Obstet Ginecol Venez. 1968; 28:507.

180. Nutritional anaemias. WHO Tech Rep Ser. 1968; 405:37.

181. Langer A, Hung CT. Hookworm disease in pregnancy with severe anemia. Obstet Gynecol. 1973; 42:564–7.

182. Pearson RD, Irons RP, Sr., Irons RP, Jr. Chronic pelvic peritonitis due to pinworm. Enterobius vermicularis. JAMA. 1981; 245:1340–1.

183. Keystone JS, Murdoch JK. Mebendazole. Ann Intern Med. 1979; 91:582–6.

184. Trussell RR, Beeley L. Prescribing in pregnancy. Infestations. Clin Obstet Gynecol. 1981; 8:333–40.

185. Reinhardt MC. Malaria, trypanosomiasis and Chagas' disease in pregnancy. J Trop Pediatr. 1980; 26:213–6.

186. Bruce-Chwatt LJ. Malaria in African infants and children in southern Nigeria. Ann Trop Med Parasitol. 1952; 46:173–200.

187. Smith AM. Malaria in pregnancy (letter). Lancet. 1972; 2:793.

188. Reinhardt MC. A survey of mothers and their newborns in Abidjan. Helv Paediatr Acta (Suppl.) 1978; 41:1–132.

189. Centers for Disease Control. Congenital malaria in children of refugees. MMWR. 1981; 30:53–5.

190. Chemoprophylaxis of malaria. MMWR. 1978; 27:81–90.

191. Lawson JB, Steward DB, eds. Obstetrics and gynaecology in the tropics and developing countries. London: Edward Arnold, 1967.

192. Koch-Weser J, Goldman P. Drug therapy: Metronidazole. N Engl J Med. 1980; 303:1212–8.

193. Main EK, Main DM, Krogstad DJ. Treatment of chloroquine-resistant malaria during pregnancy. JAMA. 1983; 249:3207–9.

194. Krick JA, Remington JS. Toxoplasmosis in the adult—An overview. N Engl J Med. 1978; 298:550–3.

195. Remington JS, Desmonts G. Toxoplasmosis. In: Remington JS, Klein JO, eds. Infectious diseases of the fetus and newborn infant. Philadelphia: Saunders, 1976:191–332.

196. Brooks RG, Remington JS. Toxoplasma and pregnancy. Infectious Disease Letters for Obstetrics-Gynecology. 1983; 5:19–24.

197. Stray-Pedersen B. A prospective study of acquired toxoplasmosis among 8,043 pregnant women in the Oslo area. Am J Obstet Gynecol. 1980; 136:399–406.

198. Alford CA, Stagno S, Reynolds DW. Congenital toxoplasmosis: Clinical, laboratory, and therapeutic considerations, with special reference to subclinical disease. Bull NY Acad Med. 1974; 50:160–81.

199. Kimball AC, Kean BH, Fuchs F. Congenital toxoplasmosis: A prospective study of 4,048 obstetric patients. Am J Obstet Gynecol. 1971; 111:211–8.

200. Wilson CB, Remington JS. What can be done to prevent congenital toxoplasmosis? Am J Obstet Gynecol. 1980; 138:357–63.

201. Fiumara NJ. The sexually transmissible diseases. DM 1978; 25(3):1–67.

202. Thomas V, Shelokov A, Forland M. Antibody-coated bacteria in the urine and the site of urinary tract infection. N Engl J Med. 1974; 290:588–90.

203. Jones SR, Smith JW, Sanford JP. Localization of urinary tract infections by detection of antibody-coated bacteria in urine sediment. N Engl J Med. 1974; 290:591–3.

25. NEUROLOGIC DISORDERS

William H. Bentley

From the brain, and from the brain only, arise
our pleasures, joys, laughter and jests, as well
as our sorrows, pains, griefs and tears . . .
—Hippocrates
The Sacred Disease

A wide variety of neurologic abnormalities are encountered during pregnancy [1,2]. Some of these disorders are recognized for the first time during gestation, while others previously known assume a special risk for the gravida and her fetus. This chapter discusses specific neurologic disorders with an emphasis on how they manifest differently because of pregnancy or adversely affect the course and outcome of pregnancy.

EVALUATION OF NEUROLOGIC FUNCTION DURING PREGNANCY

Despite the many physiologic and endocrine changes that occur throughout the course of a normal pregnancy, the nervous system remains quite stable and predictable. The clinical neurologic examination should remain unchanged. No specific mental or intellectual changes take place, although mood swings may be slightly exaggerated. Women may complain of generalized weakness or, more commonly, fatigue, but there should be no focal motor weakness or involuntary movements. Coordination, equilibrium, sensation, and the special senses remain unchanged during gestation. Deep tendon reflexes are variable in the normal population. Nevertheless, they should remain relatively constant and symmetric throughout the course of an individual pregnancy.

The most commonly used electrodiagnostic studies are safe and unaffected by normal pregnancy. Electromyography and nerve conduction studies can be useful for identification of radicular, peripheral nerve, or neuromuscular dysfunction. Electroencephalography remains the diagnostic procedure of choice for characterizing seizure disorders, since it is unaltered by normal pregnancy. Evoked potential tests, including visual, auditory, and somatosensory evoked responses are the newest of the electrodiagnostic studies. These tests can be particularly useful in the early recognition of demyelinating diseases.

Computed tomography (CT) scanning imparts the risk of radiation exposure to the fetus. When it is necessary to perform a CT scan, it is best done without administration of the iodinated contrast agent. CT scans are indicated when there is clinical evidence of a structural intracranial lesion. The most common indications for a CT scan are the onset of severe headache, altered consciousness, altered intellectual or language function, or evidence of focal motor, visual, or sensory abnormalities. Other neuroradiographic studies that can be done if necessary during pregnancy include cerebral arteriography and myelography. Arteriography is indicated for the evaluation of a possible mass lesion when the CT scan is not diagnostic or for the evaluation of a possible subarachnoid hemorrhage. Myelography can be done to evaluate spinal cord and radicular compressive lesions. However, adequate shielding of the fetus during lumbar myelography is virtually impossible.

Lumbar puncture remains a major neurodiagnostic procedure that can be safely performed during pregnancy. Throughout the course of a normal pregnancy, spinal fluid pressure and chemical and cellular composition are unchanged [3]. Lumbar puncture is indicated when there is evidence of a central nervous system infection or a subarachnoid hemorrhage. The procedure is contraindicated if there is evidence of an intracranial mass that might cause herniation, if the patient is anticoagulated, or if there is infection at the site of lumbar puncture. Complications of lumbar puncture include infection, injury to the nerve root, and delayed development of a subdural hematoma intracranially or at the site of the puncture. The latter complication is quite rare but has been reported following the administration of both spinal and epidural anesthetics during labor [4,5].

Table 25-1. Causes of spontaneous subarachnoid hemorrhage other than A-V malformation or aneurysm

Coagulation disorders
Anticoagulant therapy
Abruptio placentae with DIC

Mycotic aneurysm from bacterial endocarditis

Vasculitis

Metastatic choriocarcinoma

Eclampsia
Early—hypertensive intracerebral hematomas
Late—cerebral infarction and multiple petechial hemorrhages

Postpartum cerebral phlebothrombosis

Ruptured spinal cord A-V malformation

Source: Donaldson [2]. Original data from Locksley HB, J Neurosurg. 1966; 25:219–39.

SPECIFIC NEUROLOGIC DISORDERS
Cerebrovascular Disease
Subarachnoid and Intracranial Hemorrhage

Subarachnoid hemorrhage is an infrequent but potentially devastating event. The reported incidence of this type of hemorrhage is approximately 1 per 10,000 pregnancies [2]. The majority of spontaneous hemorrhages result from ruptured aneurysms or arteriovenous (A-V) malformations. For women under the age of 25 years, A-V malformations are a more common cause of subarachnoid hemorrhage than aneurysms [2]. When the general population including men is considered, aneurysms are a far more common cause of subarachnoid hemorrhage than A-V malformations. Approximately 10 to 15% of patients with spontaneous hemorrhage have some cause other than A-V malformation or aneurysm. These other causes are listed in Table 25-1. Clinical consideration of these other causes of hemorrhage is essential, since several of them are specifically related to pregnancy.

The overall mortality from a subarachnoid hemorrhage is approximately 30%, although mortality figures vary according to the patient's level of consciousness at the time of presentation. In patients presenting with coma the mortality can be as high as 40 to 50%, while the mortality for alert patients is approximately 10%. These figures appear not to be altered by pregnancy [6].

Aneurysms usually occur in women older than 30 years. The risk of bleeding from a cerebral aneurysm increases as gestation advances. Although aneurysms rarely rupture initially during parturition, rebleeding is common at that time [2]. There is an approximately 8 to 10% fetal death rate associated with ruptured aneurysms [7].

Hemorrhage from arteriovenous malformations tends to occur in women in their teens or early 20s. During pregnancy A-V malformations are likely to bleed initially during the second trimester or during parturition. Rebleeding from A-V malformations is more common than from aneurysms. The fetal mortality associated with hemorrhage from an A-V malformation is approximately 16% [7].

The most common presenting symptoms of a subarachnoid hemorrhage are sudden onset of severe headache, stiff neck, nausea, vomiting, and altered consciousness. A few patients may develop focal neurologic deficits. Clinical suspicion of subarachnoid hemorrhage should be confirmed by a CT scan, lumbar puncture, or cerebral arteriography. In about 85 to 90% of cases, CT scan will show blood in the subarachnoid space. Lumbar puncture is diagnostic in virtually all cases and is safe unless there is an associated intracerebral hematoma, which should be apparent on CT scan. Once the diagnosis has been made by CT scan or lumbar puncture and causes of hemorrhage other than A-V malformations or aneurysms have been excluded, cerebral arteriography is needed to delineate the exact site and cause of bleeding.

Initial treatment of subarachnoid hemorrhage includes sedation, control of blood pressure, administration of corticosteroids, and careful observation. When the patient is neurologically stable, surgical ablation of the aneurysm or arteriovenous malformation can be performed [6–8]. If surgery is technically impossible, clips can be placed on feeding vessels to reduce flow to the lesion, thereby increasing the chance of thrombosis and decreasing the chance of rupture. If the patient is comatose or unstable surgery is considered extremely hazardous, and conservative management is the treatment of choice throughout the remainder of pregnancy.

The outcome of treated subarachnoid hemorrhage in the pregnant patient is very similar to that in nonpregnant patients. If the lesion has been surgically ablated, it is felt that the pregnancy may be carried to term, and delivery may proceed without major risk to the mother or fetus. If an aneurysm has not been surgically ablated but is stable, the pregnancy may also be carried to term. In either case cesarean delivery is probably the most prudent form of delivery. In patients with surgically untreated arteriovenous malformations, there is an increased chance of rupture during labor or immediately post partum. These patients should be delivered early by cesarean delivery when the fetus is mature.

If a woman has had a surgically treated aneurysm or arteriovenous malformation, there is little neurologic reason to advise against further pregnancies. If she has had a prior subarachnoid hemorrhage from a lesion that has not been treated surgically, the patient should understand that recurrent hemorrhage is a risk during future pregnancies. This risk is much higher with arteriovenous malformations than it is with aneurysms. Because of the increased risk, a number of authors have recommended elective sterilization in women with surgically inaccessible arteriovenous malformations who have had a history of spontaneous subarachnoid hemorrhage [2,7]. Oxytocic drugs have been used safely in patients whose vascular lesions have been surgically ablated [8]. However, they should not be used in women with uncorrected lesions.

Parenchymal Hemorrhage
Another type of intracranial hemorrhage that occurs during pregnancy, though much less frequently than subarachnoid hemorrhage, is parenchymal hemorrhage. The cause of parenchymal hemorrhage may be a ruptured arteriovenous malformation or aneurysm, but often it results from chronic hypertension with or without superimposed preeclampsia. Most series report a 30 to 50% incidence of intracranial hemorrhage during eclampsia [2,9]. Patients with parenchymal hemorrhage secondary to preeclampsia complain of a sudden onset of headache accompanied by a focal neurologic deficit, alteration in level of consciousness, and perhaps seizures. CT scanning is helpful in documenting the presence of an intracranial hemorrhage from any cause and may provide useful information to guide management. In the vast majority of cases, conservative management is adequate, but depending on the size and location of the intracranial clot surgical decompression may be necessary for some patients. Conservative management includes blood pressure control, reduction of increased intracranial pressure by means of diuretics, steroids, or hyperventilation, anticonvulsants when seizures are present, and sedation. The prognosis for recovery from intracranial hemorrhage is dependent on the degree of neurologic impairment, especially the level of consciousness, and the underlying conditions responsible for the hemorrhage.

Arterial Occlusive Disease
Arterial occlusive disease is more common in pregnant women than in age-matched nonpregnant women [10,11]. One-third of all strokes that occur in women aged 15 to 45 years happen during pregnancy. Of the strokes suffered by pregnant women, there is a disproportionately large number of major arterial occlusions, involving the middle cerebral artery or the carotid artery. These arterial occlusions can occur at any time during the pregnancy and the puerperium, although they are most likely in the second half of pregnancy or the early postpartum period. The most common clinical presentation includes acute focal neurologic deficit, usually speech and motor impairment, sensory abnormalities, ataxia, and spinal cord syndromes [12]. Headache may or may not be a presenting symptom. A minority of patients will have focal or generalized seizures. Obtundation may occur and portends a poor prognosis.

Recovery from an arterial occlusion is variable, and usually follows a slow course over weeks or months. As many as 50% of survivors will have some degree of residual neurologic impairment.

The cause of arterial occlusive disease during pregnancy is complex. A relative hypercoagulable state occurs during the latter part of pregnancy and in the early puerperium [13], and this may be one of the risk factors for stroke but is certainly not the only explanation. Other risk factors include cigarette smoking, underlying atheromatous vascular disease, polycythemia and hyperviscosity, severe anemia, vasculitis, and hypertension.

The majority of arterial occlusions are thrombotic. Embolization can occur and should be suspected in patients with underlying atheromatous disease of large vessels, or in patients with underlying cardiac disease. Emboli can also derive from unusual sources, such as amniotic fluid, fat, and air. Vasculitis is another cause of arterial occlusion relatively common in this age group. Vasospasm occurs during migraine or preeclampsia and can lead to infarction [14,15].

The initial evaluation for a pregnant patient with suspected arterial occlusion may require a CT scan or an arteriogram to differentiate infarction from hemorrhage or mass. Arteriography may also be necessary in order to look for the site and the type of arterial occlusion.

Treatment includes blood pressure control, particularly in the preeclamptic patient. Cerebral edema following infarction can be managed with diuretics, corticosteroids, or hyperventilation. However, corticosteroids may not be as effective for diminishing edema due to infarction as they are with mass lesions. If focal seizures occur, anticonvulsants may be necessary, although seizures are usually transient and do not often require long-term treatment. Anticoagulation should be considered if there is evidence of a stroke in evolution. Great care must be used with anticoagulation because bland infarcts may be converted to hemorrhagic ones. Rarely, a patient is brought to a medical center soon enough following an occlusion to permit emergency endarterectomy.

Occlusive Venous Disease

Occlusive venous disease is rare in the general population but more frequent during pregnancy [11]. The exact incidence is difficult to determine since many reported studies did not have complete radiographic or postmortem confirmation. However, most large series estimate the incidence to be 1 per 3,000 pregnancies [16]. In the nonpregnant patient cerebral venous thrombosis occurs either in cortical veins or in the venous sinuses. It is most often associated with infections of the face, sinuses, mastoids, or ear, in the setting of dehydration or hypernatremia, polycythemia, hypercoagulable states, trauma, or treatment with birth control pills. There is an increased incidence of venous occlusion in preeclampsia. Some authors have suggested an association between occlusive venous disease in the pelvis and in Batson's vertebral venous plexus with the occurrence of cerebral venous thrombosis [16,17].

The cause of cerebral venous thrombosis is still poorly understood. It is felt that the cortical veins and venous sinuses are susceptible to thrombosis because of their low circulatory pressure, lack of valves, and specific anatomic arrangement with right-angle venous junctures. The hypercoagulable state that occurs during pregnancy and immediately post partum, as well as underlying endothelial damage, probably predisposes a patient to cerebral venous thrombosis. Approximately 80% of the cases of cerebral venous thrombosis occur during the last trimester or the first several weeks post partum. A few cases have been reported as late as four to five weeks post partum. The few cases reported in the first trimester were related to spontaneous or induced abortions [18]. Thromboses are most common in primigravidas, but there is a small risk of recurrent venous thrombosis in subsequent pregnancies.

Clinically, cerebral venous thrombosis is characterized by headache, focal, multifocal, or generalized seizures, and focal neurologic abnormalities. The headache may be initially mild but frequently proceeds to great severity, often accompanied by focal neurologic deficits, such as motor, speech, or visual impairment [19]. Often lower extremity defects precede or are more pronounced than upper extremity defects. Focal seizures accompany approximately 30% of cases. If the condition deteriorates rapidly over a few hours to include severe neurologic deficit, seizures, and obtundation,

the prognosis is poor. In other cases the condition may develop insidiously over days, and these patients generally do better. A few patients will have the onset of headache, followed shortly by bilateral papilledema, obtundation, and generalized neurologic dysfunction rather than focal deficits. These patients probably have sagittal sinus thrombosis. Their prognosis is extremely poor.

No single laboratory test is diagnostic. If infarction has occurred over an extensive area or has been present for several days, it can be demonstrated on CT scan. The majority of infarctions from venous thromboses are hemorrhagic, and often the blood may be seen on CT scan. Occasionally, venous sinuses that are usually evident on CT scan are absent. Electroencephalography often only confirms the clinical suspicion of focal abnormalities or generalized neurologic dysfunction. Lumbar puncture is indicated to evaluate possible intracranial hemorrhage or infection. The spinal fluid may be normal, but often there is increased opening pressure, a pleocytosis, red blood cells, xanthochromia, slightly increased protein, and normal sugar. The most definitive study for this condition is cerebral arteriography, but even it is not always diagnostic. Abnormal findings include delayed circulation with poor venous filling. The arterial phase of the arteriogram is often normal and easily seen. Unless careful attention is paid to the venous phase, the diagnosis can be missed.

Treatment of cerebral venous thrombosis during pregnancy is aimed at lowering intracranial pressure and controlling seizures. Treatment is similar to that described for occlusive arterial diseases and includes anticonvulsants, antihypertensives, and corticosteroids to reduce intracranial pressure. If a predisposing infection is identified, antibiotic therapy is necessary. There is a good deal of controversy concerning the use of anticoagulants in cerebral venous thrombosis. Some neurologists feel that anticoagulation is appropriate; nevertheless, the risk of associated hemorrhagic infarction is significant.

The overall mortality is approximately 30% in most series. Death usually occurs from massive cerebral infarction with or without brain herniation. If the patient survives, she usually has a good chance of slow return to normal neurologic function. Approximately 20% of patients with this condition will have some degree of permanent neurologic impairment.

Carotid Cavernous Fistula

This very rare condition occurs spontaneously in pregnant women more often than nonpregnant women [20]. Carotid cavernous fistula is an abnormal vascular connection between the carotid artery and the cavernous sinus. It is known to follow trauma. In pregnant women it may develop spontaneously, most commonly in the latter half of pregnancy or around the time of delivery. Patients with carotid cavernous fistulas may present with double vision, pulsating or nonpulsating exophthalmos, hyperemia, and ipsilateral vascular congestion of the conjunctiva. Often there is an audible bruit over the affected eye or temporal region. If the fistula diverts enough blood, ischemic symptoms from the affected cerebral hemisphere may develop. These symptoms include weakness, numbness, and visual or speech deficits. Onset may be slow or rapid. Diagnosis is best confirmed by carotid angiography. The angiogram should demonstrate the abnormal vascular channel connecting the carotid artery and the venous sinus as well as other associated veins. CT scan is less demonstrative.

During pregnancy, if the patient remains stable, she may be simply observed. There are a number of reported cases of spontaneous disappearance of a carotid cavernous fistula post partum. If the patient shows any signs of deterioration, surgical treatment of the fistula is indicated. This usually consists in clipping the arterial supply or embolization to the fistula or both. The procedure places both mother and fetus at risk and should be reserved for patients with progressive or serious neurologic impairment.

It is felt that a number of the spontaneous carotid cavernous fistulas that occur during pregnancy are due to abnormal dural arteriovenous fistulas in the region of the cavernous sinus that open because of the circulatory changes accompanying pregnancy. Once these physiologic circulatory changes remit, the fistula can spontaneously close. Following pregnancy, if cerebral arteriography demonstrates persistent shunting of blood through a carotid cavernous fistula and the patient remains symptomatic, corrective surgery should be considered.

Headache
Tension Headaches
Headaches are at least as common in pregnant women as they are in the general population. Approximately 60% of all headaches are classified as tension or muscular. Tension headaches are usually circumferential, posterior, or vertex, often described as a "pressure" sensation. This pressure may be either a feeling that the head is going to explode or a feeling of a constricting band. Tension headaches are often associated with contraction of posterior neck muscles and scalp muscles over the occipital and temporal regions. They commonly begin during the daytime and progress until early evening, often partially abating before bedtime. Tension headaches rarely awaken a patient from sleep and are not associated with altered mentation or level of consciousness, focal neurologic dysfunction, or significant visual problems. Occasionally, a patient with a severe tension headache may complain of vague dizziness. Patients frequently report that tension headaches have occurred daily for several years. These patients typically have consulted several physicians and have had poor response to a variety of different treatments and medications.

Evaluation of a patient with tension headaches often requires no more than a careful history and physical examination. If there are no indications from the history or physical of other neurologic problems, treatment may be initiated without laboratory studies. If other causes of the headaches are suspected, appropriate laboratory or radiographic studies are called for.

Treatment of tension headaches consists in identifying and ameliorating significant health, lifestyle, and environmental stresses. Simple physical measures, such as massage, heat, or ice treatments to the head and neck, may be helpful. Relaxation techniques—yoga, transcendental meditation, and biofeedback—may also be beneficial. A variety of medications have been used for tension headaches: minor and major tranquilizers, muscle relaxants, analgesics of varying strengths, and tricyclic antidepressants. None of these drugs is ideal for pregnancy. Nevertheless, acetaminophen and codeine may be used in moderation.

Vascular Headaches
Vascular headaches, very common in the nonpregnant patient, frequently diminish in severity and frequency during pregnancy. Several studies have reported a 70 to 80% reduction in the frequency of vascular headaches in pregnancy, usually during the second half [21,22]. Unfortunately, there is no way to identify those patients whose headaches will abate during pregnancy.

Common migraine is the most frequent type of vascular headache affecting both pregnant and nonpregnant women. Common migraines are cyclic or paroxysmal, throbbing headaches, which can be unilateral or bilateral. They can start any time but often are present on awakening. There is little prodrome other than a mild feeling of malaise and impending headache. Headaches will maximally intensify in 10 to 30 minutes and last for at least several hours. They are often associated with light and sound sensitivity, nausea, vomiting, and general malaise. Following sleep, common migraines often improve spontaneously.

Classical migraine is less frequent than common migraine. By definition, it is associated with a prodrome of visual aberrations such as visual field defects of scintillating scotomata. Other prodromes include localized weakness or numbness, speech disturbance, unsteadiness, and even changes in mentation and level of consciousness. Typically, the prodrome lasts 15 to 30 minutes. The headache begins when the prodrome abates. Classical migraines can be unilateral or bilateral but are most often unilateral. The duration of headache and associated symptoms is similar to that of common migraine.

Early administration of ergot alkaloids is the traditional treatment of classical migraine. However, ergotamine tartrate should not be used during pregnancy. This drug produces alpha-adrenergic blockade and, more important, acts on the central nervous system and directly stimulates smooth muscle. During pregnancy it can create tetanic uterine contractions. It can also cause a significant rise in blood pressure at therapeutic dosages. Fetal wastage and growth retardation in rats have occurred when ergots are administered during organogenesis. One retrospective study could show no increase in fetal deformity in women who took ergotamines during early gestation [23], but this was a poorly controlled study.

The use of daily prophylactic medications, such as propranolol, tricyclic antidepressants, phenytoin, phenobarbital, methysergide, and low-dose ergotamines, has been successful for many patients in preventing migraine. However, each of the drugs has significant potential risks during pregnancy [26]. Cyproheptadine, an antihistamine, has been successfully used to prevent migraines and is relatively safe during pregnancy [24]. There is mounting evidence that propranolol may also be used safely during pregnancy [25].

For the majority of patients, the recommended treatment for migraine during pregnancy is avoidance of known precipitating factors and symptomatic relief for each individual headache. Pain can usually be controlled with analgesics including codeine. Antiemetics and minor sedatives can also be helpful.

Pseudotumor Cerebri

Another cause of headaches during pregnancy is pseudotumor cerebri or benign intracranial hypertension [27]. This condition is characterized by increased intracranial pressure and appears to occur more commonly during pregnancy. It usually begins in the third, fourth, or fifth month but can persist throughout gestation, finally remitting post partum. Symptoms include headache, visual disturbances, nausea, vomiting, and behavioral changes. The most striking physical sign is papilledema; the neurologic exam is otherwise normal. Because of the severe headaches, visual symptoms, and papilledema, other intracranial lesions must be considered. A CT scan and other neurodiagnostic procedures are usually indicated. If these studies fail to show a localized mass or other cause for the elevated intracranial pressure, a spinal tap is in order. Except for the increased cerebrospinal fluid (CSF) pressure, analysis of the spinal fluid is unremarkable.

The natural course of the syndrome is gradual improvement. However, in some instances persistently high intracranial pressure can lead to optic atrophy. Treatment is directed at lowering CSF pressure. Diuretics and steroids can be helpful, as can weight reduction in the obese patient. Often repeated lumbar punctures to lower pressure are necessary. A lumbar-peritoneal shunt is effective in chronic cases.

Seizures

Epilepsy is the most common serious neurologic problem encountered during pregnancy. It occurs in 0.3 to 0.5% of all pregnancies. The chief concerns of the pregnant epileptic are loss of seizure control and the potential teratogenic effects of anticonvulsants.

The majority of seizures are idiopathic. When a patient has a first seizure during pregnancy, a complete neurologic evaluation should be performed. This evaluation should include a detailed neurologic history and physical exam. Laboratory studies should include serum chemistries, complete blood count, electroencephalography, CT scan, and possibly additional tests such as lumbar puncture or cardiac evaluation. A young adult who suffers an unexplained first seizure has a 50 to 60% chance of subsequent seizures [28]. A recent review by Montouris et al. reported that for patients with established epilepsy prior to pregnancy, seizure frequency was increased in 45%, decreased in 5%, and unchanged in 50% [29]. The likelihood that seizures will occur more frequently during pregnancy can be predicted from the history of seizure control during the two years prior to conception. Of women with no more than one seizure during the nine months preceding pregnancy, only 25% experienced an increased seizure frequency during pregnancy. By comparison, when the seizure frequency prior to gestation is greater than one seizure per month, more than 60% of patients will have a deterioration in control. This deterioration is most likely to begin in the first trimester. Following pregnancy, the previous seizure frequency is usually reestablished.

Evidence from several studies shows that there is an increased statistical risk of fetal malformations and complications associated with epilepsy during pregnancy [29–33]. The most common maternal complications are hyperemesis, vaginal bleeding, toxemia, and complications of delivery including poor induction and progression of labor. Fetal risks include preterm birth, intrauterine growth retardation, and a twofold to threefold increase in the frequency of fetal malformations. The increase in fetal malformation is not clearly dependent on maternal anticonvulsant therapy. The most commonly observed malformations are cleft palate, cleft lip, and cardiac defects, especially septal defects. Whether these abnormalities are due to an inherent genetic predisposition, the seizures themselves, anticonvulsant drugs, or a combination of all these factors is not clear.

Anticonvulsant Drugs

In 1979 the following recommendations were made by the American Academy of Pediatrics Committee on Drugs in collaboration with the American College of Obstetrics and Gynecology regarding the use of anticonvulsant medications [34]. They concluded:

No woman should receive anticonvulsant medication unnecessarily. When possible, a woman who has been seizure free for many years should be withdrawn from her medication prior to pregnancy. When a woman who has epilepsy and requires medication asks about pregnancy, she should be advised that she has a 90% chance of having a normal child, but that the risk of congenital malformations and mental retardation is two to three times greater than average because of her disease or its treatment. Women who seek advice later than the first trimester of pregnancy should be reassured with the foregoing figures rather than routinely urged to consider abortion. For these women, drug therapy should be continued throughout pregnancy because major anatomical malformations most likely would have taken place already, and the malformations associated with the hydantoin syndrome rarely have significant effect on the well-being of the child.

There is no reason at present to advise a woman to switch from phenytoin or phenobarbital to other anticonvulsants about which even less is known. Discontinuation of medication in a woman whose epilepsy is controlled by medicine may cause seizures, and prolonged

seizures could cause serious sequelae to her and the fetus.

Physicians are often asked for recommendations about breast-feeding for mothers on anticonvulsant medications. A review of the published literature shows that most anticonvulsants present in therapeutic levels in the mother also are present in breast milk. However, their concentration is low enough that there is little likelihood of any demonstrable effects on the infant. Thus, there is no evidence at the present time to suggest that a woman requiring anticonvulsants should either stop taking medication or avoid nursing.

Phenytoin

This is the most commonly used anticonvulsant in the treatment of grand mal seizures. It can also be effective for treating focal and complex-partial seizures. The exact risk of congenital malformations associated with the use of this drug is not known but is probably less than 10%. Nevertheless, a group of malformations has been attributed to the use of phenytoin and called the "fetal hydantoin" syndrome [35,36]. This syndrome has been characterized by craniofacial anomalies, limb defects, deficient growth, and mental retardation. The craniofacial anomalies include a low and broad nasal bridge, epicanthal folds, a short upturned nose, hyertelorism, ptosis, strabismus, prominent ears that are low set and malformed, a wide mouth with prominent lips, and variation in the size and shape of the head.

Despite these potential malformations, phenytoin remains a useful drug for control of seizures. Few neurologists or obstetricians would discontinue or withhold it when it is clearly indicated. However, a careful review of the need for phenytoin during pregnancy or, ideally, before is always worthwhile.

Normally, phenytoin is rapidly absorbed from the gastrointestinal tract. The drug can be given intravenously, but intramuscular injection should be avoided since it is painful and absorption is irregular. The usual adult maintenance dosage of phenytoin is approximately 300 to 400 mg daily. This dosage should provide serum levels in the therapeutic range of 10 to 20 μg/mL within six to ten days. If it is necessary to reach therapeutic levels more rapidly, a loading dose of 1,000 mg may be given intravenously or orally as a single dose or in divided doses. If the drug is given intravenously, cardiac monitoring is necessary and administration should not exceed 50 mg per minute.

Recent reports indicated that plasma phenytoin levels decrease during pregnancy and require close monitoring [33,37]. It was also found that small dosage changes result in disproportionate increases in plasma concentration as the therapeutic range is approached. Very high levels may occur during the postpartum period if the drug dosage is not decreased. Measurement of plasma drug levels should be done monthly, especially in the second half of pregnancy.

Phenobarbital

Phenobarbital is useful for control of grand mal, focal, and complex-partial seizures. The drug freely crosses the placenta and has been implicated as a possible teratogen, causing cleft lip, congenital heart disease, and microcephaly. Unlike shorter-acting barbiturates, phenobarbital is primarily excreted by the kidney. As glomerular filtration rate increases during pregnancy, the clearance of phenobarbital increases. The usual dosage (60–200 mg/day) may need to be increased to maintain a therapeutic plasma concentration of 10 to 40 μg/mL. Some infants born of mothers who took barbiturates during gestation have demonstrated withdrawal symptoms such as hyperexcitability, tremor, high-pitched cry, and feeding problems. This condition usually requires no specific treatment, except for one or two doses of phenobarbital in the first 48 hours of life.

Phenobarbital is excreted in breast milk, in which the concentration is 10 to 30% of that of maternal plasma. Neonatal lethargy has not been shown to result from this small exposure.

Phenobarbital and phenytoin, to a lesser extent, have been implicated in newborn hemorrhagic problems because of reduced synthesis of vitamin K–dependent clotting factors. There are several reports of major and even fatal hemorrhagic complications in newborns from anticonvulsant medication [38]. Affected newborns should receive vitamin K at the time of delivery.

Valproic Acid

This anticonvulsant is effective for the treatment of petit mal, complex-partial, and, to a lesser extent, grand mal seizures in nonpregnant patients. Current data suggest that valproic acid is teratogenic [39]. It is recommended that alternate forms of anticonvulsant therapy be used when possible [40]. Patients who were treated with valproic acid during the first trimester should be screened for neural tube defects.

Primidone

Primidone and both its major metabolites, phenobarbital and phenylethylmalonamide, have anticonvulsant activity. The drug is effective for control of grand mal, focal, and complex-partial seizures. Primidone may be useful for patients with seizures not controlled by phenytoin or phenobarbital. Concerns for its use during pregnancy are similar to those for phenobarbital. The usual adult dosage is 0.75 to 1.5 g per day given in divided doses. Primidone is excreted in breast milk in moderate amounts. If somnolence is noted in the newborn, either breast-feeding or administration of the drug should be discontinued.

Carbamazepine

Limited data are available regarding the risk of carbamazepine use during pregnancy, but to date there are no reports to suggest that its risk is any greater than that of the other major antiseizure drugs. It can be useful for control of grand mal, focal, and complex-partial seizures. The usual adult dosage is 0.6 to 1.2 g per day, given in divided doses. Therapeutic plasma levels are 4 to 12 μg/mL. Common maternal side effects are similar to those of phenytoin and phenobarbital plus a higher frequency of nausea, malaise, and lightheadedness at the initiation of therapy. Patients on maintenance therapy should have a complete blood count and liver function tests performed periodically. The drug is excreted in breast milk in small amounts [33].

Diazepam

This benzodiazepine is effective for short-term control of status epilepticus but is not used routinely for antiseizure maintenance therapy. Intermittent use of the drug during pregnancy is considered safe. Diazepam has been used to control eclamptic seizures, although magnesium sulfate is the drug of choice prior to delivery. The drug is excreted in breast milk, and its use by lactating mothers is not recommended.

Magnesium Sulfate

Magnesium sulfate has been the drug of choice for prevention of eclamptic seizures. It works by depressing neuromuscular transmission. It can be administered intravenously or intramuscularly with rapid attainment of therapeutic plasma concentrations. Deep tendon reflexes, respirations, and urine output should be monitored during administration of magnesium sulfate. When the drug is administered intravenously a loading dose of 4 g in 250 mL D_5W is given over a 20-minute period. Therapeutic levels can be maintained with 1 to 3 g per hour. The intramuscular loading dose is 5 g in each buttock (10 g total) followed by 5 g every four hours. Dosages should always be titrated by deep tendon reflexes, respiratory rate, and urinary output. Any signs of neuromuscular depression or decreased urine output should delay further administration of the drug. Pregnant women with myasthenia gravis should not ordinarily be given magnesium sulfate.

In summary, patients with previously demonstrated epilepsy or those who acquire epilepsy during pregnancy should be treated with appropriate anticonvulsants. Patients who do not clearly have seizures should not be treated unnecessarily with anticonvulsants. There is an increased risk of fetal malformations in the pregnant epileptic, but it is not entirely clear whether this increased risk is due to the epilepsy itself, associated genetic factors in epileptics, anticonvulsant medications, or a combination of these factors [30–33,41,42]. Since magnesium sulfate nearly blocks neuromuscular transmission and does not affect the primary pathophysiology of preeclampsia/eclampsia, at least one investigator has suggested that treatment consist of antihypertensive drugs, particularly vasodilators and major anticonvulsant medications (J.O. Donaldson. Address to the American Academy of Neurology, San Diego, April, 1983). There is no compelling reason to switch from one medication to another during pregnancy.

In the course of a pregnancy, plasma levels of all anticonvulsant drugs may change. Monthly anticonvulsant levels should be monitored and drug dosages adjusted to maintain efficacy and safety. Post partum, drug levels must still be monitored weekly to prevent toxicity in the mother.

Status Epilepticus

The term *status epilepticus* is applied to multiple seizures that follow each other without recovery of consciousness between attacks. Status epilepticus is associated with a high incidence of stillbirths, abortions, and fetal abnormalities [2]. Treatment requires significant dosages of intravenous anticonvulsants. Initial loading doses of 200 to 600 mg of phenobarbital or 500 to 1,000 mg of phenytoin should be given. The administration of phenobarbital may cause respiratory depression, especially if the patient has previously received diazepam. The administration of phenytoin may cause hypotension or cardiac arrhythmias. Phenytoin should be given intravenously only when the patient is under close observation on a cardiac monitor and at a rate no greater than 50 mg per minute. Occasionally, more than one anticonvulsant is needed to control status. Adequate hydration, electrolyte balance, and oxygenation should be maintained. Once status is controlled, maintenance dosages of an anticonvulsant agent should be administered and drug levels should be monitored.

Neuropathies

A variety of mononeuropathies and polyneuropathies are encountered during pregnancy [43].

The usual neuropathies seen during pregnancy are those resulting from entrapment or pressure. These neuropathies are suggested by isolated areas of numbness, tingling, weakness, or occasionally diminished reflexes. Pressure neuropathies are caused by compression in anatomic canals, presumably due to increased fluid retention, and in some cases by relaxation of ligaments. The most common entrapment and pressure neuropathies will be considered individually.

Carpal Tunnel Syndrome

Carpal tunnel syndrome results from compression of the median nerve as it crosses under the flexor retinaculum at the wrist. Typical symptoms include paresthesias and numbness in the thumb, index, and middle fingers. Symptoms most often occur at night and frequently awaken the patient. If compression is severe, there may be considerable pain as well as motor loss and atrophy in the thenar eminence. This syndrome commonly occurs in the third trimester and puerperium. Some series have reported an incidence of carpal tunnel syndrome during pregnancy as high as 20% [44]. When it occurs post partum, it is often associated with breast-feeding [45]. Examination reveals diminished sensation over the thumb, thenar eminence, and index and middle fingers, as well as a tingling sensation that radiates into this same distribution when the median nerve is percussed at the wrist (Tinel's sign). Active or passive wrist flexion can produce the same sensation in the median nerve distribution (Phalen's sign). The majority of patients with carpal tunnel syndromes have remission of their symptoms post partum, although symptoms may persist up to three months.

Initial management includes a splint worn at night that keeps the wrist in a neutral position. If this is not successful, injection of hydrocortisone into the carpal tunnel may provide temporary relief. In patients who have severe pain or significant motor loss surgical decompression is recommended. This is a very simple operation, done under local or regional anesthesia, and carries no risk to the mother or fetus. Since symptoms usually remit post partum, surgery should be delayed if at all possible.

Meralgia Paresthetica

Another common entrapment neuropathy is meralgia paresthetica or entrapment of the lateral femoral cutaneous nerve. The lateral femoral cutaneous nerve courses through the pelvis and exits beneath the inguinal ligament (Fig. 25-1). It supplies sensation to the superficial anterior and lateral thigh. The nerve is ordinarily entrapped as it courses beneath the inguinal ligament. Entrapment causes dysesthesias, numbness, and occasionally pain in the anterior or lateral thigh. Symptoms are most likely to be seen in the latter half of pregnancy and are thought to result from weight gain, pelvic pressure, and change in posture. Treatment is rarely necessary. The majority of these problems remit soon after delivery.

Bell's Palsy

Bell's palsy occurs when there is compression of the facial nerve as it courses through the bony facial nerve canal, causing paralysis of the same side of the face. The frequency of Bell's palsy appears to increase significantly during pregnancy [46]. Even though this palsy may cause complete paralysis of the face, the majority of patients recover with normal or near-normal facial function. Recovery typically takes months. Less than 10% of patients will have any serious residual motor weakness.

Management is aimed at preventing complications from lack of motor function in the involved side of the face. Patients should be instructed to massage the eye and use eye drops to keep the cornea from drying. The facial muscles should also be massaged several times a day to prevent contractures. The use of steroids is controversial. Several authors have suggested that prednisone administered during the first week of symptoms increases the chance of more rapid and complete recovery [47].

Lower Extremity Neuropathies

Postpartum footdrop can occur as a result of pressure on the lower lumbar roots and upper sacral roots where they form elements of the common peroneal nerve in the pelvis or from direct pressure on the peroneal nerve at the fibular head when the patient is in the stirrups (Fig. 25-2). In either cases, typical symptoms include weakness of dorsiflexion, eversion, and toe extension, as well as decreased sensation over the anterolateral lower leg and foot. Most of these pressure palsies improve spontaneously, although occasionally the patient may need a supporting splint to keep the foot in dorsiflexion in order to prevent shortening of the Achilles tendon while the muscles are weakened.

The obturator nerve can be compressed by the fetal head or by forceps during delivery. In this event the symptoms are weakness of thigh adduction and a small area of sensory loss over the medial thigh. Like peroneal neuropathies, this neuropathy usually resolves spontaneously post partum.

The femoral nerve is vulnerable to compression by retractors used during surgical procedures in the low abdomen. A femoral neuropathy is suggested by weakness of the quadriceps, absent or depressed knee reflex, and an area of diminished sensation over the anterior thigh. The prognosis for recovery is good.

A lumbosacral plexus neuropathy can occur with mixed motor and sensory findings throughout the lower extremity. This commonly results from pressure in the pelvis by the fetal head. Symptoms and signs are weakness of a variety of different muscles of the lower extremity, areas of sensory loss corresponding to the same radicular innervation, and correspondingly diminished knee or ankle reflexes. Specific muscle weakness or sensory loss depends on the exact location of compression in the plexus. Often, the lower lumbar

Fig. 25-1. Relationship of the fetus to the major nerve roots in the pelvis.

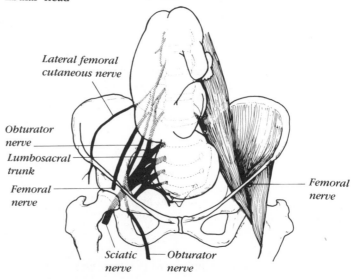

Lateral femoral
cutaneous nerve

Obturator
nerve

Lumbosacral
trunk

Femoral
nerve

Femoral
nerve

Sciatic
nerve

Obturator
nerve

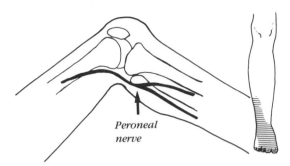

Fig. 25-2. Relationship of the peroneal nerve to the head of the fibula. Note distribution of sensory loss resulting from nerve compression.

and upper sacral roots are involved, causing foot-drop. The prognosis for recovery from a lumbosacral plexus neuropathy is good.

Lumbar Disk Syndrome

Another "neuropathy" that occurs during pregnancy is a lumbar or sacral radiculopathy due to an extruded lumbar disk [48]. This is not a true neuropathy, but it is considered here because of its clinical similarity. Relaxation of the spinal joints and accentuation of lumbar lordosis predispose pregnant women to low back pain and lumbar disk extrusion. Occasionally, nerve root compression can be seen during pregnancy secondary to a leiomyoma [49]. Pain usually radiates down the lower extremity, most commonly in the postero-lateral distribution, to the foot. The pain is generally exacerbated by sitting or standing for a long time and by the Valsalva maneuver. Some comfort is afforded by lying on one side with hips and knees flexed. There may be weakness, sensory loss, and depression of reflexes corresponding to specific nerve roots. The roots most likely to be involved are S-1 and L-5. Lumbar disk problems ordinarily occur late in pregnancy. Patients can usually be managed with bed rest and analgesics. Rarely, an acute midline disk extrusion results from labor. This is characterized by painless bladder and rectal sphincter dysfunction and is an indication for surgical decompression.

Intercostal Neuralgia

Another nerve entrapment that occurs more frequently in pregnant women or in patients with an abdominal or pelvic mass is intercostal neuralgia [50]. Their neuralgia is characterized by painful dysesthesias over the lower chest and abdominal wall. Symptoms are exacerbated by movement, straining, or standing and are relieved by lying. Physical examination is unremarkable except for

an area of diminished sensation corresponding to the area of pain. Pain is assumed to be caused by stretching of the intercostal nerves. Patients can be reassured that the neuralgia will resolve shortly after delivery.

Recurrent Brachial Neuritis

In recurrent brachial neuritis the brachial plexus becomes inflamed, causing pain that radiates from the shoulder to the entire upper extremity, often followed by numbness, tingling, and weakness in the same distribution. This condition commonly occurs in the ulnar distribution but may affect any part of the upper extremity. Recurrent brachial neuritis is often familial and can be expected in subsequent pregnancies [51]. Symptoms typically remit post partum. The condition must be differentiated from a pressure or traction brachial neuritis, which results from altered posture and breast enlargement. Often physical therapy is beneficial in hastening functional recovery.

Toxic and Metabolic Neuropathies

Toxic and metabolic neuropathies typically present as symmetric polyneuropathies affecting both sensation and motor function. The most common early symptoms are painful dysesthesias in the distal lower extremities.

Metabolic neuropathies frequently result from chronic medical illnesses such as diabetes, thyroid dysfunction, renal or liver disease, vasculitis, nutritional deficiency, alcoholism, pernicious anemia, and porphyria. The more common medications found to cause neuropathies include the sulfonamides, nitrofurantoin, isoniazid, allopurinol, glutethimide, and hydralazine. Occasionally, phenytoin or amitriptyline may cause a neuropathy. Treatment of an underlying medical problem or discontinuation of the responsible medication may stop the progression of the neuropathy and actually lead to reversal of the neuropathic findings. There is no indication for termination of pregnancy as a treatment of any of these neuropathies.

Gestational Polyneuropathy

This is a polyneuropathy caused by distal degeneration of axons, the longest axons being affected first [2]. Like the neuropathy that affects alcoholics, this condition is probably the result of malnutrition and not a specific neuropathy of pregnancy. Gestational polyneuropathy is extremely rare in developed countries. When gestational polyneuropathy does occur, it can progress to include encephalopathy. Adequate nutrition is the treatment for this neuropathy.

Guillain-Barré Syndrome

Guillain-Barré syndrome is an acute polyneuritis characterized by weakness that develops over days to several weeks. Weakness is usually symmetric and involves proximal and distal muscles. Deep tendon reflexes are usually absent. The CSF is under normal pressure and has a normal to only slightly elevated cell count; elevated protein concentration is found in most cases, but values on the first lumbar puncture in the first few days of the disease are generally normal or only slightly elevated. The simultaneous occurrence of Guillain-Barré syndrome and pregnancy is probably coincidental. Unless severe paralysis occurs, pregnancy, delivery, and the fetus are unaffected by the disease [2].

Muscle Disease

Impaired muscle function is often further exacerbated by the extraordinary demands of pregnancy. Few muscle disorders arise as a result of pregnancy, but many subclinical conditions can be unmasked by pregnancy.

Polymyositis

This inflammatory myopathy has been reported rarely during pregnancy. Several cases that appeared during pregnancy remitted in the puerperium [52,53]. The disease is generally thought to have an unfavorable course during pregnancy, possibly related to other associated maternal disease such as occult malignancy. Corticosteroids are the only available treatment.

Muscular Dystrophy

In general, patients with muscular dystrophy do not encounter any unusual complications during pregnancy. Any problems during labor and delivery result from generalized weakness. Most of the inherited muscular dystrophies are not evident at birth. Rather, they present in childhood or early adult years. The Duchenne type is a sex-linked recessive disorder presenting in early childhood and affects only males. Becker's type, also a sex-linked recessive disorder, presents later in life and progresses more slowly. Facioscapulohumeral dystrophy is an autosomal dominant disorder typically presenting in late childhood with progressive facial and proximal upper extremity weakness. The limb-girdle dystrophies probably represent a group of variably inherited, adult-onset, slowly progressive myopathies.

Myotonic Dystrophy

Myotonic dystrophy is an autosomal dominant systemic disease that involves striated muscle. It is characterized by generalized weakness and myotonia (an inability to relax muscles after a forceful contraction), frontal balding, intellectual impairment, cataracts, endocrine dysfunction, hepatic dysfunction, and cardiac dysfunction. Most women with myotonic dystrophy have been diagnosed prior to pregnancy [54,55]. Nevertheless, occasional cases are recognized for the first time during pregnancy. Impairment of muscular function can increase at any stage of pregnancy but occurs mainly during the third trimester. Spontaneous abortion and preterm labor are common in women with myotonic dystrophy. Prolongation of the second stage of labor can result from ineffective pushing and cause fetal distress.

Management of patients with myotonic dystrophy includes frequent brief rest periods. However, prolonged bed rest should be avoided since disuse of involved muscles can bring further weakening. Attention should be paid to general health, particularly early recognition and treatment of infections.

Use of anesthesia can be especially difficult in myotonic patients. A myotonic muscle infiltrated with procaine becomes flaccid. Furthermore, nerve blocks will not prevent myotonia, which is an intrinsic phenomenon of muscle. Regional or local anesthesia should be used whenever possible. Curare can be used safely. Attention must always be paid to diminished respiratory function; there is some evidence that myotonics have some degree of primary alveolar hyperventilation. Heavy sedation may lead to respiratory difficulties and should be avoided. Arrhythmias and sudden death have occurred with general anesthesia.

Myotonic dystrophy is an autosomal dominant disease with variable penetrance. Infants can develop the disease in utero. Affected infants present as floppy babies with facial diplegia and respiratory difficulties. Even in mothers with mild disease, neonatal disease can be severe.

Myasthenia Gravis

Myasthenia gravis is a disorder of neuromuscular transmission caused by circulating autoimmune antibodies to the acetylcholine receptor protein at the endplate of striated muscle. The disease occurs most frequently in young women in the childbearing age. Myasthenia is characterized by localized bulbar weakness such as ptosis, diplopia, and difficulty chewing or swallowing. It can also present as a systemic disorder with generalized muscular weakness. Typically, symptoms improve following rest and deteriorate with activity.

The course of myasthenia during pregnancy can vary from complete remission to respiratory failure. There does not appear to be any way to identify patients who will deteriorate during pregnancy [56,57].

For several decades myasthenia gravis has been managed with the use of anticholinesterase drugs, such as neostigmine and pyridostigmine. However, characterization of myasthenia as an autoimmune disease led to the use of corticosteroids and early thymectomy. Nevertheless, many patients can effectively be controlled with anticholinergics. Other general principles of management include increased periods of rest and vigilant attention to infections and exacerbations.

Exacerbation can occur at any time. The myasthenic crisis is typified by severe weakness, occasionally to the extent of hypoventilation and respiratory insufficiency. Crisis can be precipitated by a superimposed illness, infection, or drugs that block neuromuscular transmission such as aminoglycoside antibiotics or muscle relaxants. Myasthenic crisis must be differentiated from cholinergic crisis, in which the patient has been overmedicated with the anticholinesterase drugs. Cholinergic crisis is characterized by tearing, abdominal cramps, diarrhea, nausea, and generalized weakness, which may also progress to respiratory failure. The best laboratory test to differentiate these two is the administration of 2 to 10 mg of edrophonium chloride intravenously. This rapid-acting anticholinesterase will produce a transient improvement in symptoms in the myasthenic crisis and will produce transient worsening of symptoms or no change in the cholinergic crisis. If a myasthenic crisis is diagnosed, treatment involves increased amounts of anticholinesterase medications, as well as corticosteroids, and occasionally the use of ephedrine or potassium or even the consideration of plasmapheresis. If the patient is having a cholinergic crisis, treatment involves stopping all anticholinergic medications and supporting the patient until dosages can be adjusted to the appropriate level.

Parenteral neostigmine is used to control myasthenic symptoms during labor and delivery. Oral medications are absorbed poorly, and plasma drug levels can be variable. Continual observation is necessary to monitor muscle strength. Staff must be extremely vigilant to prevent respiratory depression. Sedatives, narcotics, and analgesics increase the risk of respiratory depression. Regional anesthesia is preferred. The patient with severe myasthenia may benefit from plasmapheresis prior to delivery. Improvement should be noted within 48 hours of treatment and last up to several weeks.

Treatment of the myasthenic patient with superimposed preeclampsia can be a particularly diffi-

cult task. The usual treatment for preeclampsia, magnesium sulfate, has been shown to depress muscle membrane excitation by diminishing the depolarizing action of acetylcholine and decreasing the amount of transmitter substance at the motor endplate.

For several weeks post partum the woman with myasthenia is especially vulnerable to acute and severe exacerbations. Regular periods of rest are mandatory.

Approximately 10 to 20% of offspring born to myasthenic mothers will have neonatal myasthenia. One investigator suggests this is due to circulating antiacetylcholine receptor antibodies, contributed by the mother [58]. However, there is new evidence to suggest that the occurrence of this syndrome in the newborn is not only related to the presence of maternal circulating antibody but to antibody synthesized by the newborn as well [71]. Often the onset of symptoms is not seen for several days because of the presence of circulating anticholinesterase in the newborn received from the mother in utero. Neonatal myasthenia is a transient problem, generally recognizable within the first several days of life. It is suggested by generalized weakness and difficulty with feeding and breathing. Often the babies require intensive care monitoring and ventilatory assistance, but the syndrome resolves as the antibody level diminishes. The management of neonatal myasthenia includes appropriate dosages of anticholinesterase drugs. Myasthenia in these affected infants does not persist.

There are other early-life forms of myasthenia, usually seen in children delivered of unaffected mothers who have a family history of myasthenia. These cases begin later than the neonatal myasthenia. The earliest form, congenital myasthenia, is demonstrated by ophthalmoplegia and weakness of extraocular facial muscles without generalized weakness. It is clinically different from neonatal myasthenia.

There has been some concern about whether myasthenic mothers should breast-feed their infants because of passage of the antibodies responsible for the disease and passage of anticholinesterase medications. This has not proved to be a significant problem, and there does not appear to be a clear contraindication to breast-feeding for myasthenic mothers.

MULTIPLE SCLEROSIS

Multiple sclerosis is a demyelinating disease of the central nervous system that occurs predominantly in young adults. It is characterized by an unpredictable waxing and waning course. Typical symptoms and signs of multiple sclerosis include blurred vision, diplopia, areas of numbness over any part of the body, weakness of the extremities, spasticity, ataxia, interference with normal bowel, bladder, and sexual function, and occasionally personality changes or depression. The disease can present with an acute attack, then remit for months to years, or it can begin insidiously with constant progression. The diagnosis is made by a careful neurologic history and examination suggesting lesions of white matter that occur in different sites and over a period of time. The CT scan and EEG are usually normal. Spinal fluid examination may be normal early in the course of the disease, but the gamma globulin fraction of the total protein may become elevated as the disease progresses. Recently, studies of oligoclonal banding of the CSF gamma globulin have been useful in establishing a diagnosis of multiple sclerosis. Evoked potentials are also helpful in confirming the diagnosis.

The course of multiple sclerosis can be adversely affected by physical or emotional stress or any generalized systemic illness that weakens the patient. Multiple sclerosis has been shown to worsen during pregnancy and the puerperium [59–63]. The cause for this clinical exacerbation is unknown. The increased demands of pregnancy and caring for a newborn may be enough to account for the observation. When attacks occur, they are best managed by bed rest. The use of corticosteroids has been advocated for severe exacerbations, but their efficacy remains controversial. In any case, patients should be treated with enforced rest before the use of corticosteroids is considered.

There appears to be no increased incidence of stillbirths or fetal problems associated with multiple sclerosis. The exception to this general rule is the patient who is severely debilitated by multiple sclerosis. This patient is more susceptible to infections, severe fatigue, and pulmonary difficulties. Women who are seriously debilitated by multiple sclerosis should be carefully counseled about maternal problems during gestation as well as the rigors of child rearing. Management includes adequate rest and good nutrition; physical therapy for problems of weakness, spasticity, and ataxia; and prompt treatment of infections, most commonly of the urinary tract. There are few data regarding the use of antispasticity agents such as dantrolene and baclofen during pregnancy. Their use is not recommended. Similarly, drugs used for bladder control are best avoided during pregnancy. Patients should rely on physical measures for control.

Movement Disorders

Chorea Gravidarum

Movement disorders are seen in a small percentage of pregnant patients. The most common of these is chorea gravidarum [64], a disorder that usually affects primigravidas in early pregnancy. It is characterized by involuntary, abrupt, random movements of any limb. Occasionally it is accompanied by facial grimacing and dystonias. Often there are associated mental status changes. Involuntary movements are aggravated by anxiety and ameliorated by rest.

Chorea gravidarum is thought to be a recurrence of Sydenham's chorea encountered earlier in life from a streptococcal infection. A history of Sydenham's chorea can be obtained in 50 to 60% of patients with chorea gravidarum, but associated rheumatic valvular disease is not always present. This condition is believed to result from small vessel arteritis with localized infarcts in the basal ganglia [65]. Chorea gravidarum can be successfully managed with phenothiazines or haloperidol [66].

Wilson's Disease

Wilson's disease (hepatolenticular degeneration) is an autosomal recessive disorder of copper metabolism manifested by hepatic dysfunction, rigidity, tremors, and behavioral changes. Diagnostic laboratory abnormalities include a low serum ceruloplasmin concentration, a normal or low total serum copper level, and increased urinary copper excretion. Histologic demonstration of copper in the liver confirms the diagnosis. Before this disease was controlled with D-penicillamine treatment, most women had spontaneous abortions in the third or fourth month of gestation. Theoretically, D-penicillamine poses several problems for the fetus. However, in one series reported by Walsche all infants were unaffected at birth [70].

Huntington's Chorea

This is an autosomal dominant disorder characterized by involuntary movements and behavioral changes. On rare occasions Huntington's chorea may first appear during pregnancy mimicking chorea gravidarum. Unlike chorea gravidarum, Huntington's does not remit post partum. Haloperidol may be helpful for controlling the chorea.

Restless Legs Syndrome

Restless legs syndrome is an uncomfortable anxious feeling in the legs occurring when the patient is lying down or sitting. Patients state that their legs feel better when they are moved or when the patients are standing. The etiology is unknown. It has a benign course and is not associated with any particular underlying neurologic disorder but is thought to occur in association with iron deficiency. Small amounts of benzodiazepines are usually helpful in controlling the symptoms. Occasionally iron supplements have been noted to be helpful.

Other Causes of Movement Disorders

Phenothiazine therapy, autoimmune disease [67], and thyroid dysfunction can cause involuntary movements and need to be considered when evaluating a patient with a movement disorder.

THE PARAPLEGIC PATIENT

Although paraplegic women have certainly completed successful pregnancies, special care must be given throughout gestation to prevent urinary tract infections, maintain normal bowel function, and prevent pressure sores [68,69]. Women who were paraplegic prior to pregnancy appear to have no special risk of fetal problems, although series have been too small to obtain meaningful statistics.

If the spinal cord lesion is above T-11, the patients may not be able to appreciate uterine contractures during the course of labor. They will need very close observation during late pregnancy. After the twenty-eighth week, they should be seen weekly for cervical examination. At term they should be hospitalized and evaluated for possible induction of labor. Generally, these patients can be delivered vaginally.

REFERENCES

1. Baker AB, Baker LH, eds. Clinical neurology. New York: Harper & Row, 1981.
2. Donaldson JO. Neurology of pregnancy. Philadelphia: Saunders, 1978.
3. Davis LE. Normal laboratory values of CSF during pregnancy. Arch Neurol. 1979; 36:443.
4. Jack TM. Postpartum intracranial subdural hematoma; a possible complication of epidural analgesia. Anesthesiology. 1979; 34:176–80.
5. Reynolds AF, Slavin L. Postpartum acute subdural hematoma; a probable complication of saddle block analgesia. Neurosurgery. 1980; 7:348–9.
6. Amias AG. Cerebral vascular disease in pregnancy. I. Haemorrhage. J Obstet Br Comm. 1970; 77:100–20.
7. Robinson JL, Hall CS, Sedzimir CB. Arteriovenous malformations, aneurysms and pregnancy. J Neurosurg. 1973; 41:63–70.
8. Minielly R, Yuzpe AA, Drake CG. Subarachnoid hemorrhage secondary to ruptured cerebral aneurysm in pregnancy. Obstet Gynecol. 1979; 53:64–70.
9. Beck DW, Menezes AH. Intracerebral hemorrhage in a patient with eclampsia. JAMA. 1981; 246:1442–3.
10. Cross JN, Castro PO, Jennett WB. Cerebral strokes associated with pregnancy and the puerperium. Br Med J. 1968; 3:214–8.
11. Amias AG. Cerebral vascular disease in pregnancy. II. Occlusion. J Obstet Gynecol Br Comm. 1970; 77:312–25.
12. Dunn DW, Ellison J. Anterior spinal artery syndrome during the postpartum period. Arch Neurol. 1981; 38:263. (letter.)
13. Collaborative Group for the Study of Stroke in Young Women. Oral contraception and increased risk of cerebral ischemia or thrombosis. N Engl J Med. 1973; 188:871–8.
14. Singh BM, Morris LJ, Strobos RJ. Cortical blindness in puerperium. JAMA. 1980; 243:1134. (letter.)
15. Gaitz JP, Bamford CR. Unusual computed tomographic scan in eclampsia. Arch Neurol. 1982; 39:66.
16. Carrol JD, Leak D, Lee HA. Cerebral thrombophlebitis in pregnancy and the puerperium. Q J Med. 1966; 35:347–68.
17. Gupta OP, Tewari IJ, Mital VN. Primary cerebral thrombophlebitis of puerperium. J Indian Med Assoc. 1977; 68:160–3.
18. Lavin PJ, Bone I, Lamb JT, Swinburne LM. Intracranial venous thrombosis in the first trimester of pregnancy. J Neurol Neurosurg Psychiatry. 1978; 41:726–9.
19. Beal MF, Chapman PH. Cortical blindness and homonymous hemianopsia in the postpartum period. JAMA. 1980; 244:2085–7.
20. Toya S, Shiobara R, Izumi J, Shinomiya Y, Shiga H, Kimura C. Spontaneous carotid cavernous fistula during pregnancy or in the postpartum stage. J Neurosurg. 1981; 54:252–6.
21. Massey EW. Migraine during pregnancy. Obstet Gynecol Surv. 1977; 32:693–6.
22. Somerville BW. A study of migraine in pregnancy. Neurology (Minneap.). 1972; 22:824–8.
23. Wainscott G, Sullivan FM, Volans GN, Wilkinson M. The outcome of pregnancy in women suffering from migraine. Postgrad Med J. 1978; 54:98–102.
24. Dalessio DJ. Neurologic complications. In: Burrow GN, Ferris TF, eds. Medical complications during pregnancy. Philadelphia: Saunders, 1975:642–88.
25. Rubin PC. Beta blockers in pregnancy. N Engl J Med. 1981; 305:1323–6.
26. Berkowitz RL, Coustan DR, Mochizuki TK. Handbook for prescribing medications during pregnancy. Boston: Little, Brown, 1980.
27. Greer M. Benign intracranial hypertension. III. Pregnancy. Neurology (Minneap.) 1963; 13:670–2.
28. Johnson LC, DeBolt WL, Long MT, et al. Diagnostic factors in adult males following initial seizures: a three year follow-up. Arch Neurol. 1972; 27:193–7.
29. Montouris GD, Fenichel GM, McLain LW Jr. The pregnant epileptic: a review and recommendations. Arch Neurol. 1979; 36:601–3.

30. Knight AH, Rhind EG. Epilepsy and pregnancy: a study of 153 pregnancies in 59 patients. Epilepsia. 1975; 16:99–110.

31. Nelson KB, Ellenberg JH. Maternal seizure disorder, outcome of pregnancy, and neurologic abnormalities in children. Neurology. 1982; 32:1247–54.

32. Gross-Selbeck G, Doose H (eds.). Epilepsy—Problems of Marriage, Pregnancy, Genetic Counseling. New York: Thieme-Stratton, 1981.

33. Janz D, et al. Epilepsy, Pregnancy, and the Child. New York: Raven, 1982.

34. American Academy of Pediatrics Committee on Drugs. Anticonvulsants and pregnancy. Pediatrics. 1979; 69:331–3.

35. Hanson JW, Smith DW. The fetal hydantoin syndrome. J Pediatr. 1975; 87:285–90.

36. Hampton GR, Krepostman JI. Ocular manifestations of the fetal hydantoin syndrome. Clin Pediatr. (Phila.). 1981; 20:475–8.

37. Kochenour NK, Emergy MG, Sawchuck RJ. Phenytoin metabolism in pregnancy. Obstet Gynecol. 1980; 56:577–82.

38. Bale JF, Allen RW, Hulme J, Wyman ML. Epileptic mother. Arch Neurol. 1981; 38:263–4.

39. Bjerkedal T, Cziezel A, Goujard J, et al. Valproic acid and spina bifida. Lancet. 1982; 2:1096 (letter).

40. Centers for Disease Control. Valproic acid and spina bifida: A preliminary report—France. MMWR. 1982; 31:565–6.

41. Stumpf DA, Frost M. Seizures, anticonvulsants and pregnancy. Am J Dis Child. 1978; 132:746–7.

42. Swaiman KF. Antiepileptic drugs, the developing nervous system, and the pregnant woman with epilepsy. JAMA. 1980; 244:1477. (editorial.)

43. Massey EW, Cefalo RC. Neuropathies of pregnancy. Obstet Gynecol Surv. 1979; 34:489–92.

44. Gould JS, Wissinger HA. Carpal tunnel syndrome in pregnancy. South Med J. 1978; 71:144–5.

45. Snell NJ, Coysh HL, Snell BJ. Carpal tunnel syndrome presenting in the puerperium. Practitioner. 1980; 224:191–3.

46. Adour KK, Wingerd J. Idiopathic facial paralysis (Bell's palsy): factors affecting severity and outcome in 446 patients. Neurology (Minneap.). 1974; 24:1112–6.

47. Adour KK, Wingerd J and Bell DN. Prednisone treatment for idiopathic facial paralysis (Bell's palsy). N Engl J Med. 1972; 287:1268–72.

48. O'Connell JE. Lumbar disc protrusions in pregnancy. J Neurol Neurosurg Psychiatry. 1960; 23:138–41.

49. Heffernan LP, Fraser RC, Purdy RA. L-5 radiculopathy secondary to a uterine leiomyoma in a primigravid patient. Am J Obstet Gynecol. 1980; 138:460–1.

50. Pleet AB, Massey EW. Intercostal neuralgia of pregnancy. JAMA. 1980; 243:770.

51. Taylor RA. Heredofamilial mononeuritis multiplex with brachial predilection. Brain. 1960; 83:113–37.

52. Bauer KA, Siegler M, Lindheimer MA. Polymyositis complicating pregnancy. Arch Intern Med. 1979; 139:449.

53. Katz AL. Another case of polymyositis in pregnancy. Arch Intern Med. 1980; 140:1123. (letter.)

54. Hilliard GD, Harris RE, Gilstrap LC, Shoumaker RD. Myotonic muscular dystrophy in pregnancy. South Med J. 1977; 70:446–52.

55. Webb D, Muir I, Falkner J, Johnson G. Myotonia dystrophica: obstetric complications. Am J Obstet Gynecol. 1978; 132:265–70.

56. Giwa-Osagie OF, Newton JR, Larcher V. Obstetric performance of patients with myasthenia gravis. Int J Gynaecol Obstet. 1981; 19:267–70.

57. Plauche WV. Myasthenia gravis in pregnancy: an update. Am J Obstet Gynecol. 1979; 135:691–7.

58. Ohta M, Matsubara F, Hayashi K, Nakao K, Nishitani H. Acetylcholine receptor antibodies in infants of mothers with myasthenia gravis. Neurology (Minneap.). 1982; 31:1019–22.

59. Müller R. Pregnancy in disseminated sclerosis. Acta Psychiatr Neurol Scand. 1951; 26:397–409.

60. Millar JHD. The influence of pregnancy in disseminated sclerosis. Proc R Soc Med. 1961; 54:4–7.

61. Millar JH, Allison RS, Cheeseman EA, et al. Pregnancy as a factor influencing relapse on disseminated sclerosis. Brain. 1959; 82:417–26.

62. McAlpine D, Lumsden CE, Acheson ED. Multiple sclerosis: a reappraisal. 2nd ed. London: Churchill-Livingstone, 1972.

63. Poser S, Raun NE, Wikström J, Poser W. Pregnancy, oral contraceptives and multiple sclerosis. Acta Neurol Scand. 1979; 59:108–18.

64. Willson P, Preece AA. Chorea gravidarum. Arch Intern Med. 1932; 49:471–533, 671–97.

65. Ichikawa K, Kim RC, Givelber H, Collin GH. Chorea gravidarum: report of a fatal case with neuropathological observations. Arch Neurol. 1980; 37:429–32.

66. Patterson JF. Treatment of chorea gravidarum with haloperidol. South Med J. 1979; 72:1220–1.

67. Agrawal BL, Foa RP. Collagen vascular disease appearing as chorea gravidarum. Arch Neurol. 1982; 39:192–3.

68. Robertson DN, Guttermann L. The paraplegic patient in pregnancy and labour. Proc R Soc Med. 1963; 56:381–7.

69. Robertson DN. Pregnancy and labour in the paraplegic. Paraplegia. 1972; 10:209–12.

70. Walshe JM. Pregnancy in Wilson's disease. Q J Med. 1977; 46:73–83.

71. Lefvert AK, Osterman PO. Newborn infants to myasthenic mothers: A clinical study and an investigation of acetylcholine receptor antibodies in 17 children. Neurology. 1983; 33:133–8.

The psychiatrist is the obstetrician of the mind.
—Anonymous

26. PSYCHIATRIC APPROACH TO HIGH-RISK OBSTETRICS

Steven L. Dubovsky

As many as 30 to 60% of nonpsychiatric (including obstetric) inpatients and 25 to 80% of outpatients experience significant psychological distress [1–3]. Overt depression is diagnosed in at least 10% of obstetric patients; however, since 15 to 30% of the general population suffer at least one episode of clinical depression, it is likely that this condition is underdiagnosed [4–6]. Since a pregnant patient may conceal her problems from the obstetrician in order to be considered a "good patient," depression and other disorders may be overlooked unless she is examined carefully [7,8]. Thus, while less than 1% of obstetric patients require intensive treatment by the psychiatrist, a wide range of emotional problems must be diagnosed and managed by the obstetrician [8]. This chapter outlines a practical approach to these problems.

THE DOCTOR-PATIENT RELATIONSHIP

In no setting is the physician's relationship with his patient more important than in obstetric practice. Even the most uncomplicated pregnancy arouses ambivalence, fear of death and fetal abnormalities, negative feelings about the child, anxiety, and depression, and these are accentuated in high-risk situations [9]. The obstetrician must encourage confidence and compliance while at the same time eliciting data the patient may feel too ashamed or guilty to volunteer. Several concepts are useful in understanding some puzzling interactions of obstetric patients who are reacting to the stress of pregnancy with their physicians [10–14].

Regression

Any condition that places the patient in an ongoing dependent position (e.g., hospitalization or severe illness) can revive feelings that she experienced when she was a child and was dependent on her parents. This tendency is strengthened when a patient in the latter stages of pregnancy identifies with her child and longs for the care the child will receive, or when the patient must remain in bed and cannot resume her usual adult activities. If the quality and quantity of care she received in childhood was normal and if she feels comfortable depending on others, the patient is likely to adapt to the dependent role easily. However, patients who were deprived of normal caretaking as children may experience a resurgence of chronically unmet needs with surprising force, while those who were gratified excessively may expect to have every need met again. In either case, the patient may display childlike, demanding, dependent, clinging behavior and low tolerance for pain and frustration as the childhood emotional state emerges. This return to psychological functioning that was appropriate to an earlier time in the patient's life initially may seem psychotic to the patient and her physician. Patients who are frightened of dependency may become excessively anxious or may attempt to deny that they need any caretaking.

The patient who is made anxious by regressed behavior should be reassured that it represents a time-limited reaction to hospitalization or the stress of pregnancy. It may also be necessary to treat the patient as though she were a child, telling her firmly that she must comply with the treatment regimen and setting limits on demanding, complaining behavior.

Separation Anxiety

Like small children, regressed patients are particularly vulnerable to becoming distressed when they are away from a spouse, child, physician or nurse upon whom they feel dependent. Separation anxiety is manifested by anxiety, increased complaints, and demands for attention (e.g., ringing for the nurse) whenever the patient is left alone. Some patients also develop *stranger anxiety* in response to a new physician or change of house staff or nurses.

Separation anxiety can be managed effectively by allowing unrestricted visiting by family and friends, placing the patient near the nursing station, and encouraging brief (2–5 minutes) but frequent visits by nursing staff. Stranger anxiety is reduced by minimized cross-coverage or preparing the patient in advance for changes in personnel.

Transference

Transference, the repetition of elements of a significant relationship from the past in a present interaction, is especially likely to occur in important relationships and when similarities exist between a person in the present and someone in the past. It results in behavior that is inappropriate, ambivalent, intense, and changeable. Without being aware of it, the person experiencing transference alternates between seeing individuals realistically and seeing them as though they were people she knew in the past. The doctor-patient relationship is especially likely to stimulate transference because physicians play a parental role in the lives of patients who depend on them to meet important needs. The sicker, more frightened, or more dependent the patient, the more likely she is to feel and act toward the physician as she has toward other important caretakers, particularly her parents.

Several types of transference reactions may be encountered in obstetric patients. The *eroticized* transference is characterized by the sudden appearance of intense romantic feelings toward the physician that are not justified by his behavior. Usually, an underlying chronically unsatisfied need for love or attention, as well as considerable hostility, are hidden beneath declarations of love, and demands for a sexual relationship may be presented in an unsettling manner. These feelings should be discussed openly and appropriate professional distance reestablished. Since eroticized transference represents the repetition of an ambivalent wish to be loved from some other important relationship, it does not represent a true attachment to the doctor. The patient's underlying anger at those who never gratified her sufficiently is likely to replace her apparent love, making reciprocation of her positive feelings potentially destructive to patient and physician.

Other patients who experience serious trauma in childhood may feel that they are entitled to special treatment to make up for their earlier deprivations. This may be expressed as *entitled, dependent transference*. Intensive obstetric care may remind them of how much they missed as children, especially if they are jealous of the care their own children will receive. The doctor's interest and kindness then may make them feel that it now is possible to make up for past deprivations with extra attention and caring from the physician. They may attempt to extort this care through increasing complaints, multiple phone calls at inconvenient times, or even surreptitious noncompliance designed to worsen their condition and force the obstetrician to spend more time with them. If the obstetrician responds to these demands, the patient may learn that being sick or in pain will force extra caretaking, and her complaints may increase. In addition, because the physician is seen as a substitute parent, the patient may come to believe he or she is responsible for more and more aspects of her life—for example, whether she is happy in her marriage or capable of raising her children. Questions about how to manage her pregnancy are gradually replaced with questions about how to live her life, and the physician is blamed when his or her suggestions do not work (because the patient is repeating both parts of an old relationship: a wish to be cared for and disappointment in caretakers who always fail her). If the obstetrician implicitly takes increasing responsibility for the patient's life, she learns to rely on him or her rather than to make her own decisions, decreasing the likelihood that her problems will be resolved. It therefore becomes important to help the patient take more responsibility both for her obstetric care and for her personal life, by explaining to her that she is avoiding making her own decisions and refusing to do anything for her that she can do for herself.

Denial

People often ignore some aspect of a frightening situation so that anxiety will not interfere with their capacity to cope effectively. While adaptive in many situations, the patient who attempts to reassure herself by insisting that her pregnancy is uncomplicated may not comply with obstetric care. She may refuse indicated hospitalization or other care on the grounds that she is not sick enough to need it. Attempts to convince the patient of the danger of her situation usually increase her anxiety and her denial of the need for treatment. A more effective approach involves reducing anxiety through relaxation, hypnosis, and, in carefully selected patients in their second and third trimesters, the judicious use of antianxiety drugs. The obstetrician can also avoid focusing excessively on the risks of the patient's situation, encouraging her to remain in the hospital or comply with outpatient treatment as a way of being even more certain that things will work out well.

Stimulation of Underlying Psychological Vulnerabilities

Patients with weaknesses in certain areas of psychological function are particularly likely to experience distress during pregnancy. For example, the woman whose self-esteem or sense of entitlement to love depends on her beauty may attempt to compensate for feelings of inadequacy or fear of loss of affection by behaving in an inappropriately seductive or self-important manner. If she is openly confronted, her insecurities may increase; however, if she is realistically praised for keeping herself attractive or treated in a deferential manner, she may be reassured. Similarly, patients who have not resolved grief over an important loss (e.g., of a parent, child, or fetus) are more likely to become depressed in response to perinatal loss.

Spouses have their own vulnerabilities, which may result in the development of obvious psychological distress in the husband or, more commonly, in his asking for help indirectly by covertly provoking the patient. It is therefore a good idea to include all significant others in the evaluation of an apparent psychiatric disturbance in a pregnant patient.

Countertransference

Although it might theoretically be desirable for the physician to be able to treat complex and life-threatening problems without sharing any of the patient's fears of pain, this ideal is impossible in all but the most technically oriented fields. In addition, one important means of communicating important emotions, especially if the patient is not consciously aware of them, is to induce similar feelings in the physician. For example, the patient who is reluctant to express anxiety about her pregnancy may in subtle ways make her obstetrician feel anxious, while a patient who is unaware of being angry at her husband may, through covert provocation, "get rid" of her feeling by inducing a similar state in the doctor, then remaining aware of it in the physician but not in herself. In the absence of any other explanation such as fatigue, a recent experience that aroused strong feelings, or transference (e.g., the patient reminds the physician of someone he knows), strong reactions in the obstetrician are likely to reflect the patient's emotional state. This condition may be confirmed by observing the patient closely and asking about the emotions the physician suspects may be hidden beneath the surface. Usually, the patient is relieved when these are uncovered.

HYPEREMESIS GRAVIDARUM

Although nausea and vomiting during the first trimester are seen in 50 to 88% of American women, persistent pathologic vomiting requiring hospitalization is seen in no more than 10 per 1,000 patients [15–17]. Many investigators feel that organic and psychological factors both play a role in producing hyperemesis, marked ambivalence about pregnancy and childbirth being the most commonly noted emotion along with concerns about femininity and sexuality [15–18]. Most women are ambivalent or openly negative about being pregnant at times, especially during the first trimester [9]. This reaction is likely to be much more intense in any patient who is experiencing significant persistent physical discomfort. However, the expression of emotional distress as physical symptoms seems to be common in the histories of women who develop hyperemesis [16].

Even when psychological stress is obvious to the obstetrician, many hyperemesis patients deny that they have any problems at all or that psychiatric factors could possibly be playing a role in their vomiting. They may become angry or display increased symptoms when attempts are made to uncover emotional conflict. Efforts to bring insight are usually not helpful, therefore, at least while the patient is actively ill [17].

A more supportive approach in which the patient is isolated from all potential sources of stress (Table 26-1) rapidly results in control of the patient's vomiting, possibly in part by decreasing the input of psychological stress and inducing a brief, controlled regression that allows the patient to reorganize and marshal psychic strengths. Relaxation techniques and hypnosis can obviate the need for medication and bring about significant improvement in the majority of patients in only one to three 20 to 45-minute sessions [17]. The psychiatrist can be useful in helping to determine whether a patient is likely to be a good hypnotic subject.

Although most episodes of hyperemesis can be controlled within a few days to a week or two, the physician should not be dismayed at relapses. Attempts to avoid hospitalization may cause an intensification of symptoms, while prompt readmission usually results in rapid reduction in the patient's vomiting. During each admission, the patient should gradually be reintroduced to her family and the responsibilities of everyday life as her

Table 26-1. Treatment of hyperemesis gravidarum

Hospitalize the patient.

Maintain fluid and electrolyte balance.

Place the patient in a private room.

Restrict all visitors initially no matter how much the patient seems to wish to see them.

Minimize environmental stimulation, including bright lights, loud noises, newspapers, radio, and television.

Provide a supportive, nonintrusive, caretaking atmosphere.

Employ hypnosis and relaxation techniques in suitable patients.

Avoid attempts at psychological insight.

When vomiting subsides, gradually reintroduce family members, initially for brief periods of time.

If vomiting recurs, restrict visitors and reinstitute supportive measures.

Rehospitalize when further episodes of vomiting do not respond rapidly to standard outpatient measures.

Request psychiatric consultation when the patient does not improve or to assess suitability for adjunctive techniques (e.g., hypnosis).

Table 26-2. Organic causes of sexual dysfunction

Systemic
Alcohol and drug abuse, some prescription drugs
Venereal disease
Thyroid disease
Diabetes mellitus
Multiple sclerosis
Spinal cord disease
Peripheral neuropathy
Hypertension
Liver disease
Any debilitating or painful condition that distracts from sexual interest

Genital and rectal
Female
 Lesions of vulva, introitus, vagina, cervix, or uterus
 Weakness of pubococcygeal muscles
 Chronic urinary tract and gynecologic infections
Male
 Prostate disease
 Disease of the penis
 Varicocele and hydrocele
 Peyronie's disease

Table 26-3. Psychological causes of sexual dysfunction

Ignorance and misinformation

Anger between the partners

Guilt about previous sexual activities or an extramarital affair

Other marital conflicts

Problems initiating or refusing sex openly

Belief that the partner should know one's sexual likes and dislikes without having to be told

Religious or cultural taboos about sex

Performance anxiety (worries about being unable to achieve an erection or lubricate, resulting in more attention being paid to performance than to enjoyment of sex)

Fear of injuring the fetus

symptoms decrease and she indicates an increasing interest in returning to her previous level of functioning.

SEXUAL PROBLEMS DURING PREGNANCY

Complaints of marital discord, depression, insomnia, aches and pains, and irritation with others, and requests of either spouse to meet with the physician without the other's knowledge, often indicate an underlying sexual problem [10]. Since embarrassment or uncertainty about the physician's ability to help her may prevent the patient from volunteering that she is experiencing difficulties with sex, routine questioning about changes in sexual frequency, enjoyment, or interest should be a part of routine antenatal and postnatal care. A sexual dysfunction that is uncovered during pregnancy may have been present before the patient became pregnant, or the stresses of pregnancy on the couple (especially fear of injuring the fetus, conflicts about becoming parents, and financial worries) may have produced a new problem.

In taking a sexual history, the physician should determine when the disturbance appeared and under what circumstances it is manifested. Extramarital affairs, which not uncommonly begin during a pregnancy and usually affect sexual involvement in the marriage, may be uncovered only when each spouse is interviewed separately. However, both partners must be seen together at some

point in the evaluation. A detailed description of a typical sexual encounter includes type and duration of foreplay, length of time after entry and before ejaculation, and how often and with what types of stimulation the woman reaches an orgasm. The couple's knowledge and attitudes toward sex and pregnancy (including moral and religious taboos) and their misconception should be elicited, as should the use of medications, alcohol, and nonprescription drugs.

Physical causes of sexual disorders (Table 26-2) are now known to cause 40 to 55% of cases of erectile dysfunction and a smaller number of other problems. Common psychological factors are listed in Table 26-3 [9,10,19–22].

Problems that arise for the first time during pregnancy and require education and retraining in communication of sexual needs are particularly amenable to treatment by the obstetrician. Common examples are difficulty with lubrication, reactive secondary orgasmic dysfunction (failure to achieve orgasm in a woman who was previously orgasmic), uncomplicated premature ejaculation, and reactive secondary impotence (difficulty attaining an erection in a man who has been potent). The following techniques are useful in treating these problems [10,19,20].

1. *Involve both partners.* Both individuals must be involved in the treatment of even the most uncomplicated problem. Even when the partner does not contribute actively to the problem, his or her assistance must be secured in treating it.
2. *Reassure* the couple that their problem is not uncommon and can be corrected.
3. *Educate* the couple about sexual anatomy and physiology, and correct misconceptions. Common misunderstandings are that the woman should be able to reach orgasm without direct clitoral stimulation, that intercourse will harm the fetus, and that alcohol should not affect potency.
4. *Encourage communication of sexual likes and dislikes.* When a couple thinks that each should know the other's preferences without having to talk about them, neither partner may feel free to express dissatisfaction with the other's techniques. Instead, sex may become chronically unfulfilling or may be increasingly avoided. This problem is dealt with by encouraging open discussion of each partner's sexual preferences, and the ways in which he or she would like the other person to respond.
5. *Prescribe physical pleasuring sessions.* First, a temporary ban is placed on genital contact and intercourse. The couple is instructed to touch or massage each other anywhere except the genitals. Erections or lubrication are enjoyed without any sense of obligation for intercourse, and partners take turns demonstrating to each other the ways in which they prefer to be stimulated. Gradually, the couple proceeds, under the physician's direction, to genital contact and then intercourse, avoiding intercourse again if impotence or difficulty with lubrication occurs. During pleasuring sessions, sensory awareness exercises, in which each partner's attention is distracted away from worries about not being able to lubricate or achieve an erection and to-

ward the pleasurable aspects of lovemaking, help to decrease performance anxiety.
6. *Examine for lax pubococcygeal muscles.* When orgasmic dysfunction is due to this condition, exercises to strengthen pubococcygeal muscles may provide more clitoral stimulation during intercourse.
7. *Treat premature ejaculation with the start-stop technique or the squeeze technique.* In the former method, the male first masturbates and then has intercourse in the female superior position to the point of ejaculatory inevitability (the point beyond which ejaculation cannot be prevented by conscious control). Stimulation then is halted until his erection begins to recede, at which point stimulation is restarted. In an analogous manner, the squeeze technique utilizes strong pressure of the patient's (and then the wife's) thumb on the ventral surface of the frenulum and first and second fingers on the dorsal surface of the penis until the erection recedes.

ADOLESCENT PREGNANCY

Adolescent sexual activity, particularly, among young women, has been steadily increasing throughout the world, paralleled by a startling increase in the number of teenage pregnancies [23,24]. It has been estimated that as many as 8% of girls aged 14 to 19 now have an illegitimate child, another 5% may marry because of pregnancy, and more than 20% may undergo abortions [25,26]. Twenty percent of these pregnancies occur during the first month of sexual activity, and 50% within the first six months [24].

The predominant reason for the failure of most teenagers to use contraceptives at least some of the time is the belief that they will not become pregnant, especially if they engage in intercourse "only once." Young women also may wish to avoid feeling that sex is premeditated or to assuage guilt feelings about engaging in sex, or they simply may not consider the risks of pregnancy at a moment of passion [23,24,26]. Adolescent boys, on the other hand, are more likely to either want to have their own children or not care about whether their partner becomes pregnant [24].

About one-third to one-half of teenage pregnancies end in abortion, the most commonly performed operation in the United States [27]. Teenagers who choose abortion tend to be white, younger than 15 or older than 18, more financially independent of their families and of public assistance, of higher socioeconomic status, and not as attached to the child's father, as compared to teenagers who deliver [27]. When performed under optimal surgical conditions by a concerned obstetrician, abortion does not exacerbate preexisting psychiatric disorders and does not lead to long-term psychological sequelae in the majority of patients; in fact, it may improve mental health in patients with severe conflicts about being pregnant [23,27]. However, every patient who undergoes abortion, regardless of her age, should be encouraged in an accepting and non-judgmental manner to discuss her feelings about the procedure. Guilt and ambivalence are not uncommon, and mourning for the lost child may need to be encouraged [28]. When the patient feels that her decision does not entitle her to feel bad about it, is ashamed of the abortion or of her reaction, or thinks that the physician disapproves of her, she may conceal her discomfort from him. It is therefore a good idea to ask directly about the patient's emotions at each follow-up visit while leaving sufficient time for the patient to discuss them. Younger patients, those with inadequate social support, and those who were markedly ambivalent about the procedure are most likely to experience adverse reactions to abortions.

In contrast to the low complication rate from abortion, carrying a teenage pregnancy to term is associated with a high risk of medical and psychosocial complications in mother and child [27]. Although mothers over the age of 14 are physically at no greater risk of experiencing complications than older patients, prenatal care and nutrition are likely to be inadequate, resulting in a greater morbidity and mortality in teenaged mothers and their children [24,27]. Serious psychiatric illness is also more common in this group [27].

Pregnancy is the major cause of teenaged girls leaving high school [24]. Because most of these adolescents do not return to school, the outcome is lower educational and socioeconomic status, poorer jobs, and a greater chance of requiring welfare or other public assistance [24,27]. The divorce rate in teenage marriages that are occasioned by a pregnancy is higher than in other populations, and even later second marriages of teenaged mothers are at greater risk of breaking up [23,24].

Since adolescents are less experienced and informed and under greater stress than older mothers, they are less likely to be effective parents [24,27]. As a result, their children seem to experience more behavioral problems and exhibit poorer performance on tests of motor and mental development, as well as possibly poorer performance in school. Children who receive auxiliary mothering from grandparents or other relatives or who spend a significant amount of time in day care centers appear to enjoy more favorable development [27].

The most important aspect of the management of adolescent pregnancy is primary prevention [23,26]. Since 70% of teenagers who employ contraception at their first sexual experience continue its use subsequently, early discussion of all adolescents' attitudes and misconceptions about sex is indicated [24]. The high cost of pregnancy should be described and the patient encouraged to learn about and choose a contraceptive before rather than after she thinks she may engage in intercourse. Most young women would forgo contraception—but not sex—if parental permission were required, so it is preferable to give the patient the option of whether to inform her parents that a contraceptive has been prescribed [24]. It is also useful to encourage parents to discuss sex with their teenage children, and to uncover and deal with concerns that parents may have about such discussions. Encouraging teenaged patients and their parents to talk about sexuality and the use of contraceptives will become even more crucial if laws requiring parental permission for the prescription of contraceptives are introduced.

Should a teenager become pregnant, abortion should be discussed openly and objectively. If the patient wishes to carry the pregnancy to term, extra attention should be paid to nutrition and other aspects of prenatal care. The patient should also be expected to require help in learning about parenting and infant and child development, and any resources in the family that may be available to help her with child rearing should be mobilized.

POSTPARTUM PSYCHOSES

Puerperal psychosis represents a relatively rare (1–2 per 1,000) but severe complication of pregnancy, accounting for 1 to 8% of all female psychiatric hospital admissions [29,30]. Psychotic symptoms begin suddenly in an apparently healthy patient, usually within a month of delivery and often within three to six days, and consist of agitation, hallucinations, delusions of illness or death of the child, depression, excitement, and confusion [30,31]. As a rule the psychosis resolves, and it does not recur in 40 to 50% of patients [30]. Although the risk of a subsequent psychotic episode is increased in the remainder of patients, up to 10 to 15% of puerperal psychoses become chronic, probably because an underlying schizophrenic illness was precipitated by delivery [30,31].

Rather than representing a separate diagnostic entity, postpartum psychosis represents a major

Table 26-4. Causes of postpartum psychosis

Organic brain syndrome

Mania

Depression

Schizoaffective disorder

Schizophrenia

Brief reactive psychosis*

*A psychogenic disorder producing psychotic, often paranoid symptoms lasting less than 2 weeks.

Table 26-5. Diagnostic clues to organic brain syndrome

Sudden onset

Negative past history

No family history of mental illness

Fluctuating symptoms

Diminished attention

Disorientation to time and place, but not person

Defect in short-term memory

Confused or concrete thinking

Symptoms worse at night

Slowing of the EEG

Table 26-6. Risk factors for postpartum psychosis

Unmarried

Primipara

Past history of psychosis, especially postpartum psychosis

Family history of psychosis

Excessive dependence on mother, husband or both

Failure of husband to visit or otherwise offer support, or expressions of his disappointment in the child

Severe marital discord

Marked ambivalence about pregnancy

psychiatric disorder (Table 26-4) that is precipitated by childbirth [31–33]. On the obstetric unit, the physician should determine that a complication of delivery, adverse drug reaction, or other medical illness has not produced psychotic symptoms through a direct or indirect effect on the patient's brain (organic brain syndrome). If diagnostic clues summarized in Table 26-5 are present, a thorough search for an organic cause of the patient's psychosis should be undertaken [10].

Most of the functional conditions that cause postpartum psychoses are thought to result from a combination of subtle alterations in brain neurochemistry and psychological stresses. Among the latter are an excessively close and dependent relationship with the husband or the mother or both that the new child threatens to disrupt, jealousy of the child's dependency, and ambivalence about the pregnancy and the marriage. Although many patients experience such conflicts without becoming psychotic, those at increased risk (Table 26-6) should be observed closely during the first postpartum month [8,29–31,34].

Once organic illnesses are ruled out, postpartum psychoses are treated by the psychiatrist and the obstetrician with a combination of antipsychotic (see Table 26-8) or antidepressant (see Table 26-12) medication, psychotherapy, and family therapy. Treatment is often complicated by

covert attempts by the patient's mother or husband to undo the patient's improvement in order to maintain control over her, and their visits may need to be restricted temporarily. The patient and her family may be unaware of obvious emotional conflicts and unwilling to discuss the disruption in the family's homeostasis caused by the birth of a new child.

CHILD ABUSE

Clues to child abuse potential are often present in the immediate postpartum period. Since only 10% of the abusive parents suffer from a diagnosable psychiatric illness, the obstetric team must rely on other indicators of abuse potential [35]. One well-known risk factor is impaired bonding between mother and child, which may be caused by early separation from the child due to maternal illness, prematurity, or postnatal problems in the child [35,36]. However, up to 40% of normal women initially may feel indifference or even dislike for their newborns, which is replaced by strong affection within a week [37]. Immediate absence of affection for the child is more likely to occur if the patient has undergone difficult labor or an amniotomy or has received two or more doses of analgesic. Nevertheless, most women who fail to demonstrate immediate bonding become very attached to their children and do not become abusive [37]. While no single factor may be relied on, when several of the signs listed in Table 26-7 are present, assistance from the psychiatrist and the child protection team in determining the patient's potential to become abusive should be sought [35–38].

Because patients with abusive thoughts or behavior usually feel ashamed and guilty, they are likely to give socially acceptable answers to direct, confronting questions about abuse. It is, therefore, crucial to establish rapport in a nonjudgmental manner and to avoid immediately confronting the parents. Several brief discussions focusing on the

*Table 26-7. Some factors indicating
an increased risk for child abuse*

Early separation of mother and child

Impaired bonding between mother and child

History of abuse or neglect in either parent

Psychiatric illness in the mother

Parents younger than age 21

Failure of parents to make preparations for baby's arrival
(e.g., buying clothing and diapers)

Choice of a name for only one sex

Unrealistic expectation of the child (e.g., that he soothe
the mother or become toilet-trained too early)

Baby described as difficult or disappointing

Social isolation in parents

Child colicky or fussy or with a birth defect

Excessive concern that child's appearance and behavior
must be perfect

Worries about spoiling the baby

Fears of loss of control

Postpartum depression

Failure to thrive

Any injury to infant

parents' feelings of isolation, loneliness, anger at their own parents, and high expectations of the child are more effective than a single long interview. It is also important to see the patient and her husband immediately, if briefly, when they appear for an unscheduled appointment, as they are likely to be testing the physician's interest in them. The parents should be kept fully informed about all aspects of obstetric and pediatric care, and no secrets should be kept from either parent.

When child abuse is uncovered or strongly suspected, the infant must be kept in the hospital until a thorough evaluation can be conducted. The parents usually accept continuing hospitalization for further study, and the mother too may wish to remain for a few extra days. If a child protection team is not available, a psychiatrist should evaluate the child and the parents. In many states, the law requires that child abuse be reported to the appropriate agency. Finally, if the initial investigation is inconclusive, the patient and her child should be followed closely by the obstetrician, pediatrician, psychiatrist, and child protection team until the potential for abuse can definitely be said to be low. Early intervention in the absence of definite signs of abuse can prevent further decompensation in the family, and immediate steps taken to protect the child and the mother after any suspicious injury can prevent a fatal outcome [38].

USE OF PSYCHOACTIVE DRUGS IN OBSTETRIC PRACTICE

While drugs play an essential role in the management of major psychiatric syndromes, the use of many psychotropic medications must be modified in the pregnant patient. Prescription and nonprescription centrally acting drugs are considered separately below.

Antipsychotic Drugs (Neuroleptics)

In standard doses, antipsychotic drugs (Table 26-8) can be used to treat acute schizophrenic (Table 26-9) and manic psychoses (Table 26-10), to prevent recurrent schizophrenic psychoses, and to ameliorate disability caused by chronic schizophrenic psychoses [10,32,39,40]. The latter indication is becoming more important in obstetric prac-

Table 26-8. Some antipsychotic medications

Drug	Usual daily dose in acute psychosis (mg)
Phenothiazines	
Chlorpromazine[a]	300–2,000
Thioridazine[a]	200–800[c]
Trifluoperazine[b]	10–60
Butyrophenone	
Haloperidol[b]	15–100
Thioxanthenes	
Thiothixene[b]	10–60
Chlorprothixene[a]	50–400
Other heterocyclics	
Loxapine	60–250
Molindone	50–400

[a]Tend to be used in higher milligram amounts and to be more sedating.
[b]Tend to be used in lower doses and to be less sedating.
[c]*Never* administer more than 800 mg/day of thioridazine (may cause pigmentary retinopathy).

Table 26-9. Diagnostic clues to acute schizophrenia

Continuous signs of illness for at least 6 months

Deteriorating level of functioning

Delusions, especially of being controlled by an outside force, thoughts being inserted or withdrawn from the patient's mind, any nonpersecutory or jealous delusion, or delusions of persecution or jealousy accompanied by hallucinations

Auditory hallucinations, especially voices speaking the patient's thoughts out loud, commenting on the patient's actions, or arguing about the patient

Disorganized thinking or behavior

Past history of schizophrenia

Family history of schizophrenia

Table 26-10. Diagnostic clues to mania

Pathologically elevated mood

Irritability

Increased physical activity

Rapid, pressured speech

Grandiosity

Distractibility

Poor judgment

Decreased need for sleep

Past history of mania or depression

Family history of mania, depression, alcoholism, or antisocial behavior

Table 26-11. Andidepressant medications

Drug	Usual daily dose in healthy patients (mg)
Tricyclics	
Amitriptyline[a]	150–300
Nortriptyline	50–150[b]
Protriptyline	10–60
Imipramine	150–300
Desipramine	150–250[b]
Doxepin[a]	100–200
Amoxapine	150–300
Heterocyclics	
Maprotiline	150–300
Trazodone	150–400
Lithium carbonate	900–2,400 (serum concentration = 0.5–1.5 mEq/L; toxicity at 2 mEq/L)

[a]More sedating.
[b]Therapeutic window.

Table 26-12. Diagnostic clues to depression

Symptom duration of at least two weeks

Pervasive change in mood: sadness, crying, discouragement, irritability

Hopelessness, helplessness

Lowered self-esteem

Loss of interest in usual activity

Decreased libido

Multiple somatic complaints

Suicidal thoughts

"Vegetative" signs
  Decreased appetite and corresponding weight change
  Insomnia (especially early morning awakening) or hypersomnia
  Psychomotor retardation or agitation
  Loss of energy
  Difficulty concentrating

tice as antipsychotic medications stabilize patients sufficiently to carry pregnancy to term [41]. Low doses of nonsedating neuroleptics (e.g., haloperidol, 2–10 mg/day) are also sometimes used to treat agitation caused by organic brain syndromes, while some antipsychotics (especially thioridazine) may be helpful in depression accompanied by agitation or psychotic features.

As with many of the psychoactive drugs, potential adverse effects are numerous. Anticholinergic symptoms have been reported with administration of antipsychotic medication and may be additive with other anticholinergic agents. Postural hypotension, tachycardia, acute parkinsonian symptomatology, and more rarely chronic tardive dyskinesia may follow the use of several antipsychotics. A lowered convulsive threshold and quinidine-like effects may be seen, and sudden death has been reported with thioridazine, though rarely. Neuroleptics can promote the sedative effects of other central nervous system depressants and may interfere with the action of some antihypertensives. Barbiturates may decrease effective blood levels of some antipsychotic drugs. There is no evidence that neuroleptics are associated with an increase in fetal defects or loss [41]. However, they are excreted in breast milk and may produce excess sedation and extrapyramidal syndromes in the infant, especially parkinsonism, akathisia (motor restlessness), and respiratory dyskinesias leading to respiratory distress [41,42]. It should also be borne in mind that children of schizophrenics, regardless of the family in which they are raised are at an increased rate of acquiring schizophrenia themselves [43].

Antidepressants

Antidepressants (Table 26-11) are used to treat depression, some phobias, and panic attacks [10,40]. They have also been shown to be useful in the management of migraine headaches and chronic pain. Before instituting treatment with an antidepressant, depression (Table 26-12) must be distinguished from grief, postpartum blues, and transient situational reactions [10,32]. Patients with depression with "endogenous" features (e.g., prominent guilt and lowered self-esteem, vegetative signs), family history of affective disorder, and past or family history of response to an antidepressant are more likely to respond to medication than are patients whose depression seems to be an understandable reaction to life stresses in the absence of signs of biologic dysfunction [10]. Recently, it has been shown that in the absence of medical illness or corticosteroid administration patients who fail to suppress serum cortisol below 5 mg per deciliter on the afternoon following the administration of 1 mg of dexamethasone (dexamethasone suppression test) have a high likelihood of having an endogenous depression, regardless of their actual symptoms [44]. The frequency of abnormal dexamethasone suppression tests in otherwise normal pregnant patients, however, has not yet been established.

While they are effective if prescribed in adequate doses, antidepressants are extremely dangerous when taken in overdose (they are not dialyzable), and death has been reported in patients acutely ingesting 1,200 mg (a one week's supply) and regularly in patients taking 2,000 mg [40].

Side effects are not uncommon in patients using antidepressants. Postural hypotension, sedation, weight gain, and anticholinergic symptoms may be seen. More serious but less frequent is a quinidine-like effect (especially heart block), particularly in patients with preexisting partial bundle-branch block. Rarely, sudden death has been reported in patients who have had myocardial infarction. If the patient is taking other medications, adverse drug interactions may occur. The antidepressant medications can interfere with the action of clonidine, guanethidine, and bethanidine. Barbiturates and alcohol may decrease effective blood levels of the prescribed antidepressant, and hypertension may follow administration of amphetamines, norepinephrine, phenylephrine (including cold preparations), and monoamine oxidase (MAO) inhibitors. The latter, a class of antidepressants usually prescribed by the psychiatrist for treatment-resistant or atypical depression, may cause infertility; they have been implicated in fetal reabsorption in animals and should not be used during pregnancy [41]. Symptoms of phenytoin toxicity have also been reported following concurrent administration of several antidepressant medications.

Lithium is indicated for the treatment of acute mania and the prophylaxis of recurrent attacks of mania and depression. It is probably useful in the management of some acute depressions, as well as cluster headaches and neutropenia.

Patients on lithium may experience thirst, polyuria, diarrhea, abdominal pain, nausea, vomiting, or leukocytosis. Goiter, nephrogenic diabetes insipidus, hyperparathyroidism, and irreversible renal damage have also been reported. Phenothiazines may decrease effective blood levels of lithium and indomethacin, whereas methyldopa, some heterocyclics, and sodium-wasting diuretics may elevate these levels. Succinylcholine action may be prolonged by lithium, and neurotoxicity may ensue when haloperidol is prescribed with lithium. In addition to being lethal when taken in overdose, lithium taken during the first trimester may cause severe fetal abnormalities, including limb deformities, cardiovascular anomalies, goiter, hypotonia, and cyanosis. It should be discontinued immediately in any patient who becomes pregnant, and pregnancy testing is indicated in any patient in whom lithium therapy is contemplated. However, since discontinuation of lithium in bipolar (manic-depressive) patients may be associated with an increased risk of postpartum psychosis, the drug may need to be restarted shortly after delivery. Antidepressants and lithium are excreted in breast milk; their long-term effects on the infant are unknown [41].

Antianxiety Drugs
While the use of antipsychotic drugs or antidepressants after the first trimester may be necessary in some pregnant patients with schizophrenia or severe depression, the risks of antianxiety drugs ("minor" tranquilizers) generally outweigh their usefulness. Diazepam administered during the first trimester has been associated with cleft palate; barbiturates also have been implicated in these anomalies as well as skeletal abnormalities, hypotonia, and lethargy in the infant. Women should therefore be cautioned against the routine use of antianxiety drugs and sedative-hypnotics (sleeping pills), including benzodiazepines (e.g., diazepam, chlordiazepoxide, flurazepam, temazepam), glycerol derivatives (e.g., meprobamate), and barbiturates and related compounds (e.g., secobarbital, pentobarbital, amobarbital, glutethimide, methaqualone). Insomnia in pregnancy should be managed when possible with warm milk, tryptophan, biofeedback, or hypnosis.

ALCOHOL ABUSE
Alcohol abuse is alarmingly common, occurring in up to 25% of pregnant adolescents. The fetal alcohol syndrome, which occurs in 1 to 2 per 1,000 births, is associated with abnormalities in the central nervous system (including mental retardation in 80%), stunted growth in length and head circumference, and abnormalities of the eyes, nose, mouth, and maxilla. In addition, abstinence syndromes, characterized by irritability, seizures, and opisthotonos, may develop 6 to 12 hours after birth in newborns of mothers who continue to consume significant amounts of alcohol until shortly before delivery [45]. Twenty-five percent of alcoholic women have an alcoholic partner, but

the effects of alcohol abuse in the father on the newborn are unknown [45].

Although safe levels of alcohol consumption in pregnancy are unknown, the chronic ingestion of three ounces per day constitutes a major risk to the fetus [46,47]. Pregnant women should probably be warned to consume less than one ounce of ethanol (absolute alcohol) per day, and to drink less if possible. The total amount imbibed may be less important than peak blood levels attained at any time [45–47].

NARCOTIC ABUSE

Because the narcotic addict pays little attention to obtaining adequate prenatal care, complications of pregnancy, including abruption, abortion, eclampsia, septic thrombophlebitis, and low birth weight, are common. Medical complications of addiction, especially anemia, subacute bacterial endocarditis, gestational diabetes, preeclampsia, pneumonia, venereal disease, tuberculosis, and phlebitis, can also occur during pregnancy. Neonatal narcotic abstinence syndromes usually begin 72 hours after birth (but may not start for two weeks) and last six to eight weeks. Signs and symptoms include central nervous system excitability, respiratory distress, gastrointestinal dysfunction, fever, stuffy nose, lacrimation, and inability to suck. Congenital malformations are also more common in the children of heroin addicts [45].

While avoidance of narcotics during pregnancy is preferable, increased oxygen requirements caused by withdrawal of narcotics in the mother may cause fetal distress. Withdrawal, therefore, should be attempted only in cooperative patients, and preferably only when fetal monitoring can be done and delivery would be possible. Earlier in pregnancy, substitution therapy with methadone offers an alternative. One standard protocol substitutes 30 mg per day of methadone and then adjusts the total daily dose to suppress *objective signs* of withdrawal or to a maximum daily dose of 50 mg per day [10]. Because of the patient's unreliability and the danger of fetal distress, withdrawal from narcotics should *never* be attempted outside of a hospital.

REFERENCES

1. Lipowski ZJ. Consultation-liaison psychiatry. Gen Hosp Psychiatry. 1979; 1:3–10.
2. Shevitz SA, Silverfarb PM, Lipowski ZJ. Psychiatric consultations in a general hospital. A report on 1,000 referrals. Dis Nerv Syst. 1976; 37:295–300.
3. Fisher JV. What the family physician expects from the psychiatrist. Psychosomatics. 1978; 19:523–7.
4. Molinski H. Masked depressions in obstetrics and gynecology. Psychother Psychosom. 1979; 31:283–7.
5. Cassem NH. Depression. In: Hackett TP, Cassem NH, eds. MGH handbook of general hospital psychiatry St. Louis: Mosby, 1978:209–30.
6. Klerman GJ. Overview of affective disorders. In: Kaplan HI, Freedman AM, Sadock BJ, eds. Comprehensive textbook of psychiatry III. 3rd ed. Vol. 2. Baltimore: Williams & Wilkins, 1980:1305–19.
7. McHugh MK. When everything is "fine, just fine." Nursing. 1980; 10:144–5.
8. Hatherly LI, Breheny JE, Robinson FS, et al. Psychiatric disorders in obstetrics. Obstet Gynecol Surv. 1980; 35:439–41.
9. Daly MJ. The emotional problems of patients encountered in the practice of obstetrics and gynecology. Obstet Gynecol Annu. 1980; 9:339–56.
10. Dubovsky SL, Weissberg MP. Clinical psychiatry in primary care. 2nd ed. Baltimore: Williams & Wilkins, 1982.
11. Nemiah JC. Anxiety state. In: Kaplan HI, Freedman AM, Sadock BJ, eds. Comprehensive textbook of psychiatry III. 3rd ed. Vol. 2. Baltimore: Williams & Wilkins, 1980:1483–93.
12. Strain JJ, Grossman S. Psychological care of the medically ill. New York: Appleton-Century-Crofts, 1975.
13. Kahana RJ, Bibring GL. Personality types in medical management. In: Zinberg NE, ed. Psychiatry and medical practice in a general hospital. New York: International Universities Press, 1964:108–23.
14. Dubovsky SL. Psychotherapeutics in primary care. New York: Grune & Stratton, 1981.
15. Chertok L. The psychopathology of vomiting of pregnancy. In: Howells JG, ed. Modern perspectives in psycho-obstetrics. New York: Brunner/Mazel, 1972:269–82.
16. Katon WJ, Ries RK, Bokan JA, et al. Hyperemesis gravidarum: a biopsychosocial perspective. Int J Psychiatry Med. 1981; 10:151–62.
17. Fuchs K, Paldi E, Abramovici H, et al. Treatment of hyperemesis gravidarum by hypnosis. Int J Clin Exp Hypn. 1980; 28:313–23.
18. Fairweather DVI. Nausea and vomiting in pregnancy. Am J Obstet Gynecol. 1968; 102:135–75.
19. Dubovsky SL, Weissberg MP, Johnston DA. Psychiatry. In: Reller LB, Sahn S, Schrier RW, eds. Clinical internal medicine. Boston: Little, Brown, 1979.
20. Renshaw DC. Helping patients with sex problems in the 1980's. Psychosomatics. 1982; 23:291–4.
21. Derogatis LR, Meyer JK. A psychological profile of the sexual dysfunctions. Arch Sex Behav. 1979; 8:201–23.
22. Schiavi RC, Derogatis LR, Kuriansky J, et al. The assessment of sexual function and marital interaction. J Sex Marital Ther. 1979; 5:169–224.
23. McAlpine IS. Adolescent sexuality. Aust Fam Physician. 1980; 9:555–60.
24. Phipps-Yonas S. Teenage pregnancy and motherhood. Am J Orthopsychiatry. 1980; 50:403–31.
25. Hepburn S. Adolescent pregnancy in Australia. Aust Fam Physician. 1979; 8:531–9.

26. Fielding JE. Adolescent pregnancy revisited. N Engl J Med. 1978; 299:893–6.

27. Olson L. Social and psychological correlates of pregnancy resolution among adolescent women. Am J Orthopsychiatry. 1980; 50:432–45.

28. Adler N. Emotional responses of women following therapeutic abortion. Am J Orthopsychiatry. 1975; 45:446–56.

29. Ketai RM, Brandwin MA. Childbirth-related psychosis and familial symbiotic conflict. Am J Psychiatry. 1979; 136:190–3.

30. Kaij L, Nelsson A. Emotional and psychotic illness following childbirth. In: Howells JG, ed. Modern perspectives in psycho-obstetrics. New York: Brunner/Mazel, 1972:364–84.

31. Kendell RE, Rennie D, Clarke JA, et al. The social and obstetric correlates of psychiatric admission in the puerperium. Psychol Med. 1981; 11:341–50.

32. American Psychiatric Association. Diagnostic and statistical manual of mental disorders. 3rd ed. Washington, D.C.: American Psychiatric Association, 1980.

33. Brockington IF, Cernik KF, Schofield EM, et al. Puerperal psychosis. Phenomena and diagnosis. Arch Gen Psychiatry. 1981; 38:829–33.

34. Cheetham RW, Rzadkowolski A. Psychiatric aspects of labour and the puerperium. S Afr Med J. 1980; 58:814–6.

35. Oates RK, Davis AA, Ryan MG. Predictive factors for child abuse. Aust Paediatr J. 1980; 16:239–43.

36. Cater JI, Easton PM. Separation and other stress in child abuse. Lancet. 1980; 1:972–4.

37. Robson KM, Kumar R. Delayed onset of maternal affection after childbirth. Br J Psychiatry. 1980; 136:347–53.

38. Kempe CH, Helfer RE, eds. Helping the battered child and his family. Philadelphia: Lippincott, 1972.

39. Anderson WH, Keuhnle JC. Current concepts in psychiatry: diagnosis and early management of acute psychosis. N Engl J Med. 1981; 305:1128–30.

40. Baldessarini RJ. Drugs and the treatment of psychiatric disorders. In: Gilman AG, Goodman LS, Gilman A, eds. The pharmacological basis of therapeutics. New York: Macmillan, 1980:391–447.

41. Targum SD. Dealing with psychosis during pregnancy. Am Pharm. 1979; 19:482–5.

42. Ayd FJ. Respiratory dyskinesias in patients with neuroleptic-induced extrapyramidal reactions. Int Drug Ther Newsl. 1979; 14:1–3.

43. Kinney DK, Matthysse S. Genetic transmission of schizophrenia. Annu Rev Med. 1978; 29:459–73.

44. Carroll BJ, Feinberg M, Greden JF. A specific laboratory test for the diagnosis of melancholia. Standardization, validation and clinical utility. Arch Gen Psychiatry. 1981; 38:15–22.

45. Finnegan LP. The effects of narcotics and alcohol on pregnancy and the newborn. Ann NY Acad Sci. 1981; 362:136–57.

46. Food and Drug Administration. Fetal alcohol syndrome. FDA Drug Bull. 1977; 7:18.

47. Clarren SK, Smith DW. The fetal alcohol syndrome. N Engl J Med. 1978; 298:1063–7.

INDEX

Hypoparathyroidism
  causes, 115
  in pregnancy, 114–115
  treatment, 115
Hyposensitization therapy, 232–233
Hypothyroidism
  high-risk groups for, 107
  laboratory determination of, 107–108
  in pregnancy, 107–108
  symptoms, 107
  transient occurrence in postpartum period, 112
  treatment, 108
  TSH in, 107

Idiopathic hypertrophic subaortic stenosis, 189
Idiopathic pulmonary fibrosis, 249
Idiopathic thrombocytopenic purpura, 301–302
Immune adaptations, to pregnancy, 229–230
Immune enhancement, 230
Immune globulin
  hepatitis B, 324
  hyperimmune, 324–325
  pooled, 325
  varicella-zoster, 325
Immune serum globulin, 321
Immunity
  adaptations in pregnancy, 229–230
    and beneficial effect on rheumatic disease, 263, 264
    fetal hypertrophied suppressor system, 263
    cancer chemotherapy effects on, 309
    cell-mediated, 229–230
    fetal, 230
Immunization, 321–325. See also Vaccines
  active, 321
  immune globulins, 324–325
  passive, 321
  during pregnancy, 321–325
  toxoids, 324
Immunoglobulins
  in fetus, 230
  transplacental passage of, 230
Immunosuppressive agents
  in lupus erythematosus, 273
  in rheumatoid arthritis, 269–270
Immunotherapy
  in allergic disorders in pregnancy, 232–233
  in asthma, 255
Impetigo herpetiformis, 288
Indomethacin
  adverse effects in pregnancy, 268

Indomethacin—Continued
  in lupus erythematosus, 273
Infectious arthritis, 275–276
Infectious diseases, 321–350. See also under specific infection
  antibiotics used in, 326–329. See also Antibiotics
  chorioamnionitis, 336–337
  congenital. See Fetus, infections in
  fungal, 345–346
  group B streptococcus, 336
  immunization against, 321–325. See also Immunization
  isolation procedures for, 331–332
  parasitic, 347–350
  pneumonia, 339–340
  puerperal mastitis, 337
  sexually transmitted diseases, 329–336
  teratogenic, 86. See also Fetus, infections in
  tuberculosis, 343–345
  urinary tract, 337–339
  viral, 340–343
Infective endocarditis, 189
Influenza, 343
  immunization during pregnancy, 323, 343
  mortality in pregnancy, 246–247
  pneumonia due to, 340
  safety of vaccine in pregnancy, 343
  signs and symptoms, 343
Informed consent, 14
  on abortion, 15
  on drug therapy in pregnancy, 80
  ethics of, 3–4, 7–8
  regarding continuation of high-risk pregnancy, 14
  regarding pregnancy outcome, 19
Inheritance. See Genetics
Injury, death rates due to various forms of, 91
Insect allergy, 237
Insulin, 131–133
  in diabetic ketoacidosis, 133
  during labor and delivery, 135–136
Intercostal neuralgia, 367
Intermittent positive pressure breathing (IPPB), in asthma, 259
Interstitial nephritis, and pregnancy outcome, 154
Intestinal obstruction, 221–222
  causes in pregnancy, 221
  signs and symptoms, 222
  treatment, 222
Intracranial hemorrhage, 359

Intrahepatic cholestasis, of pregnancy, 203
Iodide
  alterations in thyroid handling during pregnancy, 105
  contraindication during pregnancy, 258
  deficiency during pregnancy, 47
  fetal uptake of, 106
  radioactive, fetal exposure to, 94
  requirements during pregnancy, 42
Iron
  content in supplements, 38, 295
  deficiency in pregnancy, 291
  metabolism changes in pregnancy, 291
  pica related to deficiency of, 51
  requirements during pregnancy, 38
    effect of vegetarian diet on, 43
  serum levels during pregnancy, 100
  use in treating iron-deficiency anemia, 295
Iron-binding capacity, serum levels during pregnancy, 100
Iron-deficiency anemia, 294–295
  macrocytic anemia coexisting with, 294
Isolation procedures, 331–332

Jaundice. See also Liver disease
  drug-induced, 207
  idiopathic occurrence in pregnancy, 286

Ketoacidosis, 133
Kidney
  anatomical changes in pregnancy, 141
  biopsy in pregnancy, 146–147
  disorders in pregnancy, 141–155
    acute renal failure. See Renal failure, acute
    chronic renal disease, 151–155
      chronic interstitial nephritis, 154
      diabetic nephropathy, 133–134, 153–154
      hemodialysis and, 154–155
      hypertension effect on, 152–153
      lupus nephropathy, 153
      polycystic kidney, 154
      pregnancy effect on, 154
      primary glomerular disease, 153
      severity prior to pregnancy, 153
      urolithiasis, 154